Nutrition and
Diagnosis-Related Care

Nutrition and Diagnosis-Related Care___

SYLVIA ESCOTT-STUMP, M.A., R.D.
Director, Dietetic Services
Forbes Center for Gerontology
Pittsburgh, Pennsylvania

Third Edition

Lea & Febiger ● ● Philadelphia ● London

Lea & Febiger
200 Chester Field Parkway
Malvern, PA 19355-9725
U.S.A.
(610) 251-2230

Executive Editor: Darlene Cooke
Project Editor: Dorothy DiRienzi
Production Manager: Samuel Rondinelli

Library of Congress Cataloging-in-Publication Data

Escott-Stump, Sylvia.
    Nutrition and diagnosis related care / Sylvia Escott-Stump.—3rd
ed.
      p. cm.
    Includes bibliographical references and index.
    ISBN 0-8121-1556-2
    1. Diet therapy—Handbooks, manuals, etc. 2. Nutrition—
Handbooks, manuals, etc. I. Title.
    [DNLM: 1. Diet Therapy—handbooks. 2. Nutrition—handbooks.
WB 39 E74n]
RM216.E64   1992
615.8'54—dc20
DNLM/DLC
for Library of Congress   91-42187
                                               CIP

First Edition, 1985
Second Edition, 1988
Third Edition, 1992

PRINTED IN THE UNITED STATES OF AMERICA

Print No. 4 3

Foreword

Recognition is given to the professional dietitians and physicians who provided a review of this edition.

Credit for the initiation of this work goes to the dietetic interns of Shadyside Hospital, who recommended such a publication.

Diet counseling provides "individualized professional guidance to assist a person in adjusting his daily food consumption to meet his health needs."* Diet counseling incorporates patient interviewing, counseling, and consulting. The impact of a diet is far-reaching in consequence and must be cautiously planned by the provider.

The steps of effective nutritional intervention are as follows†:

1. Developing an appropriate diet prescription.
2. Establishing patient acceptance of the treatment plan.
3. Providing nutritional instructions. Qualitative diets, in which the mention of specific foods is avoided, are more easily followed by the patient than quantitative diets (using exchange lists).
4. Incorporating the diet into the family's eating pattern.
5. Providing long-gterm follow-up reinforcement. Follow-up visits should be continued until the patient can adhere to the new pattern comfortably.

True learning involves a behavioral change. The nutrition advisor must reassess the needs of the learner to assure such behavioral change. Learner-centered objectives are of critical importance, especially in a world designed to meet consumer needs.

---

* Guidelines for diet counseling. *JADA* 66:571, 1975.
† Willard M.: Nutritional Management for the Practicing Physician. Reading, MA: Addison-Wesley, 1982, p. 126.

Foreword to the Third Edition

Dietitians and other health professionals must keep abreast of the many new developments that impact on the quality of health care and clinical practice. This is becoming more challenging as a result of the rapid advances being made in technology, business, research, and education. Good reference books and other materials play a vital role in enabling practitioners easy access to new information that is needed to maintain competence in practice. Key information that is organized and presented concisely is a valuable resource for practitioners.

Nutrition and Diagnosis-Related Care is a highly recommended reference for all health professionals. It provides important information about the medical care of patients with various diseases, disorders, and conditions, and covers normal life-cycle conditions and dietary practices. Current guidelines for the treatment of medical problems and health concerns, including objectives of care, dietary therapy, and patient education issues, are presented succinctly and in a manner that facilitates the nutrition care planning process.

Nutrition and Diagnosis-Related Care will enable practitioners to enhance their effectiveness and efficiency in clinical practice. In so doing, this reference text will benefit the clinical skills of practitioners and thereby improve the quality of health care.

University Park, PA   P.M. Kris-Etherton, Ph.D., R.D.

Preface

Dietitians must identify all elements of patient care capable of affecting nutritional status and outcomes. With recent limitations on length of hospital stay (as directed by diagnosis-related groupings), the registered dietitian must provide nutritional care in a more practical, efficient, timely, and effective manner.

Nutrition and Diagnosis-Related Care has been developed as a tool to supplement other texts and references used by dietetic practitioners, interns, and students to quickly assimilate and implement care for numerous disorders. This manual can be used to help establish protocols and priorities in nutritional care to demonstrate transitional methods of therapy at a lower cost* than total parenteral nutrition (TPN) and to categorize disorders in which nutritional input can reduce morbidity and mortality or length of stay. Not only can adequate nutritional intervention demonstrate humane concern, but it can also result in financial savings.

1. The reader has an adequate background in nutritional science, physiology, pathophysiology, medical terminology, biochemistry, and interpretation of laboratory data.
2. An individualized drug history and review is required for all patients, since only a few popular medications are listed in this manual.
3. The Patient Education section assumes that the reader will provide appropriate diet copies. Added tips are listed in this guide to prepare the patient for independent functioning.
4. Shortened hospital lengths of stay will force dietitians to accelerate their nutritional care during hospitalizations. In addition, dietitians will find

---

* For example, oral intake may cost $15 per day, enteral tube feedings $50, and TPN $180.

new roles in ambulatory centers, extended care facilities, and private practices. Home care is also a viable alternative for many patients.

5. Fewer laboratory tests will be available for monitoring of nutritional status. The major tools (e.g., weight changes) will remain essential as the registered dietitian learns to document outcomes in a cost-effective manner.

6. A current diet manual or diet therapy text should be used to acquire complete lists of all diet modifications. Such lists are not included in this book.

7. Except where specifically noted for children, therapy plans are listed for adults over age 21.

8. Supplements can cause food-drug interactions and should only be taken in the case of a documented deficiency. Athletes, women, the elderly, and vegetarians tend to take vitamin and mineral supplements most often. Plan meals and nourishments carefully.

9. In general, the rules developed for suggesting a well-balanced, varied diet with the four food groups are the basis for all dietary plans.

10. Ethics and a concern for patients' rights should be practiced at all times.

11. Healthy persons should obtain nutrients from food, not pills, especially single-dose units. Single nutrients cannot halt the progression of acute or chronic illness.

The third edition was written to update data and to include the 1989 RDAs. Because patient care plans and goals must be created individually for each patient, the reader is encouraged to maintain current educational endeavors and to revise nutritional protocols as the literature indicates. This manual serves to provide the stimulus for improving dietetic practice and nutritional care in all settings.

Pittsburgh, Pennsylvania   Sylvia Escott-Stump

Contents

List of Figures and Tables

    Note. The reader is also referred to the table of contents for charts and tabular material in Appendix A and Appendix B.

Section 1
Normal Life-Cycle Conditions

Table 1–1.

Dietary Guidelines for Americans*

1. Maintain healthy weight.
2. Use more fiber (whole grains, legumes, fruits, vegetables).
3. Provide variety in food choices.
4. Use sugars and alcohol in moderation only.
5. Choose a diet low in total fat, cholesterol, and saturated fat.
6. Use salt and sodium in moderation.

---

* Adapted for a lifestyle designed for all Americans (U.S. Dept. of Health and Human Services, 1990).

Chief Assessment Factors

General state of health, recent surgery/hospitalizations, weight history, % IBW/HBW for height, loss of LBM, previous weight curve, fatigue, weakness, cachexia

Chills, sweating, tremors, anorexia, nausea, diarrhea, vomiting, blood pressure, temperature, pulse

Hair or nail changes, skin rashes, itching, lesions, turgor, petechiae, pallor

Headache, seizures, otitis media, glaucoma, cataracts, glasses, blurring of vision, sinusitis, altered sense of smell, nasal obstruction

Dentures, loose or missing teeth, caries, bleeding gums, oral hygiene, taste alterations, dysphagia

Chest pain, dyspnea, wheezing, cough, hemoptysis, ventilator support, blood gases, electrolyte balance, hypertension, cyanosis, edema, ascites, cardiac output, anemias, heart rate, arrhythmias, blood loss

Appetite, jaundice, constipation, indigestion, ulcers, hemorrhoids, melena, stool characteristics, special diets, TSF/MAC/MAMC, visceral proteins, BEE, wt. changes, N balance, vitamin/mineral intake, nutritional support, BS, dietary intake, alcohol intake

Hematuria, fluid requirements, specific gravity, UTIs

Hormone balance, goiter, glucose intolerance, cellular immunity, allergy, sensitivity, intolerances

Pain, arthritis, numbness, amputations, range of motion, muscular strength

Convulsions, altered speech, paralysis, gait, anxiety, memory loss, sleep patterns, depression, ETOH abuse, substance abuse, motivation

Medications, side effects, food-drug interactions, therapies, effects on nutritional status, educational background

NOTES

PREGNANCY

Usual Hospital Stay

3 days.

Notation

Gravida—pregnant woman; para—woman who has given birth. Tissue growth: breast, 0.5 kg; placenta, 0.6 kg; fetus, 3–3.5 kg; amniotic fluid, 1 kg; uterus, 1 kg; increase in blood volume, 1.5 kg; and extracellular fluid, 1.5 kg.

Objectives

1. Meet increased needs for fetus and tissues. Prevent hypoglycemia and ketosis.
2. Provide additional nutrients and calories (net cost of pregnancy, 80,000 kcal). Studies indicate needs vary from 20,000–80,000 kcal.
3. Provide adequate amino acids to meet fetal and placental growth, etc. About 950 g of protein are synthesized for fetus and placenta.
4. Provide adequate weight gain during course of pregnancy (25 to 30 lbs total). Obese women should gain 15–25 lbs; thin women 28–40 lbs. For twins, a woman should gain 35–45 lbs.
5. Encourage proper rate of gain: 2–4 lbs first trimester, 10–11 lbs second trimester, 12–13 third trimester. *More weight* should be gained if patient is below IBW prior to pregnancy; this is especially true for young women. Overweight women should gain 2/3 lb per week.
6. Promote development of an adequate fetal immune system (during first trimester).

2

Risk Assessments

Pre-pregnancy

1. Adolescence (poor eating habits, greater needs).
2. History of three or more pregnancies in past 2 years, especially miscarriages.
3. History of poor obstetrical/fetal performance.

Pre-pregnancy or During Pregnancy

1. Economic deprivation.
2. Food faddist; smoker; user of drugs/alcohol; practicer of pica with iron or zinc deficiency.
3. Modified diet for chronic systemic diseases.
4. Pre-partum weight of less than 85% or more than 120% of IBW (may reflect inability to attain proper wt. or poor dietary habits).
5. Deficient Hgb (under 11 g) or Hct (under 33%).
6. Any wt. loss during PG or gain of less than 2 lbs/month in the last two trimesters.
7. Risk of toxemia (2 lbs weight gain per week or greater).
8. Poorly managed vegetarian diets.

Dietary Recommendations

1. 1 g protein/kg body weight daily (or 10 g in excess of RDA for age). Young teens 11–14 (1.7 g/kg); 15–18 (1.5 g/kg); over age 19 (1.7 g/kg); high risk (2 g/kg).
2. First trimester, add 50–150 kcal/day. In second and third trimesters, add 200–350 kcal/day. Add more or less, activity-dependent. Usually 2300–2500 kcal/day for patients under age 35, 1800–1850 kcal/day for patients over age 35. Evaluate teens individually according to age, pre-pregnancy weight, for an average of 36–40 kcal/day; 15% protein, 55% CHO, 30% fat.
3. The diet should include 400 μg folacin; 30 mg iron (supplemental) 1200+ mg calcium, increased intake of zinc (+3 mg, as from meat sources). Encourage use of vitamin C with the iron sulfate supplement. Use adequate vitamin A; 50% more vitamins D and E. Avoid hypervitaminosis.
4. Be sure to use iodized salt. Avoid excesses.
5. Pattern of food intake; 4 cups milk (calcium, protein); 8 oz meat or meat substitute (protein, iron, zinc); one to two citrus servings (vitamin C); two servings of other fruits (vitamins A and C); vegetables (vitamin A, folacin); three servings whole grain or enriched breads/substitutes (iron, calories).
6. Omit alcohol and caffeine (or limit severely).
7. Use cereal grains, nuts, green vegetables, and seafood for added magnesium.

8. Essential fatty acids from fats like safflower oil should equal 1–2% of daily calories.
9. Vegan vegetarians will need a B_{12} supplement and perhaps calcium and vitamin D also.

Profile

Pre-PG wt	Present wt	Gravida
Desired wt at term	Ht	Para
H & H	Alb	Abortus
Urea N	BP	$\downarrow T_3$, $\uparrow T_4$
Gluc	Smoker	BUN/Creat
Use of Alcohol	Nausea	Chol (inc.)
Vomiting	Transferrin	Alk phos (inc.)
Ca^{++}, Mg^{++}	Ceruloplasmin	TIBC (inc. in late PG)

Side Effects of Common Drugs Used

1. After the fourth month, encourage use of vitamin-mineral supplements between meals for better utilization. Supplements vary greatly; read labels carefully. Iron is the only nutrient that cannot be met from diet alone.
2. Avoid taking iron supplements with antacids.
3. Avoid taking *isotretinoin* (Accutane) or *13-cis retinoic acid* for acne; they have been linked to birth defects.
4. Avoid excesses of vitamin A in the first trimester.

Patient Education

1. Describe an adequate pattern of weight gain in pregnancy. Explain the rationale for such gain.
2. Explain to the patient what to do for constipation, nausea, vomiting, and pica.
3. Encourage adequate milk and calcium intake. Discuss what to do for milk allergy/intolerance.
4. Discourage faddist behavior, junk foods, the practice of skipping breakfast. Discuss ketosis.
5. Encourage stress reduction, which has an effect on nitrogen and calcium. Encourage a good appetite.
6. Encourage breast-feeding. Explain reasons for doing so.
7. For *hyperemesis gravidarum*, hospitalization with TPN may be needed. When eating orally, liquids taken between meals, extra B-complex and vitamin C, and limited fat may be beneficial. Hyperemesis affects 20% of pregnancies. Electrolyte imbalances should be avoided. Metoclopramide (Reglan) may help some women.
8. For excessive weight gain, the goal should be to restore eating patterns

to match a normal growth curve. Severe calorie restriction should be avoided, and at least 150 g CHO will be needed.

9. Discuss fluoride and iodine intake.
10. Discuss effects of marijuana (decreased birth weight, congenital malformations) and other drugs as needed.
11. Limit intake of aspartame-sweetened foods to 3–4 servings per day (*Topics in Clin. Nutrition*, Oct. 1990).

For More Information

WIC Programs
c/o Children's Foundation, Inc.
1420 New York Ave., NW
Washington, DC 20005

March of Dimes (local chapter)

NOTES

LACTATION

Usual Hospital Stay

Varies by specific disorder.

Notation

Human milk is far better absorbed than other forms of milk. It has more PUFA, less sodium, and a proper protein ratio. It is also better digested and has more antibodies. In comparison, cow's milk has twice as much protein and ash. Breast milk yields 1 mg iron/liter with 49% absorption rate. Cholesterol content is 15–23 mg/dl regardless of maternal intake. The whey:casein ratio of 80:20 is more desirable than that of many formulas.

Objectives

1. Normalize body composition gradually so that the mother returns to ideal weight (see Comments section).
2. Provide for adequate lactation (usual secretion, 850–1200 ml/day).

Human milk provides 67 calories/dl. Good calorie intake does increase calorie production.

3. Have the mother continue breast-feeding beyond several months. The ideal time for the mother to discontinue lactation is when the infant is 1 year old, unless contraindicated.
4. Decrease nutritional risks (use of alcohol, etc.) while mother is breast-feeding. Alcohol intake inhibits let-down reflex (oxytocin).
5. Promote adequate infant growth and development, including bone mineralization.
6. Discourage excessive use of stimulants, including caffeine.

Dietary Recommendations

1. In the first 6 months, increase the mother's caloric intake to +500 over RDA for age—approximately 2200 calories for a woman of average childbearing age. In second 6 months, use +400 over RDA for age.
2. Consider the special needs of adolescents or women over age 35.
3. Increase the mother's intake of protein by 15 g (or about 65 g for average age). Encourage intake of sources of HBV protein.
4. Encourage intake of usual sources of vitamins and minerals. Intake of calcium should be 1200 mg daily. Increases of B complex (thiamine and vitamin B_6), and of vitamins A and C should be taken.
5. Increase intake of fluids.
6. Forbid the use of alcohol unless permitted by physician.
7. Adequate vitamin D will be needed if maternal intake is poor or if infant receives little sunshine exposure.
8. Beyond 3 months of lactation, mother should increase her calorie intake if her weight loss has been excessive.

Profile

Pre-pregnancy wt	Alb	Smoker
DOB for infant	Present wt	Alk phos
Goal for return to	Ht	PT
IBW	H & H	Chol, Trig
Gluc	BP	Ca^{++}, P

Side Effects of Common Drugs Used

1. Alcohol, caffeine, and most drugs are transmitted through breast milk to infants. Their use should be discouraged, unless permitted by a physician. Cigarette smoking also reduces the amount of milk produced.
2. *Cimetidine* and other drugs may be contraindicated.
3. Be careful about hypervitaminosis A and D. Read supplement labels carefully.

Patient Education

1. Explain the composition of breast milk and the benefits of breast-feeding. Show the mother how to care for nipples. Discuss stools of BF babies.
2. Explain the meaning of a balanced diet. Encourage the mother to normalize weight after delivery, but while the mother is nursing, she should not be placed in a weight loss program. Other than postpartum diuresis, average loss is .67 kg/month.
3. Explain the requirements of infant nutrition after the infant has been weaned. Refer to the WIC program, if available, for eligible children.
4. If necessary, omit chocolate, gas-forming foods, and highly seasoned foods.

Comments

Breast milk has one and one half times as much lactose as cow's milk; consequently, protein is better absorbed. The volume of milk decreases in a poorly nourished mother.

Try to maintain the mother's postpartum weight during the period of lactation. No weight loss program should be initiated until lactation has been discontinued. Infant feeding method does *not* alter weight loss; total gain does. More gain leads to greater postpartum losses.

Reasons for discontinuing lactation often include an acute infection in the mother; the mother's return to work; the mother's inability to provide 50% of the infant's needs; the presence of chronic illness (tuberculosis, severe anemia, chronic fevers, cardiovascular or renal disease) in the mother; the infant's inability (due to weakness) to nurse; and the infant's inability to nurse adequately because of oral anomalies. Women also discontinue breast-feeding because of a lack of information and support, or inadequate preparation. Working mothers may need part-time jobs, flexible scheduling and convenient daycare.

Bacterial flora of breast-fed infants are generally *Lactobacillus*, not *E. coli*, like those of formula-fed infants.

Women following vegan diets may need zinc or vitamin B_{12} supplementation. These diets may also be low in carnitine.

For More Information

La Leche International
9615 Minneapolis Ave.
Franklin Park, IL 60131

NOTES

INFANT, NORMAL (0–6 MONTHS)

Usual Hospital Stay

Varies by disorder.

Notation

The average birth weight of an infant ranges between 5.5 and 10 lbs, average being approximately 7–7.5 lbs. Normal gestation is 40 weeks.

Infants are born with a 4–6 months supply of iron, if maternal stores were adequate during gestation and if she was not anemic. Be careful not to oversupplement.

Infants are comprised of approximately 75–80% water, compared with adults (60–65% water).

Infants of vegan mothers may require calcium and vitamin B_{12} supplementation.

Some research suggests that SIDS infants have abnormally high levels of Hgb; watch iron intake levels carefully from formula and supplements. SIDS Hotline: (800) 221-SIDS.

Objectives

1. Promote normal growth and development: assess sleeping, eating and attentiveness habits. Compare infant's growth to the chart of normal growth patterns.
2. Overcome any nutritional risk factors or complications, such as otitis media or dehydration.
3. Discourage early introduction of solids and cow's milk. Evaluate use of such items.
4. Encourage the mother to use breast milk as the infant's main source of nutrition for the first 6 months.
5. If the infant is breast-fed, assess the mother's prepregnancy nutritional status and risk factors, weight gain pattern, food allergies, medical history (such as toxemia or chronic illnesses or anemia). Discuss any conditions in the present that may affect lactation.
6. If the infant is formula-fed, the mother should learn about nursing-bottle caries syndrome prevention and about potential overfeeding problems.

Dietary Recommendations

1. Fluid requirements may include: 60–80 ml/kg water in newborns; 80–100 ml/kg by 3 days of age; 125–150 ml/kg up to 6 months of age. Assess individual needs according to status.
2. Calorie needs are: 115 kcal/kg from birth to 6 months.
3. Protein needs are generally: 2.2 g/kg (13 g). A sick infant may need a ratio of 1:150 protein:nonprotein calories.
4. *If infant is breast-fed*, discourage mother from use of drugs, caffeine and alcohol. Teach parents about use of dilute fruit juice (perhaps apple) at 4 months of age. Breast-fed infants generally require 300 IU vitamin D, 0.25 mg fluoride; and sometimes iron supplements (at about 3 months of age). Mothers of infants predisposed to allergies should avoid fish, cow's milk, and nuts.
5. *Formula-fed infants*: Type: (milk-based, soy, etc.). Check list of significant ingredients and amount used for 24 hours. No calorie-containing formula should be given in bed; only water. Sweetened beverages should not be used between meals or at bedtime. Be careful in warming up bottles; folacin and vitamin C may be destroyed. Iron-fortified formula is often used after 3 months, generally using 1 mg iron/kg. No fluoride supplement is needed unless the water supply provides less than 0.3 ppm. Use 30 mg vitamin C for evaporated milk formula.
6. Enfamil and SMA have a 60:40 whey:casein ratio, which is desirable in a formula. The standard formulas provide 20 kcal/oz. Breast milk yields an 80:20 whey:casein ratio and approximately the same calories.
7. Special formulas are available for special needs—Nutramigen for cow's milk and soy allergies; Portagen & Pregestimil for MCT; Standard Vivonex for other complex problems.
8. Infants on soy formulas may need a source of carnitine, which is available from breast milk.
9. For *special conditions*, TPN may be used. 1–2% EFAs may be necessary to prevent such signs of deficiency as inadequate wound healing, growth, immunocompetence, and platelet formation. Linoleic and linolenic acids seem to be required.
10. *At 4–6 months*, introduce plain (not mixed or sweetened or spiced) strained or pureed baby cereals, then nonallergenic vegetables, then fruits. Start with 1–2 teaspoons and progress as appetite indicates. Always use a single new item for 3 days to detect any signs of food allergy. The intake of solids should not decrease breast-milk or formula intake to less than 32 oz daily.
11. Ensure that the RDAs are being met for all other nutrients for each stage of growth.

Profile

Gestational age	Birth weight	Gluc
Head circumference	Percentile weight/	Length
H & H (after 3 mos.)	length	Sucking reflex
Apgar scores	Hydration status	I & O
		P_{CO_2}, P_{O_2}

Patient Education

1. Explain the proper care of infant's teeth, including risks of nursing-bottle caries syndrome.
2. Explain the proper timing and sequence of feeding. Discuss risks related to inadequate growth.
3. Explain growth patterns: for example, the 4–6-month-old infant should double his or her birth weight.
4. Emphasize the importance of adequate bonding.
5. Explain the proper timing and sequence of solid food introduction. Avoid use of stringy foods, or foods like peanut butter that are hard to swallow.
6. Discuss the rationale for delaying introduction of cow's milk (allergy, gastrointestinal bleeding).
7. Discuss why fluid intake is essential, and explain that needs are much greater than for adults.
8. If infant is breast-fed, discuss the normalcy of 4–6 soft stools each day. Compare the normal stool with symptoms of diarrhea.
9. Discuss successful feeding: trusting and responding to cues from the infant about timing, pace, and eating capacity.

Table 1–2.
Special Problems in Infant Feeding

1. *Spitting Up.* If there is no weight loss of concern, just offer encouragement that the problem will resolve in a few months.
2. *Regurgitation.* Position the infant in an upright (40–60°) position after feeding for about 30 minutes; have the doctor rule out other problems.
3. *Diarrhea.* Replace fluids and electrolytes (for example, Pedialyte) as directed by the doctor. After an extended period of time, have the doctor rule out allergy.
4. *Pale, Oily Stools.* Check for fat malabsorption. Use an MCT-containing formula.
5. *Constipation.* The doctor will make a careful assessment and may suggest adding 1 teaspoon corn syrup (or other CHO source) to 4 oz water or formula, 1–2× daily.
6. *Colic.* Check for hunger, food allergy, incorrect formula temperature, stress, or other underlying problems. Give small, frequent feedings and

parental encouragement. Check CHO, fat and protein sources; ask about use of milk.

7. *Allergy*. Introduce new foods at the appropriate time and singly; try for 3 days and discuss any symptoms with the doctor immediately.

NOTES

INFANT, NORMAL (6–12 MONTHS)

Usual Hospital Stay

Varies by disorder.

Notation

Many of the same principles associated with infant feeding during the first 6 months will continue, with the greater use of solids. In addition, introduction of cow's milk at 12 months brings new problems and risks related to essential fatty acid deficiency if low-fat or skim milks are used.

Objectives

1. Continue to promote normal growth and development during this second stage of very rapid growth.
2. Prevent significant weight losses.
3. Avoid dehydration.
4. Correct or prevent such complications as otitis media.
5. Introduce new solids at appropriate periods of time.
6. Begin to encourage greater physical activity; prepare for walking by ensuring adequate calorie intake.
7. Continue to emphasize the role of good nutrition in the development of healthy teeth.
8. Delay allergenic foods until 12 months (corn, citrus, egg white, cow's milk).

Dietary Recommendations

1. Fluid requirements may include: approximately 125–150 ml/kg up to 1 year of age. Fluid needs may decline slightly during this stage.

2. Continue to provide breast milk or iron-fortified formula during this stage. Avoid use of sweetened beverages.
3. For calories, provide 90–100 kcal/kg body weight.
4. Protein needs are generally 14 grams.
5. Introduce more solids as indicated: egg yolk at 8–9 months; meat and cottage cheese at 9–10 months; finger foods at 10–12 months, such as peeled and cooked fruit, dry toast, vegetable bits, zwieback or arrowroot crackers.
6. Avoid raw vegetables and fruits (other than ripe banana or soft apple). Beware of foods that may cause choking (e.g., hot dogs, popcorn, nuts, seeds).
7. As tolerated, introduce coarsely ground table foods at 12 months.
8. Introduce cow's milk at 12 months, assuring that intake does not go above 1 quart daily to prevent anemia. Use whole milk.
9. Whole egg may be offered at 12 months, using caution because of egg allergy.
10. Begin to offer fluids by cup at about 9 months; try to wean at about 1 year of age. Avoid sweetened beverages at this age whenever possible.
11. Spicy foods are often not liked or not tolerated.
12. Continue use of about 6 tablespoons of iron-fortified baby cereal after 12 months of age to ensure adequate intake. Adult cereals are often inappropriate for infants and children under age 4. About 10 mg iron is required.

Profile

Age	Wt	Length
Head circumference	Percentile wt/length	Tooth development
H & H	Hydration status	I & O
Developmental stage	Gluc	P_{CO_2}, P_{O_2}

Patient Education

1. Discuss adequate weight pattern: infants generally triple birth weight by 12 months of age.
2. Discuss overfeeding, iron intake, fluid intake and other nutritional factors related to normal growth and development.
3. When child begins to brush teeth, beware of swallowing of fluoridated toothpaste.
4. Discuss role of fat-soluble vitamins and their presence in whole milk. Discuss also the role of essential fatty acids in normal growth and development of the nervous system.

NOTES

CHILDHOOD

Usual Hospital Stay

Varies according to disorder.

Notation

*Toddler (1–3 years)—autonomy. Preschooler (4–6)—initiative. School-aged (6–12 years)—industry. Teens (12–18 years)—identity. See Adolescence.

Objectives

1. Assess growth patterns, feeding skills, dietary intake, activity patterns, inherited factors, and intellectual development.
2. Monitor long-term drug therapies and their related side effects.
3. Assess nutritional deficiencies, especially iron. If possible, detect and correct pica (eating any one food to the exclusion of others—even ice chips).
4. Prevent "milk anemia."
5. Evaluate status of the child's dental health. Prevent dental decay.
6. Promote adequate response to immunizations.

Dietary Recommendations

1. Calories—55 kcal/kg 12–18 months; 25–30 kcal/kg thereafter.
2. Protein 16 grams (ages 1–3), 24 grams (ages 4–6), 1.20 g/kg (ages 7–10).
3. Provide fat as 30% total kcal.
4. 800 mg each of calcium and phosphorus.
5. Day-care meals given for a 4–8 hour stay should provide for 1/3-1/2 daily needs.
6. Give 50–60 ml/kg fluid daily.

---

*Erikson, Eric: *Childhood and Society*, 2nd ed. New York, W.W. Norton & Company, 1963.

Profile

Ht	MAMC	Gluc
Growth %, Age	Transferrin	MAC
Alb	Wt	Fe
Trig	H & H	CHI
TSF	Chol	Alk phos
		Ca^{++}

Side Effects of Common Drugs Used

1. *Nutritional supplements* are to be taken as prescribed by a physician only. The mother should be careful about using cereals fulfilling the adult recommended dietary allowances, vitamins, etc.
2. *Anticonvulsants* may cause problems with the child's growth and normal body functions.
3. *Corticosteroids* may also cause growth stunting if given over an extended time in large doses.

Suggested Pattern of Food Intake

Preschool Children. Milk, 3/4 cup four times daily; meat, 4 tablespoons twice daily; fruits and vegetables, 4 oz four times daily—check for sufficient intake of vitamins A and C; four servings bread or substitute daily.

School-aged Children. Milk, 3/4-1 cup four times daily; meat, 6–8 tablespoons twice daily; fruit and vegetables, 4–6 oz four times daily—check for sufficient intake of vitamins A and C; 1–2 servings bread or substitute four times daily.

Patient Education

1. Explain the appropriate diet for children. Fifty percent of the diet should contain HBV proteins.
2. Encourage the parents to use finger foods, snacks, iron-rich desserts. Cheese cubes are good for the teeth.
3. Encourage a relaxed atmosphere at mealtime. There should be no pressure to eat, finish, etc.
4. Explain to the parents that bribery or rewards for eating should never be used. Rewards can actually decrease acceptance.
5. Remind the parents that children have food jags, and that they also prefer single foods.
6. Encourage the parents to avoid sweetened beverages and empty-calorie foods.
7. Teach the parents about food intake and dietary practices that affect learning and problems.
8. With toddlers, continued use of iron-fortified cereal and vitamin C-fortified infant juice can be beneficial.

9. Children should be allowed to vary in their food acceptance, choices and intakes, just as adults do.
10. Children who have chronic illness fare better if parents give them responsibilities, such as meal planning and taking their own medications.
11. A proper emotional atmosphere is important to children, especially at mealtimes.
12. Parents must be careful about "control" issues; disordered eating may result in later years.
13. The 1928 Clara Davis studies have been disproven; children *do* prefer sweets and must be helped to choose balanced meals.

Comments

Hyperactive children need positive interactions, especially correlated with their attention deficits. Stimulants like methylphenidate (Ritalin) or dextroamphetamine (Dexedrine) may cause anorexia, growth stunting, nausea, stomach pain, weight loss. EFA deficiency is being researched.

In *measles*, children benefit from vitamin A supplementation.

For More Information

EPSDT
Office of Child Health
DHHS—Health Care Financing Administration
Dogwood West Bldg.
1848 Gwynn Oak Ave.
Baltimore, MD 21207

ADOLESCENCE

Usual Hospital Stay

Varies by disorder.

Notation

The growth spurt of girls occurs when they are 9 1/2–13 1/2 years old; menarche is generally at 12 1/2 years. For boys the growth spurt occurs during the age of 11 3/4–14 1/2 years. Most skeletal growth is completed by age 19. RDAs divide teens by ages 11–14, 15–18, and 19–22.

Objectives

1. Modify diet to meet the needs of an ongoing or potential growth spurt.
2. Determine the patient's sexual maturity (menarche etc.), and whether oral contraceptives or intrauterine devices are being used by girls. Alter diet accordingly.
3. Prevent or correct nutritional anemias.
4. Evaluate the patient's weight status.
5. Provide adequate nutrients: girls need approximately 2000–2500 kcal/day; boys need approximately 2500–3000 kcal/day. Protein intake should be 45–60 g/day in boys, 46 g in 11–14-year-old girls, and 44 g in 15–18-year-old girls.
6. Evaluate any use of fad diets or unusual eating patterns, or tendency toward anorexia nervosa or bulimia.

Dietary Recommendations

1. The four basic food groups: 3–4 cups milk (or equivalent source of calcium); two servings of meat, 4 oz or more per serving; four to six servings, bread group; four servings fruit and vegetable group, 4–6 oz each.
2. Adequate zinc for growth and sexual maturation; iodized salt.
3. Calcium is needed for bone growth; iron for menstrual losses. Vitamin D is also essential, as is vitamin A.
4. Calorie needs vary—boys need 200 kcal at age 7, 2400 kcal at age 11, 3500 kcal at age 16. Girls need 200 fewer kilocalories than boys at age 10, 300 kcal less at age 12, 400 kcal less at age 14, 600 kcal less at age 16.

Profile

H & H	Alk phos	Alb
Trig	RBP	Ht
Gluc	IBW/HBW	Recent changes (ht,
Wt	P	wt)
Wt/ht %	Chol	Ca^{++}

Patient Education

1. Explain the four basic food groups and the rationale behind the concept.
2. Explain the relation of diet to the needs of the adolescent athlete, as well as its influence on acne, weight control, and general appearance. Educate the patient with regard to acceptable snacks.
3. Help the family recognize the adolescent's need for independence.
4. Emphasize dental health and oral hygiene.
5. Teen diets are often low in vitamins A and C and iron. Snacks should be carefully chosen.

6. Discuss role of heroes, peer pressure, and related issues.
7. Emphasize the importance of not skipping meals, especially breakfast.
8. Discuss calcium; half of adolescent girls consume inadequate amounts.

Comments

1. *Adolescent Pregnancy.* Of all teens who deliver, 94% will keep their babies. The diet for the pregnant adolescent should provide for optimal fetal growth and maintain an optimal nutritional status during and after gestation. If patient is pregnant, add the desired increments for calories and protein to the required daily allowance for same-age nonpregnant teens, or monitor the weight gain pattern to assess the adequacy of present diet. By the end of pregnancy, the mother's desired weight gain should be between 25 and 35 lbs. Prenatal vitamins should be prescribed by the physician. Note that the dietitian may be seen as another authoritarian figure rather than as a friend; encourage the teen to see herself as having a key role in providing good nutritional support for her new family. A diet may include 5 cups milk, 3 servings of meat, 4 fruits/vegetables and 4 breads/cereals. Problem nutrients include calcium, zinc, iron, and vitamins A and C. LBW and prematurity are common. Fetuses grow more slowly in 10–16 year olds. Check gynecologic age (chronological age less age of menarche) to determine future potential growth of the mother. Discourage skipping of meals.
2. *Diet for Athletes.* An acceptable diet for the athlete would be a normal diet for age, sex, and level of activity, plus adequate intake of carbohydrates and fluids. Excessive intake of protein and inadequate replacement of electrolytes should be prevented. See Sports Nutrition entry.
3. When the teens years begin, the adolescent has 80–85% of final height, 53% of final weight, 52% of final skeletal mass. Teens may almost double their weight and can add 15–20% in height.

SPORTS NUTRITION

Usual Hospital Stay

Athletes are not generally hospitalized except for idiosyncratic chronic or emergency reasons. See specific entries.

Notation

Many athletes are runners, joggers, weight lifters, wrestlers (sports active) when they seek nutritional guidance. Some may want weight control guidance, others may have disordered eating patterns, still others may want wellness guidance. Generally, only 10% who seek help from a nutritionist have a clinical concern (N. Clark, M.S., R.D., Sports Medicine Systems, Brookline, Mass., 1987).

The primary fuel for athletic events using less than 50% maximum O_2 capacity ($\dot{V}O_{2max}$, or aerobic capacity) is *fat*. Over 70% max O_2, (as in most events like swimming or sprint running), *glycogen* is the key fuel. In long-duration events or over 70% max O_2 activities (such as long-distance running or cycling or swimming), muscle glycogen can be depleted in 100–120 min; glycogen-loading may be of benefit here.

Objectives

1. Promote healthy, safe eating habits. Promote, as well, activities that can be continued throughout life. Aerobic activity is especially beneficial.
2. Correct faddist beliefs, erroneous trends, meal-skipping and other unhealthy eating behaviors.
3. Promote improved performance.
4. Enhance overall health and fitness.
5. Help to prevent injuries, dehydration, or overhydration.
6. Prevent or correct sports anemia, stress fractures and similar complications.
7. Monitor or correct eating disorders, such as bulimia or anorexia nervosa.
8. Meet extra calorie requirements created by a higher BMR for metabolically active muscle mass.
9. Prevent or correct amenorrhea, which may result from poor protein intake.
10. Prevent osteoporosis during later years.

Dietary Recommendations

1. Use a normal diet for age and sex, with special attention to calorie needs for the specific activity and frequency. 50–60% CHO is generally a good target.
2. Protein requirements should be calculated by age and sex, with a slightly higher requirement (e.g., 1.4 g/kg in strenuous sports activity, 1 g/kg for mild and moderate activities). Avoid excesses of protein.
3. Extra riboflavin may be needed to meet muscle demands.
4. Fluid replacement may be essential, with a calculation of 1 ml/kcal used for an average. A sample beverage for a sports activity could be 1 part juice to 4 parts water.
5. Electrolytes must be carefully monitored and replaced. Products like "Exceed" from Ross Labs contain glucose polymers, with lower osmolality than sugared drinks or Gatorade.
6. Where appropriate, glucose loading may help for long-distance activities. Here, 500–600 grams CHO (70% of total kcal) can be used to replete body stores. In addition, increased starch intake can also help with glycogen storage.

7. Avoid fads, such as omission of meat from the diet. Heme iron is important, and meat is also a good source of zinc.
8. Ensure adequate calcium intake in women (i.e., 1–1.5 g/day) to prevent osteoporosis in women and to reduce muscle cramping and stress fractures.
9. Reduce total fat intake to less than 25% total calories.
10. Watch meal timing—eat during the day, diet at night. Prevent meal skipping. Breakfast is especially important in maintaining homeostasis.

Profile

Ht/Wt/IBW/HBW	Goal wt, BMI	Serum gluc
Serum insulin	H & H	Other parameters prn
Ca^{++}	K^+, Na^+, Cl^-	(BP, N, Alb)

Side Effects of Common Drugs Used

1. Steroids may affect numerous nutritional parameters. Take a careful drug history and discuss all side effects as appropriate.
2. Salt tablets should be discouraged. Water intake is generally the requirement during athletic events.
3. Discuss the fact that excessive use of vitamin-mineral supplements can lead to toxicity, especially for vitamins A and D.

Patient Education

1. Dispel such myths as "milk is for children only," "meat is bad for you," "carbohydrates are fattening," and "dieting is the key to fluid control." Discuss appropriate alternatives.
2. If the client is an adult child of alcoholic parents, he or she may need help in reducing such traits as perfectionism, compulsive or controlling behaviors, or the need for attention. Many athletes are driven by such traits and can cope more effectively with personalized counseling.
3. For weight control problems, address not only body weight but also family genetics and body type. Body fatness is another key issue. See Table 1-3.
4. Ergogenic aids are expensive and not necessary. A well-balanced diet will suffice for most athletic events.

Table 1–3.
Body Fat Standards

25% or more men, 30% or more women	Clinical obesity
15–18% men, 25–28% women	Normal levels
12–15% men, 20–25% women	Athletes
7–10% men, 12–18% women	Top athletes
5% men, 11% women	Essential for life

5. Pre-event diets should be eaten 3 1/2–4 hours before the activity. Complex carbohydrates should be consumed, using less fat and protein because of their impact on digestive processes. The meal may contain 300–1000 calories.
6. Discuss how to obtain a high-calorie, high-complex-carbohydrate diet, with attention to the individual's preferences. 3000–6000 kcal may be needed in vigorous training programs.
7. Caffeine and alcoholic beverages do nothing to promote performance and may impact negatively on neurological and cardiac systems.
8. The habit of eating candy before a game can cause an insulin overshoot, leading to hypoglycemia. A balanced diet is more practical.

For More Information

Women's Sports Foundation (800) 227-3988

Sports Medicine Systems c/o Nancy Clark, R.D. (617) 731-5800

NOTES

ADULTHOOD

Usual Hospital Stay

Varies by disorder.

Notation

The period of young adulthood is from 18 to 40 years. The period of middle adulthood is 40 to 65 years; family is the primary concern in the middle years.

Objectives

1. Maintain quality of nutrition while compensating for lowered caloric needs.
2. Alleviate obesity resulting from a sedentary lifestyle (where prevalent).
3. Prevent or delay the onset of medical conditions—hypertension, osteoporosis, cardiovascular disease, renal disorders, oncologic conditions. Treat those problems that do exist.
4. Promote adequate bone mass density, which peaks at 25–30.

Dietary Recommendations

1. Ensure intake of the four basic food groups: milk group, two or more servings; meat group, two or more servings; vegetable and fruit group, four or more servings; bread group, four or more servings. Fats, oils, sugars, and sweets are to be controlled as needed to increase or decrease caloric intake. P:M:S fat ratio should be 1:1:1.
2. Modify diet as needed for special medical conditions—it may be that sodium and fat intake should be controlled to prevent future difficulties. In addition, after age 23, only underweight persons need to gain weight.
3. Calorie needs: females 35 kcal/kg IBW; males 40 kcal/kg IBW—vary by sedentary or active status.
4. For most healthy adults, 0.8–1 g protein/kg will suffice.
5. Use more fish and fiber. Encourage nonmeat entrees (dry beans, peas, nuts).
6. A careful sodium:potassium balance should be maintained, along with adequate calcium and magnesium.
7. Adequate vitamins A, C, and E and selenium should be consumed to reduce risks of cancer.

Profile

Ht	Mg^{++}	Wt
IBW/HBW	Ca^{++}	H & H
Alb	Na^+	Gluc
BUN	Creat	BP
K^+	Alcohol use	Chol
Trig	Smoking	

Side Effects of Common Drugs Used

Women. Contraceptive steroids decrease serum levels of vitamins B_6 and B_{12}, folic acid, and vitamin C and increase serum levels of vitamin A, copper, and lipids. Adjust diets accordingly. Users of *intrauterine devices* should increase their intake of iron and vitamin C to counteract increased menstrual losses.

Men. Adequate supplementation with vitamin C (1 g/day) has helped some couples overcome problems with *infertility* (see *JAMA* 249:2747, 1983).

Other medications may have nutritional side effects and should be assessed individually.

Patient Education

1. Explain the benefits of weight control and exercise for the adult.
2. Describe the effects of the "business lunch" and alcohol on nutritional status. Average daily alcohol intake equals 300 kcal.
3. Help the patient plan a diet in accordance with his or her own lifestyle.

Nutrient density and food cost, as well as safe food handling and sanitation, should be explained.
4. Discuss calcium alternatives for people who exclude milk products.
5. Discuss fiber, nonmeat vegetarian meals, cooking methods for nutrient preservation.
6. A normal female has 26–28% body fat, suitable for normal reproduction. Beware either too much or too little body fat.

Table 1–4.
Special Nutrition-Related Concerns of Women*
Recommendations:

1. Eat a variety of foods from all major food groups.
2. Maintain healthy body weight (HBW).
3. Exercise 3 days per week on an average.
4. Limit total fat to 33% of total kcals; use a variety of saturated/monounsaturated/polyunsaturated fats.
5. Eat at least 50% daily kcals from carbohydrates, especially complex CHOs.
6. Eat a variety of fiber-rich foods.
7. Include plenty of iron-rich foods.
8. Limit intake of salt and sodium-rich foods.
9. Limit alcohol to 1–2 drinks daily.
10. Rely on foods, not always supplements.
11. Include 3–4 servings of calcium-rich foods daily.
12. Avoid smoking.
13. Adjust health behaviors to personal concerns.

---

* American Dietetic Association (*JADA* 86:1663, Dec. 1986).

Premenstrual Syndrome (PMS)

Women should omit alcohol and caffeine and excesses of chocolate from their diets 7–14 days before menstruation if they suffer from PMS. A balanced diet with adequate protein and vitamin B_6 should be consumed. Six small meals may be better tolerated. A general multivitamin/mineral capsule may be recommended by the doctor. Adequate magnesium may be helpful. PMS symptoms include edema, hypoglycemia, migraines, hypothyroidism and slightly elevated prolactin levels. For some, spironolactone by prescription may be helpful. PMS Hotline: (800) 222-4767.

Fibrocystic Breast Disease

Decreased caffeine intake has generally been recommended. Postum and some herbal teas may be acceptable substitutes. Vitamins A, C, and E as well as B-complex, iodine and selenium have been suggested. Fish and fish oils may also be beneficial.

Menopause

Exogenous estrogens may be a concern in the development of adenoma of the endometrium. Postmenopausal osteoporosis may lead to bone fractures. Encourage regular physical examinations.

NOTES

GERIATRIC NUTRITION

Usual Hospital Stay

Varies by disorder. Only 4–5% of the elderly are in nursing homes. About 48% of medical and 50% of surgical hospital admissions may have malnutrition as a complication.

Notation

Persons over age 65 now comprise 10% of the U.S. population.

Two thirds of persons 75 years old have no teeth. Decreased salivation and absorption, as well as declining taste and smell, should be considered. BMR declines 2% each decade of life; LBM declines 6% each decade, replaced by fat. The oldest age attained by humans seems to be 114 years; calorie deprivation/control may play a part.

Objectives

1. Provide proper nutrition for weight control, healthy appetite, and prevention of illness/complications (e.g., osteoporosis, fractures, anemias, obesity, diabetes, heart disease and CA).
2. Correct existing nutritional deficiencies. Malnutrition may be caused by poverty, ignorance, or mental or physical disability.
3. Provide foods of proper consistency by status of dentition. Dentures increase bitter and sour taste sensations. In addition, the elderly have fewer taste buds, especially for sweets.
4. Evaluate laxative abuse and alcohol abuse. Recommend suitable alternatives.

5. Provide a diet that excludes hard, sticky foods that are difficult to chew and swallow.
6. Choose an appropriate regimen: "If the gut works, use it."
7. Investigate all major shifts in body weight. Ensure adequate hydration.
8. Assess the environment. (Who cooks, who shops, how are finances, how many meals are eaten away from home?)

Dietary Recommendations

1. Diet should reflect the patient's age and provide the four basic food groups. Adults need the same nutrients throughout life.
2. Diet should provide adequate intake of protein (1 g/kg body weight— 63 g for men, 50 g for women), 800 mg calcium, the B-vitamins, 10 mg iron, 12–15 mg zinc, RDAs for other nutrients according to the patient's age and sex. Consider liver and renal impairments.
3. Calories (See Comments section): RDA for age or $1.2 \times$ BEE. If patient has cardiovascular disease, ensure that intake of fat is low and use a NAS (4g) diet. Average 75-year-old female needs 1900 kcal; males need 2100 kcal if mobile. Less would be needed for nonambulatory persons. See Comments.
4. The consistency of the food should be altered (ground, strained, chopped) as required.
5. Adequate fiber and fluid intake is necessary. Prudent increases in fiber (e.g., from prunes and bran) can reduce laxative abuse. Dehydration is a common cause of confusion.
6. Adequate amounts of vitamin C, folic acid, and iron are needed—these nutrients are frequently deficient in the diets of the elderly.
7. When taste sensations are weak, the diet should provide adequate intake of zinc and vitamin B_{12}.
8. Increased thiamine may be needed because of decreased metabolic efficiency. Men are especially susceptible.
9. Reduce intake of simple sugars; poor glucose tolerance and insulin resistance are common over age 65.
10. If early satiety is a problem, having the main meal at noon may help. Taste-related nutrients include zinc, folate, vitamin B_{12} and vitamin A.
11. Encourage socialization at mealtimes.

Profile

Wt	Ht	Difficulty in chewing
Recent wt changes	Urinary N	or swallowing
Transferrin	K^+	Decubiti
TLC	H & H	TSF, MAC, MAMC
Ca^{++}	Chol	IBW/HBW
Trig	Gluc	BP

Dentition	Alb (may be	Clinical signs of
Eyesight and hearing changes	deceptively high in dehydration)Gluc	malnutrition
		BUN, creat

Side Effects of Common Drugs Used

1. Many drugs affect the nutritional status of the patient. A thorough drug history is needed.
2. Use of *mineral oil* as a laxative should be discouraged because it decreases absorption of fat-soluble vitamins and calcium.
3. Evidence exists that a long-term, high-carbohydrate, low-protein diet may be undesirable with drug therapies of many types. Drug metabolism is slowed down, a potentially dangerous occurrence.
4. Drug metabolism and detoxification require adequate methionine, vitamins A, C, and E, choline, folacin, selenium, other sulfur amino acids, and vitamin B_{12}.
5. *Sulfonamides* decrease levels of vitamin K and the B-complex.
6. *Diuretics* can decrease serum levels of potassium, magnesium, calcium, and zinc.
7. *Cimetidine* can decrease vitamin B_{12} levels.
8. *Aspirin* decreases serum folate, vitamin C and iron.
9. *Estrogens* (Premarin) may cause nausea, vomiting, weight changes.

Patient Education

1. Emphasize the need to consume adequate amounts of calcium and iron.
2. Be aware of income limitations when planning a menu—less expensive protein sources may be necessary. Discuss shopping and meal preparation tips.
3. Prevent excessive use of coffee and tea, which inhibit iron absorption.
4. Ensure that the diet uses sources of fluid and fiber to alleviate constipation. Discuss exercise also.
5. Determine whether the patient is using alcohol since multiple deficiencies may result, especially thiamine, B_{12}, folacin and zinc.
6. Encourage participation in Meals-on-Wheels, Food Stamps, or Congregate Feeding Programs.
7. Ensure adequate fluid intake, where permitted.

Comments

Aging involves a progression of physiological changes with cell loss and organ decline ($\downarrow$ GFR, $\downarrow$ HCl, $\uparrow$ constipation, $\downarrow$ glucose tolerance, $\downarrow$ cell-mediated immunity can occur). Because of these changes, RDAs may eventually be separated for ages 50–70, and 70$^+$. Intake of calories can decrease 10% for ages 50–70; 20–25% less thereafter. After age 70, body weight declines; physical activity can prevent loss of LBM.

For More Information

Administration on Aging
330 Independence Ave., SW
Washington, DC 20201

Section 2
Dietary Practices and Miscellaneous Conditions

CULTURAL FOOD PATTERNS

Objectives

1. Provide individualization for cultural patterns that differ from the standard in the region. Do not assume that each person fits the typical pattern, but be prepared to understand the differences from a "typical American" diet.
2. Determine which habits, if any, are detrimental for healthy lifestyles. In addition, review any patterns or food intakes that aggravate existing or predisposing chronic or àcute conditions for each person.
3. Correct the diet for deficits—such as calcium and riboflavin in dietary patterns where milk is excluded or not tolerated.

Dietary Patterns

1. *Chinese Patterns*. The diet may be low in calcium and riboflavin because milk is often not tolerated or consumed. Encourage use of tofu, green vegetables and fish containing small bones. The diet can be high in sodium if MSG and soy sauces are used. "Hot" and "cold" foods may be used during pregnancy or illness, but these have nothing to do with food temperatures.
2. *Mexican/Puerto Rican Patterns*. Milk again may be used only rarely, but cheese is a common additive to meals. Fruits and vegetables may be viewed as luxuries, but chili peppers, mangos and avocado are com-

mon. The main starch is corn or flour tortilla. The diet may be high in sugar and saturated fat (lard). Beans with rice is a common main dish. Salsa or sofrito seasonings are used frequently. Obesity may be a problem.

3. *Southeast Asian/Vietnamese Patterns.* Again, milk is seldom used and calcium may be a problem. Fish and pork are common entrees. A highly salted fish sauce is used. Snacking is rare in the family diet. As in the Chinese patterns, hot-cold patterns are sometimes observed.

4. *Southern/Soul/Cajun Patterns.* Broccoli, greens and evaporated milk often constitute the calcium source. Pork, ham, black-eyed peas, beans, and nuts are typical protein sources. Rice, cornbread, and hominy grits make up the starches in addition to bread. High sodium salt pork and bacon are used as seasonings. Milk is often not tolerated or consumed. Problems may include obesity, hypertension, diabetes and heart disease.

Adapted from: Holman, S.: *Essentials of Nutrition for the Health Professional.* Philadelphia, J.B. Lippincott, 1987.

NOTES

VEGETARIANISM

Usual Hospital Stay

Varies by disorder.

Notation

There are three major categories of vegetarianism: *vegan*, a very strict vegetarian food pattern ("pure" vegetarianism); *lacto*, a vegetarian food pattern using milk; and *lacto-ovo*, a vegetarian food pattern using milk and eggs.

Objectives

1. Encourage use of a wide variety of foods, in adequate quantity and balance of amino acids.
2. Provide nutritionally adequate menus with sufficient calories for weight maintenance/idealization. Discourage the excessive use of sweets.

3. Monitor fiber intake, since excesses interfere with absorption of calcium, zinc, and iron.
4. Monitor the diet carefully if the patient is an infant, child, pregnant woman, or lactating mother. In addition, monitor elderly persons following a vegetarian diet.
5. Prevent or correct anemia.

Dietary Recommendations

1. Followers of a *lactovegetarian diet* should be watched for deficiencies in iron, phosphorus, potassium, B-complex, and protein. Followers of a *vegan diet* should be watched for deficiencies in calcium, iron, iodine, vitamin B_{12}, vitamin D, protein, riboflavin, and zinc.
2. Beware of the limiting amino acids in typical protein foods: wheat (lysine), rice (lysine and threonine); corn (lysine and tryptophan); beans (methionine); and chickpeas (methionine).
3. Use iodized salt.
4. Stress the need for vitamin D. Spending time in the sun or supplementation should be recommended for children, infants, pregnant women, and the elderly.
5. Suggest dark, leafy greens for calcium, riboflavin, and iron. Watch for the presence of oxalates in spinach, rhubarb, kale, and chard.
6. Recommend a fortified cereal or a supplement (as needed) to maintain proper levels of vitamin B_{12}. Fortified soy milk may be used.
7. Ensure adequate calorie intake.
8. For zinc, use of foods like legumes, hard cheese, soy products, nuts and seeds will help.
9. For calcium, tofu and soy milk provide sources for vegans.

Profile

Ht	Wt	Serum B_{12}
IBW/HBW	Alb	Ca^{++}, Mg^{++}
H & H, MCV	Chol, Trig	Serum Fe
Transferrin	Gluc	

Patient Education

1. Explain patterns of food intake that provide complementary amino acids.
2. Emphasize the importance of a balanced diet.
3. Describe the role vegetarian diets play in lowering serum cholesterol, triglycerides and glucose.
4. Soy milk should be fortified with calcium and vitamin B_{12}.
5. Counsel about use of herbal teas, especially regarding toxic substances.
6. Counsel about appropriate products for infants and children (e.g., fortified soy formula). Protein may be the biggest problem.

Comments

1. *Complementary Protein Relationships.** Different food combinations provide essential amino acids that produce higher quality proteins.

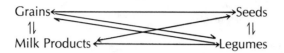

⇌ means "complementary between several items in each group."
↔ means "complementary between a few items in each group."

> EXAMPLES. *Grains and milk:* bread and milk; rice and cheese; pasta and cheese. *Grains and legumes:* rice and beans; bread and beans; corn and beans. *Seeds and legumes:* garbanzos and sesame (as in dips); seeds and beans (as in roasted snacks). *Vegetables* with nuts, dairy products, rice, sunflower seeds or wheat germ.

2. *Vegetarian diets* can improve obesity, constipation, coronary heart disease, diabetes, hypertension and diverticular disease. They may also reduce incidence of breast cancer, colon cancer and gallstones. Vegetarians also tend to have less appendicitis, hiatal hernia, irritable bowel syndrome, hemorrhoids and varicose veins.

3. The National Cancer Institute recommends intake of 25–35 g of fiber a day (28 g = 1 oz). Vegetarian diets can easily provide this level.

---

* From Lappe, F.: *Diet for a Small Planet*, 2nd ed. New York, Ballantine Books, 1983.

NOTES

KOSHER DIETARY PRACTICES (KASHRUTH)

Usual Hospital Stay

Varies by specific disorder.

Notation

The term "kosher" applies to foods "fit, proper and in accordance with the Kashruth." Pareve is a term for foods made without milk or meat or their derivatives. A Kosher diet forbids all foods not in accordance with Mosaic Law.

Objectives

1. Observe dietary practices as followed by the kosher laws of Judaism: meats are limited to cud-chewing animals with cloven hooves. Pork, shellfish and scavenger fish are forbidden.
2. Separate utensils are to be used for preparation and eating, and especially for separating meat and milk foods.
3. Remember that the kosher diet tends to be high in cholesterol and saturated fats, as well as sodium.
4. Reduce lactose and sodium in sensitive individuals.

Dietary Recommendations

Meat and dairy dishes are eaten separately.

1. *Meat.* No pork, rabbit, shellfish, or eel may be eaten. Eggs are pareve foods.
2. *Dairy.* Milk may be consumed before a meal, but once meat is eaten, 3–6 hours must pass before dairy products can be consumed.
3. *Kosher products must be used.* On food labels "U" or "K" means a kosher food. "Pareve" indicates that the food is neutral.
4. Fruits, vegetables and grains can be used, except that breads made with milk products are forbidden with meat meals.
5. Leavened (raised) bread is forbidden during Passover.
6. Omit lactose if necessary; provide other sources of calcium and riboflavin.

Profile

Ht	Wt	K^+
Gluc	BP	Ca^{++}
Chol	Trig	Alk phos
IBW/HBW	Na^+	

Patient Education

1. Show the patient how to limit foods high in cholesterol/fat if weight and elevated lipid levels are a problem.
2. Discuss sodium and obesity in relationship to hypertension, as appropriate. Recommend other herbs, spices and cooking methods.
3. Low-fat cheeses should be substituted for high-fat cheese, such as cream cheese.

DENTAL DIFFICULTIES AND ORAL DISORDERS

Usual Hospital Stay

4 days.

Notation

Cell turnover is very rapid for tongue and oral mucosa; therefore, one of the first areas where signs of systemic disease appear is the oral cavity. Changes in the oral/dental health of a patient should be checked. In *dental caries*, a chronic infectious disease leads to progressive destruction of tooth substances from interactions between bacteria and organic tooth compounds. *Streptococcus mutans* and *Lactobacillus* are common culprits. Acid forms 20 sec–30 min after contact.

Objectives

Edentulism. Provide proper consistency to allow the patient to eat.

Broken or Wired Jaw. Provide adequate nourishment to allow healing while reducing jaw movement. Decrease fever, nausea and vomiting. Prevent excess weight loss (usually 10%).

Mouth Ulcers. Lessen mouth soreness to increase dietary intake.

Tongue Disorders. Provide adequate nourishment despite disability.

Dental Caries. Alter dietary habits; deprive bacteria of substrate; reduce acid; keep pH at 7.0.

Dietary Recommendations

Edentulism. A chopped, ground, strained, or pureed diet should be followed as required.

Broken or Wired Jaw. A diet of pureed and strained foods, as well as liquids of high protein/calorie content, is necessary. Adequate amounts of vitamin C should be taken to aid healing. Monitor food temperatures carefully. 6–8 meals are needed. Follow meals with salt-water rinse.

Mouth Ulcers. Foods low in acid should be taken (e.g., citrus juices are not allowed). Supplement the diet with vitamin C, protein, and calories to speed the rate of healing.

Tongue Disorders. If the patient is unable to chew, tube feeding is necessary. Liquids may be added to the diet as tolerated.

Dental Caries. Decrease sucrose and sticky starches, as well as the frequency of snacking. Use a balanced diet, eating sweets or starches *with* meals. Cheese, raw fruits and vegetables, peanuts and cocoa are anticariogenic. Fluoride intake should be adequate.

Profile

Ht	lacerations	teeth
IBW/HBW	H & H	Sore or bleeding gums
Wt	P	Dentures, especially
Alb	TSF, MAMC, MAC for	poorly fitted
Ca^{++}	wired jaw	Taste alterations
Recent wt changes	Caries	
Mouth or tongue	Missing or loose	

Nutrients Needed for Proper Oral Tissue Synthesis and Dental Care

1. *Vitamin A.* Necessary for epithelial tissue and enamel.
2. *Vitamin C.* Enables connective tissue cells to elaborate intercellular substances. Deficiency can lead to easy bleeding or swelling of gums, and gingivitis.
3. *Calcium, Phosphorus, Vitamin D.* Necessary for dentin and bony tissue synthesis. Poor mineralization occurs with deficiency.
4. *Fluoride.* Reduces susceptibility of teeth to caries formation. Drinking water should contain 1 ppm. Toothpaste, mouth rinses and topical treatments also help.
5. *B-complex Vitamins.* Deficiencies show a bright scarlet tongue and stomatitis in niacin deficiency; magenta tongue, cheilosis and angular stomatitis in ariboflavinosis; smooth tongue in vitamin B_{12} deficiency, etc.
6. *Protein.* Needed for healthy tissue growth and maintenance.
7. *Folacin.* Needed for a healthy blood supply.

Patient Education

1. If needed, blended foods and/or tube feedings should be prepared.
2. Provide the patient with creative ideas for the seasoning and flavoring of foods. Discuss choices from restaurant options.
3. Ensure that fluoride is provided in some way by the diet, and by the water supply.
4. Encourage good habits in oral hygiene and diet: detergent foods (raw fruits and vegetables) should be recommended rather than sticky or impactant foods (soft cookies, bread, sticky sweets, dried fruits, etc.).
5. Read milk labels to ensure vitamin D fortification.
6. Use cheese after meals or sugary snacks to normalize pH.

Comments

Erosion of tooth enamel may occur in patients who chronically consume acidic beverages and/or keep such beverages or foods in the mouth for a period of time (e.g., sucking lemons, chewing vitamin C tablets, chewing lemon hard candies).

Some tooth problems are age-specific. Infants should be monitored for the *nursing-bottle caries syndrome*; dental decay often occurs during the growth spurts of adolescents; and elderly patients should be monitored for changes in eating habits, use of an inadequate diet, caries. Keep in mind also that poor oral hygiene can increase the likelihood of gingival abnormalities in scorbutic conditions.

For More Information

American Dental Association
211 East Chicago Ave.
Chicago, IL 60611

SELF-FEEDING PROBLEMS

Usual Hospital Stay

Varies by other conditions.

Notation

Four areas of concern are considered here: blindness, coordination problems, chewing problems, and dysphagia. Where appropriate, these factors are also mentioned in relation to specific disorders in other sections.

Objectives

1. Promote independence in self-feeding, where possible.
2. Address all nutritional deficiencies and complications individually.
3. Promote overall wellness and health.
4. Increase interest in eating.
5. Prevent malnutrition and weight loss.
6. Decrease instances where constipation or anorexia or other problems affect nutritional status.
7. Increase pleasure associated with mealtimes.

Dietary Recommendations

Blindness:

1. Provide special plate guards, utensils, double handles, compartmentalized plates with foods placed in similar locations at each meal.
2. Work with OT or family to practice kitchen safety and to determine ability to have independence at mealtimes
3. Create a feeling of usefulness by delegating appropriate tasks related to mealtime, such as drying dishes, assisting with simple meal tasks that are safe for the person.

Coordination Problems:

1. Self-feeding requires—ability to suck, to sit with head and neck balanced, to bring hand to mouth, to grasp cup and utensil, to drink from a cup, to take food from a spoon, to bite, to chew and to swallow.

2. Each person should be assessed individually to determine which, if any, aspects of coordination have been affected by his or her condition. Adjust self-feeding accordingly.

Chewing Problems:

1. Decrease texture in foods as necessary (e.g., use a mechanical soft, pureed or liquid diet as needed). Season as desired for individual taste.
2. If needed, use a tube feeding.
3. For some persons, a straw may be helpful. For others, it is not useful.
4. Liquid or blenderized foods may be beneficial.
5. Protein foods such as tofu, cottage cheese, peanut butter, eggs, cheese and milk products can be used when meats or nuts cannot be chewed.

Dysphagia:

1. Watch for signs such as drooling. See CVA entry as well.
2. Swallowing requires 5–10 seconds and three phases for completion— oral phase, pharyngeal phase and esophageal phase. All must be adequate to prevent choking.
3. Prevent aspiration by careful selection of foods, such as thick, soft, pureed foods instead of liquids. Progress back to liquids when possible.
4. Crushed bran on cereal or Enrich products can help to alleviate constipation.
5. Tube feed or use gastrostomy when necessary.
6. Thicken foods with special products, such as Thick-It.

Patient Education

1. Discuss the importance of various therapies and medications for recovery.
2. Discuss the role of nutrition in health, weight control, recovery or repair processes.
3. Provide instruction on simplified meal planning and preparation.
4. Refer to agencies such as Meals-on-Wheels, etc.

Comments

In *Ophthalmology*, key nutrients include vitamins A (for healthy cornea and conjunctiva), B_6 (for healthy conjunctiva), and C (for healthy conjunctiva and vitreous humor), zinc (for healthy retina and optic nerve), riboflavin (for corneal vascularization), vitamin B_{12} (for retina and nerve fibers) and thiamine (for normal retinal and optic nerve functioning). Niacin is also important.

For More Information

American Council for the Blind: (800) 424-8666

PERIODONTAL DISEASE

Usual Hospital Stay

4 days.

Notation

Periodontal disease is a painless, chronic inflammatory disease, generally caused by dental plaque and microbial flora.* A poor diet and inadequate dental hygiene can also cause destruction of the jawbone. Periodontal disease is evident about 10 years before osteoporosis; it most commonly manifests as *pyorrhea alveolaris*. In the United States, periodontal disease affects 75% of the population. At risk in particular are pregnant women, diabetics, alcoholics, smokers, and persons on certain medications.

Objectives

1. Reduce inflammation.
2. Promote healing.
3. Correct poor nutritional habits that can produce conditions such as chronic subclinical nutritional deficiencies in levels of vitamin C, amino acids, riboflavin, folacin, vitamin A, zinc, and calcium.
4. Prevent further decline in status of bones and gums.

Dietary Recommendations

1. Ensure adequate intake of calcium, protein, and phosphorus, as well as a proper calcium:phosphorus ratio.
2. Vitamin D fortified milk should be used.
3. Ensure adequate intake of vitamin C, fluoride, vitamin A and zinc.
4. Use high detergent foods (firm, fresh fruits and raw vegetables).
5. If needed, a weight control diet should be planned.

---

* Usually dental caries and peridontal disease are not present in the same patients because microbial flora differ.

Profile

Alb
Ht
IBW/HBW
H & H
Wt

Gums—color,
  friability
Oral exam for tooth
  mobility, calculus

Presence of dental
  caries, missing teeth
Overall nutritional
  status

Side Effects of Drugs Commonly Used

Oral contraceptives may lower serum levels of folate and vitamin C, thereby jeopardizing gingival health.

Patient Education

1. Encourage a proper diet, especially a correct calcium:phosphorus ratio and RDAs for age.
2. Recommend meticulous oral hygiene and regular dental exams to maintain dental hygiene.
3. Encourage pregnant women, diabetics and leukemia patients to pay special attention to oral hygiene.

Comments

Tissues that support teeth in the jaws are collectively known as the periodontium (gums, alveolar bone, periodontal membrane). Any abnormality that leads to a visual change or loss of integrity of any component of the supporting tissue is listed as a periodontal disease. Examples:

1. *Gingivitis*—minor inflammatory change; it may be acute or chronic, local or generalized. Vitamin C deficiency has been implicated.
2. *Acute necrotizing ulcerative gingivitis* (Vincent's disease or trench mouth) is an acute ulceration affecting marginal gingiva with inflamed or necrotic interdental papillae. The onset is abrupt and painful, with slight fever, malaise, excess salivation, and fetid breath. It can be caused by systemic disease. A bland diet may be useful.
3. *Periodontitis* involves a gross breakdown of supporting tissues with progressive loosening and loss of teeth; it is a major cause of tooth loss in adults.
4. *Periodontoclasia* involves destruction of tissues around the teeth.

For More Information

American Academy of Periodontology
Suite 924, 211 East Chicago Ave.
Chicago, IL 60611

TEMPOROMANDIBULAR JOINT DYSFUNCTION (TMJ)

Usual Hospital Stay

4 days.

Notation

TMJ disorders result from local or systemic causes, such as RA or osteoarthritis or connective tissue disorders. Each TMJ is a diathrosis with moving elements (mandible) and fixed elements (temporal bone). With this dysfunction, overuse or abuse of any part of normal action affects the mastication process. Women between the ages of 30–60 years account for 75% of all cases.

Signs and symptoms include pain, clicking noise, stiffness of neck, face, or shoulders, locking of affected joint, trismus, mandibular deviation—often from repetitive overloading (stress or habit such as gum chewing, grinding), from functional masseter muscle coordination problems, or from incorrect occlusion (as with missing teeth).

Objectives

1. Reduce repetitive overloading by use of a splint or by breaking bad habits, such as grinding.
2. Reduce stress with relaxation techniques.
3. Relieve pain and muscle spasms.
4. Prevent or correct malnutrition or weight loss.
5. Ensure adequate intake of fiber.
6. Reduce any existing inflammation.
7. Prevent complications, such as mitral valve prolapse.

Dietary Recommendations

1. Use a normal diet, with soft foods to prevent pain on chewing.
2. Cut food into small, bite-size pieces.
3. Avoid opening mouth widely, as for large and thick sandwiches.
4. Avoid chewy foods such as caramel, nuts, toffee, chewy candies, gummy bread and rolls.
5. Grate vegetables (e.g., carrots) to reduce chewing.
6. Use adequate sources of vitamin C for adequate gingival health.

Profile

Ht	Alb	H & H
Wt	Gum status	Chol
IBW/HBW	Gluc	Trig

Patient Education

1. Discuss the role of dental care in maintaining adequate health.
2. Monitor gum soreness; advise the dentist if necessary.
3. Physical therapy may be needed to correct functioning of muscles and joints.
4. Nail-biting, gum-chewing, use of teeth to cut thread, or similar habits should be stopped.

Comments

Structural problems are treated by surgery (e.g., fusion can be treated by removing the area of fused bone and replacing it with silicon rubber). Sometimes an artificial joint is the answer. Surgery is recommended, however, for only a very few patients. Undue muscle tension causes the majority of TMJ, with some other problems stemming from inadequate bite (as from a high filling or from a malocclusion).

Most people with TMJ will benefit most from a visit to their dentist, with secondary visits to other specialists (e.g., ear-nose-throat specialists) as appropriate.

NOTES

SKIN DISORDERS

Usual Hospital Stay

3–6 days.

Notation

The skin often reflects internal problems—GI problems, alcoholism, or general inanition. Eczema is a skin condition manifested by itching, blistering, oozing, and scaling skin rash.

Objectives

1. Reduce inflammation and edema if present.
2. Apply nutritional principles according to the particular condition.

Dietary Recommendations

1. *Acne.* Encourage intake of adequate zinc (this condition is hormone-dependent). Adequate vitamin A is also key.
2. *Psoriasis.* Hormonal vitamin D $(1, 25 - (OH)_2 - D_3)$ has proven recently to be of some benefit. Studies have been conducted at Boston University. Increase use of zinc from meats, seafood, and whole grains. Psoriasis may precede arthritis by months or years.
3. *Chronic urticaria.* Reduce salicylates and aspirin use, or penicillin and food molds. Berries and dried fruits are high in salicylates, as are herbs and spices.
4. *Infantile eczema.* A familial tendency may be noted for this condition, which may result from hypersensitivity to milk, egg albumin, or wheat. Control caloric excess in obese infants.
5. *Acrodermatitis enteropathica.* Supplement with zinc, as absorption of zinc is impaired in this condition. Use adequate HBVs, decrease excess fiber.
6. *Dermatitis herpetiformis.* A gluten-free diet is quite successful in treating this condition.
7. *Hypercarotenemia.* Reduce dietary and supplementary carotene (carrots, tomatoes, etc.).
8. *Nickel dermatitis.* Avoid canned fish, tomatoes, corn, spinach, other canned vegetables, and nuts. Do not cook with stainless steel utensils.

Profile

Ht	Serum zinc	Trig
Growth pattern in infants/children	Histamine	IBW/HBW
	Wt	Serum carotene
Alb (dec. in exfoliative dermatitis)	H & H	RBP
	Gluc	Uric acid (inc. in chronic eczema)
	Chol	

Side Effects of Common Drugs Used

1. *Topical corticosteroids* usually have a mild effect on the nutritional status of the patient. Stronger brands or dosage may impact like oral steroids.
2. *Isotretinoin* (Accutane) may be used for acne or psoriasis. Watch for decrease in HDL and an increase in triglycerides and avoid vitamin A supplementation. Dry mouth can occur. Avoid during pregnancy.
3. *Tetracycline* should not be taken with milk or calcium supplements. Excesses of vitamin A can cause headaches, HPN. Use more riboflavin, vitamin C and calcium in the diet. Beware of a general protein and iron malabsorption. Diarrhea is the major GI effect.

Patient Education

1. Encourage the patient to read food labels.
2. Explain good sources of protein, vitamin A, zinc, vitamin C.
3. Help the patient modify his or her diet as specifically indicated by the condition.
4. Encourage adequate fluid intake, but not excess.
5. Discuss use of sunscreens, avoidance of topical or specialty products, and roles of nutrients in skin care.

For More Information

Help-line: (800) 222-SKIN

Acne Hotline: (800) 235-ACNE

American Academy of Dermatology
P.O. Box 3116
Evanston, IL 60204-3116

American Society for Dermatologic Surgery: (800) 441-ASDS

NOTES

DECUBITUS ULCER

Usual Hospital Stay

8–9 days.

Notation

Decubitus ulcer is a pressure sore usually occurring in the elderly. It is caused by a lack of oxygen and nutrition to the area, especially among patients with PCM, or bedridden or paralyzed patients. Decubitus ulcers often occur over bone or cartilaginous prominences (hip, sacrum, elbow, or heels). Risk factors include immobility, poor circulation, infection, poor nutritional status, prolonged pressure, drugs, and serum albumin below 3.0 g/dl.

Objectives

1. Restore normal protein and nutrient status. Correct PCM.
2. Heal the decubitus ulcer and prevent further tissue breakdown.
3. Improve low-grade infections, fever, diarrhea, and vomiting.
4. Assess intake via calorie counts.

Dietary Recommendations

1. Provide a high protein/high calorie diet.
2. Feed by tube if necessary.
3. Supplement diet with multivitamins, especially vitamins A and C, and thiamine. Include zinc as well.
4. Provide small, frequent feedings if oral intake is poor, 4–6 times daily.

Profile

Ht	Alb, RBP ($\downarrow$)	Anorexia
IBW/HBW	N balance	Vomiting
BUN, creat	Gluc	Diarrhea
H & H	Stage of Ulcer	Transferrin
Wt	Wt loss	TLC
TP ($\downarrow$)		

Patient Education

1. Instruct nursing personnel and patient's family about the importance of adequate nutrition for healing of tissues.
2. Discuss importance of maintaining healthy, intact skin.

Comments

Table 2–1.
Stage of Ulcer*

Stage I—redness and warmth
Stage II—shallow ulcer with distinct edges
Stage III—full-thickness loss of skin
Stage IV—involvement of fascia, connective tissue, muscle, and bone
Stage V—area covered with black eschar

---

* Derived from: Durr, E.D.: Nutritional intervention for patients with pressure sores. *Nutrition Support Services* 6:28, 1986; and Hunan, K., and Schesle, L.: Albumin vs. weight as a predictor of nutritional stutus and pressure ulcer development. *Ostomy/Wound Manag.*, 33:447, 1991.

NOTES

VITAMIN DEFICIENCIES (VITAMIN A, BERIBERI, SCURVY, RIBOFLAVIN, PELLAGRA)

Usual Hospital Stay

2–5 days.

Notation

Deficiencies may be primary (self-induced by inadequate diet) or secondary to disease process. They are especially common in diet faddists, in alcoholics, in people who live alone and eat poorly.

Objectives

1. Replenish the deficient nutrient and restore normal serum levels.
2. Prevent side effects of nutrient deficiency:

Vitamin A. Reduced growth, night blindness leading progressively to xerophthalmia, changes in epithelial tissue, failure of tooth enamel and/or degeneration, loss of taste and smell.

Thiamine. Impairment of cardiovascular, nervous, and gastrointestinal systems.

Riboflavin. Magenta tongue, angular stomatitis, and cheilosis.

Niacin. Dermatitis, diarrhea, depression, and (sometimes) death.

Vitamin C. Changes in oral cavity (gums, teeth), easy bruising. Anemia may also be a common finding, with petechiae and circulatory problems as well. Delay in wound healing can also occur.

Dietary Recommendations

Vitamin A Deficiency. Use a diet including foods high in vitamin A and carotene: carrots, sweet potatoes, squash, apricots, collards, broccoli, cabbage, dark leafy greens, liver, kidney, cream, butter, and egg yolk.

Beriberi. Use a diet including foods high in thiamine: pork, whole grains, enriched cereal grains, legumes, green vegetables, fish, meat, fruit and milk in quantity. A high protein/high CHO intake should be included.

Riboflavin Deficiency. Use a diet including foods high in riboflavin: milk, eggs, liver, kidney, heart. Caution against losses resulting from cooking and exposure to sunlight.

Pellagra. Use a diet including foods high in niacin and other B-vitamins: yeast, milk, meat, peanuts, cereal bran, and wheat germ.

Scurvy. Use a diet high in citrus fruits and tomatoes.

Profile

Ht/Wt
IBW/HBW
Signs of malnutrition (hair, eyes, skin, tongue, teeth).
Neurological changes
Serum levels of specific nutrients
SGOT (decreased in beriberi)

Side Effects of Common Drugs Used

Vitamin A. Aquasol A is the trade name of one supplement drug. Absorption of vitamin A depends on bile salts in the intestinal tract. Also, beware of doses greater than 1000–3000 IU per kg body weight/day. This is especially true for children. Controlled 25,000 IU/day doses may be prescribed.

Thiamine. Anorexia and nausea may be common at the beginning of treatment. Intravenous therapy may be better tolerated. A common dose is 5–10 mg thiamine/day.

Riboflavin. Achlorhydria may precipitate a deficiency, and may preclude successful correction. Riboflavin is destroyed by alkaline substances.

Niacin. Treatment with niacin may cause flushing. Niacinamide is a better choice. 200–400 mg niacin or niacin equivalents may be used. Nicotinic acid can cause nausea, vomiting, and diarrhea.

Vitamin C. Excesses can cause false-positive glucosuria tests. Cevalin or Cevita are drug sources. 50–300 mg/day may be given to correct scurvy.

Patient Education

1. Explain where sources of the specific nutrient may be found.
2. Demonstrate methods of cooking, storage, etc. that prevent losses.
3. Help the patient to plan a menu incorporating his or her preferences.

Comments

Vitamin D deficiency—see Osteomalacia entry; nutritional rickets in children is rare. Treatment consists of giving adequate vitamin D_3 and ensuring adequate exposure to sunlight. Calderol, Rocaltrol, Hytakerol, and Calciferol are common drug sources.

Vitamin E deficiency—very, very rare; problems can occur with fat malabsorption (especially in children). Abetalipoproteinemia is the most severe deficiency and occurs mainly in premature and sick children. Aquasol E has no adverse side effects, if used within RDA dosage.

Vitamin K deficiency—rare except in intestinal problems and short gut syndromes. Vitamin K can be made by intestinal bacteria in the gut. Synkayvite, Mephyton and Konakion are trade name sources.

Folacin and vitamin B_{12} deficiencies—megaloblastic anemias can result. Peripheral neuropathy and a positive Schilling test are needed to indicate B_{12} deficiency. Treat both conditions with adequate vitamin supplementation. See anemias.

Vitamin B_6 deficiency—deficiency decreases conversion of tryptophan to niacin. It can occur after surgery or as a result of poor diet. Vitabee 6 is a pyridoxine hydrochloride drug.

Pantothenic acid deficiency is rare. Pantholin is a drug which is prescribed as needed.

NOTES

FOOD ALLERGY

Usual Hospital Stay

Allergic reactions, 2–3 days.

Notation

True food allergy is an immune response, generally from IgE, with a reaction usually within 2 hours. A food allergy results from hypersensitivity to an antigen of food (usually protein) source. The manifestations of the allergy are caused by the release of histamine and serotonin. The most common results of food allergies are GI related—(70%): diarrhea, nausea, vomiting, cramping, abdominal distention and pain; 24% are skin-related; 4% are respiratory; 2% are from other body system responses.

Objectives

1. Exclude or avoid the offending allergen. If it is not known, use the Rowe elimination diet to discover what is causing the allergy.
2. Monitor the onset of the reaction, which may be delayed or immediate. If delayed, onset of the reaction may take as long as 5 days. An im-

mediate response is more common with raw foods; patient history may include diarrhea, urticaria, eczema, rhinitis, asthma. Cooking may alleviate some allergenic properties.

3. Treat nutritional deficiencies or insure adequate supplementation.
4. For patients with *asthma*, use a normal diet with small meals. Nothing should be eaten after dinner, to reduce GI reflux.
5. Keep food diaries to determine food reactions.

Dietary Recommendations

1. For the elimination diet, use an unflavored elemental diet as a hypoallergenic base to which other foods are added as test challenges.
2. Read labels of foods served to the patient. Check all menus served to the patient. Monitor food preparation methods to exclude possible contact with the allergen.
3. Monitor nutrient needs.
4. The most common allergens in infants are milk, eggs, wheat, citrus, chocolate, and fish. For children, cow's milk, eggs, legumes, wheat, tree nuts (filberts, cashews), and fish are often a problem. For adults, common allergens include shellfish, peanuts, nuts, and grains.
5. For infants, exclusive breast-feeding is best. Breast milk is generally nonallergenic. Mothers may need to omit cow's milk from their own diets, as well as eggs, fish, and nuts.
6. Infants allergic to cow's milk and soy may need Nutramigen or another hydrolyzed formula.

Profile

Ht	Histamine
Recent changes	Alb
H & H	IqE levels
Chronic complaints (GI distress,	Skin tests (not 100% effective, but
rashes, diarrhea, rhinitis, asthma)	most reliable—follow with food
IBW/HBW	challenge)
Wt	RAST testing

Side Effects of Drugs Commonly Used

Benadryl should be taken with food. It contains sodium sulfite. Dry mouth, constipation, or GI distress may occur.

Most Common Allergens and Possible Nutritional Consequences

Milk. Check for deficiencies in protein, riboflavin, vitamin A, vitamin D, and calcium. Be wary of early introduction of cow's milk in infancy.

Eggs. Check for iron deficiency. Egg albumin is used in marshmallows, frozen dinners, and many other food mixes. Yolks are generally tolerated.

Wheat. Check for B-vitamins and iron. Read labels on packaged soups, sauces.

Fish. Spoiled sources, even before taste change occurs, are especially high in histamine.

Shellfish (Crab, Lobster, Shrimp).

Tomatoes. Usually an allergenic reaction to tomatoes is linked to the frequency of use in the diet.

Citrus Fruits. Persons allergic to citrus fruits can easily become deficient in vitamin C.

Cola, Chocolate.

Legumes (Peanuts, Soybeans, Peas, Lima Beans). Watch labels for lecithin and other soy additives.

Corn. Hidden sources of corn include cornstarch, corn syrup, corn oil, frozen yogurt, baking powder, paper plates, etc.

Nuts. Avoid nut butters also. Aflatoxins can cause a reaction.

Spices. Cinnamon is a common allergen.

Artificial Food Dyes. It may also be necessary to eliminate aspirin and salicylates. Many drugs contain tartrazine (FD&C No. 5 yellow dye).

Molds. This category includes penicillin. Use a diet low in milk and milk products (watch out for deficiencies in calcium and riboflavin), mushrooms, cheese, sour cream, bacon, jams and jellies, spices.

Sulfites. Salad bars, wine, beers, colas, dried fruits and vegetables, maraschino cherries, dried or frozen potatoes may contain sulfites.

Patient Education

1. Encourage the patient to keep a food diary and to read all labels.
2. Persons with a milk allergy can add vanilla or honey flavoring to soy milk.
3. Explain to those patients taking goat's milk that it has less lactalbumin, vitamin D, and folacin than cow's milk has, and that supplements may be required.
4. Persons with milk allergy can use greens, broccoli, clams, oysters, shrimp, and salmon to provide sufficient levels of calcium.
5. Natural sources of histamine include Chianti wine, bleu and Parmesan cheeses, spinach, eggplant, and Burgundy wine. These foods may distort serum levels during testing for allergies.
6. Some persons who are sensitive to milk are also sensitive to beef.
7. Food/plant sensitivities are common (e.g., melon/ragweed; carrot/potato; apple/birch; wheat/grasses). Be wary of herbal teas.
8. Recipe books are available from formula companies, industry, and from area dietitians.
9. Cytotoxic testing, sublingual testing and brain allergy theories should be refuted.
10. Bee pollen does not prevent allergies and may, in fact, cause asthma,

urticaria, rhinitis, or anaphylaxis after eating plants that cross-react with ragweed, such as sunflowers or dandelion greens (*JAMA*, 10/6/89).

For More Information

The Asthma and Allergy Foundation of America
1717 Massachusetts Ave., Suite 305
Washington, DC 20036
(202) 265-0265

American College of Allergists (312) 359-2800

NOTES

CHINESE RESTAURANT SYNDROME

Usual Hospital Stay

Varies.

Notation

An allergic response to monosodium glutamate (MSG) is the cause of the Chinese restaurant syndrome, which results in a temporary burning sensation in the neck and forearms, chest tightness, and headache.

Objectives

1. Avoid sources of MSG. This chemical is often used in the preparation of foods in Chinese restaurants.
2. Low sodium diets should include only limited amounts of MSG, which is 14% sodium.

Dietary Recommendations

1. Eliminate MSG in home-prepared foods.
2. Read labels and avoid MSG. All commercially prepared products except mayonnaise, salad dressings, or French dressings *must* list MSG on the label.

Profile

BP
Burning sensation

Histamine
Food intake history

Patient Education

1. Encourage the patient to read food labels carefully. Omit MSG (Accent, etc.).
2. Patients on diuretic therapy must avoid large amounts of MSG.

Comment

There is some evidence that this syndrome is more common in individuals with vitamin B_6 deficiency.

NOTES

FOOD POISONING

Usual Hospital Stay

3–5 days.

Notation

Food poisoning is a gastrointestinal insult resulting from contaminated beverages or food. Millions of cases occur annually, but only a few hundred are reported. Children under 6, people with chronic illnesses, and the elderly are most at risk.

Objectives

1. Allow the GI tract to rest.
2. Progress as tolerated.
3. Prepare and store all foods using safe food handling practices and good personal hygiene.

Dietary Recommendations

1. Feed with IV glucose (NPO) until progress has been made.
2. Start with bland or soft foods, then progress to a normal diet.
3. Prepare and hold all foods at proper temperatures.

Profile

HT, wt, IBW/HBW	illness
Usual wt	K^+, Na^+
Cl^-	Vomiting, Diarrhea
Weight loss/changes during	

Types of Food Poisoning

Salmonella or Staphylococcus aureus. Symptoms include mild to severe vomiting, headache, diarrhea, cramps, and fever. The illness is caused by ingestion of meat, poultry, fish, eggs, dairy products (salmonella) or creamed foods (staphylococci). Salmonella reacts within 12–36 hrs, lasting 2–7 days. Staph poisoning begins within 2–8 hrs, lasting 24–48 hrs.

Clostridium perfringens. Symptoms include nausea with vomiting, diarrhea, signs of acute gastroenteritis lasting 1 day. Illness usually results from the ingestion of canned meats or from ingestion of contaminated dried mixes.

Clostridium botulinum. Symptoms include dizziness, headache, double vision, followed by paralysis and respiratory and cardiovascular failures. Illness is caused by improperly sterilized, nonacidic foods (meat, corn, peas, green beans, mushrooms, beets) or acidic foods that have grown moldy. The toxin causes an illness 12–48 hrs after ingestion. It may also be found in honey or corn syrup.

Yersinia enterocolitica. Symptoms include diarrhea, fever, headache, severe abdominal pain. The illness is caused by postpasteurization contamination of chocolate milk, reconstituted dry milk, pasteurized milk and tofu. Cold storage does not kill the bacteria.

Listeria monocytogenes. Symptoms include a mild fever, headache, vomiting, severe illness in pregnancy. Postpasteurization contamination of cheese, milk and commercial cole slaw has been implicated.

Campylobacter jejuni. Diarrhea and abdominal cramping are the key symptoms. It may be caused by drinking raw milk or by eating raw or undercooked meat, shellfish or poultry. Some people develop antibodies to it, others do not. It is safer to drink only pasteurized milk. The bacteria may also be found in tofu or raw vegetables. Symptoms can start 2–5 days after eating/drinking a contaminated item and can last 2–7 days.

Patient Education

1. Encourage safe methods of food handling. Keep hot foods above 140° F, cold foods below 40° F.

2. Demonstrate safe food preparation techniques. For example, discard cracked eggs and cook home-canned foods appropriately. Heat foods to 180–185° F.
3. Keep pet foods and utensils separate from those for human use.

For More Information

USDA Meat and Poultry Hotline: (800) 535-4555

MIGRAINE HEADACHE

Notation

Migraine involves paroxysmal attacks of headache, vasospasm, and increased coagulation preceded often by visual disturbances. Approximately 8% of the population is affected. Vasodilators, which are found in some foods, cause blood vessels to swell and contribute to migraine headaches in sensitive persons. Reactions are often within 24 hours after the food has been consumed.

Objectives

1. Reduce or eliminate use of migraine-causing foods.
2. Encourage adequate meal spacing to prevent fasting or skipping of meals.

Dietary Recommendations

1. Promote regular mealtimes. Adequate relaxation is also crucial.
2. Foods implicated in migraine headaches include the following:
   Tuna, mackerel, swiss cheese—contain histamine
   Fermented foods—cheese, yogurt and beer contain tyramine
   Alcohol—red wine contains both histamine and tyramine
   Hot dogs and luncheon meats—contain sodium nitrate
   Coffee, tea, and cola—can trigger caffeine-withdrawal headache from methyl xanthines (18 hrs after withdrawal)
   Chocolate—contains phenylethylamine
   Nuts—some contain vasodilators
   Monosodium glutamate—can cause "Chinese restaurant syndrome" in susceptible persons.
3. Magnesium and fish oils have been recommended for some cases.

Profile

Symptoms and duration	History of similar reactions	Na^+, K^+ Ca^{++}
Foods eaten in past 24 hours	Histamine PT	Mg^{++}

Patient Education

1. Teach patient how to incorporate changes in his or her dietary pattern.
2. Teach the importance of not skipping meals, since fasting can increase a migraine headache.
3. Teach the patient how to complete accurate food records.
4. Monitor drugs taken in correlation with foods/migraine.
5. Research about omega-3 fatty acids is not yet conclusive, but some evidence suggests that they can prevent migraines.

Side Effects of Drugs Commonly Used

1. *Cafergot* contains 100 mg caffeine/tablet. It can cause nausea, vomiting, drowsiness,a nd edema.
2. *Sansert* contains tartrazine. Reduce sodium intake. Nausea, vomiting, indigestion, and weight changes are common.
3. *Sedatives, tranquilizers, antidepressants, and diuretics* may be used. Alter diet accordingly.

For More Information

Headache Hotline: (800) 843-2256.

NOTES

MENIERE'S SYNDROME

Usual Hospital Stay

3 days.

Notation

A rare disease of unknown origin, Meniere's syndrome affects the inner ear and causes disturbed balance.

Signs and symptoms include rapid onset, recurrent deafness, tinnitus with roaring sensation, vertigo, nausea and vomiting, and blurred vision. Patient may have a history of otitis media, smoking, allergies, leukemia or athero-sclerosis. Attacks may last from a few hours to several days.

Objectives

1. Correct nausea and vomiting; replace any necessary electrolytes.
2. Avoid or decrease edema.
3. Decrease fluid retention, which can aggravate an attack.
4. Omit any known food allergens from the diet.

Dietary Recommendations

1. Low sodium diet as tolerated may be necessary.
2. Restrict fluid to reduce pressure on the labyrinth.
3. Use supplements as necessary: vitamins A and C, riboflavin and niacin may be low.
4. Provide a diet that is free of known allergens, specific for the individual.

Profile

Ht, wt	IgE; known allergies	BP
IBW/HBW	Temp	Electrocochleography
Chol	Trig	

Side Effects of Common Drugs Used

1. *Diuretics* are often used to reduce edematous states.
2. *Atropine or epinephrine* may be used.
3. *Diazepam*
4. *Anticholinergics*
5. *Antihistamines*
6. *Vasodilators*

Patient Education

1. Discuss how a balanced diet can affect general health status.
2. Discuss sources of sodium and hidden ingredients that could aggravate the condition.

Section 3
Special Pediatric Conditions

Chief Assessment Factors

Birth data (wt., length, head, GA, size)

Chronic illnesses

Congenital or chromosomal abnormalities

Recent trauma, surgery, hospitalizations and illnesses

Medications

Chemotherapy, radiation, etc.

Feeding modality

Food intake and preferences

Gastrointestinal functioning, nausea, vomiting, diarrhea, and constipation

Growth and development milestones (greatest for infants)

Protein-calorie malnutrition (approximately 1/4–1/3 of hospitalizations in children)

For More Information About Birth Defects

March of Dimes
Birth Defects Foundation
Box 2000
White Plains, NY 10602

For Feeding Problems

American Occupational Therapy Association, Inc.
1383 Piccard Drive
P.O. Box 1725
Rockville, MD 20850-4375

For More Information About Rare Disorders

National Information Center for Orphan Drugs and Rare Diseases:
(800) 336-4797

NOTES

Ross Laboratories now carries Pedia-Sure as a complete enteral formula for children 1–6. It contains 237 kcal/250 cc and is free of lactose and gluten.

ADRENOLEUKODYSTROPHY (ALD)

Usual Hospital Stay

6 days.

Notation

ALD is an X-linked disorder characterized by demyelination, adrenal insufficiency and accumulation of saturated very-long-chain fatty acids (VLFA), especially hexacosanoate (C26:0). Onset is usually in childhood, with a rapid, progressive demyelination of the CNS.

Recent studies at Duke University and at the Medical College of Virginia suggest an enzymatic defect in VLFA oxidation (very abundant in sphingo-myelin). An adult form is usually manifested as an adrenomyeloneuropathy (AMN).

Objectives

1. Decrease rapid progression of demyelination of CNS.
2. Prevent or lessen complications of the disorder.
3. Alter type of dietary fat to limit progression of the disease.
4. Overall, maintain total VLFA levels while altering sources.

Dietary Recommendations

1. Increase endogenous VLFA synthesis of monounsaturated fatty acids by restricting exogenous (dietary) VLFA (C26:0) to less than 3 mg and by increasing oleic acid (C18:1). The typical American diet yields 35–40% total calories from fat, with 12–40 mg C26:0 daily.
2. Use the VLFA C26:0- restricted diet, with the addition of 60 ml glyceryl trioleate (GTO) oil for oleic acid. GTO is available from Capital Cities Products, Inc., P.O. Box 569, Columbus, OH 43216. The GTO can be used in cooking, as a supplement in juice, or as an oil consumed directly. GTO replaces oils, margarine, butter, mayonnaise and shortening in food preparation.
3. If patient requires tube feeding, a formula can be developed that contains nonfat milk, GTO, corn syrup or sugar, and a vitamin-mineral supplement.
4. Studies are not conclusive regarding vitamin E, selenium, and carnitine requirements.

Profile

Ht, Wt
IBW or Growth chart
Fatty acid profile

Plasma
  phosphatidylcholine
Chol

Plasma sphingomyelin
Trig

Patient Education

1. The whole family can be instrumental in accepting the diet; it can be adapted for everyone.
2. Restaurant dining can be a problem. Some special meals may have to be developed for travel.
3. If nausea occurs, the oil can be taken in an emulsion.

Comments

C26:0 is present in fatty foods and in cutin (outer layer of plants, fruits, vegetables and nuts).

GTO is similar to olive oil (87% C18:1, 4.8% linoleic acid), but lacks measurable fatty acids with a chain length greater than C20.

United Leukodystrophy Association
Sycamore, IL

NOTES

BILIARY ATRESIA

Usual Hospital Stay

4–5 days.

Notation

Biliary atresia, a serious condition also called neonatal hepatitis, has an unknown etiology. Complete degeneration or incomplete development of one or more of the bile duct components, due to arrested fetal development, occurs in this condition. It results in persistent jaundice, liver damage, and portal hypertension, with pale stools, dark urine and swollen abdomen. It is evident 2–6 weeks after birth.

Objectives

1. Correct malabsorption and alleviate steatorrhea from decreased bile.
2. Prevent hemorrhage from high blood pressure.
3. Correct malnutrition of fat-soluble vitamins.
4. Prepare for potential surgery (Kasai procedure removes damaged tubes) or transplantation.
5. Postoperatively, promote normal growth and development.

Dietary Recommendations

1. Use a low total fat diet. Supplement with oil high in medium-chain triglycerides. Add EFAs for age and body size.
2. Use Portagen as a formula for infants. Tube feed if recurrent or prolonged bleeding occurs.
3. Control intake of protein. Carefully elevate levels without precipitating hepatic coma.

4. When edema exists, restrict the intake of sodium to 1–2 grams. Hydralyte, Pedialyte, or Lytren can be worked into a pattern of food intake, with caution.
5. Decrease fiber intake to prevent hemorrhage.
6. Schedule small, frequent feedings.
7. Supplement with vitamins A, D, E, and K. Intravenous supplementation may be necessary, or water-miscible forms can be used.

Profile

Ht	Steatorrhea	Edema
Growth %	Birth wt	Transferrin
Alb	Jaundice	Prealbumin
BUN	H & H	SGOT, SGPT
Dark urine	Cholesterol	PT
		Trig

Side Effects of Common Drugs Used

1. *Antacids* may be helpful for biliary atresia.
2. *Phenobarbital* and *cholestyramine* are often used to control the hyperlipidemia of this disorder, as well as pruritus.
3. *Diuretics* may be used; monitor carefully.

Patient Education

1. Teach parents about proper feedings and supplements.
2. If bile flow improves after surgery or transplantation, a regular diet may be used.

Comments

If a donor is available, the patient may be a candidate for a liver transplant. Drugs would then be used to overcome organ rejection.

For More Information

American Liver Foundation (Support Groups): (800) 223-0179

NOTES

CEREBRAL PALSY

Usual Hospital Stay

3–4 days.

Notation

Cerebral palsy is a neurologic dysfunction resulting from brain damage to motor centers before, during, or after birth. It causes physical and mental disabilities. Types of palsy include spastic paralysis (difficult movement), chorioathetosis (involuntary movement), ataxia (impaired coordination and balance), and flaccidity (decreased muscle tone).

Objectives

1. Alleviate malnutrition resulting from the patient's inability to close lips, suck, bite, chew, or swallow.
2. Promote independence through use of special feeding devices.
3. Assess appropriate caloric needs.
4. Promote mealtimes in a quiet, unhurried environment.
5. Correct nutritional deficits.

Dietary Recommendations

1. For the specific problems below, follow the directions given.
   Chewing. Eliminate coarse, stringy foods.
   Vomiting. Assess actual intake (take a calorie count).
   Dribbling. Add cereal or yogurt to fluids.
   Constipation. Use laxative foods and bran in the diet. Provide extra fluids.
   Swallowing. Tube feed if necessary.
2. Reduce caloric intake for the spastic patient. Increase caloric intake (45–50 kcal/kg) to accommodate the added movements of the athetoid patient.
3. Supplement with B-complex vitamins and a general multivitamin complex.

Profile

Ht	Wt	IBW/HBW
Skull x-ray	Seizures	Growth %
Alb	H & H	
Transferrin	LBW	

Patient Education

1. Remind patients to keep lips closed to avoid losing food from their mouths as they try to chew.
2. Fortify the diet with dry or evaporated milk, wheat germ, and other foods when intake is inadequate.
3. If special training is needed for a specific feeding procedure (e.g., a preemie nipple for poor suck), it should be provided.
4. Help parent or caretaker with problems relating to dental caries, drugs, constipation, pica or weight.

For More Information

United Cerebral Palsy Association, Inc.
66 East 34th Street
New York, NY 10016
(212) 481-6344

NOTES

CLEFT PALATE

Usual Hospital Stay

Surgical, 3 days; medical, 2 days.

Notation

Cleft palate is a congenital malformation occurring during the embryonic period of development. It results in a fissure in the roof of the mouth, which may be unilateral or bilateral. Some cleft palates are complete; some are incomplete.

Objectives

1. Compensate for the patient's inability to suck.
2. Prevent choking, air swallowing, coughing, and fatigue as much as possible.
3. For surgery, allow extra calories and protein for healing; use a multivitamin supplement.

Dietary Recommendations

1. Provide a normal diet in accordance with the patient's age (RDAs should be fulfilled, etc.).
2. For feeding, use a medicine dropper or plastic bottle with a soft nipple and enlarged hole. Release formula or milk a little at a time, in coordination with the infant's chewing movements. Burp the infant frequently to release swallowed air.
3. When the infant is 6 months old, begin to use solids in the diet. Pureed baby foods can be used with milk in the bottle; or the infant can be spoon fed, with milk used to dilute the baby foods.
4. Avoid fruit peelings, nuts, peanut butter, leafy vegetables, heavy cream dishes, popcorn, grapes, biscuits, cookies, and chewing gum.
5. Feed the infant in an upright position.
6. If irritating, avoid spicy, acidic foods.

Profile

Growth %	Length
Wt	Wt changes
Head circumference	H & H
Alb	Palate type

Patient Education

1. Explain how to feed the infant with a special nipple.
2. Indicate at what age the infant may be fed solids.
3. Tell parents to supplement the infant's diet with vitamin C if citrus juices are not taken well.
4. Have parents use small amounts of liquid when they are feeding the infant. To prevent choking, slow swallowing should be encouraged.

For More Information

"Feeding Young Children with Cleft Lip and Palate"—booklet for $1.50
Minnesota Dietetic Association
1821 U. Avenue, Suite S-280
St. Paul, MN 55104

Forward Face Support Group
NYU Medical Center
Institute of Reconstructive Plastic Surgery
New York, NY
(212) 263-8209

NOTES

CONGENITAL HEART DISEASE

Usual Hospital Stay

3–4 days.

Notation

Persons born with congenital heart disease may have associated noncardiac anomalies (25%). A small percentage (6%) are small for gestational age at birth. Usually some developmental defect occurred between weeks 5 and 8 of pregnancy, e.g., from rubella.

Objectives

1. Support normal growth and weight gains. These infants or children tend to have growth failure, especially with associated CHF.
2. Improve oral intake. Poor suck may occur in infants.
3. Lessen fatigue associated with mealtimes.
4. Meet caloric needs from increased metabolic rate and from need for catch-up growth, without creating excessive cardiac burden.
5. Avoid excessive renal solute overload.

Dietary Recommendations

1. Use calorie needs for age (e.g., 100 kcal/kg in second year of life, etc.). See RDA tables. For infants, a formula containing 90–100 kcal/dl can be used, while carefully monitoring adequacy of fluid ingestion. Most formulas contain 67 kcal/dl.
2. Formulas with a lower mineral:protein ratio may be needed (e.g., partially demineralized whey).
3. Calories should contain approximately 10% protein (avoid overloading); 35–50% fat as vegetable oils known to be readily absorbed; and 40–55% CHO.
4. Sodium intake should be approximately 6–8 mEq daily, dependent on diuretic use and cardiopulmonary status.
5. Continuous 24-hour NG tube feeding may be useful.

Profile

Ht, Wt	I & O	K$^+$
Growth profile	Urinary Osm	BUN
BP	Na$^+$	Creat
Wt changes		

Side Effects of Common Drugs Used

Drugs are specific to the individual patient's requirements.

Patient Education

1. Discuss the role of nutrition in achieving adequate growth and in controlling heart disease.
2. Discuss growth patterns and goals.

NOTES

CYSTIC FIBROSIS (MUCOVISCOIDOSIS)

Usual Hospital Stay

5 days.

Notation

Cystic fibrosis (CF) is an autosomal recessive inherited disease manifested by general dysfunction of mucus-producing exocrine glands, high levels of sodium and chloride in the saliva and tears; high levels of electrolytes in the sweat; and highly viscous secretions in the pancreas, bronchi, bile ducts, and small intestine. Meconium ileus is a classic sign in the newborn with CF. Death often results from malnutrition, bronchopneumonia, lung collapse, and cor pulmonale. Genetic research suggests that a calcium defect in the kidneys may be implicated (*NEJM* 8/88).

CF affects 1/2000 live births. Pancreatic insufficiency occurs in 80–90% and 85% show growth retardation. Average life span is 24 years, but is improving, even up to 30–40 years.

Objectives

1. Achieve desirable body weight. Correct anorexia from respiratory distress.
2. Provide optimal amounts of protein for growth, development, and resistance to infection. Increase lean body mass if depleted.
3. Spare protein by providing up to twice the normal amount of calories.
4. Decrease electrolyte losses in vomiting and steatorrhea. Replace lost electrolytes.
5. Provide adequate nutrition despite excessive losses from maldigestion and malabsorption, and modify intake as required.
6. Provide essential fatty acids in tolerated form.
7. Correct edema, diarrhea, anemia, azotorrhea, and steatorrhea.
8. Prevent progressive pulmonary disease or complications such as glucose intolerance, intestinal obstruction, and cirrhosis.

Dietary Recommendations

1. For persons with acute disease, starch may not be well tolerated unless adequate pancreatic enzymes are provided.
2. Protein should be 30–35% of total calories (4 g/kg infants; 3 g/kg children; 2 g/kg teens; 1.5 g/kg adults).
3. Supplement the diet with two times the normal recommended daily allowances for vitamins A, D, and E (use water-miscible sources), and iron (if needed). Use 4–6 g of sodium to replace perspiration losses. Use riboflavin for cheilosis. MCTs and safflower oil may be beneficial.
4. Lactose intolerance is common, as is intolerance for gas-forming foods and concentrated sweets. Until tolerance is seen in the patient, condiments should be used sparingly. Fats may not be tolerated as well— e.g., gravies, dressings, peanut butter, chips, fried foods, pastries, creamed foods, excesses of margarine or butter. Check use of enzymes in adequate amounts.
5. Calorie intake should be 150 kcal/kg in children, 200 kcal/kg in infants or 150% RDA for age and sex.
6. Fluid intake should be liberal, unless contraindicated.
7. Replace zinc and vitamin K as needed; check weekly.
8. Omit milk during periods of diarrhea if lactose intolerance occurs.
9. Infants can tolerate most formulas (may need 24 kcal/oz); or commercial products such as Nutramigen, Probana, Pregestimil, or Portagen. Intake of protein should be higher; that of fat, lower. *Do not add pancreatic enzymes to formula*—the desired amount may not be totally consumed, or the enzymes may block the opening of the nipple.
10. Nocturnal tube feeding may be appropriate, especially with growth failures. Pulmocare or Ensure Plus may be beneficial.
11. Elemental feedings like Vivonex do not necessitate use of pancreatic enzymes.

12. Salt should be added to commercial baby foods; monitor carefully, especially for cor pulmonale.
13. Decrease simple sugars if glucose intolerance develops.
14. Soft foods may be useful if chewing fatigues the patient.
15. Increase fat:CHO ratio with respiratory distress. Pulmocare (Ross) may be used.
16. Encourage fish intake, for omega-3 fatty acids.
17. Carnitine may be useful to correct fatty liver.

Profile

Growth chart for ht and wt	H & H	P_{CO_2}, P_{O_2}
pH	Pancreatic enzymes	BEE
Chol	Cl	IBW/HBW
K^+	WBC	Serum Carotene levels
Na^+	PT	Fecal fat study
Alb	Gluc	Mg^{++}

+ Pilocarpine iontophoresis sweat test

Side Effects of Drugs Commonly Used
(Up to 40–60 pills daily are common)

1. *Pancreatic Enzymes.* Pancreatic granules (Viokase or Cotazym) are used to help improve digestion/absorption. Give with meals or snacks. If too much is given, anorexia and constipation may result. Return of a voracious appetite and increase in stool bulk suggest an inadequate dosage. Pancreatic enzyme therapy interferes with oral iron therapy. Enteric preparations (Pancrease) act in the duodenum.
2. *Potassium iodide* liquefies secretions.
3. *Antibiotics* are needed during infections. Check magnesium levels.
4. *Bronchodilators* are used to open passages.
5. *Mucolytics* are needed to liquefy secretions.

Patient Education

1. Diet must be periodically re-evaluated to reflect growth and disease process.
2. New foods may be introduced gradually.
3. To liquefy secretions, adequate fluid intake should be ensured.
4. Bronchopulmonary drainage three times daily may be required. Plan meals for one hour preceding or after therapy.
5. Assure that all foods and beverages are nutrient-dense.
6. Discuss signs of dehydration.
7. If the patient is a teen, discuss issues related to fertility (CF males are often infertile, but not females).

8. Discuss the fact that pancreatic enzymes should not be chewed.
9. In adults with CF, 40% have some glucose intolerance.

Comment

IV fat emulsions may be useful to reduce inflammatory processes.

For More Information

Cystic Fibrosis Foundation
6931 Arlington Road
Bethesda, MD 20814

NOTES

CYSTINOSIS (FANCONI'S SYNDROME)

Usual Hospital Stay

4–5 days.

Notation

A hereditary disorder of amino acid metabolism, cystinosis occurs when crystals of cystine are deposited throughout the body. The infantile form leads to renal disease. Toxic accumulations of copper in the brain and kidney account for neurologic symptoms. Manifestations are also seen in hereditary fructose intolerance. Cystinosis may be caused by lead poisoning; the enzyme defect is unknown. The syndrome may be a preneoplastic state.

Objectives

1. Prevent bone demineralization.
2. Correct hypokalemia.
3. Adapt to swallowing dysfunction.

Dietary Recommendations

1. Provide sufficient fluid intake. Input and output should be checked by standards for age.

2. Supplement with vitamin D and calcium as appropriate.
3. Provide sufficient sodium and potassium replacements.
4. Use a diet low in cystine, with Product 80056 (Mead Johnson). Amino acids can be added separately.
5. Alter consistency (liquids, solids) as needed.

Profile

Birth wt; present wt	CO_2	Dehydration
Growth %	Length	I & O
H & H	Patchy brown skin	Uric Acid (dec.)
Ca^{++}	Alb	BUN
P (dec.)	Serum vitamin D	Creat
Na^+	Alk phos	Ceruloplasmin
	K^+ (dec.)	Dysphagia

Side Effects of Common Drugs Used

1. *Sodium bicarbonate or citrate* should be used to correct acidosis.
2. *Cysteamine*, administered orally, can halt glomerular destruction.

Patient Education

1. Emphasize the importance of correcting fluid and electrolyte imbalances.
2. Discuss any necessary changes in consistency.

NOTES

DOWN'S SYNDROME (MONGOLISM)

Usual Hospital Stay

7 days.

Notation

A congenital defect, Down's syndrome is caused by trisomy of chromosome 21. There is a direct correlation between the incidence of the syndrome and maternal age. Children with this condition are often short and overweight and have mental retardation.

Objectives

1. Provide adequate calories and nutrients for growth.
2. Assist with feeding problems.
3. Prevent emotional problems that may lead to overeating.
4. If the patient is inactive, compensate by reducing caloric intake.
5. Counteract constipation and UTIs.

Dietary Recommendations

1. Tube feed if the patient is unable to eat orally. Gradually wean to solids when possible.
2. Supply adequate amounts of calories and protein for age. Prevent further brain impairment. 1–1.5 g protein/kg (age-dependent) may be needed.
3. Monitor for pica, overeating, and idiosyncrasies.
4. Supplement diet with additional vitamin A, vitamin B_6, and zinc.
5. Provide feeding assistance if needed.
6. Provide extra fluid for losses in drooling or spillage.
7. Encourage complex CHOs, prune juice, etc. if constipation is a problem.

Profile

Birth weight	Length	Present wt
Growth %	Prematurity hx	IBW/HBW
Eye slant	Large tongue	I & O
Hyperextensibility of	Endocardial defects	Chol
joints	Gluc	Trig
Plasma Zn	Uric acid (inc.)	

Patient Education

1. Explain feeding techniques.
2. Help control or increase caloric intake in the diet.
3. Discuss use of self-feeding utensils.
4. Never rush mealtime.
5. Encourage socialization.

For More Information

National Down's Syndrome Society
121 Fifth Avenue
New York, NY 10010
(800) 221-4602

NOTES

FAILURE TO THRIVE

Usual Hospital Stay

3–4 days.

Notation

The growth percentiles of an infant who fails to thrive are far below the norm for weight and length of infants the same age. Other indices include a small head circumference, muscular wasting, apathy, and weight loss. Organic FTT is caused by some disease state; nonorganic FTT is from another cause. Learning failure can occur (slow to talk, behavior problems).

Objectives

1. Provide optimal nutrition compatible with normal growth pattern. Achieve daily gains (30 g infant, 60–90 g older child).
2. Correct causes, which include decreased intake, increased nutrient losses, increased metabolic demands, and decreased growth efficiency. Determine if malnutrition is *primary* (from faulty feeding patterns or dietary inadequacy) or *secondary* (from disease process interfering with intake). Primary FTT is also called nonorganic.
3. Teach caretaker how to properly feed and how to determine needs.
4. Provide adequate schedule of feeding for infant's age.
5. Support catch-up growth.

Dietary Recommendations

1. Calculate diet according to infant's age for kcal and protein. Begin with 150 kcal/kg body wt.; protein 8% total kcal.
2. Check RDAs for nutrients and provide adequate zinc and vitamin B_6, as determined by the infant's age.
3. Evaluate the infant's nutritional history and growth in comparison to the percentiles of normal infants. Discuss with caretaker.
4. Determine a calorie count for hospital food intake.
5. Monitor growth (weights) and feeding behaviors.
6. If the infant is in a state of dehydration, provide adequate amounts of water.

Profile

Ht	Apgar scores	Gluc
Percentiles	Wt	IBW/HBW
Skinfold thickness	Head circumference	Chol, Trig
H & H	Alb	BUN
Birth wt		Goal wt

Patient Education

1. Describe the appropriate nutritional intake according to age of the infant. Describe the predisposing organic conditions, where appropriate.
2. Encourage the use of growth charts at home to monitor success.
3. Explain proper use of over-the-counter vitamin-mineral supplements.
4. Develop progress chart for developmental milestones.
5. Offer simple, specific instructions.
6. Practical suggestions should be offered regarding emotional support for the child.
7. Follow-up should be provided at outpatient clinics or by home visits.

Comments

Failure to thrive is another term for protein-calorie malnutrition in children. In many pediatric centers, one third of the referred children are malnourished. Vitamin-mineral depletion is also found with protein-calorie malnutrition. Adequate hydration is needed.

Growth failure plus FUO and anemia in older children or teens may suggest the onset of Crohn's disease.

NOTES

FETAL ALCOHOL SYNDROME (FAS)

Usual Hospital Stay

3 days.

Notation

Generally noted from shortly after birth, fetal alcohol syndrome is a syndrome in infants of developmental delay, anomalies, LBW, tremors, and retardation of intellect with microcephaly. FAS is the third leading cause of mental retardation in the United States.

Objectives

1. Promote effective family coping skills.
2. Prevent additional retardation and developmental delays, blindness, etc.
3. Improve intake and nutritional status.
4. Prevent or correct vomiting and other problems.
5. Improve cardiac symptoms.
6. Promote effective parental bonding.
7. Encourage normal growth patterns.

Dietary Recommendations

1. Provide a diet appropriate for age and status (see LVW entry).
2. Ensure adequate protein and calories for catch-up growth.
3. If necessary, provide tube feeding or TPN while hospitalized. Some infants may require additional attention in the home setting to promote normalized development.

Profile

Birth wt., length	Growth %	Gluc
Alb	Head circumference	Seizures
Other parameters as available	H & H	

Side Effects of Common Drugs Used

Anticonvulsants may be needed to correct seizures.

Patient Education

1. Encourage mother's participation in alcohol rehabilitation if needed.
2. Discuss appropriate feeding techniques for age of infant.
3. Discuss importance of diet in aiding normal growth and development.

For More Information

FAS Resource Coalition
7802 S. E. Taylor St.
Portland, OR 97215
(503) 246-2635

NOTES

INBORN ERRORS OF CARBOHYDRATE METABOLISM

Usual Hospital Stay

4–5 days.

Notation

A defective gene that prevents a normal step in carbohydrate metabolism is the cause of these disorders.

Objectives

1. Eliminate the nutrient that cannot be digested.
2. Alter other nutrient intakes to promote growth and maintenance.
3. Read labels carefully.
4. For persons with *galactosemia*, correct diet to prevent physical and mental retardation, cataracts, portal hypertension, cirrhosis.
5. For persons with *glycogen storage disease*, maintain glucose homeostasis, prevent hypoglycemia, promote positive nitrogen balance and growth, correct or prevent fatty liver.
6. *Sucrose intolerance* occurs rarely as a genetic defect or temporarily after GI flu or irritable bowel distress. Sucrase deficiency may be combined with maltase deficiency. Eliminate the carbohydrate(s) in order to decrease osmotic diarrhea.
7. *Fructose intolerance* is rare and can cause GI discomfort, nausea, malaise, and growth failure.

Dietary Recommendations

Fructosemia results from a defect in the enzyme converting fructose to glucose; therefore, the diet must exclude fructose, sucrose, sorbitol, invert sugar, maple syrup, honey, and molasses.

Galactosemia results from a lack of galactose-1-phosphate uridyl transferase. Use a galactose-free diet: no milk, milk products, soybeans, peaches, lentils, liver, brains, or breads or cereals containing milk or cream cheese. For infants with the condition, try soy-based formulas, such as Nutramigen or ProSobee; meat-based formulas; or caseine hydrolysate. Supplement with calcium, vitamin D, and riboflavin.

Glycogen storage disease, type 1 (Von Gierke's disease), is caused by a deficiency of glucose-6-phosphatase, which normally converts glycogen to glucose. Increase protein intake; use small, frequent feedings; and, if steroids are used in treatment, use 2 g of sodium in the diet. Avoid excessive calorie intake; lactose or sucrose should be excluded from the diet. Glucose, as provided in Pregestimil, may be given. Provide nocturnal Vivonex, or cornstarch.

Sucrose/maltose intolerance requires omission of sucrose and maltose from the diet. For nongenetic form, add these sugars back gradually to the diet.

Profile

Wt	Trig (inc. in Von Gierke's)
Growth %	Urinalysis
Uric acid	Jaundice
Infections	Head circumference
N & V	Chol (inc. in Von Gierke's)
Urinary & serum galactose	Alb
IBW/HBW	Edema
Length	Gluc
	Acetone

Side Effects of Common Drugs Used

1. For persons with *galactosemia,* eliminate drugs containing lactose and supplement with calcium and riboflavin.
2. Sucrose and maltose are added to many drugs; check carefully.
3. All vitamin-mineral supplements must be free of the nontolerated carbohydrates.

Patient Education

1. Explain which sources of carbohydrate are allowed, specific to the disorder.
2. In *galactosemia,* galactose can often be reintroduced later in life.
3. Read labels carefully. Many foods contain milk solids, galactose (e.g. luncheon meats, hot dogs), and other sugars. Omit according to the disorders.
4. For *glycogen storage disease,* giving uncooked starch at night may help the liver to maintain a normal blood glucose level (sometimes allowing omission of parenteral nutrition). A multivitamin supplement with iron and calcium may be needed. Fruits and milk are limited; concentrated sweets may be restricted.
5. Contact formula companies regarding special products.

NOTES

HIRSCHSPRUNG'S DISEASE (MEGACOLON)

Usual Hospital Stay

4 days.

Notation

Megacolon in infancy is a congenital malformation due to segmental absence of parasympathetic ganglion cells in the mesenteric plexus. This results in interference with normal mass peristalsis and causes functional obstruction. Treatment includes enemas and laxatives for chronic constipation. Surgical removal may be required, and may be followed by a colostomy.

Objectives

1. Replace electrolytes and fluids.
2. Compensate for poor absorption.
3. Provide adequate nutrition for the patient's age and development.

Dietary Recommendations

1. Use a high calorie/high protein diet. Enteral products (e.g., Ensure) can be used if required.
2. Monitor levels of potassium if laxatives are used.
3. Provide total parenteral nutrition if large sections of the bowel are removed. Gradually progress to soft/bland foods at a proper time.
4. Provide fluids adequate for the patient's age.

Profile

Birth wt	Length	Present wt
Growth %	Temp	IBW/HBW
FTT	V	Na^+
Diarrhea	Dehydration	Gluc
Alb	H & H	K^+

Side Effects of Drugs Commonly Used

Laxatives can deplete numerous nutrient reserves; monitor carefully.

Patient Education

1. Teach patient about sources of protein, calories and potassium from the diet.
2. Discuss wound healing if surgery was completed.

NOTES

HOMOCYSTINURIA

Usual Hospital Stay

4–5 days.

Explanation

Homocystinuria is caused by an autosomal recessive trait (IEM) in which cystithionine enzyme is missing. It may also be due to deranged vitamin B_6 metabolism or low levels of reductase enzyme (methionine to crystine conversion). If untreated, it leads to mental retardation, seizures, poor growth, hepatic disease, osteoporosis, thromboses, glaucoma or cataracts.

Objectives

1. Reduce methionine in the diet.
2. Prevent further mental retardation and growth delays.
3. Prevent cardiovascular complications (arterial and venous thrombosis).
4. Supplement with essential nutrients.

Dietary Recommendations

1. Use a low protein diet with a supplement of cystine to supply sulfur. Reduce intake of methionine in the diet: no meat, poultry, fish, or eggs. Soy products (Isomil, ProSobee, Soyalac) can be used. Maxamaid (XMET) or Product 3200-K (Mead Johnson) are also useful.
2. Large doses of vitamin B_6 (e.g., 250–500 mg) may be prescribed by the doctor. Supplement as well with folic acid. Monitor needs carefully.
3. Increase fluid intake.

Profile

Birth wt
Growth %
Hepatomegaly
Plasma methionine
(inc.)

Pale complexion
Serum and/or urinary
homocystine
Length

FTT
Seizures
Present wt
IBW/HBW
SGOT, SGPT
Gluc

Side Effects of Drugs Commonly Used

Dipyridamole may be used to decrease thrombosis.

Patient Education

Emphasize the importance of controlling the diet, snacks, etc.

LARGE-FOR-GESTATIONAL-AGE INFANT (LGA)

Usual Hospital Stay

5 days with complications.

Notation

High birth weight (3300–4000 grams+) at 40 weeks is termed "large for gestational age." These infants are considered to be over the 90th percentile of appropriate weight for gestational age. They are often born to diabetic mothers, multipara, or mothers with genetic predispositions for excessive birth weight.

Signs and symptoms often include hypoglycemia, respiratory distress, aspiration pneumonia, bronchial paralysis or facial paralysis. Infants of diabetic mothers may also have macrosomatia.

Objectives

1. Allow adequate growth rate and development.
2. Prevent hypoglycemia.
3. Maintain calorie level at lowest possible level while allowing adequate growth to prevent obesity and its consequences.
4. Monitor serum lipid levels as deemed necessary.

Dietary Recommendations

1. Feed often or with larger amounts, as indicated by infant's appetite.
2. Control source of calories, avoiding excessive glucose intake if infant shows signs of hyperglycemia.
3. Alter intake of fat as determined by a lipid profile.

Profile

Length and birth weight	Growth pattern	Head circumference
H & H	Respirations	I & O
Serum gluc	Urinary acetone	Serum insulin
Chol	Trig	
	BP	

Side Effects of Common Drugs Used

Insulin may be necessary to control hyperglycemia. Beware of any excesses, which could aggravate hypoglycemia.

Patient Education

1. Signs of hyperglycemia and hypoglycemia should be discussed.
2. Discuss normal growth patterns as appropriate for the larger infant.
3. Review risks inherent in another pregnancy, especially if mother has diabetes.

NOTES

LOW-BIRTHWEIGHT INFANT

Usual Hospital Stay

13–17 days, with prematurity or complications.

Explanation

Low-birthweight (LBW) infants weigh less than 2500 g or 5.5 lbs (below 10th percentile for gestational age) at birth. Premature infants are infants less than 36 weeks old, gestational age. The usual gestational age is 40 weeks. LBW infants are 6–7% of all live births; 20% are born to mothers under 15. They may be small for date, or have intrauterine growth retardation or dysmaturity. Typical problems include hypoglycemia, hypothermia, jaundice, dry skin, decreased subcutaneous fat. Admission to neonatal ICUs is common. VLBW infants (under 1300–1500 g) are especially prone to nutritional deficits.

Objectives

1. Begin feedings of distilled water or colostrum as soon as possible for infants without respiratory distress.
2. Encourage the mother to breast-feed, especially to provide milk with the higher preterm protein level.
3. Supplement the infant's diet as needed with formula or medium-chain triglycerides; ensure intake of EFAs.
4. Gradually increase calories and protein to meet needs of rapid growth.
5. Promote normal growth and development. Prevent illness, rickets, RDS, hypoglycemia or hyperglycemia, NEC, infections, obstructive jaundice, and tyrosinemia.
6. Ensure proper whey:casein ratio.
7. Include amino acids in proper amounts, especially cysteine, taurine, tyrosine, glycine. American McGaw makes IV Trophamine for PN.

Dietary Recommendations

1. While the infant is in the radiant warmer, feed the infant 60–80 ml/kg BW/day of water. Gradually increase to 150 ml/kg body weight. Add Na^+, Cl^-, K^+ on at least the second day.
2. Day one—breast-feed or give glucose at 6–8 mg/kg/min. Progress to special formulas like Similac Special Care 24, SMA "Preemie," Enfamil Premature Formula (24 kcal/oz) to yield 120–150 ml/kg up to 180–200 ml/kg/day. Use TPN if not fed by day 3.
3. By the second week, the diet should provide 120–150 kcal/kg body weight daily. Carbohydrate should be 40–45% total kcal (10–30 g/kg). Protein should be age-specific. Nonprotein:protein kcals should be 150–200:1.
4. If poor sucking or swallowing instincts exist, the infant may need gavage feeding. Feed every 2 hours.
5. Feeding style: if infant weighs 1000–1750 g, feed more vigorously; if infant weighs 1750 g or more, feed as a normal term infant.
6. The nutrient needs of an LBW infant may be as follows: high levels of calcium, 25 IU of vitamin E (water-soluble) daily, 2.5 mg iron/100 kcal in formula (necessary only if stores are depleted), 300–500 IU of vitamin D, adequate folic acid, adequate sodium (3 mEq/day) to avoid hyponatremia, 30–50 mg vitamin C/day. Other nutrients should be provided according to the RDAs for the newborn: vitamin A, magnesium, zinc, and copper may be low.
7. Soybean oil can give EFAs in linoleic acid form (maximum dose 3 g/kg/day; usually 0.5–1 g/kg). *Exogenous carnitine* may be needed to take EFAs into the mitochondria. Total fat should be 1–2 g/kg, 1–2% EFAs.
8. With TPN, use up to 3 mg/kg/day lipid infused continuously, or early enteral feeding, to prevent cholestatic liver disease.

Profile

Birth wt	Birth length	Alb
Gestational age	% wt/length	Ca^{++}
H & H	Sucking reflex	RDS
Swallowing reflex	Gluc	Prealbumin (7 days
TLC	Bilirubin	half-life)
Temp (often dec.)	I & O	Transferrin (8 days
Lecithin:sphyngo-	Apgar scores	half-life)
myelin ratio (L:S		SGOT, SGPT
ratio)		

Nutritional Deficits in the Premature or Low-Birth-Weight Infant

1. Marginal nutrient stores at birth: fat, glycogen, minerals such as calcium and phosphorus.
2. Limited ability to consume adequate amounts of nutrient, caused by delayed oral neuromuscular development and small gastric capacity.
3. Immaturity at the cellular level, with consequent alteration of biochemical needs.
4. Higher metabolic demands and rate of growth.
5. Malabsorption from underdeveloped digestive/absorptive abilities.
6. Risk from poor nutritional intake of the mother, where relevant. Mothers who are folate-deficient are more likely to give birth to low birth weight infants.
7. Risk of *EFA deficiency*, with less growth, more renal and lung changes, fatty liver, impaired water balance, erythrocyte fragility, and dermatitis.

Patient Education

1. Teach caretaker or parent about increased nutrient needs of infant. Special formulas have 80 kcal/dl compared to the usual 67 kcal/dl, and have MCT, extra protein, calcium, phosphorus, and sodium.
2. Emphasize the normal progression of infant feeding once the infant achieves adequate growth pattern and weight. Catch-up is common by 2–3 years.
3. Emphasize the importance of zinc, vitamin B_6, and vitamin E in small infants (for growth).
4. Monitor for the tendency to aspirate, for lactose intolerance, and for other problems.
5. Decrease use of supplements once 300 kcal/day can be consumed.
6. Follow-up clinic or home visits are recommended.
7. The child may benefit from the WIC Program where available.

Comments

1. *Enteral Needs (Preemie)* basal
	basal	40–50 kcal/kg
	+ activity	5–15 kcal/kg
	+ cold stress	0–10 kcal/kg
	+ fecal losses	10–15 kcal/kg
	+ SDA	10 kcal/kg
	+ growth	20–30 kcal/kg
		85–130 kcal/kg

2. *Special needs:* extra calories may be needed for fever (12% per °C elevation); for cardiac failure (15–25%); for major surgery (20–30%); for severe sepsis (40–50%); for PCM (50–100%); for burns (100%); or for growth failure (60%).
3. *TPN needs* are similar to EN needs.
4. *Tube Feeding Initiation*   3 kg—start @ 10–15 ml/hr @ 1/4 strength
            5 kg—start @ 15 ml/hr @ 1/2 strength
       10 kg—start @ 25 ml/hr @ 1/2 strength
       Progress as tolerated.

MYELOMENINGOCELE

Usual Hospital Stay

9 days.

Notation

This condition is a congenital CNS defect with myelodysplasia and cystic distention of the meninges. Patients are usually wheelchair-bound, or will wear braces or be on crutches. Obesity is, therefore, common because of decreased active muscle tissue. Obesity can increase decubiti and make ambulation and surgery more difficult.

See also Spina Bifida and Neural Tube Defects.

Objectives

1. Control weight; metabolic rate may only be 50% usual rate for age.
2. Prevent or heal decubiti.
3. Promote any and all possible ambulation or activity.
4. Correct infections; prevent or correct sepsis.

Dietary Recommendations

1. Decrease calories to control weight. If patient is very young, allow growth to stabilize weight.
2. Low calorie snacks should be the only between-meal snacks allowed.

3. For healing of any debubiti, zinc, vitamins A and C and adequate protein are required.
4. Be cautious with use of zinc and iron supplements (especially PN) with infections or sepsis.

Profile

Ht, wt	Temp	Gluc
IBW	Wt changes	TSF
H & H	Alb	Other parameters as needed

Side Effects of Common Drugs Used

No specific drugs are used in this condition. Monitor individual orders.

Patient Education

1. Behavior modification, low-calorie food and snack preparation, rewards, and activity/exercise factors should be reviewed with parent/caretaker.
2. Food lists with green "go" foods, red "stop" foods, and yellow "caution" foods have been used with some success.
3. Parental/caretaker motivation and attitude are important.

MAPLE SYRUP URINE DISEASE

Usual Hospital Stay

4–5 days.

Explanation

Maple syrup urine disease (MSUD) results from an autosomal recessive trait, causing an inborn error of metabolism in which branched-chain amino acids (BCAAs—leucine, isoleucine, valine) are not degraded through decarboxylation to simple acids. If the disease is left untreated, it leads to retardation. Thiamine is the coenzyme for BCAAs. Onset of disease occurs in children aged 1 to 8 years. The name of the disease reflects the maple syrup odor of the urine and sweat of affected children.

Objectives

1. Feed despite difficulty with sucking and swallowing reflexes.
2. Replace needed electrolytes if prolonged vomiting occurs.
3. Control intake of BCAAs for life. Add individually as the child grows, in a controlled manner.
4. Prevent tissue catabolism. Support normal growth and development.

Dietary Recommendations

1. Restrict intake of BCAAs in the diet. Use Mead Johnson's maple syrup urine disease powder or Ross Lab's Maxamaid MSUD. Use the latter with Product 80056 (Mead Johnson) because it contains no cholesterol or fat.
2. Use patient support to alleviate feeding problems.
3. Use small amounts of milk in the diet to support growth.
4. Gelatin, a form of protein low in BCAAs, may be used in the diet.
5. Replace needed electrolytes.
6. Large doses of thiamine for those children who are thiamine-responsive may be prescribed by the doctor.
7. Provide adequate caloric intake to spare protein.

Profile

Birth wt, Present wt	Length
Growth %; IBW/HBW	Urinary odor
Grand mal seizures	Hypertonicity
Plasma leucine, isoleucine, valine	Alb
Urinary excretion of ketoacids	Globulin
	Uric acid (inc.)

Patient Education

1. Tell the patient that the diet must be maintained for life.
2. Make sure that the diet's total calorie and protein intake is appropriate for the patient's age and stage of development.
3. Cow's milk contains 350 mg leucine, 228 mg isoleucine and 245 mg valine per 100 ml.

NOTES

NECROTIZING ENTEROCOLITIS

Usual Hospital Stay

2–3 days.

Notation

Necrotizing enterocolitis (NEC) involves ischemia of the intestinal tract and invasion of the mucosa with enteric pathogens. It occurs more often in small and asphyxiated preterm infants, after exchange transfusions, or with Hirschsprung's disease.

Symptoms and signs include a distended abdomen, lethargy, respiratory distress syndrome, pallor, hyperbilirubinemia, vomiting, diarrhea, and sepsis.

Objectives

1. Allow bowel to rest; avoid stimulants. These measures are usually temporary.
2. Prevent or correct starvation diarrhea and further malnutrition.
3. Prepare patient for bowel surgery and for wound healing if surgery becomes necessary, as for perforation.
4. Prevent or correct hypoglycemia.

Dietary Recommendations

1. *Acute:* NPO with IVs and TPN as appropriate.
2. *Recovery:* Use 2× RDA of protein; 25% more kcal than normal for age; frequent feedings.
3. If formula is used, review intolerances. Some predigested formulas are available (such as Pregestimil or Nutramigen). Simple nutrients may be required if digestive tract has not recovered fully.
4. Omit milk if lactose is not tolerated. Provide a replacement for calcium and riboflavin if milk will be omitted for an extended period of time.
5. Ensure adequate intake of iron, but not in excess while infection is extensive (especially parenteral iron). Zinc is also to be monitored during acute stages, as it also contributes to bacterial nutriture.

Profile

Ht/length	Blood in stools	Platelets (dec.)
H & H (dec.)	Na^+ (dec.)	K^+ (inc.)
PT (inc.)	Head circumference	Glucose
Wt/birth wt		

Side Effects of Common Drugs Used

Antidiarrheal medications may be used, as appropriate for age.

Patient Education

1. Promote continuation of breast-feeding, where possible.
2. Monitor weight and stool changes; advise physician when necessary.

3. Assure that parent/caretaker understands the differences between ready-to-feed and concentrated formula (i.e., hypertonicity of the solution).

Comments

1. Hypoxia------------------------shunting of blood away from GI tract

Ischemic mucosal lesions

BF infants receive lactobacillus antibodies and immunoglobins leading to more rapid recovery.

Formula-fed infants may develop gram-negative sepsis, leading to *NEC.*

Fig. 3–1. One Source of NEC.

2. Oral administration of IgA-IgB may prevent development of NEC in low birthweight infants (*NEJM 319:1,* 1988.

NOTES

CHILDHOOD OBESITY

Usual Hospital Stay

Varies.

Notation

Up to age 6, the number of fat cells increases (hyperplasia). After age 6, the size of fat cells increases (hypertrophy). Obesity involves skinfold thickness greater than 2 standard deviations above the normal range. Infants who are obese are generally overfed. Later, genetics and environment both play a role.

Objectives

1. *Gradually* reduce excess food intake and increase activity. Allow the child to "grow" into his or her weight.
2. Discourage the use of sweets and foods to reward behavior.
3. Determine the extent of dental caries; offer appropriate suggestions.

4. Evaluate the types of entrees used, as well as use of vegetables, sweets, snacks, and milk in the daily diet.
5. Counsel family about good nutrition in general and, in particular, the caloric needs for different age groups. Avoid the "clean plate" theory.
6. Help the child "find" the right body for him/her.
7. Be wary about withholding food; it can have the opposite effect.

Dietary Recommendations

1. Determine the recommended dietary allowances for the child's age group: kcal _____, protein _____, other nutrients _____. Protein should be 20%, fat under 30%, CHO 50%.
2. Ensure that the family has adequate fluoride protection.
3. Decrease the use of sweets as snack foods, or as dessert. Decrease fatty or fried foods.
4. Plan a diet with basal calories. Do not provide a reduction diet per se. The diet should be calculated according to the patient's age, required needs, activity, growth spurt.
5. Check for anemia; correct diet accordingly.
6. Limit milk to a reasonable amount daily; use low fat or skim milk after age 2.
7. Good snacks include: fresh fruit or vegetables, plain crackers, pretzels, plain popcorn, cooked egg slices, unsweetened fruit or vegetable juices, low-fat cheese cubes.
8. Serve small portions and limit additional helpings.

Profile

Birth weight	H & H	Present wt
Wt hx	Chol	Ht
Ideal wt/Healthy wt	Gluc	Alb
Fe	Birth length	Trig
Family hx CHD	Family hx HPN	Ca^{++}, P
	Alk phos	O_2, CO_2

Side Effects of Common Drugs Used

Discourage the use of drugs for weight loss in childhood.

Patient Education

1. Explain to parents that obese parents tend to "beget" obese children. Discuss hereditary and environmental factors.
2. One fourth of children who enter adolescence overweight will be unable to achieve ideal body weight as an adult.
3. Help the family to carefully monitor menu planning, snacking patterns. Encourage regular meals; limit unplanned snacking.

4. Encourage activity. Demonstrate the relationship of food, weight, and energy balance.
5. Discourage risk-filled weight control schemes or practices.
6. Try to eliminate one "problem food" per visit, such as regular soda pop. Offer an acceptable alternative.
7. While weight loss is occurring, maintain the child's self-image through positive reinforcement. Stress non-food related achievements; do not nag.
8. A good example should be set in the home by the parent/caretaker.
9. Between meals, ice water should be offered as a special beverage instead of soda pop or fruit drinks.
10. A system for "traffic light" foods can be used—green "go" foods, yellow "caution" foods, red "stop" foods.
11. Responsibilities should be shared—parents are responsible for a proper emotional setting and for *what* is *offered*; the child is responsible for *what* is *eaten* and for *how much* is eaten. (Ellyn Satter, Ellyn: *Child of Mine*, 2nd ed., Bull Publishing, Palo Alto, CA, 1986).
12. Parents who practice restrained eating with their children tend to be overly indulgent later (fast/feast), with chronic anxiety resulting. Eating can become very controlled, inconsistent and emotional.

Comments

The preferred weight gain history in childhood is as follows: year 1, three times the child's birth weight; year 2, 3.5–4.5 kg gain; year 3, 2–3 kg; and annually thereafter, 2–3 kg. About 10% of all children ages 10–14 in the U.S. are obese.

NOTES

PHENYLKETONURIA

Usual Hospital Stay

7 days.

Notation

Phenylketonuria is caused by an inborn error of metabolism in which absence or inactivity of phenylalanine hydroxylase occurs. As a result, phenylalanine is metabolized in other pathways besides tyrosine. The disorder is caused by an autosomal-recessive trait. Infants are tested for this disorder after the first feeding and again after 2–4 weeks.

Objectives

1. Establish the child's daily requirement for phenylalanine,* protein, and calories according to age.
2. Prevent mental retardation. Promote normal intellectual development.
3. Provide a diet aiding growth and development.
4. Provide adequate protein-sparing.
5. Introduce solids and textures at usual ages. Encourage self-feeding when it is possible for the infant to do so.
6. Provide increased phenylalanine during febrile periods.
7. Allow intellectually normal PKU patients to develop a normal social life.
8. Develop a positive attitude toward the diet in parent or caretaker and in the child.

Dietary Recommendations

1. Use a diet low in phenylalanine. The average diet provides 5% phenylalanine in a protein food. The Lofenalac formula, Phenyl-free or Maxamaid XP can be used.
2. Use large amounts of sugar, fruits, some vegetables. Omit meat, fish, poultry, bread, milk, cheese, legumes and peanut butter. Use Lofenalac for 85 to 100% of the infant's needs.
3. Initially, the infant's tolerance must be assessed individually, and progress in treatment must develop accordingly.
4. Some milk and Lofenalac formula should be used to provide for the infant's needs. Flavors can be added to the formula.
5. Supplement the diet with zinc, manganese, and niacin, as synthetic powders are low in these nutrients.
6. Introduce solids and textures at appropriate age.
7. Subtract phenylalanine requirement in formula from total needs (the difference is that which is provided by solid foods).
8. To add calories, try jam, jelly, sugar, honey, molasses, syrups, cornstarch and oils, which are phenylalanine-free.

---

* Desirable levels of phenylalanine are always less than 20 mg/dl. Normal range is 3–7 mg/dl; the range seen in patients with phenylketonuria is often 15–30 mg/dl.

Profile

Birth wt, present wt
Growth %; IBW/HBW
Urinary phenylalanine
Mental retardation
Mousy odor in urine and sweat

Length
Plasma phenylalanine
Eczema
EEGs
Plasma tyrosine

Patient Education

1. Because initial acceptance of Lofenalac may be poor owing to its strong taste, the mother should be careful not to express her own distaste. Recommend appropriate recipes and cookbooks.
2. Monitor the presence of phenylalanine in the diet.
3. Avoid items sweetened with aspartame (Nutra-Sweet or Equal).
4. Self-management should begin by age 7–8, at least for formula preparation. By age 12, the child should begin calculating own intake of phenylalanine from foods.

Comments

The appropriate phenylalanine intake for age is as follows: infants, 0–3 months, 60–90 mg/kg; 4–6 months, 40 mg/kg; 7–9 months, 35 mg/kg; 10–12 months, 30 mg/kg; children 1–2 years, 25 mg/kg; children 2–5 years, 20 mg/kg body weight; children over 5 years, 15 mg/kg body weight.

Inadequate intake of phenylalanine can result in anorexia, fever, vomiting, lethargy, bone changes, and stunted growth.

Lofenalac contains 454 calories in 100 g powder: protein, 15 g; CHO, 60 g; fat, 18 g. A milk substitute, it is made from casein hydrolysate, corn oil, corn syrup, tapioca starch, minerals, and vitamins.

Phenyl-free is unable to provide total nutritional needs.

NOTES

PRADER-WILLI SYNDROME

Usual Hospital Stay

3–4 days.

Notation

The Prader-Willi syndrome is a genetic disorder (possibly a defect in chromosome 15) in which obesity is caused by hyperplasia. Its cause is unknown, but it is thought that there is a defect in the regulation of lipogenesis. Onset occurs in children aged 1–4 years. Signs and symptoms include truncal obesity, small hands, feet, and genitalia, short stature, and insatiable appetite. These children often had poor suck and floppy muscle tone as infants.

Objectives

1. Reduce weight.
2. Maintain RDAs for all nutrients and protein to promote growth and development.
3. Provide feeding assistance if needed.
4. Prevent complications like CHD, HPN, DM, and pneumonia.

Dietary Recommendations

1. Use a low calorie diet to reduce weight. Monitor for age. 1000 kcal + 100 kcal for each year until age 10 is common.
2. Ensure that the diet provides adequate protein and nutrients. Check RDAs for age.
3. Gavage feeding should be used as needed.
4. Consider gastric bypass if hyperphagia becomes a problem.

Profile

Birth wt	Present wt	IBW/HBW
Ht	Small head	BP
Mental retardation	Gluc	Chol, trig
H & H	Alb	P_{CO_2}, P_{O_2}

Patient Education

1. Encourage the patient to be active. Help the patient lose weight with behavior modification techniques.
2. Main elements of concern in the diet are sugars and fats.
3. Discuss good feeding practices plus activity factors.
4. Some systems promote green/yellow/red traffic light system of food choices (go/caution/stop).
5. Record-keeping and calorie-counting are generally better than use of exchange systems.
6. Control is the main issue.

For More Information

Prader-Willi Association
6490 Excelsior Blvd., E–102
St. Louis Park, MN 55426
(612) 926-1947

NOTES

RICKETS, NUTRITIONAL

Usual Hospital Stay

4–5 days.

Notation

This disorder is caused by vitamin D deficiency, a rare problem but usually seen in children or infants (often premature). The condition may also occur in breast-fed infants who do not receive adequate supplementation, exposure to sunlight or vitamin D-fortified milk. It can also occur secondary to malabsorption or steatorrhea, anticonvulsant use, renal failure, or in biliary cirrhosis.

Objectives

1. Correct status; prevent further problems and deformity.
2. Prevent or correct tetany, hypocalcemia and other complications.

Dietary Recommendations

1. Use a balanced diet, appropriate for age and sex.
2. Use milk if no milk or lactose intolerances exist; increase appropriately while monitoring serum values.
3. There may be additional use of such calcium-containing foods as cheeses, yogurt, ice cream, etc. if milk is not tolerated.

Profile

Ht	Alk Phos ($\uparrow$)	as appropriate
Wt	Ca^{++}	Phosphorus
IBW or Growth %	Other parameters	

Side Effects of Common Drugs Used

1. *Calciferol.* 1500–3000 IUs daily by mouth helps in 2–4 weeks; some maintenance doses may also be required over time. Monitor use with dietary calcium.
2. *Vitamin D.* 2000–5000 IUs may be given upon diagnosis, with long-term usage given according to causative factors. Be wary of toxic effects of vitamin D (hypercalcemia, nausea, vomiting, anorexia, malaise, renal problem or hypertensive problems).

Patient Education

1. Discuss needed alterations of the diet in conjunction with drug therapy.
2. Discuss the role of sunlight in vitamin D metabolism.

SPINA BIFIDA AND NEURAL TUBE DEFECTS

Usual Hospital Stay

9 days.

Notation

Spina bifida is a birth defect involving damage to the spine and nervous system, causing a lack of union between the laminae of the vertebrae. The lumbar section is generally affected. Club foot, dislocated hip, scoliosis and other musculoskeletal deformities may also be present.

Myelomeningocele is a more severe malformation that includes external protrusion of meninges, spinal fluid and cord, as well as nerve roots. See the entry for Myelomeningocele.

Spina bifida occulta is seen in about 10% of children and adults, with the defect discovered accidentally on x-ray. Spina bifida cystica is more severe.

Objectives

1. Control side effects (i.e., hydrocephalus and possibly sepsis).
2. Increase independence and self-care potentials.
3. Improve nutritional status.
4. Achieve and maintain IBW for age.
5. Preserve brain function, as far as possible, with hydrocephalus.
6. Initiate treatment or surgical intervention, as appropriate.
7. Correct constipation, decubitus ulcers, etc.

Dietary Recommendations

1. Individualize diet for proper nutrition to achieve a desirable weight and monitor carefully.

2. Provide adequate protein, calories, B-complex, zinc and other nutrients for age. Folic acid has been implicated in etiology, but the evidence is not clear.
3. Provide adequate nutrients for wound healing if surgery has been performed.

Profile

Ht	Temp	Gluc
Wt	TLC	Alb
IBW or Growth	Serum folic acid	H & H
Percentile	I & O	

Side Effects of Common Drugs Used

Antibiotics may be required if patient develops sepsis.

Patient Education

1. Family counseling may be needed in preparation for future pregnancies.
2. Referral to a local March of Dimes may be beneficial.

For More Information

Spina Bifida Association of America
343 South Dearborn St., Suite 310
Chicago, IL 60604
(312) 663-1562 or (800) 621-3141

NOTES

TYROSINEMIA

Usual Hospital Stay

4–5 days.

Notation

Tyrosinemia is a hereditary disorder in which a deficiency of parahydroxy-phenyl-pyruvic acid oxidase blocks the conversion of tyrosine to homogentisic acid. This condition results in liver failure or severe nodular cirrhosis with renal tubular involvement. Tyrosine accumulation can be aggravated by vitamin C deficiency, a high protein diet, and liver immaturity.

Objectives

1. Restrict phenylalanine and tyrosine from the diet.
2. Promote normal growth and development for age.
3. Provide adequate vitamin C for conversion processes.

Dietary Recommendations

1. Initially, low amount so phenylalanine/tyrosine hydrolysate should be fed to infants with small amounts of milk added to provide the minimum requirements of tyrosine and phenylalanine. Mead Johnson product 3200-AB or Ross Maxamaid XPHEN, TYR can be used.
2. If blood methionine levels are elevated, try Product 80056 (Mead Johnson). Use carbohydrate supplements like Polycose plus vitamins and minerals.
3. Supplement with vitamin C appropriate to the patient's age.

Profile

Birth wt, present wt	Length
Growth %, IBW/HBW	Abdominal distention
FTT	Hyperpigmentation
Phosphate	Dermatitis
Gluc	"Cabbage-like" odor
Alb	H & H
Plasma phenylalanine	Plasma tyrosine
Methionine	Urinary levels

Patient Education

1. Provide sources of tyrosine and phenylalanine in the diet.
2. Adjust intake of calories and nutrients according to the patient's age.

NOTES

WILSON'S DISEASE (HEPATOLENTICULAR DEGENERATION)

Usual Hospital Stay

4–5 days.

Notation

An inborn error of metabolism, Wilson's disease causes abnormal transport and storage of copper, resulting in hepatolenticular degeneration, neurologic damage, and damage to the kidney, brain, and cornea. Onset may occur from ages 5 to 40 years.

Objectives

1. Keep optimal balance of copper in patient.
2. Decrease serum copper levels, generally with drug chelation.
3. Prevent or reverse damage to body tissues and liver.
4. Watch caloric intake to prevent obesity.
5. Monitor changes in gag reflex or dysphagia.

Dietary Recommendations

1. A normal diet provides 2–5 mg per day of copper. A low copper diet (1–2 mg) may be needed.
2. The diet must limit liver, kidney, shellfish, nuts, raisins and other dried fruits, dried legumes, brain, oysters, mushrooms, chocolate, poultry, and whole-grain cereals.
3. Control calories, food textures, and other nutrients if necessary.
4. Increase fluid intake, but avoid alcoholic beverages.

Profile

Ceruloplasmin (often low)	difficulty	Easy bruising
	Serum P	SGOT
Ht	Wt	SGPT
Alb	PT	Alk phos
H & H	Serum Cu (inc.)	Kayser-Fleischer ring
BUN/Creat	Liver tests	
Swallowing	Urinary Cu	

Side Effects of Common Drugs Used

1. *D-penicillamine* (Cuprimine or Depen), a copper chelating agent, should be taken orally before meals. A vitamin B_6 supplement is needed with this drug, usually a dose of 25 mg. Zinc may also be necessary.
2. Laxatives or stool softeners may be needed.

Patient Education

1. Teach the patient about the copper content of foods.
2. Explain that breast milk has higher copper levels than cow's milk.
3. Help the patient with feeding at mealtimes if poor muscular control is demonstrated.
4. Discuss effective coping mechanisms, community resources, genetic counseling.

For More Information

Foundation for Study of Wilson's Disease, Inc.
5447 Palisade Ave.
Bronx, NY 10471

Comment

Copper is essential for promoting iron absorption for hemoglobin synthesis, as well as for formation of bone and myelin sheath. In hepatic tissues, 90% of the copper in the copper-albumin complex is converted to ceruloplasmin. In Wilson's disease, tissue deposition occurs rather than formation of ceruloplasmin.

Section 4
Neurological and Psychiatric Conditions

Chief Assessment Factors

loss of consciousness, seizures

dizziness, vertigo

weakness, drowsiness

headaches, memory loss

numbness

paralysis

bowel or bladder dysfunction

disturbed taste, smell, vision

hallucinations

confusion

tremors, tics

nervousness, irritability

pain

Table 4–1.

Goals in Treatment of Psychiatric Patients

Positive approach	Team-concept treatment
Prevention of malnutrition	Restoration of feeding abilities and satisfaction

Table 4–2.

Conditions Impairing Ability to Self-Feed—Central Nervous System and Neuromuscular States*

Severe mental retardation	Spasticity
Organic brain syndrome	Ataxia
Cerebral palsy	Other dyskinesias
Altered consciousness	Paresis or paralysis from stroke
Some psychotic states	Other cerebral lesions
Tremor	Peripheral neuropathy
Motor weakness from demyelinating and related diseases	Muscular weakness from myopathies

* Willard, M.: *Nutritional Management for the Practicing Physician*. Reading, MA, Addison-Wesley Publishing, 1982, p. 26.

Table 4–3.

Food and Brain Functioning

The substrates of neuronal communication are called neurotransmitters. Those neurotransmitters subject to dietary manipulation include serotonin, norepinephrine, and acetylcholine. Increases or decreases in dietary precursors will affect nervous tissue functioning—i.e., tryptophan will affect serotonin production, choline will affect acetylcholine production, tyrosine will affect norepinephrine production. Different combinations for meal content and/or drugs will alter substrate availability for neuron activity. Tryptophan can induce sleep from high CHO meals while high protein meals increase alertness.

A normal brain weighs 45 ounces, with steady growth up to age 20, then loss of weight for the rest of life.

Table 4–4.

Brain Parts

Medulla oblongata (8–12th cranial nerves here)
Midbrain
Cerebellum (3–5th cranial nerves here)
Cerebrum
Pons (6th cranial nerve here)

For More Information

Brain Research Foundation
343 South Dearborn Street
Chicago, IL 60604

ALZHEIMER'S DISEASE AND DEMENTIA

Usual Hospital Stay

7 days.

Notation

Alzheimer's disease involves a progressive deterioration of intellect, memory, personality and self-care, leading to severe dementia from degeneration of nerve cells in the cerebral cortex (sometimes as a result of hypothyroidism or brain tumor). The acetylcholine-containing neurons are especially affected. Alzheimer's causes 50% of dementias.

Chronic Organic Brain Syndrome (OBS) can be caused by Alzheimer's, CVA, neurological diseases, mental retardation or head trauma. Prognosis in Alzheimer's is poor, with death from renal or pulmonary or cardiac complications.

Objectives

1. Prevent weight loss or excessive gains from altered activity levels and eating habits.
2. Avoid constipation or impaction. Promote continence as long as possible.
3. Encourage self-feeding at mealtimes.
4. Nourish by appropriate methods (tube, if necessary).
5. Prevent or correct dehydration.
6. Monitor dysphagia and aspiration.
7. Protect patient from injury; provide emotional support.

Dietary Recommendations

1. Ensure an adequate diet, including protein and calories, for age, sex, and activity, especially for "wanderers."
2. Adequate vitamin E is essential (*Lancet* 3/22/86); perhaps selenium, fluoride, and choline will also be identified as essential in this disorder.
3. Offer one course at a time (first salad, then entree, etc.) to prevent confusion.
4. Because sweets are well-liked, prepare nutrient-dense desserts to offer.
5. Tube feed or use thick pureed foods if needed.
6. Use of foods like soybeans or eggs will provide choline in the form useful to the body; lecithin tablets do not necessarily increase acetylcholine levels adequately.
7. Adequate fluid intake is essential. Be careful not to give excesses at night.

Profile

Ht, wt	Creat	I & O
IBW/HBW	H & H	Acetylcholine levels
K$^+$	Wt changes	EEG
BUN	Alb	

Side Effects of Common Drugs Used

1. *Laxatives* may be used to control constipation. Offer fiber foods whenever possible. Ensure adequate fluid intake.
2. Monitor side effects of other medications.

Patient Education

1. Encourage routines, such as regular mealtimes, good mouth care, etc.
2. Refer family or caretakers to support groups.
3. Aluminum toxicity studies are still controversial; discuss with empathy how research studies require much time. Avoid acidic foods stored/cooked in aluminum cookware.
4. If patient needs to be spoon-fed, holding his or her nose will force open the mouth.
5. Products like Carnation Instant Breakfast can add extra calories and protein without excessive expense.

For More Information

Alzheimer's Hotline: (800) 621-0379

NOTES

AMYOTROPHIC LATERAL SCLEROSIS

Usual Hospital Stay

9 days.

Notation

Also known as motor neuron disease, progressive spinal muscular atrophy, or Lou Gehrig's disease, amyotrophic lateral sclerosis is a progressive neuron disease of adult life that ultimately causes death. Men are more often affected than women; the disease strikes 2–7/100,000 persons, usually after age 40. Symptoms and signs include muscular wasting and atrophy, drooling, loss of reflexes, respiratory infections or failure, spastic gait, and weakness.

Objectives

1. Maintain good nutrition to prevent further complications.
2. Reduce difficulties in chewing and swallowing. Monitor gag reflex.
3. Reduce the patient's fear of aspiration: test swallowing reflexes with water and feed slowly.
4. Minimize the possibility of urinary tract infection and constipation.
5. Correct negative nitrogen balance and nutritional deficiencies that exist.
6. Ease symptoms to try to maintain independence.

Dietary Recommendations

1. Use a soft diet. Progress to tube feeding (gastrostomy better tolerated for a long time) when dysphagia becomes severe. Provide adequate roughage in the diet.
2. The diet should include 2–3 liters of water daily.
3. Place food at side of mouth and tilt head forward to facilitate swallowing, where possible.
4. Caloric intake should be normal to high. Five to six small meals should be scheduled daily. Increase protein intake to counteract wasting.
5. Diet and supplemental feedings should provide an adequate intake of zinc, magnesium, potassium, amino acids, phosphorus, and vitamin E.

Profile

Ht	Difficulty in	N balance
IBW/HBW	swallowing	Temp
H & H	Wt changes	I & O
K$^+$	Alb	Gag reflex
Wt	BUN	

Table 4–5.
Cranial Nerves Affecting Mastication and Swallowing

Nerve	Function
Trigeminal (V)	Controls some tongue and jaw muscles
Facial (VII)	Controls facial muscles
Glossopharyngeal (IX)	Controls muscles of pharynx; affects taste
Hypoglossal (XII)	Controls tongue muscles

Patient Education

1. Tell the patient about adding fiber to the diet to prevent constipation. Explain which foods have fiber.
2. Encourage the planning of small, adequately balanced meals.
3. Carefully monitor the patient's weight loss. A weight loss of 10% is common.
4. Lightweight utensils are beneficial. A referral to an occupational therapist is recommended.
5. Minimize chewing, but avoid use of baby food, which can be insulting. Puree adult foods, especially preferred foods.
6. Discuss care plan in front of patient; include the patient as much as possible.
7. In Guam, flour made from the cycad nut has caused fatal ALS. No known direct causation has been determined in the United States.

For More Information

ALS Society of America: (213) 476-6451

National ALS Foundation, Inc.: (212) 679-4016

NOTES

ANOREXIA NERVOSA

Usual Hospital Stay

8 days.

Notation

Anorexia nervosa is a condition in which the patient severely rejects food, causing extreme weight loss, low basal metabolic rate, and exhaustion. Death occurs in extreme cases. Anorexia nervosa is ten times more common in girls; it is especially common in girls just after the onset of puberty. This condition usually involves the relentless pursuit of thinness and the misperception of body image. Amenorrhea often results. Bulimia and self-induced vomiting may also occur. See Bulimia entry.

Onset is usually under age 25, peaking at 12–13 and 19–20 years. Symptoms and signs include intense fear of becoming fat, not diminishing as weight loss progresses; no known physical cause, weight at 75% former wt.; amenorrhea; disturbed body image. 6–15% of the population is affected.

Objectives

1. Check growth chart and determine % difference, as well as future goals. Promote weight gain of 1–2 lbs weekly to reach a wt closer to HBW.
2. Restore normal physiologic function by correcting starvation and its associated changes, including electrolyte imbalance.
3. Obtain diet history to assess bulimia, vomiting, use of diuretics or laxatives.
4. *Do not force feedings.* Rejection of food is part of the illness. Promote normal eating behavior.
5. Gradually increase intake to a normal or high calorie diet in order to reduce excessive edema.
6. Reduce preoccupation with weight and food; promote adequate self-esteem.

Dietary Recommendations

1. Serve attractive, palatable meals in small amounts observing food preferences.
2. Beware of bulky foods in early stages of treatment. Gastrointestinal intolerance may exist.
3. Diet should be called a "low calorie diet for anorexia nervosa" in order to convince the patient of the counselors' good intentions.
4. Gradually increase intake to 3000+ calories; caloric intake should be age-dependent. Increasing the caloric intake must be done *slowly!* Start at basal needs +300–400 kcal.
5. Use tube feeding if this is necessary. This is not a preferred method of feeding. Tube feed only if patient is 40% IBW or lower.
6. Have the patient measure and record food intake at first; then gradually lessen the emphasis on food.
7. Help the patient resume normal eating habits. Assure the patient that constipation will be alleviated.
8. A "no added salt" diet can reduce fluid retention.
9. Avoid caffeine because of stimulant/diuretic effect.
10. A vitamin-mineral supplement may be needed (zinc, etc.)

Profile

Former wt	BP	Leukopenia
Recent wt	Chol	K^+, Na^+, Cl^-
Present wt	Gluc	Cortisol

% changes	H & H	Hx of bulimia or
IBW/HBW	TSH	laxative abuse
LH (dec.); FSH	Amenorrhea	
Estrogen	Lanugo hair	
Alb	Edema	

Patient Education

1. Help the patient become an effective, independently functioning person. Convey principles rather than rigid "rules" to avoid reinforcing the patient's compulsive rituals and preoccupation with food. Positive, regular habits should be encouraged.
2. Encourage the patient to follow a balanced diet. Discuss weight gain, weight maintenance, and snacks.
3. Discuss nutritional hunger signs.
4. Include family members in positive nutrition education.
5. Assertiveness training or transactional analysis theories may be helpful when the patient is ready.
6. For patients with IDDM, see the appropriate entry.
7. Neuropeptide-Y may someday be useful in treatment. Research is not yet conclusive.

For More Information

American Anorexia/Bulimia Association, Inc.
133 Cedar Lane
Teaneck, NJ 07666
(201) 836-1800

Anorexia Nervosa and Related Eating Disorders (ANRED)
PO Box 5102
Eugene, OR 97405
(503) 344-1144

Comments

Two possible long-term sequelae include Cushing's disease and osteoporosis.

NOTES

BULIMIA

Usual Hospital Stay

6 days.

Notation

Criteria for diagnosis include—recurrent episodes of binge eating; ingestion of high calorie foods during binges; inconspicuous eating during a binge; termination from pain, sleep, social interruption or induced vomiting; weight fluctuations greater than 10 lbs; inability to stop; depression and self-depreciation; no physical causation. Of the 5–30% of the population with bulimia, 85% are college-educated women. Bulimia patients are more likely than non-bulimics to experience loneliness, irritability, passivity, sadness, and suicidal behavior. Usually 60–70% have had overweight mothers; eating may have been taught as a coping mechanism for stress. Mothers may also have been more domineering, with excessively high expectations of their children. Bulimics are often at normal weight or slightly above normal. They may be at higher risk for chemical abuse. Bulimia is also a medical term for gorging.

Objectives

1. Stabilize fluid and electrolyte imbalances.
2. Assess patient thoroughly and create an individualized care plan. Include such factors as weight history, dieting behaviors, binge-eating episodes, purging behaviors, eating patterns, exercise patterns.
3. Promote effective weight control while altering life-stress management. Establish a target weight in accordance with standard ht./wt. tables, present weight, time frame for recovery and related factors.
4. Correct or prevent edema.
5. Prevent any or additional tooth enamel decay or erosion from vomiting and poor eating habits.

Dietary Recommendations

1. Provide basal energy needs plus 300–400 calories above present intake.
2. Utilize controlled portions of a regular diet, with usually 3 meals and 2 snacks.
3. Decrease sugar intake overall, stressing importance of other key nutrients.

Profile

Ht	K^+	Chol, Trig
Usual wt & changes	Cl^-	Gastrin
Alb	IBW	
Wt	Na^+	

Side Effects of Common Drugs Used

1. *Laxative* abuse and diuretic abuse can cause cardiac arrest and other problems.
2. *Phenytoin* (Dilantin) is sometimes given to patients with abnormal EEGs.

Patient Education

1. Self-help groups, such as Overeaters Anonymous, or group therapy can help.
2. Information can also encourage improved habits, as from basic nutrition texts.
3. Help the patient rediscover the ability to be alone without giving in to the urge to binge.
4. Assertiveness training may be of great benefit.
5. Discuss the outcomes of electrolyte imbalance: muscle spasms, kidney problems, or cardiac arrest.
6. Assert that there is "no such thing as a forbidden food."
7. Discuss the vicious cycle of bulimia: hopelessness or anxiety leading to gorging leading to fear of fatness leading to vomiting or drug abuse leading to release from fear leading to guilt, etc.

Comments

"Bulimia nervosa" is a term describing a powerful urge to eat and preoccupation with food. The person with this condition has a morbid fear of fatness.

For More Information

Bulimia Anorexia Self-Help Hotline: (800) 762-3334

NOTES

CEREBRAL ANEURYSM

Usual Hospital Stay

6 days.

Notation

A cerebral aneurysm may involve the dilation of a cerebral artery resulting from a weakness of the blood vessel wall.

Symptoms and signs include altered consciousness, drowsiness, confusion, stupor, sometimes coma, headache, facial pain, eye pain, blurred vision, vertigo, tinnitus, hemiparesis, elevated blood pressure, and dilated pupils.

Objectives

1. Omit fluids if necessary to reduce cerebral edema.
2. Avoid constipation and straining at stool.
3. Lower hypertension if possible.
4. Prevent further complications or problems.

Dietary Recommendations

1. NPO unless otherwise ordered. Appropriate IVs will be utilized.
2. Upon verification of progress, the physician will order a diet appropriate for condition. Assist with self-feeding measures.
3. Restrict sodium and dietary cholesterol if deemed necessary.
4. Alter dietary fiber intake, as appropriate.

Profile

Ht/Wt/IBW/HBW	CT scan results	Gluc
Chol	Trig	Na^+, K^+
Alb	H & H	
I & O	BP (inc.)	

Side Effects of Common Drugs Used

Cardiovascular drugs are usually ordered according to significant parameters. Adjust dietary intake accordingly.

Patient Education

1. Discuss fiber sources from the diet. Foods such as prune juice or bran added to cereal can be helpful in alleviating constipation.
2. Counsel regarding self-feeding techniques.
3. Discuss role of nutrition in preventing further cardiovascular problems.

NOTES

COMA

Usual Hospital Stay

4 days. Often transferred to a rehabilitation facility.

Notation

Coma is an unconscious state in which the patient is unresponsive to verbal or painful stimuli. A Glasgow coma scale may be used by the staff to determine levels of unconsciousness and prognosis.

Objectives

1. Maintain standards for primary condition.
2. Elevate head to prevent aspiration during feeding process.
3. Assess daily calorie and fluid requirements.
4. Prevent or treat decubitus ulcers, constipation, and other complications of immobility.

Dietary Recommendations

1. Tube feed (increased calories and protein as appropriate) every 2–3 hours or as ordered by the physician. Parenteral fluids may also be appropriate at this time.
2. TPN or use of IV fat solutions can be appropriate for some persons, dependent on evaluations of original disorder, sepsis, or other complicating factors.
3. A product like Enrich or Susta II can be helpful in preventing or easing constipation because of added fiber content.
4. Progress as possible to oral feedings.

Profile

Ht/Wt/IBW	Serum lipids	Glasgow coma scale
BP	Alb	(4–7 = coma;
P_{CO_2}	Gluc	measures eye
P_{O_2}	BUN	opening, motor &
Wt. changes (bed scale)	Creat	verbal responses)

Side Effects of Common Drugs Used

1. *Anticonvulsants*, such as phenytoin (Dilantin), may aggravate folic acid metabolism and cause decreased serum levels over time.
2. *Steroids* may be used, with side effects like increased sodium retention, increased potassium, calcium, and magnesium losses, increased nitrogen depletion.

3. *Antacids* may be needed to prevent stress ulcers.
4. *Cathartics* are often used.

Patient Education

1. Discuss with caretaker or family any necessary measures that are completed to provide adequate nourishment. Explain importance of prevention of complications, such as aspiration.
2. Evaluate self-feeding potentials over time.

NOTES

DEPRESSION

Usual Hospital Stay

6 days.

Notation

Good physical health, including nutrition, is an adjunct to psychiatric treatment. *Exogenous/reactive* depression involves an unrealistic and inappropriate reaction to some event or internal conflict. *Endogenous* depression involves multiple factors leading to intrapsychic conflict; this is a major depression that requires antidepressants or psychotherapy. Signs and symptoms include poor appetite with reduced intake and weight loss, or increased appetite with weight gain; poor sleep pattern; change in usual activity; loss of interest; fatigue; and diminished concentration.

Objectives

1. Provide adequate nutritional intake—e.g., shock therapy requires increased caloric intake.
2. Monitor weight weekly to evaluate progress.
3. Detect complications as suggested by weight loss. Determine whether weight loss is caused by inadequate calorie and nutrient intake.
4. Assess usual eating habits and related problems, which may include loneliness, difficulty in activities of daily living, boredom, lack of hobbies and interests, and poor sleep habits.
5. Monitor calorie intake if overeating; counsel appropriately.

Dietary Recommendations

1. Use a diet providing HBV proteins and a high calcium intake. Emotional stress lowers nitrogen and calcium levels.
2. Watch out for inadequate protein intake, which may lower levels of iron, thiamine, riboflavin, niacin, and vitamins B_6 and B_{12}.
3. Use a tyramine-restricted diet for patients given monoamine oxidase inhibiting drugs. Such a diet excludes aged cheese, beer, red wine, ale, pickled herring, chicken liver, broad bean pods, canned figs, sausage, salami, pepperoni, commercial gravies, ripe avocado, fermented soy sauce, ripe banana, yeast concentrates, and pickled or smoked fish.
4. If overeating, limit access to food and provide a low-calorie diet.

Profile

Ht	Wt	Serotonin
Alb	N balance	I & O
Serum Ca^{++}	BP	Mg^{++}
H & H	Food pica	Transferrin
IBW/HBW	K^+	Constipation
Na^+	Gluc	T_4

Side Effects of Common Drugs Used

1. *Monoamine oxidase inhibitors* [tranylcypromine (Parnate), phenelzine (Nardil), isocarboxazid (Marplan)] require a tyramine-restricted diet to prevent hypertensive crisis. Tyramine is a pressor amine. Spoiled, overripe and aged products are the most problematic. Beware of Chianti wines.
2. *Tricyclic antidepressants* [imiprimine (Tofranil), amitryptyline (Elavil), amoxapine (Asendin)] may cause dry mouth. Some may cause an increase in appetite, with potential for excessive weight gain. Others may cause nausea, vomiting, SIADH, constipation, anorexia, or stomatitis.
3. *Lithium carbonate* (Lithane, Lithobid, Lithotabs) requires a constancy in sodium intake. Weight gain, metallic taste, nausea, vomiting, and diarrhea may occur. Limit caffeine intake.
4. *Nortriptyline* (Aventyl, Pamelor) may cause increased appetite for sweets, GI distress, vomiting, and diarrhea.

Patient Education

1. Teach creative menu planning.
2. Teach the patient how to moisten foods for the dry mouth syndrome resulting from certain medications. Sugar-free candy may help.
3. Limit caffeine-containing foods and beverages in the late evening.

Comments

1. 40% of persons with depression may have a deficiency of brain *serotonin*. A mixed diet of protein/CHO should provide a balance of tryptophan, a precursor of serotonin.
2. Studies at Rush-Presbyterian/St. Luke's Medical Center in Chicago suggest the use of *phenylalanine* with mild manic-depressive illness. Conclusions are not final.

NOTES

EPILEPSY/SEIZURE DISORDERS

Usual Hospital Stay

3–4 days.

Notation

Epilepsy, a paroxysmal disturbance of the nervous system, results in recurrent attacks of loss of consciousness, convulsions, motor activity, or behavioral abnormalities. The seizures result from excessive neuronal discharges in the brain. A *grand mal* seizure involves an aura, a tonic phase, and a clonic phase. A *petit mal* seizure involves momentary loss of consciousness. There are many forms of epilepsy, each with its own symptoms. No structural abnormality is found in 2/3 of cases. A single seizure does not imply epilepsy. Incidence is 2–6/1000 people. It is common with cerebral palsy and spina bifida.

Objectives

1. Minimize seizures via medications or lesionectomy surgery.
2. Provide a well-balanced diet that avoids excess of food or fluid intake.
3. If drug therapy does not work (as in the case of intractable myoclonic or akinetic seizures of infancy), a *ketogenic diet* may be used to produce ketosis. Ketosis stabilizes convulsions by decreasing restlessness and irritability. Reverse the usual ratio of cholesterol and fat. Beware of changing the diet abruptly; a gradual approach is preferred. This approach works best for children ages 2–5.
4. Monitor need for key nutrients.

Dietary Recommendations

1. Provide a normal diet reflecting the patient's age and activity.
2. A ketogenic diet is unpalatable. The diet follows a ratio of 3:1 or 4:1 fat to carbohydrate and protein. Medium-chain triglycerides are more ketogenic, having more rapid metabolism and absorption. If used in this way, medium-chain triglycerides would provide 60% of kcal (the rest of the diet would consist of 10% other fats, 10% protein, and 20% carbohydrates). Protein should meet basal needs (1 g/kg body weight).
3. Stimulants such as tea, coffee, colas, and alcohol are not permitted.
4. Supplements may be needed, especially for calcium, vitamin D, folacin, and vitamins B_6 and B_{12}.

Profile

Ht	Wt	Chol, trig
Urinary acetone (a.m. levels)	Alb	IBW/HBW
	CT scan	Skull x-ray
EEG	Alk phos	BP
Serum Ca^{++}	I & O	

Side Effects of Common Drugs Used

1. *Anticonvulsant therapy* can cause interference with vitamin D metabolism, leading to a calcium imbalance and possibly rickets or osteomalacia. Therapy with 25-hydroxy vitamin D is recommended.

   Carbamazepine (Tegretol) causes dry mouth, vomiting, nausea and anorexia.

   Ethosuximide (Zarontin), trimethadione (Tridione), and *primidone* (Mysoline) can cause gastrointestinal upset and weight loss. Take with food or milk.

   Phenytoin (Dilantin) causes gum hyperplasia and carbohydrate intolerance. It also binds serum proteins and decreases folate and vitamin B_{12} absorption. Patients will also need more vitamin C and magnesium. Be careful with vitamin B_6; excess supplementation can reduce effectiveness.

   Phenobarbitol depletes vitamins D, K, B_{12}, B_6, folate, and calcium. Nausea, vomiting and anorexia may also occur.
2. *Cough syrups, laxatives and other medications* contain a high CHO content; monitor drug-drug actions.

Patient Education

1. Ketogenic diets cause nausea and vomiting. Orange juice can help relieve the symptoms. Regular monitoring of the diet is crucial.
2. An ID tag is recommended, such as Medic-Alert.
3. Alcohol should be avoided. A balanced diet is needed.

4. To alter fats, the following tips may be helpful:
    a. To increase LCT—add sour cream, whipped cream, butter, margarine, or oils to casseroles or desserts or other foods.
    b. To use MCT—add to salad dressings, fruit juice, casseroles, and sandwich spreads.

For More Information

Epilepsy Foundation of America
4351 Garden City Drive
Landover, MD 20785

Epilepsy Hotline: (800) 426-0660

NOTES

GUILLAIN-BARRÉ SYNDROME

Usual Hospital Stay

7 days.

Notation

This condition is also known as acute postinfectious polyneuritis and is a neurological syndrome of increasing weakness, numbness, pain and paralysis, often following a recent viral infection or even following immunization.

Symptoms and signs include muscular weakness of lower extremities progressing to arms, trunk, face, and head; respiratory failure; paralysis of lower extremities or quadriplegia; unstable blood pressure; aspiration; dysphagia; difficulty in chewing; impaired speech; muscular pain; low-grade fever; tachycardia; weight loss; anorexia; UTIs; or personality changes.

Objectives

1. Prevent or correct weight loss and resulting malnutrition.
2. Adjust diet for chewing and swallowing problems.
3. Meet added calorie requirements from any fever.
4. Wean, as possible, from ventilator dependency.
5. Improve neurological functioning and overall prognosis.

Dietary Recommendations

1. *Acute.* IV fluids will be required. Tube feeding or TPN may be necessary while patient is acutely ill over a period of time. Increased calories and protein may be necessary. Alter fat intake as appropriate to reduce production of carbon dioxide, especially on ventilator.
2. *Progression.* When tolerated, a soft diet or general diet can be used as tolerated by the individual. For some, a thick pureed diet may be beneficial with dysphagia.
3. Supplement oral intake with frequent snacks, such as shakes or eggnogs.
4. A vitamin-mineral supplement may be beneficial if intake has been poor.

Profile

Ht/wt/IBW/HBW	Wt changes	CSF protein levels
CBC	BP	Temp
H & H	Alb	Gluc
P_{CO_2}	P_{O_2}	Dysphagia, etc.

Side Effects of Common Drugs Used

1. *Antibiotics* may be needed if UTIs or other problems are identified.
2. *Analgesics* are used to reduce pain and inflammation.
3. *Steroids* are used to reduce inflammation and swelling; their effects can be deleterious over time.
4. *Vasopressors* may be used.

Patient Education

1. Encourage self-feeding if possible.
2. Maintain adequacy of calorie and protein intake to improve weight status and nutritional health.
3. Avoid upper respiratory infections and exposure to other illnesses.
4. Arrange for special feeding utensils if needed by the individual.
5. Avoid constipation through use of fruits, vegetables, crushed bran, prune juice, and adequate fluid intake.

NOTES

HUNTINGTON'S CHOREA

Usual Hospital Stay

9 days.

Notation

An autosomal dominant hereditary disease, Huntington's chorea develops in middle to late life, with involuntary spasmodic, irregular movements. Cerebral degeneration occurs. Behavioral changes begin 10 years before movement disorder begins at ages 35–42. Duration is generally 17–30 years before death.

Objectives

1. Promote normal nutritional status, despite tissue degeneration.
2. Encourage the patient to self-feed until this is no longer possible.
3. Improve brain levels of dopamine and acetylcholine, which tend to be low.

Dietary Recommendations

1. Provide a high calorie, high protein diet.
2. Tube feed when necessary.
3. Feed slowly to prevent choking.
4. Provide adequate fiber (e.g., prune juice) for normal elimination.

Profile

Ht	Chewing or	H & H
IBW/HBW	swallowing	Acetylcholine levels
Wt	difficulties	Dopamine levels
Ability to feed self	BUN/creat	I & O

Patient Education

1. Semisolid foods may be easier to swallow than thin liquids.
2. Provide genetic counseling—each child of affected parent has 50% chance of inheriting the disease.
3. Teach family or caretakers about the Heimlich maneuver.

Comments

Huntington's chorea differs from Alzheimer's disease in that there is loss of control of voluntary movements.

MULTIPLE SCLEROSIS

Usual Hospital Stay

7–8 days.

Notation

Multiple sclerosis involves the loss of myelin sheath, causing progressive or episodic nerve degeneration and disability. Reduced levels of linoleic acid and lecithin are noted. It is possible that the disease is caused by a virus. Other symptoms and signs include fatigue, sensory impairment, loss of position sense, respiratory problems. Onset is usually between 20 and 40 (average age, 27); women have MS 3:2 more often than men. After diagnosis, 70% are as active as previously.

Objectives

1. During the active phase of the disease, corticosteroids are used to decrease symptoms. Alter diet accordingly.
2. During the chronic phase of the disease, treatment centers around reducing the incidence of respiratory and urinary tract infections, managing bowel problems, controlling muscle spasms, and preventing contractures and decubitus ulcers.
3. Adjust caloric intake to avoid excessive weight gain, if this becomes a problem.
4. Prevent or correct constipation or fecal impaction.
5. Maintain good nutritional status.
6. Reduce fatigue associated with mealtimes.

Dietary Recommendations

1. No special diet is necessary, although some persons suggest use of a low-fat diet (under 30 grams), with 10 g saturated fats, normal protein levels, and adequate carbohydrates to complete caloric needs. (See *AJCN 48*:1387, 1988.)
2. As swallowing difficulties increase and as coordination decreases, foods may need to be liquefied or provided in tube feeding.

3. Laxative foods and liquids may ease constipation.
4. Reduce sodium intake during use of steroid therapy. Otherwise, sodium plays a role in lipid/protein transport in myelin tissues.
5. Provide adequate intake of vitamin C and multivitamins, especially B complex.
6. Small frequent meals may be better tolerated than large meals.

Profile

Ht	Trig	Temp
IBW/HBW	BP	Wt
Alb	Gluc	H & H
Chol	CSF (WBC, gamma	EEG
K$^+$	globulin are	I & O
Edema	increased)	L:S Ratio

Side Effects of Common Drugs Used

1. *Corticosteroids* require controlled sodium intake while these drugs are being used. Glucose intolerance, negative nitrogen balance, and decreased serum zinc, calcium, and potassium may occur.
2. *Antispasticity drugs* such as baclofen (Lioresal) may cause nausea, diarrhea, and constipation.
3. Muscle relaxants may be used.

Patient Education

1. Teach the patient how to control caloric intake.
2. Teach the patient about sources of PUFAs in the diet.
3. Describe the role of fat in myelin sheath formation/maintenance.
4. Teach the patient about foods high in fiber.
5. Avoid total inactivity.
6. Utensils with large handles may be useful in food preparation and self-feeding.
7. At a restaurant, foods may need to be cut before serving.
8. Use table-top cooking methods and equipment to avoid lifting.
9. Maintain optimism.

Comments

Table 4–6.
Courses of MS*
Benign—few, mild early exacerbations with normal life expectancy and minimal disability—20% of cases

---

* Scheinberg, L.: *MS: Guide for Patients and Families.* New York, Raven Press, 1983.

Exacerbating/Remitting—more frequent early attacks with less complete clearing; long periods of stability, some disability—25% of cases.

Chronic/Relapsing—fewer and less complete remissions after attacks; greater disability which may plateau after many years—20% will be ambulatory, 20% nonambulatory

Chronic/Progressive—onset is more insidious and more slowly progressive than chronic/relapsing—15% of cases

For More Information

National Multiple Sclerosis Society
205 East 42nd Street
New York, NY 10017

MYASTHENIA GRAVIS

Usual Hospital Stay

6–7 days.

Notation

Myasthenia gravis results from a fluctuating weakness of some voluntary muscles. It is related to a defect in transmission of nerves at the neuromuscular junction. This may be caused by the inadequate synthesis or release of acetylcholine, the result of an autoimmune response. Etiology is not known, but some patients benefit from removal of the thymus gland. Symptoms and signs include fatigue, general weakness, dysphagia, weak voice, inability to walk on heels, and pneumonia.

Objectives

1. Increase the likelihood of obtaining adequate nutrition through altering the consistency of the foods. This is necessary when the muscles used in chewing and swallowing are weakened.
2. Feedings should be small to reduce fatigue.
3. Prevent permanent structural damage to the neuromuscular system.
4. Allow adequate time to complete meals.

Dietary Recommendations

1. The diet should include frequent, small feedings of easily masticated foods.
2. Provide tube feeding when needed.
3. Provide adequate potassium supplements.

4. If corticosteroids are part of treatment, use a 2 g sodium diet.
5. Use a high protein/high carbohydrate diet.
6. The use of lecithin and choline has been successful in some cases, but has not been consistently documented.
7. Avoid giving medications with coffee or fruit juice; give with milk and crackers or bread.

Profile

Ht	Wt	BP
Alb	H & H	Acetylcholine levels
K$^+$	IBW/HBW	
Wt changes	Tensilon test	

Side Effects of Common Drugs Used

1. Short-acting *anticholinesterase* compounds [neostigmine (Prostigmin) or pyridostigmine (Mestinon)] or corticosteroids (prednisone, etc.) may require limiting sodium intake. Anorexia, abdominal cramps, diarrhea and weakness may result from use of these drugs.
2. Long-term use of *antacids* negatively affects calcium and magnesium metabolism.

Patient Education

1. Show patient how to prepare foods with the use of a blender, if that is necessary.
2. Indicate how to take medication with food or milk. Discuss potential side effects.
3. Avoidance of alcohol is important.
4. Food and utensils should be arranged within reach of the patient.

NOTES

NEUROLOGICAL TRAUMA (SPINAL CORD INJURY)

Usual Hospital Stay

7 days—depends on location and extent of injury.

Notation

Spinal cord injury (SCI) is often from traffic accidents, diving accidents, sports injury or gunshot wounds. Partial vs. total self-care deficits depend on resulting hemiplegia, diplegia, paraplegia (thoracic or lumbar cord) or quadriplegia (cervical cord).

The nervous system of a patient with neurologic trauma is vulnerable to glucose and oxygen variations, as well as variations in other nutrients.

Objectives

1. Control acid-base and electrolyte balances. Assess needs on admission, daily thereafter.
2. Reduce the danger of aspiration by avoiding oral feedings if patient has been vomiting.
3. Ensure adequate fluid intake to prevent urinary calculi.
4. Increase opportunities for rehabilitation by monitoring weight changes. Weight loss of 10–30% in first month is common.
5. Prevent UTIs, paralytic ileus, pneumonia, malnutrition, decubitus, constipation, peptic ulcer, and fecal impaction.

Dietary Recommendations

1. Provide patient with intravenous solutions as soon as possible after injury. Check blood gas measurements and chemistries. Once peristalsis returns, patient may be tube fed. Elevate head of bed 30–45°, if possible, to prevent aspiration.
2. Ensure adequate intake of thiamine, niacin, and vitamin B_6, as well as amino acids. Monitor iron stores and adjust diet as needed.
3. Paraplegics initially need 1.5–1.7 g protein/kg. Progression to more normal intake can occur when nitrogen balance returns, such as 1.2–1.5 g/kg.
4. Monitor weight: male paraplegics should be 10% to 15% below IBW; male quadriplegics 15–20 lbs below IBW. Calculations for women are equivalent. Ensure adequate CHO and fat intake, including 1–2% EFA.
5. Encourage adequate fluid and fiber. Be careful about gas-forming foods; monitor tolerance.

Profile

Ht	Wt	Myelogram
H & H (dec.)	BUN	P_{CO_2}, P_{O_2}
Alb	IBW/HBW	PT
K^+	Gluc	Ca^{++}, Mg^{++}
Creat (eventually dec.)	BP	N balance
	Serum Fe	I & O

Side Effects of Common Drugs Used

1. *Analgesics* for pain relief (e.g., aspirin/salicylates) can prolong bleeding time. Gastrointestinal bleeding may eventually result. An increased intake of vitamin C and folacin is needed.
2. *Laxatives* may be used; encourage fiber and fluid instead.

Patient Education

1. Provide weight control measures for rehabilitation.
2. Teach patient about good sources of iron in the diet, as well as vitamins and protein.
3. Help promote a structured feeding routine. Feed slowly (over 30–45 min). Bites of food should be small.
4. Seat belts should be promoted to prevent future vehicular injury.
5. Discuss long-term risks of heart disease.

For More Information

National Spinal Cord Injury Foundation
369 Eliot Street
Newton Upper Falls, MA 02164

American Paralysis Association: (800) 225-0292

PARKINSON'S DISEASE

Usual Hospital Stay

6–7 days.

Notation

A neuromuscular disorder resulting from diminished levels of dopamine at the basal ganglia of the brain, Parkinson's disease causes tremor, rigidity, abnormal gait, and difficulty in chewing, speaking, or swallowing. L-dopa must be provided. Men are affected slightly more often than women. The disease is more common after age 60 and life expectancy is 12.5 years after diagnosis. About 24 conditions are categorized as Parkinson's disorders.

Objectives

1. Supply dopamine to the brain with drugs. Monitor diet therapy accordingly.
2. Maintain optimal physical and emotional health.
3. Improve the patient's ability to eat. Use semisolid foods rather than fluids if sucking/swallowing reflexes are reduced. Drooling may also be a problem. (See CVA entry regarding dysphagia.)

4. Provide adequate calories to prevent weight loss, but obesity should be prevented as well.
5. Avoid constipation.
6. Preserve functioning; prevent disability as long as possible.

Dietary Recommendations

1. A high intake of protein diminishes the effectiveness of levodopa. Use high biologic value proteins, 35 g (or 0.5 g/kg body weight), and limit intake of vitamin B_6 to RDA levels.
2. The following foods provide vitamin B_6 in the diet: dry skim milk, peas and beans, sweet potatoes, yams, avocado, fortified cereal, bran, oatmeal, wheat germ, yeast, pork, beef organs, tuna, and fresh salmon.
3. Cut, mince, or soften foods as required. Use small meals if needed.
4. Add crushed bran to hot cereal; prune juice may be needed.

Profile

Ht	H & H	I & O
IBW/HBW	K^+	Dysphagia
BP	Alb	Depression, anorexia
Na^+	Dopamine	BUN, creat
N balance	Norepinephrine	SGOT, SGPT
Wt	levels	Gluc
		Uric acid

Side Effects of Common Drugs Used

1. Patients being treated with *levodopa* (Dopar, Larodopa) should restrict their intake of protein, vitamin B_6, alcohol, and caffeine. Increase intake of B_{12} and vitamin C-rich foods. Nausea, dry mouth, and vomiting can occur.
2. *Carbidopa* (Sinemet) is not affected by protein, vitamin B_6 and alcohol. Nausea is common; dry mouth and vomiting are not as common.
3. *Trihexyphenidyl* (Artane) causes dry mouth.
4. *Tricyclic antidepressants* may be ordered.
5. *Benztropine* (Cogentin) can cause dry mouth, dysphagia, anorexia, and constipation.
6. Univest Technologies Ltd. in New York has formulated a vitamin-mineral supplement without vitamin B_6, called *Unilife Formula 1*. For more details on availability, call (212) 832-1203.
7. *Amantadine* (Symmetrel) can cause nausea, vomiting, and dry mouth.

Patient Education

1. Explain how to blenderize food.
2. Help patient to control weight, which may change owing to reduced mobility and/or inability to ingest sufficient quantities.

3. Check the patient's multivitamins to avoid high vitamin B_6 content. Discuss good food sources as well.
4. Place all foods within easy reach of the patient.
5. Braces may help the patient control severe tremors at mealtime.

Comments

1. Tyrosine may be useful, since it is a precursor of dopamine and nor-epinephrine.
2. Yale University School of Medicine studies suggest omission of protein foods until 5 pm, then eating protein allowance for the day (levodopa can be decreased by 41%). This allows some normal daily functioning. Benefit is noted within one week.

For More Information

Parkinson's Disease Foundation, Inc.
William Black Medical Research Building
Columbia University Medical Center
640 W. 168th Street
New York, NY 10032

American Parkinson's Disease Association
147 East 50th Street
New York, NY 10022

NOTES

PSYCHOSIS

Usual Hospital Stay

8–9 days.

Notation

Psychosis is a condition in which an individual loses contact with reality; it can be either episodic or chronic and result in irrational behaviors. It is usually best treated in a hospital setting where the afflicted persons are less likely to hurt themselves or other people. Organic forms can cause a dazed expression, confused speech, visual hallucinations, bizarre or withdrawn behavior, low self-esteem, and appetite or sleep disturbances.

Objectives

1. Provide adequate nourishment to prevent significant weight changes.
2. Correct any nutritional deficits.
3. Promote a normal pattern of dietary intake and routines.
4. Develop a trusting relationship; make expectations clear to the patient.
5. Prevent or correct constipation or impaction.

Dietary Recommendations

1. A normal diet for age and sex can be used, unless other dietary/medical problems exist.
2. Adjust calories up or down according to goal weight for patient and medications.
3. Reduce potential accidents by avoiding glass containers and serving dishes.
4. Vitamin C levels tend to be low in persons with schizophrenia; encourage improved and adequate intake accordingly.

Profile

Ht/Wt/IBW/HBW	Wt changes	Na^+
I & O	K^+	H & H
BP	CPK (elevated in acute	Gluc
Alb	episodes)	

Side Effects of Common Drugs Used

1. *Tranquilizers* are generally used.
2. *Laxatives* or stool softeners may be required. Discuss potential use of higher fiber foods, fluids, etc.
3. Other *antidepressants* and medications may be used; evaluate specific drugs accordingly.
4. *Antipsychotics* (Mellaril, Prolixin, Haldol) may cause dry mouth, weight gain, edema, nausea, or vomiting.
5. *Chlorpromazine* (Thorazine) contains sulfites. It may cause dry mouth, constipation, or weight gain.
6. In a few persons, drugs can cause psychiatric symptoms. The symptoms are rare, but may include confusion [acyclovir, propoxyphene (Darvon), and cimetidine (Tagamet)]; depression [oral contraceptives, ibuprofen, metronidazole (Flagyl), barbiturates, cimetidine (Tagamet) and diazepam (Valium)]; insomnia [acyclovir and alprazolam; paranoia (amphetamines, ibuprofen, cimetidine (Tagamet), and tricyclic antidepres-

sants]; excitement, hyperactivity or agitation [alprazolam, amphetamines, barbiturates, metronidazole (Flagyl), and diazepam (Valium)]; anxiety, mania, hallucinations, suicidal thoughts and bizarre behavior may result from various other medications. The doctor should be contacted.

Patient Education

1. Teach nutrition principles as far as possible.
2. Encourage self-care.
3. Successfully terminate client relationship when independence is possible.
4. Provide follow-up, especially with any stages of regression.

Comments

Schizophrenia. Group of disorders manifested by mood and behavioral disturbances (can be simple, catatonic, schizoaffective, paranoid, hebephrenic).

Organic Brain Syndrome. From cerebral arteriosclerosis, chemical or toxic trauma, senile dementia or other states.

Delusions. Can involve control, persecution, infidelity or other abnormal fears.

Hallucinations. Perceptions of an external stimulus without a source in the external world.

NOTES

SUBSTANCE ABUSE AND WITHDRAWAL

Usual Hospital Stay

2–3 days.

Notation

Abuse of chemical substances may be chronic or acute, and may involve abuse of alcohol, prescription or over-the-counter drugs, or illicit drugs. Physiological problems that result are definite, and are usually specific to the substance abused. Social, emotional, vocational, and legal problems may arise as a result of the abuse.

Persons with substance dependency tend to have type A personalities and are prone to perfectionism and depression. Some studies suggest that abnormalities in the metabolism of dopamine, serotonin, and norepinephrine may contribute to the cause of substance dependency; in some cases, use of antidepressant medication has helped to alleviate the dependency.

Objectives

1. Protect during withdrawal (e.g., alcohol detoxification may cause tremors, hallucinations, seizures, and delirium tremens). Of persons with delirium tremens 20% may die, even with therapy; care must be taken to prevent death.
2. Normalize brain levels of neurotransmitters.
3. Correct fluid and electrolyte imbalances or dehydration.
4. Modify diet for such problems as liver failure, cirrhosis, pancreatitis, GI bleeding, esophageal varices, renal impairment, ascites, or edema. See appropriate entries.
5. Maintain homeostasis; prevent physical complications.
6. Reorient to reality; develop trusting relationships between patient and care providers.
7. Promote abstinence and long-term substance-abuse treatment.
8. Improve nutritional status and outcome.
9. Prevent or correct any related eating disorders (approximately 50% of this group).

Dietary Recommendations

1. According to I & O values, adjust fluid intake. Offer beverage favorites.
2. Encourage nutrient-dense foods.
3. Adequate intake of protein without overloading (as with hepatic failure) will be essential. Include adequate calories, especially since patients often become hypoglycemic during detoxification.
4. Adequate intake of B-complex vitamins, L-tryptophan and L-tyrosine, and other depleted nutrients may be beneficial during recovery, but use food sources of tryptophan rather than supplements.
5. See other sections for specific diagnosis-related problems.
6. Adjust diet as appropriate to reduce excess sweets, since many chemical abusers tend to substitute sweets for their dependency drug.
7. Adequate fiber intake may be useful to correct or prevent constipation.

Profile

Ht/Wt/IBW/HBW	I & O	Alb
Na^+	Ca^{++}	Mg^{++}
Wt changes	K^+	Cl^-
Prolactin levels	BP	Gluc
	H & H	Serum folate

Side Effects of Common Drugs Used

1. *Tricyclic antidepressants* (imipramine, desipramine) are often beneficial, with some side effects, such as dry mouth.
2. *Bromocriptine* may also be used for some drug-recovery patients.
3. *Stool softeners* may be beneficial if constipation results after withdrawal, as with cocaine abuse.
4. *Antabuse*, when mixed with alcohol, can cause severe nausea, vomiting, low BP, and flushing.
5. *Amino acid/vitamin supplements* containing phenylalanine, glutamine, tryptophan, and B_6 (SAVE) are reported to reduce alcohol craving (*JAMA* 4/91, p. 464).

Patient Education

1. Help the patient accept responsibility for his or her own actions.
2. Help plan adequate discharge planning, follow-up, family therapy, or other support group interactions.
3. Help with maintenance of abstinence.
4. Avoid discussion of unanswerable questions, such as "why" substances have been abused.
5. Help dispel myths.
6. Discuss issues regarding personal "control."
7. Include patient in decision-making to increase self-esteem and confidence.

Comments

Alcoholism—the most consistent predictor of alcohol dependency is alcoholism in a biological parent. Three predisposing factors exist: constitutional lability (biochemical); personality factor (psychological vulnerability);' and social factor (environmental conditioning). Alcoholics have 2.5 times the normal death rate in similar age groups, especially from stroke or cirrhosis. An estimated 3 million children between ages 14–17 are problem drinkers.

For More Information

National Institute on Drug Abuse: (800) 662-HELP

NOTES

TARDIVE DYSKINESIA

Usual Hospital Stay

8 days.

Notation

Tardive dyskinesia (TD) is a condition that imitates other neurological disorders and is caused by long-term use of antipsychotic drugs. It occurs in 20–40% of all patients receiving long-term antipsychotic drugs. Patients are usually elderly, chronically institutionalized (often brain damaged), following extended use of such drugs as reserpine, chlorpromazine (Thorazine), thioridazine (Mellaril), haloperidol (Haldol), thiothixene (Navane), lidone, fluphenazine (Prolixin), and trifluoperazine (Stelazine). In some cases, an acetylcholine deficiency is speculated, and brain dopamine receptors may become supersensitive with chronic use of neuroleptic drugs.

Signs and symptoms include abnormal, involuntary movements (chorea, athetosis, dystonia, tics, facial grimacing). Tongue, face, neck, lung muscles and extremities are usually involved.

Objectives

1. Prevent or correct malnutrition, weight loss and other problems.
2. Identify and assist with feeding problems. Some patients have problems with sucking and puckering of the lips and difficulty in eating.
3. Restore eating capacity as far as possible.
4. Alter textures as necessary (eating problems are rare or occur late in the condition).
5. Prevent stress, which aggravates supersensitivity psychoses.

Dietary Recommendations

1. Offer the usual diet, with soft textures to reduce chewing as needed.
2. Decrease calories if obese; increase if underweight.
3. Decrease caffeine intake because of the effects of drug therapy.
4. Carbohydrate craving is common from drugs that block histamine receptors; watch overall intake of sweets or offer nutrient-dense varieties.
5. Increase dietary choline from foods such as eggs, soybeans, peanuts, and liver.
6. Moisten foods with gravy, sauces and liquids if dry mouth is a problem.
7. Alter fiber intake if needed to prevent or correct constipation.

Profile

Ht/Wt/IBW/HBW	Serum prolactin (often	Gluc
H & H	increased)	Alb
	Acetylcholine levels	

Side Effects of Common Drugs Used

Drug therapy usually includes the same medications as normal, otherwise withdrawal symptoms may be exacerbated—with a greater impact on overall signs and symptoms of TD.

Patient Education

Diet instructions should be offered directly to the patient unless this is not possible. Discuss major issues related to nutrition, self-feeding practices, moistening of foods, etc.

For More Information

American Psychiatric Association
1700 18th St., N.W.
Washington, DC 20009

NOTES

TRAUMATIC BRAIN INJURY (TBI)

Usual Hospital Stay

9 days.

Notation

TBI may result after car or industrial accidents, falls, fights, explosions, gunshot wounds (with 40% involving alcohol use). Also called head trauma, any sudden impact or blow to the head (with or without unconsciousness) is involved in TBI.

Symptoms and signs include dyspnea, vertigo, altered consciousness, seizures, vomiting, altered blood pressure, weakness or paralysis, aphasia, problems with physical control of hands, head, or neck with resulting difficulty in self-feeding.

Objectives

1. Assess regularly the substrate needs (calories, protein, etc.). Prevent malnutrition and cachexia.
2. Monitor hydration; prevent dehydration and overhydration.
3. Correct any self-feeding problems; breathing and swallowing problems; other conditions affecting self-care.
4. Provide adequate protein for improving nitrogen balance (serum albumin tends to be low, especially if comatose, and urinary losses may be as high as twice normal).
5. Prevent aspiration pneumonia, meningitis, sepsis, UTIs, SIADH, hypertension, decubiti, and Curling's ulcer.
6. Prevent or reduce seizure activity, convulsions, and intracranial edema.
7. Prevent cerebral edema and fluid overload with TPN.

Dietary Recommendations

1. Patient will be NPO for 24 hours, progressing to clear liquids if tolerated. The need for surgery or ventilation will have an impact on the ability to progress to any oral intake.
2. Tube feeding (especially grastrostomy) and TPN may be required for a period of time.
3. Patient may require 1.5–2 g protein/kg BW; 35–50 kcal/kg; and a kilocalorie:nitrogen ratio of 85–100:1 because of nitrogen losses. Monitor carefully.
4. IV lipid may be needed if patient is on TPN for an extended period of time.
5. Patients who are immobile for a long period of time may have a decrease in weight by 10%, perhaps from lowered metabolic rate. Calorie intake may need to be varied accordingly.
6. Progress, when possible, to oral intake (perhaps using a thick pureed diet with dysphagia).

Profile

Ht/Wt/IBW/HBW	CBC, TLC	BUN
P_{CO_2}	Temp	I & O
P_{O_2}	Transferrin	CAT scan, skull x-rays
Alb	Na^+	K^+
Gluc	SGOT (inc. with brain	BP
Serum ETOH levels	necrosis)	Creat
Glasgow coma scale	Intracranial pressure	

Side Effects of Common Drugs Used

1. *Steroids* used to reduce swelling—used less frequently today.
2. *Analgesics* are used for pain.

3. *Anticonvulsants* may be needed to reduce seizure activity. Watch folic acid levels and other affected nutrients.
4. *Albumin replacement* may be needed to raise serum levels.
5. *Psyllium laxative* (Metamucil) is often helpful in alleviating constipation.
6. *Antacids* may be used to reduce stress ulcer activity.

Patient Education

1. Chew and swallow slowly, if and when able to eat solids.
2. Gradually relearn self-feeding techniques.
3. Be wary of food temperatures, especially if patient has become less sensitized to hot and cold.
4. Preparation of colorful and attractive meals is crucial to acceptance.
5. The team approach is beneficial, with OT, speech therapist, psychologist and physical therapist helping the dietitian with treatment plans.
6. Use of a helmet to prevent future accidents may be suggested.

Comments

1. Hypothalamic lesions can aggravate hyperphagia.
2. Lateral lesions can aggravate aphagia and cachexia.

For More Information

National Head Injury Foundation
333 Turnpike Road
Southborough, MA 01772
(617) 485-9950

TRIGEMINAL NEURALGIA (TIC DOULOUREUX)

Usual Hospital Stay

1 day.

Notation

This condition involves a disorder of the 5th cranial nerve, characterized by paroxysms of excruciating pain of a burning nature. The painful periods alternate with pain-free periods. The disorder is rare before age 40, and is more common in women. The right side of the face is more often affected.

Objectives

1. Control pain with medications, especially before meals.
2. Provide appropriate counseling and assistance with consistency of meals (foods and beverages).
3. Individualize for preferences and tolerances.
4. Maintain body weight within a desirable range.

Dietary Recommendations

1. Use a normal diet as tolerated—perhaps altering to soft or pureed foods as needed.
2. Small, frequent feedings may be better tolerated than large meals.
3. Liquids may be preferred if given by straw. Individualize!
4. Avoid extremes in temperature.
5. Use nutrient-dense foods if weight loss occurs.

Profile

Ht/Wt/IBW/HBW	H & H	Dysphagia
Alb	BP	Temp
I & O	BUN	Creat

Side Effects of Common Drugs Used

1. *Phenytoin* (Dilantin) may be given for seizure activity.
2. *Carbamazepine* (Tegretol) may be used.
3. *Sedatives or narcotics* may be used to reduce pain.

Patient Education

1. The importance of oral and dental hygiene should be stressed, even with pain. Use pain medications as directed.
2. The patient should be encouraged to avoid eating when tense or nervous.
3. Relaxation therapy may be beneficial.

NOTES

Section 5
Pulmonary Disorders

Chief Assessment Factors

cough

pain (chest, abdominal)

wheezing

shortness of breath

poor exercise tolerance

fever or chills

rapid breathing

dizziness

sweating

flaring nostrils

red, swollen nose

cyanosis (lips, nail beds)

pallor

ashen or gray coloring

confusion

orthopnea

clubbing of nail beds

engorged eye veins

altered respirations

anorexia

elevated blood pressure

For More Information

National Jewish Center for Immunology
and Respiratory Medicine
1400 Jackson Street
Denver, Colorado 80206
(800) 222-LUNG

American Lung Association
1740 Broadway
New York, NY 10019

Table 5–1.
Factors Contributing to Malnutrition in Patients with Hypoxic Cardiopulmonary Disease*

Factors Affecting Dietary Intake	Metabolic Factors	Abnormal Losses of Nutrients	Drug Side Effects
Anorexia of chronic illness	Increased mechanical work of breathing	Therapeutic removal of body fluids	Anorexia, nausea
Gastric hypomotility	Increased cardiac work	Malabsorption; decreased xylose tolerance associated with degree of hypoxemia	Increased sympathetic tone
Difficulty in eating during continuous dyspnea	Mildly elevated body temperature		
Aerophagia	Febrile complications		
Depression, apprehension, chronic debility	Increased sympathetic tone		
Unpalatable diet	Metabolic inefficiency due to cellular hypoxia		
Concurrent vitamin deficiency			
Concurrent fasting ketosis	Hypermetabolism		

* From Willard, M.: Nutritional Management for the Practicing Physician. Reading, MA, Addison-Wesley, 1982, p. 28.

NOTES

134

BRONCHIAL ASTHMA

Usual Hospital Stay

6–7 days.

Notation

Asthma involves paroxysmal dyspnea accompanied by wheezing and is caused by spasm of the bronchial tubes or swelling of their mucous membranes. Two types are recognized: allergic (formerly called extrinsic), and nonallergic (intrinsic or infectious). Asthma appears to be inherited in 2/3 of cases.

Signs and symptoms include respiratory distress, audible wheezing, decreased breath sounds, tachycardia, cyanosis, hypotension, anxiety, pulmonary edema, dehydration, hard and dry cough, and distended neck veins. Chronic poor control can lead to a serious condition, *status asthmaticus*, which generally requires hospitalization and is considered to be life-threatening.

Objectives

1. Prevent distention of stomach from large meals, resulting in distress and perhaps aggravation of asthmatic state.
2. Promote improved resistance against disease, especially for nonallergic type.
3. For allergic asthma, identify and control allergens in the environment.
4. Promote adequate hydration, to liquefy secretions.
5. Ensure adequate nutritional intake and good nutritional status.
6. Encourage a health-maintenance program.

Dietary Recommendations

1. Provide balanced, small meals that are nutrient-dense (high quality protein, calories, vitamins and minerals), especially to reduce risk of infections and poor state of health.
2. Highlight foods rich in vitamins A, C, and B_6 and zinc. Other nutrients that support immunocompetence should be addressed.
3. For allergic asthma, omit food allergens as identified. Only 4% of adult asthmatics will have food allergies; the common foods to omit are milk, eggs, seafood and fish. Sulfites may also need to be carefully assessed. Salicylates are rarely a problem, but may aggravate asthma in 2% of patients.
4. Force fluids unless otherwise contraindicated.

Profile

Ht/Wt/IBW/HBW	H & H	Transferrin
BP	Temp	I & O

Gluc	Po$_2$	Serum lipids
Pco$_2$	Serum theophylline	Uric Acid
Alb	levels (as needed)	Bilirubin

Side Effects of Common Drugs Used

1. *Bronchodilators*—nausea and vomiting can be a problem for some types of these drugs. With *theophylline*, avoid extreme changes in protein and CHO intake; avoid extreme changes in usual intakes of caffeine-containing foods. *Metaproterenol* (Metaprel, Alupent) may alter taste and cause nausea or vomiting.
2. *Antibiotics*—long-term use can cause diarrhea and other problems. Penicillin should not be taken with fruit juices.
3. *Epinephrine* may be required for emergencies.
4. *Potassium iodide*, an expectorant, may affect existing thyroid problems.
5. *Corticosteroids* have many side effects, such as depleting serum potassium and retaining excess sodium, causing hyperglycemia and other problems. Monitor carefully, especially if needed over a long period of time.

Patient Education

1. Mild chronic asthma can be a warning that, if untreated, can lead to an acute exacerbation.
2. All medications should be taken as directed by the physician.
3. Insect bites that cause asthmatic attacks generally have no correlation with diet, although in some persons, use of thiamine hydrochloride can reduce biting of mosquitoes. Check with a physician regarding any over-the-counter or home remedies for asthma.
4. Work with patient/family to avoid precipitating events or triggers. Discuss exercise, rest, and nutrition.

Comments

For Children

Mothers of Asthmatics, Inc. (M.A. Report)—Newsletter
5316 Summit Drive
Fairfax, VA 22030

National Asthma Center
1999 Julian Street
Denver, CO 80204

NOTES

RESPIRATORY DISTRESS SYNDROME

Usual Hospital Stay

5 days.

Notation

This condition is a secondary lung state that develops in patients who have sepsis, or are critically ill, in shock, or severely injured. Patients often have pulmonary edema, but have normal left atrial and pulmonary venous pressures.

In infants, RDS often occurs in low-birthweight babies, and the condition may be called hyaline membrane disease. Such babies are often born to mothers who have diabetes.

Objectives

1. Promote rapid recovery.
2. Prevent relapse.
3. Counteract side effects of medications as ordered.
4. Replace essential fatty acids, carnitine and other nutrients as indicated.
5. Restore normal oxygenation of bloodstream and tissues.
6. Prevent or correct malnutrition. [CNS output for ventilatory drive may be depressed. Starvation decreases desire to breathe, causing abnormal breathing pattern, pneumonia, and atelectasis. Muscle mass (including diaphragm) varies with body weight. Refeeding may take 2–3 weeks.]
7. Prevent overfeeding (hepatic dysfunction, fatty liver, and CO_2 overproduction) or underfeeding (morbidity, mortality, and decreased response to therapy).

Dietary Recommendations

1. Provide parenteral fluids as ordered. Progress when possible to oral feedings.
2. Increased fat may be required to normalize respiratory quotient (RQ). Fat also adds extra calories and palatability to the diet.
3. Ensure adequate provision of EFA and fat-soluble vitamins in appropriate forms. Low linoleic acid status in critically ill RDS infants may require IVs with a fat emulsion added.

4. Be careful with TPN-induced changes in CO_2 production.
5. For weight maintenance, use $1-1.2 \times$ BEE. For anabolism, use $1.4-1.6 \times$ BEE. NPC should be 50% glucose, 50% lipid.

Profile

Ht/Wt/IBW/HBW or growth profile	CBC	BP
	Temp	P_{CO_2}
I & O	Alb	P_{O_2}
H & H	Prealbumin	K^+
Transferrin	RQ	Na^+
Indirect calorimetry		

Side Effects of Common Drugs Used

1. *Corticosteroids* may be used, with many side effects if prolonged use is required.
2. *Diuretics* are used in cases of pulmonary edema. Monitor serum electrolytes accordingly.

Patient Education

Discuss the role of fat intake on respiratory requirements. Fat decreases CO_2 production.

ACUTE RESPIRATORY FAILURE

Usual Hospital Stay

5–6 days; 8–9 days with ventilator support.

Notation

ARF involves sudden absence of respirations, with confusion or unresponsiveness and failure of pulmonary gas exchange mechanism. Chronic pulmonary disease (or injury) can cause instances of acute pulmonary failure, which require the use of mechanical ventilation. Other causes include drug OD, Guillain-Barré syndrome, myasthenia gravis, muscular dystrophy, massive obesity, adult RDS, pneumonia, asthma, and pulmonary embolism.

Objectives

1. Promote normalized nutritional intake, despite hypermetabolic status of the patient and the prohibition of oral intake due to endotracheal tubes. Relieve breathlessness; decrease CO_2 production.

2. Monitor sensations of hunger as patients are unable to communicate their hunger, as well as thirst.
3. Prevent respiratory muscle dysfunction by ensuring that the patient is properly nourished. Maintain weight. Note: not all patients are malnourished.
4. Counteract hypotension due to positive pressure ventilation, acidosis, or both.
5. Provide nutritional substrates that will not greatly increase CO_2 production, while maintaining surfactant production and keeping LBM.
6. Prevent atelectasis, pulmonary infection, sepsis, glucose or lipid intolerance, MOSF, and aspiration.
7. Adjust goals as appropriate; maintain flexible, patient-specific approaches.

Dietary Recommendations

1. Begin feeding the patient as soon as possible in order to wean the patient from the ventilator. Tube feedings of low osmolality are needed. Watch use of total parenteral nutrition because of high calorie loading and increased carbon dioxide production. Essential fatty acids should also be provided two to three times weekly; soy or safflower oil may be used as the nutrient source.
2. The diet should be high in calories, with equal amounts of fat and carbohydrate (carbohydrates are metabolized to produce large amounts of carbon dioxide). A diet with 35–50% CHO and 30–50% lipid calories is common. Watch total parenteral nutrition for this reason. Adults need a daily diet of at least 25–35 kcal/kg maintenance, or 35–45 kcal/kg anabolism. BMR increases by 60%. Protein needs may be 2 g/kg IBW.
3. Patients with *pulmonary edema* should have their sodium intake reduced as needed. Include adequate amounts of protein in the diet to prevent additional fluid retention from lowered colloidal osmotic pressure.
4. Supplement diet with multivitamins, especially vitamins A and C.
5. Phosphorus should be provided if depleted, at 2.5–5 mg/kg BW.
6. Start any TF slowly to avoid gastric retention or diarrhea. Add blue food coloring to feedings to detect problems in tracheal secretions. Advance gradually; use continuous administrations unless contraindicated.

Profile

Ht	H & H	Urinary gluc
IBW/HBW; BEE or REE	BP	CHI
Alb (dec.)	K^+	Transferrin
Na^+	Fever	P (dec. can cause
I & O	P_{CO_2}, P_{O_2}	ARF)

TLC (dec.)	RQ*	pH (acidemia below
Respiratory rate	Indirect calorimetry	7.4, alkalemia
Wt	Chol, trig	above 7.4)

Patient Education

1. A daily calorie count may be needed to assess the patient's nutritional status.
2. The greatest danger in using enteral nutrition is aspiration. Low osmolarity products are essential, as well as elevation of the head of the bed.
3. Discuss early satiety, bloating, fatigue, dyspnea, etc. as related to food or TF intake.

Comments

Skeletal muscle mass and muscle strength are affected by anabolic and catabolic hormones, muscle work, and nutritional status. Substrate and muscle work stimulate protein synthesis. Hypermetabolic patients have at least 30% increase in oxygen use. IV fat emulsions may help reduce inflammation.

In starvation, respiratory muscles are catabolized to meet energy needs. Refeeding helps ventilatory response.

---

* $RQ = \dfrac{V_{O_2}}{V_{CO_2}}$

RQ from fat = 0.7
RQ from protein = 0.8
RQ from CHO = 1.0

Table 5–2.
Ventilator-Dependency Feeding Stages*

1. Acute repletion—replenish muscle glycogen stores and reverse catabolism.
2. Preweaning—maintain positive nitrogen balance, improve visceral protein stores, improve CHI, promote weight gain.
3. Weaning—provide energy substrates to cover needs of respiratory muscles that are working harder; minimize CO_2 production
4. Postweaning—maintain nutrient needs despite anorexia or dysphagia; support anabolism.

---

* Adapted from Irwin, M., and Openbrier, D.: A delicate balance—strategies for feeding ventilated COPD patient. *Am. J. Nurs.* 85:274, March, 1985.

NOTES

BRONCHIECTASIS

Usual Hospital Stay

7 days.

Notation

Chronic dilation of the bronchi (or a bronchus) occurs in this condition, with secretion of a large amount of purulent sputum.

Symptoms and signs include an early morning, paroxysmal cough; profuse, foul and purulent sputum; decreased breath sounds; weight loss; fatigue; anorexia; pneumonia; and fever.

Objectives

1. Promote recovery.
2. Avoid fatigue associated with mealtimes.
3. Prevent or correct dehydration.
4. Improve weight status, where necessary.
5. Reduce fever.

Dietary Recommendations

1. Use a high protein/high calorie diet, appropriate for age and sex.
2. Small, frequent feedings may be better tolerated.
3. Fluid intake of 2–3 L daily may be offered, unless contraindicated.
4. IV fat emulsions may be indicated (eicosanoids are inflammatory modulators, and thromboxanes and leukotrienes tend to be potent mediators of inflammation). Evidence is still being compiled.

Profile

Ht/Wt/IBW/HBW	Temp	Resp. rate
BP	Gluc	H & H
Alb/RBP	Na^+	Transferrin
Po_2	K^+	I & O
Pco_2		

Side Effects of Common Drugs Used

1. *Antibiotics* are used if the condition is bacterial in origin.
2. *Analgesics* and *antipyretics* may be used. Monitor side effects according to the specific drugs used.

Patient Education

1. Discuss the role of nutrition in health and recovery; emphasize quality proteins and nutrient-dense foods, especially if the patient is anorexic.
2. Emphasize fluid intake, perhaps recommending juices or calorie-containing beverages instead of water.

NOTES

BRONCHITIS, ACUTE

Usual Hospital Stay

5–6 days.

Notation

Bronchitis is caused by inflammation of the air passages. The acute form may follow a cold or other upper-respiratory infection, producing hemoptysis, sore throat, nasal discharge, slight fever, cough, and back and muscle pain. The chronic form—believed due mostly to cigarette smoking and air pollution—can produce breathing difficulty, wheezing, blueness, fits of coughing, and sputum. (See COPD entry.)

Objectives

1. Normalize body temperature (decrease fever).
2. Replenish nutrients used in respiratory distress.
3. Prevent further complications such as dehydration, otitis media, etc. Avoid further infections.
4. Allow ample rest before and after feedings.
5. Prevent dehydration.

Dietary Recommendations

1. Provide a regular or high-calorie diet.
2. Limit intake of milk only if the milk tends to thicken mucus, a point unproven by research.
3. Provide adequate amounts of vitamin C.
4. Increase the intake of fluids, 2–3 liters unless contraindicated.
5. Appropriate fatty acid intake may be beneficial to reduce inflammation.

Profile

Ht	Wt
IBW/HBW	K^+
H & H	Alb
I & O	Edema
Na^+	TLC

Side Effects of Common Drugs Used

1. *Bronchodilators* can cause gastric irritation. They should be taken with milk, food, or an antacid.
2. *Theophylline* can be toxic if a diet high in carbohydrates and low in protein is used. Avoid large amounts of stimulant beverages, namely coffee, tea, cocoa, and cola, unless the physician permits them.
3. *Antibiotics* may be used. Avoid taking penicillin with fruit juice.

Patient Education

1. Explain to the patient that adequate hydration is one of the best ways to liquefy secretions.
2. Maintain body weight within IBW/HBW.

BRONCHIAL PNEUMONIA

Usual Hospital Stay

5–6 days.

Notation

Pneumonia involves inflammation of the alveolar spaces of the lung. Lung tissue is consolidated as alveoli fill with exudate. Many types exist, such as bacterial (from those normally present in mouth/throat), viral, chemical, hypostatic (in bedridden persons, usually elderly), aspiration (from swallowing a foreign substance), and allergic (as from sensitivity to dust or pollen).

Signs and symptoms include difficult, painful respirations; shortness of breath; rales; rhonchi; tachypnea; chills and fever (102–106°F); delirium; anorexia; malaise; abdominal distention; restlessness; cyanosis of nail beds; tachycardia; atelectasis; anxiety; and a productive cough that is painful and incessant (generally with green/yellow sputum that progresses to a pink or rust coloration).

Objectives

1. Prevent dehydration.
2. Relieve breathing difficulty.
3. Prevent weight loss from hypermetabolic state.
4. Avoid infections; prevent sepsis.
5. In convalescent stage, avoid constipation.

Dietary Recommendations

1. If not contraindicated, offer 3–3.5 L fluid daily to liquefy secretions, and to help lower temperature.
2. Progress as tolerated to a high calorie/soft diet. If overweight, allow normal calorie intake for age and sex.
3. Frequent small meals may be tolerated better.
4. A multivitamin/mineral supplement may be beneficial, especially including vitamins A and C.
5. When possible, add more fiber to prevent constipation.

Profile

Ht/wt/IBW/HBW	Bronchoscopy	Na^+
Temp	Alb	BP
TLC	RBP	H & H
P_{CO_2}	I & O	Transferrin
K^+	P_{O_2}	Gluc

Side Effects of Common Drugs Used

1. *Antibiotics* are used in bacterial conditions.
2. *Analgesics* are used to reduce pain.
3. *Antipyretics* are used to lower temperature.

Patient Education

1. Discuss the role of diet and fluid intake in recovery.
2. In hypostatic pneumonia, suggest greater activity (within restraints of complicating disorders).
3. Fruit and vegetable juices add calories, fluid and sometimes fiber to the diet and can be available at bedside.

NOTES

CHRONIC PULMONARY DISEASES (EMPHYSEMA, CHRONIC BRONCHITIS, CHRONIC OBSTRUCTIVE PULMONARY DISEASE)

Usual Hospital Stay

6–7 days.

Notation

COPD can result from a history of emphysema, asthma, chronic bronchitis, etc. with persistent airway obstruction.

Emphysema is characterized by distention and destruction of pulmonary air spaces caused by smoking and air pollution. Wheezing, SOB and chronic cough result.

COPD is the sixth leading cause of death in the United States. Symptoms and signs include dyspnea on exertion, frequent hypoxemia, decreased forced expiratory volume in one second, and destruction of alveolar capillary bed. In COPD, total air quantity is blown out much sooner.

Objectives

1. Correct malnutrition. As there is less oxygen available for ATP formation, the patient is less able to be active, and there is less blood flow to the gastrointestinal tract and muscles. Malnutrition increases likelihood of infections.
2. Overcome anorexia resulting from slowed peristalsis and digestion. Patient lethargy and poor appetite and gastric ulceration result from inadequate oxygen to gastrointestinal cells.
3. Improve ventilation before meals with intermittent positive pressure breathing.
4. Lessen work efforts by losing weight if needed, or prevent excessive losses, which can increase morbidity.
5. Prevent respiratory infections or respiratory acidosis from decreased CO_2 elimination. Decrease excess CO_2 production.
6. Alleviate difficulty in chewing or swallowing from shortness of breath.
7. Prevent or correct dehydration, which thickens mucus.
8. Avoid constipation and straining at stool.

Dietary Recommendations

1. A high protein/high calorie diet is necessary to correct malnutrition. Use 1.2–1.5 g protein/kg and BEE × 1.5 for anabolism. Promote weight loss through a calorie-controlled diet for obese patients. Diets should be 40–55% CHO, 30–40% fat, 15–20% protein.
2. A soft diet (no tough or stringy foods) is recommended, as well as an anti-reflux regimen. No gas-forming vegetables are allowed, unless tolerated well.
3. Supplement diet with vitamins A and C to allow healing and formation of tissue. B-complex may also be needed for energy metabolism.
4. Use small, concentrated feedings at frequent intervals to lessen fatigue. Eggnogs and shakes may be helpful.
5. Fluid intake should be high, especially if the patient is febrile. Use 1 ml/kcal as a general rule.
6. For patients with *peripheral edema*, restrict intake of sodium and increase levels of potassium.
7. Fiber should be gradually increased, perhaps through use of crushed bran, prune juice, and extra fruits and vegetables.
8. Chicken soup clears the respiratory tract better than plain water; monitor effectiveness.
9. If necessary, moderate CHO is needed to avoid overload.

Profile

Ht	Wt	Respirations
IBW/HBW	K^+	Ascites
Alb	H & H	RQ (CHO = 1,
Marasmus or	I & O	protein = .8, fat =
kwashiorkor	BP	.7)
Temperature	TLC	pH
Na^+	Chest x-ray	P_{CO_2}, P_{O_2}

Side Effects of Common Drugs Used

1. *Bronchodilators* are used to liquefy secretions, treat infections, and dilate the bronchi. They can cause gastric irritation and ulceration.
2. *Antibiotics, steroids, expectorants, antihistamines,* and other drugs may be used. Monitor accordingly.

Patient Education

1. Explain how to conserve energy while preparing meals at home.
2. Explain how to concentrate protein and calories in small feedings.
3. Encourage rest periods before and after meals. Encourage slow eating.
4. Encourage the patient to make small, attractive meals.
5. Explain that excessively hot or cold foods may cause coughing spells.

Comments

1. Nutritional depletion is significantly greater in patients who have emphysema than in those who have chronic bronchitis. Dyspnea plays a significant role. Serious weight loss can occur from anorexia that is secondary to shortness of breath and GI distress. Starvation can cause emphysema, even without any smoking!
2. *Emphysema.* "Pink puffer"—thin, wt. loss; no heart failure, generally; tissue destruction.
3. *Chronic bronchitis.* "Blue bloater." No wt. loss; cardiac enlargement with failure is common.

Table 5–3.
FOOD TIPS TO ADD CALORIES OR PROTEIN TO A DIET

To Add Calories to a Diet From Fat and Carbohydrate

Fats can be used, including butter or margarine, cream, sour cream, gravies, salad dressings, and shortening. Mix butter into hot foods such as soups and vegetables, mashed potatoes, cooked cereals, and rice. Serve hot bread with lots of melted butter and jelly.

Mayonnaise can be added to salads or sandwiches.

Sour cream or yogurt can be used on vegetables such as potatoes, beans, carrots, and squash. Try sour cream or yogurt in gravy or salad dressings for fruit.

Peanut butter (1 tablespoon = 90 kcal plus some protein) can be spread on crackers, apples, celery, pears, and bananas.

Spread honey on toast, in tea, or on the morning cereal.

Whipping cream has 60 kcal per tablespoon. Add it to pies, fruits, pudding, hot chocolate, gelatin, and other desserts.

Add marshmallows to hot chocolate.

Fry the entree (chicken, meat, fish). The caloric value of fried foods is higher than that of baked or broiled foods.

Have snacks ready to eat: nuts, dried fruits, candy, buttered popcorn, crackers and cheese, granola, ice cream, popsicles.

Drink milk shakes with lots of ice cream added. These will be high in calories and protein.

To Add Protein to a Diet

Protein can be added to many foods without having to increase the number of foods eaten.

Add skim milk powder (2 tablespoons) to the regular amount of milk* used in recipes or for a beverage. Or add 1 cup dry powder to 1 quart fluid milk, allow to sit overnight. This adds 286 kcal, 15 g protein.

---

* This beverage is often called "double-strength" milk.

147

Add milk powder to hot or cold cereals, scrambled eggs, mashed potatoes, soups, gravies, ground meats (meat patties, meatballs, meatloaf), casserole dishes, and baked goods.

Use milk or half-and-half instead of water when making soups, cereals, instant puddings, cocoa, canned soups.

Add diced or ground meat to soups and casseroles.

Add grated cheese or cheese chunks to sauces, vegetables, soups, and casseroles.

Choose dessert recipes that contain egg, such as sponge or angel cake, egg custard, bread pudding, or rice pudding.

Buy instant breakfast mixes and use them instead of milk with meals, or as snacks. One 8-oz glass provides 280 kcal.

NOTES

CHYLOTHORAX

Usual Hospital Stay

7 days.

Notation

Chylothorax involves accumulation of clear lymph (chyle) in the pleural or thoracic space. It may be spontaneous, or caused by invasion of that thoracic space. Etiologies may also include amyloidosis, congenital chylothorax, CABG, violent coughing after heavy meals, cancer, complications of neck surgery including a radical dissection, spontaneous accumulation, thoracic cage compression after CPR, thoracic duct trauma from thoracotomy tubes, thoracic surgery affecting the heart, lungs, or esophagus, thrombosis of the subclavian vein during TPN, TB, or violent vomiting after heavy meals.

Objectives

1. Offer continuous chest-tube drainage to decrease pleural chyle.
2. Lessen consequences of a nutritional or immunological nature from drainage (e.g., sepsis, PCM, decreased TLC and other parameters).
3. Replace fat, protein and micronutrient losses from exudates.
4. Achieve a positive nitrogen balance.

Dietary Recommendations

1. Decrease enteral fat intake (using Vivonex, for example, instead of Osmolite or Compleat) in tube-fed patients. In fed patients, reduce total fat intake.
2. In patients without sepsis, TPN may be indicated, with care not to aggravate the condition.
3. In fed patients, a low fat diet may be used. It may be used alone or with a product like Vivonex T.E.N.
4. Replace exudate losses of such nutrients as vitamin A and zinc. Check serum levels and replace with 5–10x RDA as necessary.

Profile

Ht/wt/IBW/HBW	Wt changes	TLC (dec.)
Alb & RBP	Transferrin	Gluc
H & H	Chol/trig	I & O

Side Effects of Common Drugs Used

Medications are given as appropriate for the etiology. Monitor side effects accordingly, especially in such conditions as TB or cancer where numerous side effects are created from the drug therapies.

Patient Education

Discuss the importance of adequate nutrition in recovery.

COR PULMONALE

Usual Hospital Stay

3–4 days.

Notation

A heart disease following disease of the lung (emphysema, silicosis, etc.), cor pulmonale strains the right ventricle, creating hypertrophy and eventual failure. It may be acute, subacute or chronic. Signs and symptoms include hypoxia, wheezing, cough, fatigue, weakness, cyanosis, and clubbing of the extremities.

Objectives

1. Improve the patient's capacity to eat meals without straining the diaphragm.
2. Correct malnourished status.
3. Reduce or prevent fluid retention and edema.
4. Prevent further damage to cardiac and respiratory tissues.

Dietary Recommendations

1. Recommend small, frequent meals.
2. Use a high calorie diet with concentrated protein sources: double-strength milk, foods with milk powder added to them, etc.
3. To reduce fluid retention, intake of fluids may be restricted to 500 ml plus amount of the previous day's fluid intake. Sodium restriction may also be necessary.
4. Use soft or bland foods to reduce gastric irritation and reflux.
5. Provide adequate potassium intake, unless fluid retention elevates levels excessively.

Profile

Ht	Wt	Chest x-ray
IBW/HBW	Edema	P_{CO_2} (inc.)
Alb	H & H	P_{O_2} (dec.)
K^+	BP	RUQ pain
I & O	BUN	Hepatomegaly
Na^+		

Side Effects of Common Drugs Used

1. *Corticosteroids* can cause sodium retention, negative N balance, etc. Monitor carefully.
2. *Diuretics* can cause potassium depletion with diuresis.

Patient Education

1. Plan small, attractive meals that are nutrient-dense.
2. Emphasize the importance of eating slowly.
3. Recommend snacks that are high in calories and protein, but that do not provide excessive amounts of sodium.

NOTES

PULMONARY EMBOLUS

Usual Hospital Stay

8–9 days.

Notation

Pulmonary embolus is caused by a blood clot from another part of the body that has found its way to the lung. The condition can be life-threatening. Sudden substernal pain, SOB, cyanosis, pallor, faintness, fever, hypotension and wheezing can occur, sometimes followed by right heart failure.

Objectives

1. Normalize body temperature if fever exists.
2. Replenish nutrients depleted by respiratory distress.
3. Stabilize prothrombin time (PT) if warfarin (Coumadin) is used.
4. Eliminate edema if present.
5. Prepare for possible surgery (embolectomy).

Dietary Recommendations

1. Use a regular or high-calorie diet.
2. Use a 2 g sodium diet for patients with edema.
3. Increase fluid intake.
4. Restrict vitamin K from diet if PT is not stabilized.
5. Small meals may be needed.

Profile

Ht	IBW/HBW	PT
Na^+	Temp (Fever)	P_{CO_2}, P_{O_2}
Edema	K^+	LDH (inc.)
Wt	I & O	WBCs (inc.)
Alb	Chest x-ray	Bilirubin (inc.)

Side Effects of Common Drugs Used

1. *Anticoagulants.* Warfarin (Coumadin) increases clotting times by thinning blood. If problems in stabilizing the PT exist, the diet may need to be restricted in vitamin K.
2. *Antibiotics, cardiotonic drugs, diuretics,* or *antiarrhythmics* may be used.

Patient Education

1. Explain sources of vitamin K in the diet.
2. Discuss relaxation techniques, especially related to mealtimes.

NOTES

PULMONARY TUBERCULOSIS

Usual Hospital Stay

7–8 days.

Notation

Tuberculosis is caused by a tubercle bacillus invading the lungs and setting up an inflammatory process. Healing occurs with a calcification of the tubercular cavity. Tuberculosis causes tissue wasting, exhaustion, hemoptysis, cough, fever, and expectoration. The *acute* form resembles pneumonia. The *chronic* form causes low-grade fever.

Objectives

1. Maintain weight (or prevent losses).* Reduce fever.
2. Normalize calcium levels in serum.
3. Replace losses from lung hemorrhage, if present.
4. Promote healing of the cavity.
5. Counteract neuritis from isoniazid (INH) therapy, where used.
6. Stimulate appetite.
7. Prevent dehydration.

Dietary Recommendations

1. Use a well-balanced diet containing liberal amounts of protein and adequate calories (approximately 3000 kcal).
2. Ensure that the diet provides sufficient calcium without excess. Vitamin D is needed in controlled amounts.
3. Ensure that the diet provides iron and vitamin C for proper hemoglobin formation and wound healing.
4. Ensure that the diet provides the vitamin B-complex, especially vitamin B_6, to counteract isoniazid (INH) therapy.
5. Alcohol should not be used as a calorie replacement.

---

* The basal metabolism rate is 20 to 30% above normal to counteract fever of 102.2°F and above.

6. Use supplemental vitamin A as carotene is poorly converted.
7. Use adequate fluids (2 liters are common) unless contraindicated.

Profile

Ht	Wt	Mg^{++}
IBW/HBW	H & H, Serum Fe	TB skin test
Alb, RBP, prealbumin	N balance	Chest x-rays
TLC	I & O	Transferrin
Temp, fever	Chol (dec.)	BUN, creat
Serum pyridoxine	Ca^{++}	LFTs (for meds)
	Serum folate	

Side Effects of Common Drugs Used

1. *Isoniazid (INH)* can cause neuritis by depleting vitamin B_6. Its bad taste can be disguised in pureed fruit or jam to make it palatable, especially for pediatric patients. Niacin, calcium, B_{12} are also depleted. Nausea, vomiting, and dry mouth are common.
2. *Rifampin* has side effects, such as anorexia and GI distress.
3. *Aminosalicylic acid* interferes with vitamin B_{12} and folate absorption. Nausea and vomiting are common.
4. Chemotherapy can increase serum Ca^{++} levels.

Patient Education

1. Add nonfat dry milk to beverages, casseroles, soups, and desserts to increase protein and calcium intake, unless contraindicated.
2. Encourage the preparation of appetizing meals.
3. Plan rest periods before and after meals.
4. Discuss anxiety related to weight loss, night sweats, loss of strength, high fever, and abnormal chest x-rays.
5. Discuss communicability of TB. Family members should have x-rays and other testing.
6. Promote adequate rehabilitation if patient is an alcoholic.

SARCOIDOSIS

Usual Hospital Stay

6 days.

Notation

Sarcoidosis is a rare disease in which tiny patches of inflammation occur in almost any organ. Etiology is unknown. Pulmonary effects are most common. In most cases it is benign; in 10% the condition becomes chronic.

Symptoms and signs may include weight loss, fever, anorexia, weakness, aching joints, abdominal pain, lymphadenopathy, bone cysts in hands & feet; pulmonary hypertension, cor pulmonale, clubbing of fingers, dyspnea, cough, hypoxemia; iritis, glaucoma, blindness; chest pain, shortness of breath, or CHF.

Objectives

1. Reduce heart failure, bronchiectasis and related problems.
2. Correct weight loss, anorexia, fever, abdominal pain.
3. Improve ability to breathe and eat normally.
4. Prevent further deterioration of organ functions, with any and all affected organ systems.

Dietary Recommendations

1. Restrict salt; 2–3 g sodium diet may be beneficial.
2. Use a diet containing adequate to high potassium (unless medications are used).
3. As needed, decrease calcium and vitamin D if bone involvement is suggested; monitor use of supplements accordingly.

Profile

Ht/Wt/IBW/HBW	Chest x-ray	Kveim test
H & H (anemia	Transferrin	Serum Fe
common)	Globulin (inc.	Ca^{++} ($\uparrow$)
Alb (dec. common)	common)	K^+
Alk phos	Ca^{++} in urine ($\uparrow$)	PO_4
BP	Na^+	
N balance	Uric acid (inc.)	

Side Effects of Common Drugs Used

1. *Corticosteroids.* May need to watch Na^+/K^+ levels and N-balance.
2. *Isoniazid* (INH) may be ordered for pulmonary status. Watch use of vitamin B_6; increase intake accordingly of high vitamin B_6 foods to prevent neuritis.
3. *Calcium-chelating agents* may be used if hypercalcemia exists.

Patient Education

1. If the patient is using steroids, antacids could be taken as well to reduce GI side effects. Check with M.D.
2. Discuss the role of diet in maintaining immunocompetence and in improving tolerance for other therapies.

NOTES

THORACIC EMPYEMA

Usual Hospital Stay

6 days.

Notation

Thoracic empyema involves accumulation of pus in the pleural cavity, often as a complication of pneumonia.

Signs and symptoms may include dyspnea, orthopnea, constant localized chest pain, productive cough, malaise, fatigue, fever, tachycardia, tachypnea, weight loss and anorexia.

Objectives

1. Lessen fatigue; promote improved well-being.
2. Reduce fever. Prevent sepsis.
3. Correct weight loss.
4. Control and reduce anorexia.

Dietary Recommendations

1. Provide diet as ordered. Patient may need high calorie/high protein foods served at frequent intervals.
2. 2–3 L of fluid may be needed daily, unless contraindicated.
3. Meals should be served in an attractive manner to stimulate appetite.

Profile

Ht/Wt/IBW/HBW	I & O	Temp
BP	Alb	Pleural exam
Transferrin	H & H	Gluc
P_{O_2} (often decreased)	P_{CO_2}	

Side Effects of Common Drugs Used

Antibiotics are often provided. Monitor side effects accordingly.

155

Patient Education

1. Discuss the role of nutrition in illness and recovery, especially as it relates to immunocompetence.
2. With family, discuss signs to observe for future problems or relapses.

NOTES

Section 6
Cardiovascular Disorders

Chief Assessment Factors

ascites, edema

chest pain

blood pressure

obesity

cholesterol or lipid profiles

angiograms

ECGs

electrolyte balance

age, especially over 40

sex (males, or women after menopause)

smoking hx

diabetes

exercise patterns

family hx heart disease

Type A personality, stressful lifestyle

xanthomas

pancreatitis, other complications

medications

alcohol use

LDH, CPK levels

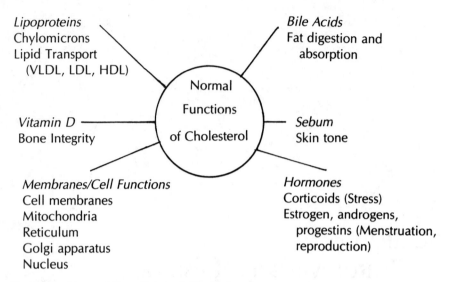

Fig. 6–1. Normal Functions of Cholesterol.

Cholesterol is readily made from acetate in all animal tissues. It has many roles in the body, but an excess can place added stress on the heart tissue. The major goal of dietary treatment of heart diseases is to maintain weight control at ideal body weight. Reduction of total fat intake, adding fiber, decreasing excess calories, and increasing exercise can all help to achieve this goal.

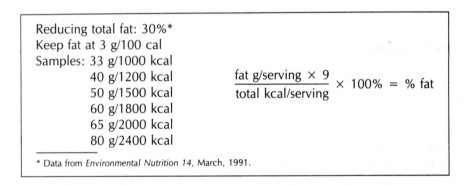

Reducing total fat: 30%*
Keep fat at 3 g/100 cal
Samples: 33 g/1000 kcal
40 g/1200 kcal
50 g/1500 kcal
60 g/1800 kcal
65 g/2000 kcal
80 g/2400 kcal

$$\frac{\text{fat g/serving} \times 9}{\text{total kcal/serving}} \times 100\% = \% \text{ fat}$$

* Data from *Environmental Nutrition 14*, March, 1991.

For More Information

Association of Heart Patients
P.O. Box 54305
Atlanta, GA 30308
(800) 241-6993

American Heart Association
205 East 42nd Street
New York, NY 10017

Heartlife (heart disease, pacemakers): (800) 241-6993

ANGINA PECTORIS

Usual Hospital Stay

4 days.

Notation

This condition involves chest pain or discomfort from decreased blood flow to the myocardium from decreased oxygen supply (often during exertion). The pain is frequently correlated with hypertension or with coronary artery disease, but may also occur as a result of anemia, hyperthyroidism, aortic stenosis, or vasospasm.

Besides chest pain, other signs and symptoms include shortness of breath, sweating, nausea and vertigo.

If newly diagnosed, the chance of living 10–12+ years is at least 50%.

Objectives

1. Increase activity only as tolerated or prescribed.
2. Maintain adequate rest periods.
3. Maintain weight or lose weight if obese.
4. Avoid constipation with straining.
5. Improve circulation to the heart.

Dietary Recommendations

1. Small, frequent feedings rather than 3 large meals are indicated.
2. Increase fiber as tolerated; include an adequate fluid intake.
3. Restrict saturated fats, cholesterol, and sodium as necessary.
4. Restrict caffeine intake to less than 5 cups of coffee or equivalent daily.
5. Promote calorie control if overweight; modify by age and sex.

Profile

Ht/Wt/IBW/HBW	H & H	Transferrin
ECG	BP	Na^+
Angiogram	Gluc	K^+
Chol	Serum Fe	I & O
Recent wt. changes	TIBC	Ca^{++}
(e.g. gain)	Trig	Mg^{++}
LDH	SGOT/SGPT	Alk phos

Side Effects of Common Drugs Used

1. Calcium channel blockers [*verapamil, nifedipine,* or *diltiazem (Cardizem)*]—nausea or edema or constipation may be side effects. Take on an empty stomach.
2. *Dipyridamole* (Persantine)—nausea or vomiting may occur. This drug contains tartrazine.
3. *Nifedipine* (Procardia)—nausea, weakness, dizziness, and flatulence may occur. Take after meals.
4. *Nitroglycerin* (Nitro-BID, Nitrostat)—take with water on an empty stomach; watch for headaches, nausea, vomiting, or dry mouth.
5. *Isosorbide* (Isordil) may cause nausea, vomiting, or dizziness. Take on an empty stomach.

Patient Education

1. The patient will require stress management, activity and proper eating habits education.
2. Discuss the role of nutrition in maintenance of wellness and in cardiovascular disease. Discuss in particular: fiber, total fat intake, potassium and sodium, calcium and other nutrients; caffeine.
3. Discuss the importance of weight control in reduction of cardiovascular risks.

NOTES

ARTERITIS

Usual Hospital Stay

4–5 days.

Notation

Temporal *arteritis,* also called cranial or giant-cell arteritis, yields chronically inflamed temporal arteries with a thickening of the lining and a reduction in blood flow. Women over 55 are twice as likely to have the condition as other persons.

Signs and symptoms include a dull, throbbing headache on one or both sides of the forehead. The artery may be red, swollen, and painful. Anorexia, weight loss, mild fever and muscular aches may also persist.

Objectives

1. Prevent stroke and blindness, which are potential complications.
2. Reduce inflammation.
3. Promote increased blood flow through the affected vessels.
4. Modify intake according to requirements and co-existing problems, such as hypertension.

Dietary Recommendations

1. Diet as usual, with increased calories if patient is underweight or decreased calories with obesity.
2. Reduce excess sodium and total fat intake; monitor regularly.
3. Patient may need to include carnitine in the diet.
4. With steroids, decreased sodium intake with higher potassium intake may be needed; adequate to high protein may also be necessary. Monitor for glucose intolerance.

Profile

Ht/Wt/IBW/HBW	K^+	H & H (often dec.)
Na^+	Alb	Serum B_{12}, folate,
Biopsy	Transferrin	ferritin
WBC (inc.)	Temp	Gluc
BP	Chol/trig	

Side Effects of Common Drugs Used

Steroids may be used, with numerous side effects, especially with long-term use. A gradual tapering is needed, and the patient must not discontinue the medication independently.

Patient Education

1. Discuss the role of nutrition in the maintenance of health for cardiovascular disease.
2. Discuss the effects of medications on nutritional status and appetite.

NOTES

ATHEROSCLEROSIS, HYPERCHOLESTEROLEMIA, CORONARY ARTERY DISEASE, AND ISCHEMIC HEART DISEASE

Usual Hospital Stay

5 days.

Notation

Coronary artery disease involves plaque build-up in the arteries of the heart.
Ischemia is a local and temporary deficiency of blood caused by obstruction (from lipids, etc.).

There are two types of *arteriosclerosis*: in arteriosclerosis proper, arteries thicken and lose elasticity because of mineral and fibrous deposits. *Atherosclerosis*—much more common and serious, and usually what is meant when hardening of the arteries is referred to—involves fatty-deposit accumulations with normal blood flow. Most often affected are the heart, brain, and leg arteries.

For each 1% reduction in serum cholesterol, there is a 2% reduction in CHD risk.

Objectives

1. Lower elevated serum lipids, especially cholesterol over 200 mg/dl, triglycerides over 250 mg/dl.
2. Initiate and maintain weight loss if patient is obese.
3. Observe prudent heart diet guidelines—less sucrose, more vitamin C, more fiber and chromium, less fat and cholesterol, less sodium, more copper and potassium.
4. Improve HDL cholesterol levels. Prevent formation of new lesions.

Dietary Recommendations

1. Restrict saturated fats to 10% of total fat and increase monounsaturated fatty acids and PUFA. Limit cholesterol to 250 mg or less per day. Total fat should be controlled at 30% total kcal. P:M:S ratio = 1:1:1.
2. Use a calorie-controlled diet with increased content of complex CHO rather than concentrated sweets and simple sugars.
3. In hypertensive patients, the restriction "No added salt" may be needed. For patients with ischemia, 2 g sodium may be needed.
4. The diet should include fewer animal proteins and more legumes and vegetables. Fish and shellfish should be used 3–4 × weekly, especially omega-3 sources.
5. Patient should take less than 5 cups of coffee a day to reduce stimulant intake.
6. Diet should include an adequate high soluble-fiber intake. Oat bran, apples and legumes should be used often.

7. Provide vitamin C and chromium in adequate amounts; copper and vitamin E also.
8. Garlic should be encouraged, with parsley as a breath freshener.

Profile

Ht	*Lipoprotein	K^+, Na^+
IBW/HBW	analysis-HDL,	Ca^{++}
Trig	LDL, VLDL	Mg^{++}
H & H	Chol (inc.)	Gluc
Wt	BP	

Side Effects of Common Drugs Used: "Diet First, Then Drugs"

1. *Cardiovascular preparations* such as digitalis, digoxin (Lanoxin), etc. require the patient to avoid excessive amounts of vitamin D or natural licorice. In addition, a low potassium intake should be avoided, as these drugs could become toxic. Avoid high-fiber meals; take drugs 30 min. before meals. Avoid herbal teas.
2. *Antihyperlipemics* such as Atromid-S may cause weight gain, nausea, and diarrhea. Colestipol (Colestid) requires supplements of fat-soluble vitamins to be added to the diet. Patients taking Cholestyramine (Questran) should have an increased fiber intake to alleviate constipation. Folate also needs to be added to the diet.
3. *Psyllium laxative* (Metamucil) lowers LDLs without affecting HDL levels.
4. *Lovastatin* (Mevacor) inhibits cholesterol production by the liver.
5. *Colestipol* and *niacin* can be effective.
6. *Lecithin* has a role in bile acid metabolism and has a small role in intestinal cholesterol absorption.

Patient Education

1. There is no cholesterol in foods of plant origin.
2. Explain which foods are sources of saturated fats and which foods are sources of polyunsaturated fats, as well as monounsaturated fats (olive and peanut oils).
3. Encourage the reading of labels: "free, low, reduced" cholesterol, etc.
4. Help the patient to creatively include iron-rich foods in the diet while lowering intake of animal proteins.
5. Discuss the roles of heredity, exercise, habits. BP, cholesterol, obesity and diabetes are affected by dietary patterns; some control is possible.
6. Note that some hearing losses and cataracts in the elderly are associated with ASHD.

---

* Goal: HDL 20–25% total
 LDL 60–70% total—over 5 mg/dl = high risk

7. Although the only sterol in shellfish (lobster, crab, shrimp) is cholesterol, intake of shellfish is no longer prohibited.
8. Omega-3 fatty acids are found in salmon, herring, and mackerel.
9. Water-soluble fibers are found in legumes (gum), fruits (pectin); and products like oat bran.
10. Relaxation, as well as exercise, should be part of the daily routine for all persons, under medical guidance.

For More Information

National Cholesterol Education Program Information Center
4733 Bethesda Ave., Suite 530
Bethesda, MD 20814-4820

NOTES

CARDIAC TAMPONADE

Usual Hospital Stay

4–6 days.

Notation

This disorder yields an accumulation of fluid or blood within the pericardial sac. Decreased heart sounds, distended neck veins with inspiratory rise in venous pressure (Kussmaul's sign), decreased blood pressure, and abdominal pain may occur.

If uncontrolled, this condition may lead to heart failure or arrest, or to shock.

Objectives

1. Care for ongoing disease process; prevent complications and acute states.
2. Prepare for possible surgery.
3. Improve any poor appetite that exists.
4. Normalize fluid balance.

Dietary Recommendations

1. For first day, patient is likely to be NPO with IVs.
2. The diet is progressed as tolerated to the usual diet (perhaps reducing or increasing sodium and potassium as appropriate for the condition).
3. Small, frequent feedings may be better tolerated.
4. If surgery is required, provide an adequate diet for wound healing and for prevention of infection.
5. Restrict fluids only if necessary.

Profile

Ht/wt/IBW/HBW	BP	K^+
H & H	TLC	P_{CO_2}
Alb	P_{O_2}	
I & O	Na^+	

Side Effects of Common Drugs Used

1. *Analgesics* may be utilized for pain relief.
2. *Antiarrhythmia* medications may be necessary; alter diet as needed. *Quinidine* (Quinaglute) should be taken with food or milk. Avoid citrus juice.

Patient Education

1. Discuss the role of nutrition in cardiovascular disease—explaining fluid and nutrient balance.
2. Provide food lists for foods to eat or avoid, as appropriate for the condition.

NOTES

CARDIAC TRANSPLANTATION

Usual Hospital Stay

Up to 20 days, medical. Surgical, 32 days.

Notation

Transplantation is usually done for terminal CHF, often after cardiomyopathies. Screening includes evaluations for chronic, co-existing illness, psychosocial stability, normal or reversible cardiac status. The best candidates are under 55 with normal hepatic and renal functioning, free of diabetes mellitus and pulmonary problems, peptic ulcers, and peripheral heart disorders.

Usually the transplant will be a Jarvik-7 or a live donor heart.

Objectives

1. Normalize heart functioning; prevent morbidity and death.
2. Prevent infection or sepsis.
3. Decrease potential of graft rejection/failure; increase survival rate.
4. Protect against further ASHD, which usually recurs within a few years of transplant.
5. Prevent complications, such as hypertension, hepatic or renal failure, and diabetes mellitus.
6. Control side effects of steroid and immunosuppressive therapy.
7. Promote adequate wound healing; prevent or correct wound dehiscence.
8. Maintain or improve nutritional status and fluid balance.

Dietary Recommendations

1. Control calories, protein, sodium, potassium, fat and cholesterol as appropriate for specific underlying condition (see appropriate sections). Keep in mind the role of nutrients needed for wound healing, including adequate calories.
2. Include appropriate levels of calcium, magnesium, and fiber.
3. Avoid alcohol, which can aggravate cardiomyopathies.
4. Increase use of garlic, fish and fish oils, and fiber (such as oat bran) when tolerance permits.
5. Reduce cardiac stimulants until fully recovered (e.g., caffeine).
6. After transplantation, increase diet as tolerated and as appropriate for status. Alter as needed.
7. For TF, use a low-sodium product and advance gradually.

Profile

Ht/wt/IBW/HBW	CBC	ECG
Na^+	BUN/Creat	BP
K^+	SGOT/SGPT	Chol/Trig
H & H	P_{CO_2}	Gluc
Transferrin	Alb	Other parameters prn
Edema	Ca^{++}, Mg^{++}	

Side Effects of Common Drugs Used

1. *Immunosuppressive drugs*, such as cyclosporine, have side effects affecting fluid balance and nitrogen balance.
2. *Steroids* may also be used. Monitor sodium-potassium balance and other nutrient status; prevent depletion of nitrogen.
3. *Analgesics* are also used to reduce pain. Long-term use may affect such nutrients as vitamin C and folacin; monitor carefully for each specific medication.
4. Antihypertensive, antilipemics, diuretics, and potassium supplements may be used. Monitor side effects accordingly.

Patient Education

1. Discuss the role of nutrition in wound healing, immunocompetence, and cardiovascular health.
2. Discuss how exercise affects the use of calories.
3. Discuss, as appropriate, fiber intake and sources of fat and cholesterol. Highlight the importance of maintaining an adequate diet to reduce risks of further heart disease and complications.

NOTES

CEREBROVASCULAR ACCIDENT (STROKE)

Usual Hospital Stay

4–5 days.

Notation

A cerebrovascular accident (stroke) is caused by damage to a portion of the brain resulting from loss of blood supply resulting from a blood vessel spasm, clot, or rupture. Unconsciousness, paralysis, and other problems may occur depending on the site and extent of the brain damage. Of all fatalities 10% involve CVAs. Right hemisphere CVA often affects speech; left CVA affects sight and hearing more commonly.

Objectives

1. *Immediate treatment* consists of maintaining fluid-electrolyte balance for life-saving measures.
2. *Ongoing treatment* consists of improving residual effects (such as dysphagia, hemiplegia, aphasia) and correcting side effects (constipation, UTIs, pneumonia, renal calculi, and decubitus ulcers).
3. If the patient is excessively heavy, weight reduction is necessary to lower elevated blood pressure and lipids and lessen workload of the cardiovascular system.
4. Chewing should be minimized and choking prevented—beware of stringy meats, unboned fish, crisply cooked vegetables, mashed potatoes (for some patients), soft bread, etc. Avoid use of straws.
5. Lower serum cholesterol if above 200 mg%.
6. Promote self-help, self-esteem, and independence.

Dietary Recommendations

1. Initial treatment—NPO, with IV fluids for 24–48 hours. Watch for overhydration. Tube feeding or TPN may be needed—especially gastrostomy or jejunostomy.
2. Treatment should progress from clear liquids to full liquids.* Following this, thick pureed liquids, and a mechanical soft diet may be used. If the patient is comatose, nasogastric feeding will be necessary. Elevate head of bed to prevent aspiration.
3. Limit intake of cholesterol, sodium, and saturated fats as needed. Use more olive oil and fish. Increase potassium, pending use of diuretics. Adequate potassium may reduce stroke mortality.
4. Provide adequate calories (patient's weight should be checked frequently). Watch the patient's activity levels. 45–45 kcal/kg; 1.2–1.5 g protein/kg may be needed.
5. Six to eight cups of fluids are needed daily. They should be given at the end of the meal to prevent interference with food intake.*
6. The diet should provide adequate fiber from prune juice, bran, etc.
7. Vitamin C intake should be adequate.
8. At first, use easy-to-chew foods and spoon rather than fork foods. Progress should be made slowly.
9. Adequate magnesium should be provided.

* *Textures* can cause problems. Liquids may not be swallowed normally, resulting in aspiration. Coughing is a danger sign. Liquids can be thickened with gels. Start always with small amounts of food.

Profile

Ht	Wt	CSF
IBW/HBW	Ca^{++}	CPK
Trig	Chol—HDL, LDL	Mg^{++}

Na$^+$	BP	Temp
Chewing ability	K$^+$	PT
Hand to mouth	Gag reflex absent?	I & O
coordination	Gluc (often inc.)	

Side Effects of Common Drugs

1. *Reserpine* causes cramping and diarrhea, which can be treated by using less fiber and fewer spices. Use fewer sodium-containing foods.
2. *Anticoagulants* like warfarin (Coumadin)—use a controlled amount of vitamin K; check TF products, supplements.
3. *Anticonvulsants, antifibrinolytics, antispasmodics* may be needed.
4. *Stool softeners* may be used. Prune juice can be added to a TF or oral regimen.

Patient Education

1. Help the patient simplify meal preparation. Arrange food and utensils within reach.
2. Explain which sources of adequate nutrition do not aggravate the patient's condition. Discuss fat, cholesterol, sodium, potassium, calcium, magnesium, and other nutrients.
3. Help the patient make mealtime safe and pleasant.
4. Encourage small bites of food, slow and adequate chewing.

Comments

1. Patients with a right hemisphere or bilateral or brain stem cerebrovascular accident have significant problems with feeding and swallowing of food. Neurogenic deficits may include *motor deficits* (muscle weakness of the tongue and lips, nerve damage with resulting lack of coordination, apraxia), *sensory deficits* (inability to feel food in the mouth), or *cognitive deficits* (difficulty sustaining attention, poor short-term memory, visual field problems, impulsiveness, aphasia, judgment problems such as not knowing how much food to take or what to do with the food once it reaches the mouth). (Seminar at Harmarville Rehabilitation Center, Pittsburgh, Pennsylvania, November 1983.)
2. For *dysphagia*, avoid foods which cause choking or which are hard to manage (e.g., tart juices and foods, dry or crisp foods, fibrous meats, bony fish, chewy meats, sticky peanut butter and bananas, thinly pureed foods that are easily aspirated, foods of varying consistency, excessively sweet drinks or fruits that aggravate drooling).

    Moisten foods with small amounts of liquid for people with decreased saliva production. Use thickeners to make semisolids out of coffee, soup, beverages, juices, shakes. Test swallowing periodically. When ready, use of a syringe or training cup is useful.

For More Information

American Rehabilitation Foundation
1800 Chicago Ave.
Minneapolis, MN 55404

Thick-It (Milani Foods: (800) 333-0003)

NOTES

CONGESTIVE HEART FAILURE

Usual Hospital Stay

4–7 days.

Notation

Congestive heart failure (CHF) results in reduced heart pumping efficiency in the lower two chambers, with less blood circulating to body tissues, congestion in lungs or body circulation, ankle swelling, and breathing difficulty. It can be caused by a coronary or other heart disease, lung disease, severe anemia, or low thyroid function. Right-sided CHF yields edema of extremities, fatigue. Left-sided CHF affects the lungs, with pulmonary edema and dyspnea. Although often seen in obese patients, it can also occur with *cardiac cachexia* (anorexia and fat and muscle wasting with edema). Decreased renal flow is common; BUN may be increased. Treatment may include hormone therapy, implantation of a pump, or cardiac transplantation.

Objectives

1. Promote rest to lessen demands on the heart. Restore hemodynamic stability.
2. Eliminate or reduce edema.
3. Avoid distention and elevation of diaphragm, which reduces vital capacity. Prevent excessive refeeding.
4. Attain IBW to decrease O_2 needs and tissue demands for nutrients. Replace LBM if needed.
5. Limit cardiac stimulants.

6. Prevent cardiac cachexia, low blood pressure, listlessness, weak pulse from K^+-depleting diuretics, anorexia, nausea and vomiting, and sepsis.
7. Correct any nutrient deficits.
8. Prevent decubitus ulcers.

Dietary Recommendations

1. Restrict sodium (500 mg at first; then progress to 1000 mg as edema subsides). Not all patients require the strict limitations; 4–6 g sodium may be satisfactory.
2. Diet should provide adequate potassium to replace potassium losses. Monitor potassium supplementation also.
3. Provide 5–6 small meals a day, with no more than 3 L fluid a day. Patients with refractory edema should receive only 0.5 ml/kcal.
4. If patient is obese, a calorie-controlled diet is necessary.
5. Restrict caffeine intake—at first no caffeine is allowed; later, coffee intake should be limited to 4–5 cups of coffee a day.
6. Use bland, low-roughage foods to lessen heartburn, distention, flatulence.
7. Use soft textures to reduce the amount of chewing. Add soluble fiber from apples or oat bran if tolerated.
8. If TPN is used, ensure adequate nutrient intake (including selenium, etc.). For TF, use a low-sodium product and increase volume gradually.
9. If fat intolerance occurs, try MCT.

Profile

Ht	Wt	Alk phos
IBW/HBW	Edema	ECG
BP	Chol	Alb, Prealbumin
Trig	GFR	BUN, Creat
Na^+, Cl^-	K^+	PT
Pco_2, Po_2	Gluc	LDH (inc.)
SGOT, SGPT	H & H	I & O
Temp	Mg^{++}, Ca^{++}	N balance
Specific Gravity (↑)	Serum zinc	Uric acid

Side Effects of Common Drugs Used

1. *Thiazide diuretics* (Esidrix, Oretic, HydroDiuril) deplete potassium, which must be replaced, either orally or by medication. *Furosemide* (Lasix) depletes K^+ and Mg^{++}. Glucose tolerance may decline; anorexia, nausea, or vomiting may occur. Use a low-sodium diet.
2. *Salt substitutes* generally contain KCl, and their use could lead to hyperkalemia if potassium-sparing diuretics such as spironolactone (Aldactone) or triamterene (Dyrenium) are part of treatment; ACE inhibitors also.

3. *Digitalis* can deplete potassium, especially when taken with furosemide. Beware of excesses of wheat bran, which can decrease serum drug levels. Anorexia or nausea may occur.
4. *Anticoagulants* are sometimes used with bedridden patients.
5. *ACE* inhibitors (captopril, enalapril, lisinopril) decrease production of angiotensin and aldosterone. Monitor for hyperkalemia.

Patient Education

1. A poor appetite may be caused by a congested feeling. Ensure that the patient takes smaller, more appetizing, and more frequent meals. Never force patient to eat. Allow rest before and after meals.
2. Check the water supply for use of softening agents. Also have the patients evaluate sodium-containing medications, toothpastes, mouthwashes.
3. Help patient plan fluid intake over waking hours, usually 75% from meals, 25% with medications and for thirst between meals.
4. Alcohol should be avoided.
5. Discuss spices and seasonings as salt alternates.

Comments

Sodium Content of Typical Items:

item	mg sodium per teaspoon
salt	1938
soda	821
baking powder	339
MSG	492

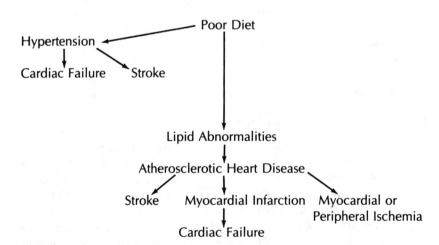

Fig. 6–2. Impact of Diet on Cardiac Failure.

CARDIAC CACHEXIA

Usual Hospital Stay

6 days.

Notation

Cardiac cachexia involves heart failure of such severity that patients cannot eat adequately to maintain weight. The condition usually follows CHF (moderate to severe), with some valvular heart disease. Nutritional insults generally affect the heart muscle severely, and the insult may be highly impacting.

Signs and symptoms include increased total body fluid (which occurs in an effort to improve heart function), supraclavicular and temporal muscle wasting, weight loss, anorexia, and malabsorption with steatorrhea or diarrhea.

Objectives

1. Improve hypoxic state and heart functioning.
2. Correct malnutrition, malabsorption and steatorrhea.
3. Optimize heart function through balance of medications, fluids, and electrolytes.
4. Meet hypermetabolic state with adequate calories.
5. Prevent infection or sepsis, especially if tracheostomy is required.
6. Provide gradual repletion to prevent overloading in a severely depleted patient.
7. Treat constipation or diarrhea as necessary.

Dietary Recommendations

1. Provide small, frequent meals to prevent overloading with high glucose or with rapid fat infusion.
2. Provide as many preferred foods as feasible to improve appetite and intake.
3. The prudent heart diet may be appropriate to reduce cardiac effects of diet.
4. Diet may need to be high in folate, magnesium, thiamine, zinc, and iron (depending on serum levels).

5. Calorie intake may be calculated at 1.5 × BEE, with a calorie:nitrogen ration of 150:1.
6. Sodium may need to be restricted to 1–2 g daily; modify potassium intake as appropriate for serum levels.
7. Protein should be calculated at a rate of 1.0–1.5 g/kg, increasing or decreasing, dependent on renal or hepatic status.
8. Offer tube feeding or parenteral nutrition if appropriate. Sometimes, tube feedings are not well tolerated because of access to the thoracic cavity, and because of reduced blood flow to the GI tract.

Profile

Ht/wt/IBW/HBW & dry wt	BP	Transferrin
Chol/trig	H & H	Fecal fat (in steatorrhea)
Edema	TLC	Ca^{++}, Mg^{++}
Na^+	K^+	BP
Gluc	Serum insulin	
	Alb, RBP	

Side Effects of Common Drugs Used

1. *Diuretics*—side effects may include potassium depletion; review types used and alter diet accordingly.
2. *Insulin* may be needed if patient has diabetes or becomes hyperglycemic.
3. *Digoxin*—monitor potassium intake or depletion carefully, especially when combining with diuretics. Avoid excessive intakes of fiber and wheat bran.

Patient Education

1. Balance medications, fluid, and electrolytes carefully.
2. Supplements may be beneficial between meals to improve total calorie intake, such as sherbet shakes.
3. Importance of diet in cardiovascular health should be addressed.

Comments/Notes

Products like Magnacal, Ensure Plus, Osmolite, Sustacal HC, Isocal HCN have a low volume with high density of calories. They are appropriate for persons with a fluid limitation, but need to be monitored with renal or hepatic difficulty.

NOTES

HEART VALVE DISEASES

Usual Hospital Stay

3–4 days, medical.

Notation

The heart has 4 valves (tricuspid, pulmonary, aortic and mitral). Inflammation of any or several of these valves can cause stenosis with thickening (which narrows the opening), or incompetence (with distortion and inability to close fully).

Mitral stenosis can cause lung congestion; breathlessness after exercise or while lying down; hemoptysis; bronchial infections; chest pains. In this problem, right heart failure can occur. 60% of persons with rheumatic heart disease later have heart valve problems; 75% of these persons have mitral stenosis. See Rheumatic Heart Disease (Section 15).

Aortic stenosis can give symptoms of angina, vertigo, fainting on exertion. Left heart failure is common here.

Tricuspid stenosis increases the risk of heart failure. *Pulmonary stenosis* is rare and occurs in only 2% of all valve disorders.

Objectives

1. Prevent heart failure (R- or L-sided); bacterial endocarditis; emboli or atrial fibrillation.
2. Prepare if necessary for valve replacement.

Dietary Recommendations

1. Avoid excesses of calories, sodium, and fluid (as appropriate for the patient).
2. If weight loss has taken place, add extra calories and snacks to return to a more desirable body weight.

Profile

Ht/wt/IBW/HBW	Wt changes	BUN, creat
Alb	BP	Na$^+$

| H & H | ECG | K$^+$ |
| Cardiac cath. | Chol, trig | Gluc |

Side Effects of Common Drugs Used

1. *Anticoagulants* are commonly used. Monitor vitamin K-rich foods carefully.
2. *Diuretics* may be used if fluid overload occurs. Monitor potassium and sodium intake carefully.

Patient Education

1. Careful use of all prescribed medications will be essential, with adequate return visits to the physician at appropriate intervals.
2. Alternative food preparation methods may be suggested to reduce sodium intake or to alter calorie levels.
3. Persons with a history of heart valve abnormalities may require antibiotic therapy to prevent infections, especially prior to surgery or dental work.

HYPERLIPIDEMIA/HYPERLIPOPROTEINEMIA

Usual Hospital Stay

4–5 days.

Notation

In *hyperlipoproteinemia* (HLP), increased levels of lipids are attached to serum proteins. Lipoproteins are combinations of proteins and triglycerides, phospholipids, and cholesterol. *Hyperlipidemia* refers to elevated serum triglycerides or cholesterol. Although used less often, Frederickson's categories (types I–V) are still utilized to identify some HLP diagnoses.

Objectives

1. All—normalize body weight. Keep cholesterol below 200 mg/dl, triglycerides below 250 mg/dl.
2. *Type I.* Minimize chylomicron formation. Lower triglycerides. Prevent abdominal pains resulting from fat ingestion. MCTs are tolerated.
3. *Type IIa.* Lower intake of saturated fats. Lower serum cholesterol.
4. *Type IIb or III.* Reduce weight. Lower serum cholesterol.
5. *Type IV.* Reduce weight. Restrict intake of carbohydrate and alcohol. Intake of cholesterol should be moderate.
6. *Type V.* Reduce weight. Modify intake of cholesterol. Keep fat intake low.

Dietary Recommendations

1. NIH Step-One diet:
   Total fat below 30% kcal.
   Saturated fat below 10%.
   PUFA up to 10%.
   MUFA 10–15%.
   Cholesterol below 300 mg.
   CHO 50–60%.
   Protein 10–20%.
2. NIH Step-Two Diet:
   Total fat below 30% kcal.
   Saturated fat below 7%.
   PUFA up to 10%.
   MUFA 10–15%.
   Cholesterol below 200 mg.
   CHO 50–60%.
   Protein 10–20%.
3. In general, use more soluble fiber (Apples, oat bran, legumes). Olive and peanut oils can be used (as MUFA).
4. Egg yolks should be limited to 3–4 per week; liver and organ meats once per month.
5. Shellfish and fish are recommended.

Profile

Ht	Pancreatitis (I)	Mg^{++}
IBW/HBW	Wt	Ca^{++}
Chol—ideal: 20–30% HDL, 60–70% LDL	Trig, fasting (I, V)	Lipid profile—HDL, LDL, VLDL, chylomicrons
BP	BUN, creat	
Uric acid (V)	GTT (II, IV, V)	K^+, Na^+
Xanthomas (V)	Carotenoids (may be inc.)	Alk phos

Side Effects of Common Drugs Used

1. *Antilipidemic Agents* such as *clofibrate* (Atromid-S) in the treatment of type IV hyperlipidemia can cause weight gain, diarrhea, nausea. *Probucol* (Lorelco) may cause nausea, vomiting, and anorexia.
2. *Colestipol* (Colestid). Add fat-soluble vitamins.
3. *Cholestyramine* (Questran). Use increased fiber to alleviate constipation. Provide folate supplement. Vitamins A, D, E and K may become deficient.
4. *Oral contraceptives* may increase lipid levels.
5. *Nicotinamide* can have undesirable flushing as a side effect. *Nicotinic acid* (Nicobid, Nico–400) reduces glucose tolerance and may cause nausea, vomiting, diarrhea, and ↑ LFTs.

6. *Lovastatin* lowers LDL cholesterol.
7. *Fish oil capsules* can cause hypervitaminosis A and D. Avoid use in children and pregnant or lactating women. Recommend fish instead.
8. *Thiazides, propranolol,* and *estrogens* raise plasma lipids.

Patient Education

1. Diets very low in fat may be dry and unpalatable. Teach new ideas for moistening foods without adding excess fat.
2. Monitor intake of fat-soluble vitamins and iron.
3. Describe food sources of saturated and PUFAs, cholesterol. Help the patient make suitable substitutions. Discuss fish, olive oil and peanut oils, and fiber (guar gum, pectin).
4. Encourage the reading of food labels.
5. Help the patient follow a calorie-controlled diet if that is necessary.
6. Discuss types of cholesterol (LDL, HDL, etc.). Chylomicrons contain the most triglycerides and are lightest, HDLs are the heaviest and contain the most protein.
7. Some cataracts may form in hypercholesterolemic patients over 40; corneal infiltration is a problem. Assure adequate intake of vitamin C.
8. Discuss coping skills, motivational factors, and environmental factors.

Comments

Table 6–1.
Lipid Alterations
Secondary Causes of Hyperlipidemia
    Weight gain in adults
    Pregnancy
    High CHO/high calorie diets
    High saturated fat diets
    Alcohol excess
    Steroids, estrogens, thiazides, oral contraceptives
    IDDM or NIDDM
    Hypothyroidism
    Nephrosis
    Chronic renal failure
    Obstructive jaundice
    Porphyria

Hypertriglyceridemia
    Very high VLDL levels—from obesity, DB, or renal disease
    Can lead to pancreatitis if over 500 mg/dl
    Can hide hypercholesterolemia or DM if over 250–500 mg/dl
    Use a high fish diet—salmon, mackerel, haddock, trout

Recommendations for Adults*

1. Total cholesterol below 200 mg/dl—general diet; retest in 5 years.
2. Total cholesterol 200–239 mg/dl, no CHD, fewer than 2 risk factors—Step 1 diet; repeat tests annually.
3. Total cholesterol over 240 mg/dl, LDL 130–159 mg/dl—Step 2 diet.
4. Total cholesterol over 240 mg/dl, LDL over 160 mg/dl—Step 2 diet and evaluation.

---

* National Cholesterol Education Program.

NOTES

HYPERTENSION

Usual Hospital Stay

4–5 days.

Notation

Hypertension results from a sustained increase in arterial diastolic or systolic pressure (160/95 mm or higher). It occurs in 15% to 50% of Americans. Blood pressure generally increases with age. OC users and alcoholics may have BP 15–20% above normal.

Symptoms include frequent headaches, impaired vision, shortness of breath, chest pain, dizziness, failing memory, and GI distress. If dyspnea occurs on exertion, left-sided heart failure must be prevented. If edema of extremities occurs, right-sided heart failure must be prevented. Untreated HPN can result in stroke, CHF, renal disease or MI. Untreated malignant HPN can be fatal within 6 months. *Essential* HPN has an unknown etiology and affects 95% of all persons with HPN.

Objectives

1. Control blood pressure to lessen the likelihood of congestive heart failure or stroke.
2. Induce negative sodium balance in the body only when this is absolutely required to lower blood pressure rapidly. The average diet contains 6–15 g of sodium.

3. Help the patient lose weight if obese. In men, there is a 6.6 mm rise in blood pressure for every 10% weight gain. Each lb requires 200 miles of new capillaries for nourishment!
4. Reduce excessive intake of caffeine and alcohol, which increase blood pressure.
5. Increase calcium, magnesium, and vitamins D and K appropriately. Allow at least 2 months to monitor outcomes.
6. Force fluids unless contraindicated.

Dietary Recommendations

1. To rapidly drop blood pressure, reduce intake of sodium to 200–250 mg. If diuretics are used, a diet of 2 g of sodium is sufficient. The most practical home diet provides 2–4 g of sodium daily. Be careful—sodium restriction decreases blood volume. Only 15% of all persons are sodium-sensitive; monitor carefully!
2. Use a calorie-controlled diet if weight loss is needed.
3. Use 50% of calories as carbohydrates, preferably complex carbohydrates like beans, oat bran, and apples (soluble fiber).
4. Use HBV proteins in the diet, but not to excess. Tyrosine may play a role in lowering blood pressure.*
5. Fat intake should be moderately low. Olive oil can be substituted for some saturated fats.
6. Diet should include adequate amounts of potassium, calcium, and magnesium. (Sodium:calcium ratio should be 1.4:4.1).
7. Limit caffeine-containing beverages to 2–3 cups per day.
8. Severely restrict alcoholic beverages.
9. Use sources of omega-3 fatty acids several times weekly (mackerel, haddock, salmon, etc.).

---

* Some studies indicate that tyrosine, the dietary precursor of norepinephrine, can be used to lower the blood pressure of some patients.

Profile

Ht	Wt	Alk phos
IBW/HBW	BP pattern	PT
Alb	BUN	Mg^{++}
I & O	K^+	Gluc
Na^+	Urine creatinine	Urinary Ca^{++}
Chol (HDL:LDL ratio)	Trig	Plasma renin
	PTH	PO_4
Ca^{++}	ECG	Uric acid
LDH	SGOT, SGPT	Cl^-

Table 6–2.

Samples of Salt Substitutes and Their Sodium and Potassium Content (per 1/2 tsp.)*

Brand Name	mg Na$^+$	mg K$^+$	mEq K$^+$
Morton's	—	1250	32
Adolph's	—	1205	31
McCormick's	—	1170	30
Diamond Crystal	—	1104	28
Co-Salt	—	987	25
Adolph's Seasoned	—	849	22
Morton's Lite Salt	488	650	16

* Questions readers ask. *Nutrition and the M.D.* 11:6, June 1985.

Side Effects of Common Drugs Used

1. *Diuretics*. Spironolactone (Aldactone) is potassium-sparing, whereas thiazides [e.g., furosemide (Lasix)] deplete K$^+$ and require supplementation. Diarrhea can occur. Avoid natural licorice.
2. *Antihypertensives*. Reserpine (Serpasil) requires reduced levels of Na$^+$; consequently, a sodium-restricted diet is useful. Take hydralazine with food; use a low-sodium/low-calorie diet.
3. *Captopril* (Capoten) can alter BUN/creatinine; take 1 hour before meals. Reduce calories and sodium.
4. *Propranolol* (Inderal), *rauwolfia* (Raudixin), and *metoprolol* (Lopressor) should be taken with a low calorie/low sodium diet.
5. *Estrogens* and *OCs* can increase BP.
6. *Amiloride* (Moduretic) is an antihypertensive with diuretic. A low calorie/low sodium diet is important.
7. *Clonidine* (Catapres) requires a low sodium/low calorie diet. Dry mouth, vomiting, nausea, and edema can occur.
8. *Prazosin* (Minipress) may cause nausea, weight gain, anorexia, diarrhea, or constipation.

Patient Education

1. Encourage patience. It takes 6–8 weeks to see the results of the diet.
2. Encourage the adequate intake of fruits and vegetables.
3. Remove the salt shaker from the table. Have the patient taste food before salting further.
4. Interesting food flavors are often hidden by salt. Discuss other seasonings and recipes.
5. Discuss caffeine sources (coffee, tea, colas, chocolate).

Comments

1. The normal adult needs only one tenth of a teaspoon of sodium (200 mg) per day. Only in hot, humid conditions or during lactation (or other

salt-losing states) are greater amounts of salt required. In such conditions 2000 mg of salt would be sufficient.
2. Salt substitutes and medications should be carefully monitored in regard to potassium content to prevent hypokalemia or hyperkalemia.
3. A University of Chicago study (5/91) suggests that celery can help reduce BP; studies are underway.

For More Information

National High Blood Pressure Education Program
120/80 National Institutes of Health
Bethesda, MD 20892

Alberto-Culver
Melrose, IL 60160
(708) 450-3000

(Papa Dash Lite Salt: 180 mg Na^+ per 1/2 tsp. and .03 mg K^+ per 1/2 tsp.)

NOTES

MYOCARDIAL INFARCTION, ACUTE

Usual Hospital Stay

9 days.

Notation

Myocardial infarction (MI) is necrosis in the heart muscle caused by inadequate blood supply or O_2 deficit.

A *coronary occlusion* is defined as the closing of a coronary artery feeding heart muscle by fatty deposits or blood clot. Commonly called a "heart attack," a coronary occlusion manifests with heavy squeezing pain, nausea and vomiting, weakness. Rest does not relieve symptoms. Stages last from 1st 48 hours (critical), to acute from 3–14 days, to convalescent up to 3 months.

An *arrhythmia* is a variation from normal heartbeat rhythm. Among its many forms is a slowing of the heart beat to under 60 beats per minute, a speedup to over 100 beats a minute and premature or "skipped" beats.

Objectives

1. Promote rest to reduce heart strain. Avoid the distention of heavy meals.
2. Prevent arrhythmias by serving food at body temperature.
3. Avoid both constipation and flatulence.
4. Avoid heart stimulation from caffeine.
5. Reduce elevated levels of lipids* and excessive weight.
6. Prevent death from arrhythmia or asystole.
7. Decrease energy required to chew, prepare meals, etc.
8. Initiate healing and promote convalescence.

Dietary Recommendations

1. Initially, use clear to full liquids to promote rest while reducing the dangers of aspiration or vomiting. Reduce caffeine intake to that recommended by the physician. Patient may also need fluid restriction.
2. As treatment progresses, the diet should include soft, easily digested foods that are low in saturated fats or cholesterol. The diet should exclude gas-forming foods. Limit the diet to 2 g of sodium, or take away salt from the food tray. Schedule three to six small meals daily. Avoid stimulants such as caffeine.
3. The diet of a patient whose condition has been stabilized, or who is at home, should be: carbohydrates, 50%; protein, 20%; fat, 30% (to be taken mostly in the form of PUFAs). Salt should be taken away from the table. If needed, use a low-calorie diet to reduce the heart's workload.
4. Increase fish, apple, oat bran, and olive oil use (see *Lancet*, Wood et al., *1*:122, 1/17/87).
5. Adequate calcium, magnesium, and potassium will be needed.

Profile

Ht	Na$^+$	CBC
IBW/HBW	PT	BP
SGOT	Wt	K$^+$
Cu (inc.)	ECG	BUN
LDH (inc.)	CPK	Mg^{++}
Trig (often inc.)	Chol—HDL,	I & O
Sedimentation rate	LDL	

Side Effects of Common Drugs Used

Appropriate drugs are provided according to needs established by the profile (elevated blood pressure, serum cholesterol, etc.). Review specific drugs given to the patients and treat accordingly.

---

* Keep cholesterol below 210–230 mg/dl, triglycerides below 250 mg/dl, HDL 20–30%/LDL 60–70%.

1. *Morphine*. Used for relief of pain, morphine should be used in minimal amounts to prevent hypotension.
2. *Anticoagulant and Thrombolytic Therapy*. Warfarin (Coumadin) or heparin may be given in some cases—e.g., when bleeding tendencies do not exist. Watch for the excessive intake of foods high in vitamin K (lettuce, fish, etc.) because they may alter PT values.

Patient Education

1. Position patient and arrange utensils to avoid or lessen fatigue.
2. If needed, use a weight-control diet.
3. Encourage relaxation, especially at mealtimes.
4. Discuss roles of fats, cholesterol, sodium, potassium, calcium, magnesium, and fiber in the diet.
5. Avoid simple sugars and alcohol, especially with diabetes or HLP.
6. Discuss convalescence—retarding progression of atherosclerosis, preventing CHF, working with cardiac rehabilitation.

Comment

Table 6–3.
Risk Factors for MI
1. Family history of heart disease
2. Patient history of heart disease
3. Diabetes
4. Hypertension
5. Advancing age
6. Stress, smoking, sedentary lifestyle, compulsive personality
7. Poor diet ($\uparrow$ kcal, $\uparrow$ Na$^+$, $\uparrow$ alcohol, $\uparrow$ fat, $\downarrow$ potassium, $\downarrow$ magnesium, and $\downarrow$ calcium).

NOTES

PERICARDITIS

Usual Hospital Stay

4–5 days.

Notation

Pericarditis is the inflammation of the pericardium due to viral infection, trauma, neoplasm, chronic renal failure, or systemic lupus. Substernal chest pain that is severe, dyspnea, shortness of breath, fever, chills, diaphoresis, nausea, fatigue and anxiety are common symptoms for the *acute stage*. The *chronic stage*, often resulting from TB, may involve ascites, CHF, edema of the extremities, and shrinkage of the pericardium.

Objectives

1. Maintain bed rest during acute stages.
2. Promote improved cardiac function.
3. Prevent sepsis.
4. Decrease fever and inflammation, which may last 10–14 days in acute form.
5. Reduce nausea and anorexic state.

Dietary Recommendations

1. Maintain an adequate diet as needed for any underlying conditions; increase protein and calories if tolerated and if needed to prevent loss of LBM.
2. Increase fluids unless contraindicated.
3. Small, frequent feedings to reduce nausea may be indicated.
4. Thiamine for the heart muscle, and potassium may be especially necessary. Monitor diet and supplements adequately.

Profile

Ht/Wt/IBW/HBW	Wt changes	K^+
H & H	Alb	Na^+
Transferrin	BP	WBCs
ECG	Temp	

Side Effects of Common Drugs Used

1. *Nonsteroidal* anti-inflammatory drugs are often used.
2. *Analgesics* of other composition may also be used.

Patient Education

1. Discuss the importance of avoiding fatigue.
2. The patient should plan rest periods before and after activities and meals.
3. The importance of nutrition in immunocompetence should be highlighted.

PERIPHERAL VASCULAR DISEASE

Usual Hospital Stay

5–6 days.

Notation

PVD is plaque build-up in the extremities, such as the hands and feet.

Complications of peripheral vascular disease can include gangrene with potential amputation. Numbness, tingling in lower extremities, pain, difficult ambulation, and gangrene can occur. Causes include heavy smoking, arterial embolism, poor circulation, or ASHD.

Objectives

1. Reduce symptoms and side effects: leg cramps on walking, ulcerative disease, gangrene of lower extremities or toes, slow-healing foot ulcers, cold extremities, paresthesias.
2. Attain desirable body weight.
3. Prevent blood poisoning.

Dietary Recommendations

1. If patient is obese, use a low-calorie diet. Use a low fat, high soluble fiber diet.
2. Diet should provide adequate intake for wound healing, where ulcers exist. Vitamin E is also suggested, as is nicotinic acid.
3. Diet should provide adequate protein, especially from fish.

Profile

Ht	Wt	Smoking hx
IBW/HBW	Trig	Gluc
CHOL—HDL, LDL	Na$^+$	Ulcerations, gangrene
K$^+$	BP	

Side Effects of Common Drugs Used

1. *Isoxsuprine* (*Vasodilan*) may be used to dilate the vessels.
2. *Antibiotics* may be used to control infections.

Patient Education

1. Emphasize the importance of weight control.
2. Reduce alcohol consumption, especially if triglycerides are elevated.
3. Fish and meatless meals should be used 3–4 × weekly.
4. Hyperbaric oxygen treatments may be needed to heal lesions. Oxygen permeates the flesh, and anaerobic bacteria cannot survive.
5. Encourage a stop-smoking program.

NOTES

THROMBOPHLEBITIS

Usual Hospital Stay

4–5 days.

Notation

Phlebitis is inflammation of a vein, usually caused by infection or injury. Blood flow may be disturbed, with blood clots (thrombi) adhering to the wall of the inflamed vein. This condition usually occurs in leg veins, especially in varicose veins.

Signs and symptoms include pain, redness, tenderness, itching, and hard and cord-like swelling along the affected vein.

Objectives

1. Reduce inflammation and swelling; reduce fever where present.
2. Prevent septicemia, deep vein thrombosis and related complications.

Dietary Recommendations

1. No special diet is warranted, but weight control diet may be needed if patient is obese.

2. Sodium restriction may be beneficial for persons with a generally high salt or sodium intake. Monitor carefully.

Profile

Ht/wt/IBW/HBW	Recent wt changes	BP
Temp	H & H	Na$^+$
Alb	Gluc	K$^+$
Chol/trig	TLC	I & O
WBCs		

Side Effects of Common Drugs Used

1. *Warfarin* (Coumadin) may be used, with side effects that alter vitamin K utilization. Monitor intake carefully.
2. *Antibiotics* are generally used in bacterial infections.
3. *Aspirin* or *acetaminophen* may be utilized to reduce fever or pain.

Patient Education

1. Bed rest may be important during acute stages. Leg and foot elevation may be required. Monitor side effects of immobility if patient will be immobilized for a long period of time.
2. Zinc ointment may relieve itching.

Section 7
Gastrointestinal Disorders

Chief Assessment Factors

painful oral tissues, tongue

dysphagia

anorexia, weight loss

indigestion, heartburn

nausea, vomiting, reflux

painful or cramping abdomen

easy fatigue

change in eating or bowel habits

change in stools

constipation or diarrhea

hemorrhoids

edema of extremities

feeding modality

antacids, stool softeners, diuretics, laxatives, cimetidine, other medications

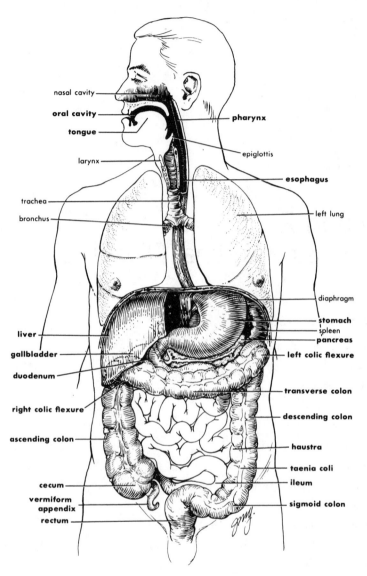

nasal cavity	
oral cavity	pharynx
tongue	
larynx	epiglottis
	esophagus
trachea	left lung
bronchus	
	diaphragm
	stomach
liver	spleen
	pancreas
gallbladder	left colic flexure
duodenum	
	transverse colon
right colic flexure	descending colon
ascending colon	
	haustra
	taenia coli
cecum	ileum
vermiform appendix	sigmoid colon
rectum	

Fig. 7–1. The Digestive System: Absorption Sites.

Stomach
water, ethanol

Duodenum
glucose, galactose, iron, magnesium, calcium, zinc, some vitamins, sodium

Jejunum
vitamins (fat- and water-soluble), sucrose, maltose, lactose, fatty acids, amino acids, chloride, peptides (mostly proximal—distal after resection or disease), cholesterol

Ileum
vitamins K and B_{12}, sodium potassium, chloride, water, bile salts
Intrinsic factor from stomach reacts with vitamin B_{12} in small intestine

Colon
Vitamin K, short-chain fatty acids, water, sodium, chloride, potassium, biotin, gases, nutrients from soluble fiber

190

Table 7–1.

Gastrointestinal Diseases Predisposing to Malnutrition*

Mechanical Function	Conditions Causing Fear of Eating
Esophageal stricture or obstruction	Ill-fitting dentures
Achalasia or esophageal hypomotility	Dental disease
Tracheoesophageal fistula	Esophageal spasm
Pyloric stenosis	Reflux esophagitis
Adynamic ileus	Gastritis
Bowel obstruction	Flatulence
Hirschsprung's disease	Peptic ulcer
Infantile achalasia	Postgastrectomy dumping syndrome
	Acute or chronic pancreatitis
	Cholelithiasis or other biliary disease
	Food allergy
	Lactose intolerance
	Irritable bowel syndrome
	Diverticuli coli
	Rectal fissures

---

* From Willard, M.: Nutritional Management for the Practicing Physician. Reading, MA, Addison-Wesley, 1982, p. 27. With permission.

Table 7–2.

Digestion and Absorption Issues

Digestion	Processes which physically and chemically break down food in preparation for absorption. Digestion begins with mastication and mixing of food with salivary fluid and enzymes (*oral phase*). In the *gastric phase*, pepsin, gastric acid, salivary amylase and lipase begin to work. Chyme is then delivered to the small intestine for mixing with pancreatic and biliary juices; *pancreatic phase* involves pancreatic amylase and lipase, proteases and phospholipase; *intestinal phase* involves disaccharidases (maltase, lactase, sucrase), peptidases, cholecystokinin for bile salts.
	Maldigestion involves the interference at any of these stages, including abnormal emptying of the stomach, steatorrhea, etc.
Absorption	Passage of molecular nutrients into the cells from bloodstream, mostly starting in the duodenum, with monosaccharides, amino acids and small peptides, monoglycerides and free fatty acids. Water is also absorbed to maintain isotonicity. Bile and fat are needed to absorb fat-soluble vitamins A, D,

E and K. Water-soluble C and B-complex are usually absorbed in the intestinal mucosa with some storage in the liver.

Malabsorption can involve any of the above process steps.

Entire process of digestion/absorption takes 24 hours.

Villi cells have a rapid turnover rate of 2–5 days.

To test absorptive capacity, Shils recommends testing with 25 g d-xylose (urinary xylose values of 1.2–1.6 g suggest that enteral feeding is possible).

EN is important to maintain GI integrity and host defense. For example, glutamine (an AA needed in stress/sepsis) requires GI processing to become effective.

Small intestine	about 3.8 cm in diameter and 4.8 m long, covered with villi projections to increase absorptive surface.
Large intestine	about 5 cm in diameter and 1.5 m long, with 2 sections (colon and rectum), forming a frame around a highly convoluted small intestine. Rectum is approximately 12 cm long. The area is susceptible to polyps and tumors.
Concerns	Problems are significant when over 70% of the bowel is resected, unless terminal ileum and ileocecal valve remain.

ESOPHAGEAL STRICTURE, ESOPHAGEAL SPASM, OR ACHALASIA

Usual Hospital Stay

3–4 days.

Notation

Achalasia is caused by failure of the cardiac sphincter to relax normally. Food fails to pass normally into the stomach. In addition, the esophagus does not demonstrate normal waves of contraction after swallowing. Signs and symptoms include dysphagia, substernal pain after meals, weight loss, regurgitation, and halitosis. *Stricture* is normally due to chemical ingestion, sliding hiatal hernia, neoplasm or reflux esophagitis. In *spasm*, segmented, concentric contractions occur simultaneously in the lower 2/3 of the esophagus.

Objectives

Esophageal Stricture. Avoid large boluses of food. Provide adequate nutrition. Prevent weight loss. Remove cause or dilate, if necessary.

Esophageal Spasm. Avoid either very cold or very hot foods or beverages. Monitor dysphagia.

Achalasia. Individualize diet according to patient tolerances and preferences. Monitor chronic dysphagia. Avoid aspiration.

Dietary Recommendations

Esophageal Stricture. Begin with liquid diet and progress to soft diet as tolerance increases. Adequate calories are needed. Gastrostomy may be needed. Antireflux regimen (no alcohol, wt loss) may be helpful.

Esophageal Spasm. Use diet as tolerated with modified temperatures for foods and beverages.

Achalasia. Provide large volume of fluids with each meal, unless dysphagia prevents appropriate swallowing of liquids.

Profile

Ht	Gastrin	Cl^-
IBW/HBW	BP	Na^+, K^+
I & O	H & H	UGI exam
Alb	Heartburn	Esophagoscopy
Wt	Specific symptoms	Cine esophagography

Side Effects of Common Drugs Used

1. *Antacids.* Check the label for aluminum, calcium, magnesium, or sodium if other medical problems exist. Beware of long-term side effects.
2. Specific medications for other conditions may affect nutritional intake significantly.
3. *Nitroglycerin* often helps spasm.

Patient Education

1. Emphasize the importance of spacing meals, achieving relaxation. Recommend intake of food at moderate temperature only.
2. Elevate head of bed for 30–45 minutes after meals, and at bedtime.
3. Encourage fluids at mealtimes.
4. Avoid foods that aggravate dysphagia (see CVA entry).
5. Bland foods are only needed if an individual prefers them.

NOTES

ESOPHAGEAL TRAUMA

Usual Hospital Stay

2 days (surgical).

Notation

Esophageal trauma is a major traumatic condition which affects the esophagus, often from chemical burns, foreign bodies, or injury.

Symptoms and signs include nausea, vomiting, loss of consciousness, dysphagia, respiratory distress, shock, and esophageal perforation.

Objectives

1. Emergency care is given as needed, such as adequate ventilation or shock therapy.
2. Allow esophagus to rest and heal.
3. Prepare for esophageal surgery, as necessary.
4. Keep adequately hydrated.
5. Improve swallowing capacity as rapidly as possible; prevent aspiration.
6. Prevent malnutrition, weight loss, sepsis, constipation, fluid loss from exudates, and other complications.

Dietary Recommendations

1. NPO as needed. Provide TPN, gastrostomy or jejunostomy feedings as appropriate for patient's condition.
2. Calculate needs at approximately 1.5 × BEE with 2 g protein/kg if tolerated. Watch hepatic and renal status.
3. Progress over time to a soft/bland diet. Avoid alcoholic beverages, extremely hot liquids and beverages, caffeine and spicy foods.
4. Force fluids unless overhydration is a problem, or unless dysphagia prevents use of thin liquids.
5. If patient has dysphagia, use thick purees until swallowing ability improves.

Profile

Ht/Wt/IBW/HBW	Wt changes	Temp
Barium swallow	I & O	Alb
Gluc	H & H	Transferrin
TLC	Dysphagia	

Side Effects of Common Drugs Used

1. Liquid topical *anesthetizing agents* (such as lidocaine) may be used before meals to reduce pain.
2. *Antibiotics* may be used in bacterial infections.

Patient Education

1. When patient can swallow, discuss the need to chew well and swallow carefully. The patient should also learn to eat slowly to prevent aspiration.
2. Discuss the appropriate food textures for different stages of progress.

NOTES

ESOPHAGEAL VARICES

Usual Hospital Stay

1 day.

Notation

Small esophageal veins become distended and may rupture due to increased pressure in the portal system. This condition is usually due to cirrhosis and portal hypertension.

Signs and symptoms include respiratory distress, aspiration of emesis, shock, hemorrhage, confusion, abdominal distention, melena, jaundice, hepatic coma. Death can also occur if condition worsens.

Objectives

1. Promote healing, recovery. Prevent worsening of symptoms.
2. Prevent constipation and straining with stool.
3. Prevent or correct hepatic encephalopathy or coma. See appropriate disorder sections, such as Cirrhosis and Hepatic Encephalopathy.

Dietary Recommendations

1. Generally, unless comatose, the patient can tolerate 5–6 small meals or soft, low-fiber foods.
2. Alter carbohydrate, protein and fat intake according to hepatic function and state of consciousness.
3. Provide adequate fluid as allowed or controlled.
4. To prevent constipation and straining, foods like prune juice or Enrich can help normalize bowel function.

Profile

Ht/wt/IBW/HBW	Wt changes	UGI bleeding
Esophagoscopy	Ascites	BP
Edema	Na^+, K^+, Cl^-	PT
H & H	Transferrin	TLC
BUN	Melena	Other parameters prn

Side Effects of Common Drugs Used

1. *Antacids* may be beneficial to buffer gastric acidity. Extended use can cause problems with pH, altered mineral and nutrient utilization and other imbalances.
2. *Antibiotics* may be used in infections.
3. *Vitamin K* may be needed to help with adequate clotting.
4. *Vasopressin* may be used.

Patient Education

1. The role of alcohol in the disease process should be discussed with the patient and family.
2. The importance of good nutrition in adequate consistency should be addressed.

HEARTBURN, HIATAL HERNIA, OR ESOPHAGITIS

Usual Hospital Stay

3–4 days.

Notation

Hiatal hernia is caused by protrusion of part of the stomach above the diaphragm muscle, which separates the chest from the abdomen. This results in the enlargement of a diaphragm opening (hiatus) through which the esophagus passes to joint the stomach. Hiatal hernia may show no symptoms or may cause heartburn, swallowing difficulty, reflux, or vomiting of blood.

Esophagitis results from gastric juice being forced into the esophagus from the stomach.

Objectives

1. Normalize reflux into esophagus, when that problem exists.
2. Achieve and maintain IBW to improve mechanical and postural states.
3. Neutralize gastric acidity, where this is possible.
4. Avoid large meals, which increase gastric pressure or LES pressure, both of which allow reflux. The LES normally limits aspiration of gastric contents.

5. Provide an individual diet reflecting patient needs. Assess intake of fat, alcohol, spices, caffeine, etc.

Dietary Recommendations

1. During acute episodes provide small, frequent feedings of soft or bland foods.
2. Avoid intake of food within 2 hours before bedtime. If needed, elevate head of the bed.
3. The diet should be high in protein to stimulate gastrin secretion and to increase lower esophageal sphincter pressure.
4. The diet should be low in fat: less fried food, cream sauces, gravies, fatty meats, pastries, nuts, potato chips, butter and margarine, etc.
5. Avoid foods that decrease lower esophageal sphincter pressure, including chocolate, regular and decaffeinated coffee, peppermint, onions, garlic, spearmint, after-dinner liqueurs, and alcohol. Have the patients limit or stop smoking.
6. Avoid irritating foods that produce spasm: citrus juices, tomatoes, and tomato sauce.
7. Other spicy foods are to be eliminated according to individual experience.
8. If needed, a low calorie diet should be used to promote weight loss.
9. Fluids can be taken between meals if consumption with meals causes distention.

Profile

Ht	Wt	Transferrin, TIBC
IBW/HBW	Gastrin	UGI exam
H & H	Alb	Esophagoscopy
Gluc	Chol	Manometry
Trig		

Side Effects of Common Drugs Used

1. *Antacids.* Used to decrease esophageal sphincter pressure and to neutralize gastric contents, antacids destroy thiamine and may provide excess sodium for the body. *Check labels carefully.* If the antacid contains calcium (e.g., Tums, which contains calcium carbonate), excess calcium may cause decreased levels of magnesium and phosphorus. Aluminum hydroxide (Maalox) depletes phosphorus, which is acceptable for patients with certain types of renal diseases, but which otherwise must be observed. When used as an antacid, sodium bicarbonate can decrease iron absorption and cause sodium retention. Caution!
2. *Cholinergic blocking agents (cimetidine).* Used to reduce amount of

197

gastric secretions, cholinergics can cause malabsorption if used for long periods.
3. *Reglan* may be used.

Patient Education

1. Encourage the patients to avoid late evening snacks.
2. Teach the proper measures for controlling weight, including small, frequent feedings.
3. Tell the patient to maintain an upright position for 2 hours after eating.
4. Patients with heartburn should probably not sleep in a waterbed.

NOTES

DYSPEPSIA/INDIGESTION

Usual Hospital Stay

Varies according to underlying disorder.

Notation

Indigestion may be secondary to other systemic disorders such as atherosclerotic heart disease, hypertension, or renal disease. Dyspepsia is not necessarily synonymous with gastritis.

Objectives

1. Determine whether the problem is psychogenic or organic in etiology.
2. Do not oversimplify the patient's discomfort.

Dietary Recommendations

1. The diet should make use of well-cooked foods, adequate in amount but not overly seasoned.
2. A relaxed atmosphere is helpful.
3. Small meals are best tolerated.
4. If the dyspepsia is organic in etiology, a soft, low fat diet may be helpful. A bland diet is often useful.

5. If the dyspepsia is psychogenic in etiology, removing the cause often results in the disappearance of the dyspepsia.

Profile

Ht	Nausea	Alb
IBW/HBW	Heartburn	Gluc
Anorexia	I & O	BUN/creat
Wt	H & H	

Side Effects of Common Drugs Used

Antacids. Beware of nutritional side effects resulting from dependency. See Heartburn entry for more information.

Patient Education

1. Encourage the patient to eat in a relaxed atmosphere.
2. Alter intake of seasonings, as appropriate.

NOTES

GASTRIC RETENTION

Usual Hospital Stay

3–4 days.

Notation

Gastric retention is caused by partial obstruction at the outlet of the stomach or the small bowel.

Objectives

1. Use liquids or foods that liquefy at room temperature, so that they are able to pass by a partial obstruction before or during absorption.
2. Bypass or correct obstruction, or other causes of retention.

Dietary Recommendations

1. The diet should use full liquids. Feedings should be small and frequent.
2. For patients with a lesser obstruction, use a mechanical soft diet. For patients with greater obstruction, use a low residue diet or tube feed. Check residuals frequently.

Profile

Ht	Wt	Gastrin
IBW/HBW	Alb	Cl^-
H & H	Gluc	Na^+, K^+
BUN	Creat	I & O

Patient Education

Help the patient determine a specific dietary regimen.

NOTES

GASTRITIS OR GASTROENTERITIS

Usual Hospital Stay

3–4 days.

Notation

Gastritis involves the stomach and intestinal lining. *Gastroenteritis* is an inflammation of the stomach. It can be caused by alcohol, food allergy, food poisoning, intestinal virus, cathartics, and other drugs. It produces malaise, nausea, vomiting, intestinal rumbles, diarrhea, and sometimes fever and prostration.

Objectives

1. Allow the stomach and GI tract to rest, but relieve thirst.
2. Empty the stomach to permit the mucous lining to heal.
3. Omit lactose if not tolerated in GE.
4. If hemorrhage occurs, it is a medical emergency.
5. Monitor for maldigestion with idiopathic gastritis.

Dietary Recommendations

1. *Acute gastroenteritis.* Patient will be NPO or on PPN/TPN for the first 24–48 hours to rest stomach. Use crushed ice to relieve thirst. Progress to a soft diet, or bland diet if desired. Alcohol is prohibited. Omit lactose if needed.
2. *Chronic gastroenteritis.* Use small, frequent feedings of bland foods. Progress with larger amounts and greater variety of foods as tolerated. Restrict fat intake, which depresses food motility, and alcohol intake. Monitor lactose intolerance.
3. *Gastritis.* Omit foods poorly tolerated. Provide adequate hydration. If chronic, mucosal atrophy can lead to nutritional deficits (pernicious anemia, achlorhydria, and functional pancreatitis). Alter diet accordingly.

Profile

Ht	Wt	Gluc
IBW/HBW	H & H	Alb
K^+	Na^+	Ca^{++}, Mg^{++}
Cl^-	I & O	Hydrogen breath test
Gastric biopsy	Serum B_{12}	

Side Effects of Common Drugs Used

1. *Antacids.* Watch for constipation caused by aluminum and calcium agents. Watch for diarrhea caused by magnesium agents. See Heartburn entry for other tips.
2. *Antibiotics* in excess over a long time may cause or can aggravate GE. Monitor carefully.

Patient Education

1. Omit offenders in chronic conditions: alcohol, caffeine, aspirin.
2. Assess vitamin B_{12} status of patients with chronic gastritis; atrophy of the stomach and intestinal lining interferes with vitamin B_{12} absorption.
3. Discuss calcium and riboflavin sources if dairy products must be omitted.

Comment

Types of gastritis include *idiopathic* (acute or chronic), *specific* (acute or chronic, as in granulomatous or postirradiation), *allergic*, or *embolic* (Palmer: *Hospital Medicine* 2/89).

HYPERTROPHIC GASTRITIS (MENETRIER'S DISEASE)

Usual Hospital Stay

3–4 days.

Notation

Menetrier's disease is a pathological condition with massive enlargement of the gastric mucosa with hyperplastic cells. An increased loss of plasma proteins occurs, resulting in hydrolysis by the proteolytic enzymes of the gut. The hydrolyzed proteins are then reabsorbed as amino acids. Edema may occur if the liver cannot produce enough albumin rapidly enough.

Objectives

1. Replace protein; maintain adequate nitrogen balance.
2. Reduce edema.
3. Spare protein for tissue synthesis and repair.
4. Promote normal dietary intake with a return to wellness.

Dietary Recommendations

1. Use a high protein/high calorie diet. The protein level should be approximately 20% total kcal unless contraindicated for other renal or hepatic problems.
2. Sodium should be maintained at 4–6 g to help normalize edematous tissues.
3. Omit any food intolerances.

Profile

Ht, Wt	Na^+	H & H
IBW/HBW	K^+	BUN
Alb	N balance	Creat
Globulin	Transferrin	Gastroscopy
A:G ratio	Pepsin levels	Gastric biopsy

Patient Education

1. Elimination of aggravating foods specific to the patient is warranted.
2. Teach the patient about HBV proteins to replenish serum protein levels.

NOTES

PERNICIOUS VOMITING

Usual Hospital Stay

3–4 days.

Notation

Uncontrolled vomiting may occur in any of several disorders, including pregnancy. Nutritional deficits are possible.

Objectives

1. Eliminate oral intake until vomiting ends.
2. Prevent weight loss.

Dietary Recommendations

1. For patients with acute condition, NPO for 24–48 hours with IV glucose is common.
2. As patient progresses, toast, crackers, jelly, simple carbohydrates may be given. Avoid fluids at mealtime; give them between meals. Gradually have the patient resume a normal diet, but decrease fats if they are not tolerated.

Profile

Ht	Alb	N balance
Wt changes	Wt	IBW/HBW
Na^+	K^+	Gluc
Cl^-	BUN	H & H

Patient Education

1. Explain why fluids should be taken between meals.
2. Discuss the role of carbohydrates in maintaining blood glucose levels.

Comments

For *Hyperemesis gravidarum*, see entry for Pregnancy (Section 1).

NOTES

PEPTIC ULCER

Usual Hospital Stay

6 days, with complications.

Notation

An ulcer is an area of GI tract that is eroded by gastric acid and pepsin, leaving exposed nerves. Of ulcers, 15% are gastric (often later correlated to stomach cancer) and 85% are duodenal, usually in the first 25–30 cm.

There is no evidence that bland ulcer diets affect the healing of an ulcer or the decrease in gastric acid secretion. There may be short-term benefits psychologically, but there are no long-term advantages. Some research suggests that *Heliobacter pyloridis* may play a role in etiology.

Objectives

1. Rest during healing stages. Reduce pain.
2. Avoid distention of large meals.
3. Dilute stomach contents and provide buffering action.
4. Assess and modify detrimental habits (e.g., rushed meals; excessive use of alcohol and caffeine; and cigarette smoking, which decreases the normal pancreatic bicarbonate buffer system).
5. Correct anemia, if present.
6. Monitor steatorrhea, bone disease, dumping syndrome, other problems.
7. Prevent other complications, such as perforation and obstruction.

Dietary Recommendations

1. Use small feedings, frequently if preferred. Include some protein and vitamin C to speed healing.
2. Avoid personal intolerances.
3. Omit gastric stimulants: caffeine, alcohol, black pepper, garlic, cloves, and chili powder. These prohibitions alone constitute the "liberal bland diet."
4. Use fewer saturated fats, more polyunsaturated fats if increased lipid levels are found. Arachidonic acid metabolites play a role in PUD.
5. If needed, a "restricted bland diet" can be used. Such a diet includes soft, smooth, nonirritating foods, but may be low in iron and vitamin C.
6. Avoid frequent feedings of milk—protein first buffers, then stimulates acidity.
7. Acidic juices (orange, grapefruit, and tomato) may not be tolerated. Assess individually.
8. Increases in fiber (e.g., wheat bran) help reduce recurrent duodenal ulcer symptoms (*JADA*, 1987).

Profile

Ht	Amylase (if perforated,	Ca^{++}
IBW/HBW	inc.)	Serum B_{12}
RBCs	H & H	Alk phos (↑)
Chol	Fe	TIBC
BUN	Trig	Na^+, K^+
Alb	PT	Cl^-
SGPT	SGOT	Serum gastrin (↑)
Wt	Transferrin	GGT
Blood guaiac	Blood loss	Creatinine

Side Effects of Common Drugs Used

1. *Antacids.* Aluminum hydroxide (Mylanta) may cause nausea, vomiting, and lowered vitamin A, calcium and phosphate absorption. Milk of magnesia (magnesium hydroxide) is a laxative-antacid, and can deplete phosphorus and calcium over time. Magaldrate (Riopan) decreases serum vitamin A, but can be used on a low Na^+ diet.
2. *Cimetidine (Tagamet).* Take cimetidine with food. This drug can elevate SGOT/SGPT and may cause confusion in the elderly. It can also cause diarrhea or constipation, urticaria, and increased creatinine.
3. *Analgesics* and *Corticosteroids.* When taken over a long time, analgesics and corticosteroids may cause gastrointestinal bleeding and ulceration. They should always be taken with food.

4. *Ranitidine* (Zantac) can cause nausea, constipation, vitamin B_{12} malabsorption.
5. *Vitamin B_{12}* may be needed as an injection, in some cases.
6. *Antibiotics* may be used if *Heliobacter pyloridis* is found.
7. *Sodium bicarbonate*, used as an antacid, can precipitate milk-alkali syndrome if taken with calcium-containing drugs and food.
8. *Aluminum hydroxide* (Amphojel) should be taken between meals, followed by water. It binds with phosphate and may lead to constipation and anorexia. *Gaviscon* contains magnesium as well as aluminum and may decrease absorption of thiamine, phosphate, and vitamin A. *Gelusil* contains magnesium, aluminum, and simethicone; it may have side effects similar to those of Gaviscon.
9. *Omeprazole* may heal ulcers by inhibiting acid secretion completely.

Patient Education

1. Discuss the relationship between personality and disease, how tension, perfectionism, and a high-strung personality may increase the pain of ulcer.
2. Discuss the risks of coronary heart disease (elevated lipids, low PT).
3. Discuss the role of any fluid in increasing gastric acidity and the flow of pepsin, as well as the importance of not skipping meals.

Comment

Table 7–3.

Typical Caffeine Content of 6 oz. Servings

Coffee, instant—60 mg	Coffee, brewed—85 mg
Tea, black—50 mg	Tea, instant—30 mg
Pepsi, Coke—18 mg	Ovaltine—0 mg

For More Information

Center for Ulcer Research and Education Foundation
11661 San Vincente Blvd., Suite 304
Los Angeles, CA 90049
(213) 825-5091

NOTES

GASTRECTOMY AND/OR VAGOTOMY

Usual Hospital Stay

8–9 days.

Notation

Gastrectomy and vagotomy are surgical procedures used when medical management for peptic ulcer no longer works. Sometimes these procedures are used for gastric carcinoma.

Billroth I. Anastomosis between stomach and duodenum after removal of distal portion of the stomach.

Billroth II. Anastomosis between stomach and jejunum after removal of two-thirds and three-fourths of the stomach. Iron loss can occur.

Vagotomy. Cutting of the vagus nerve to reduce pain. Much less nutritional intervention is required.

Objectives

Preoperative

1. Empty stomach and upper intestines.
2. Ensure high calorie intake for glycogen stores and weight gain.
3. Maintain normal fluid and electrolyte balance.
4. Ensure adequate nutrient storage to promote postoperative wound healing.

Postoperative

1. Prevent distention and pain. Reduce the likelihood of the *dumping syndrome:* nausea, vomiting, abdominal distention, diarrhea, malaise, profuse sweating, hypoglycemia, hypotension, increased bowel sounds, and vertigo.
2. Compensate for loss of storage/holding space and lessen dumping of large amounts of chyme into the duodenum/jejunum at one time.
3. Overcome negative nitrogen balance from surgery. Restore nutritional status.
4. Overcome effects of decreased hormonal output (secretin, pancreozymin, cholecystokinin) from changes in chyme and timing.
5. Prevent or correct iron malabsorption (Billroth II): weight loss; steatorrhea; calcium malabsorption; and vitamin B_{12} or folacin anemias.

Dietary Recommendations

Preoperative

1. Use a "restricted bland diet" that is high in calories with adequate protein, and vitamins C and K.
2. Progress to full liquids, then NPO after midnight.

Postoperative

1. Intake of complex carbohydrates such as bread, rice, and vegetables should be liberal (50–60%). To lessen hyperosmolar load, use only 0–15% simple sugars (sucrose, fructose, glucose). A total calorie increase will be needed for repletion.
2. Lactose intolerance is common in patients with these conditions; use less milk or omit if needed. Monitor calcium intake carefully.
3. Moderate fat intake (30% of total kcal). Use less cholesterol. MCTs may be beneficial.
4. The diet should provide less than 3 g sodium daily; salt draws fluid into the duodenum.
5. Fluids should be taken between meals rather than with meals.
6. Avoid extremes in the food temperature.
7. The diet should provide frequent, small meals.
8. The diet should provide adequate fiber, chromium, vitamin B_{12}, riboflavin, iron and folacin.
9. In a child's diet, intake of calories is age-dependent (1000 kcal at 12 months, plus 100 kcal per additional year).

Profile

Ht	Wt	Transferrin
IBW/HBW	GTT	Serum B_{12}
Gluc	Hgb A_1C	Ca^{++}
Urine acetone	BUN	Serum folate
H & H	Alb	TIBC
Chol	Trig	Prealbumin
PT	BP	RBP
K^+, Na^+, Cl^-	Amylase	Blood guaiac

Side Effects of Common Drugs Used

1. *Cholinergic blocking agents* may cause dry mouth. Rinse mouth with water before meals.
2. Drugs that slow GI activity should be taken before meals.
3. *Antibiotics* may be used to control bacterial overgrowth.

Patient Education

1. Stress the importance of self-care and optimal functioning—what to do for illness, stress, eating away from home, and how to read labels.
2. Discuss the use of artificial sweeteners.
3. Instruct the patient to eat slowly and to lie down after meals to relax.
4. Discuss the social significance of food and alcohol with the patient.
5. Help the patient to overcome reluctance and the fear of pain with eating.
6. Discuss dumping syndrome and its effects on nutrient absorption if untreated.

DIARRHEA OR ACUTE ENTERITIS

Usual Hospital Stay

3–4 days.

Notation

Diarrhea is a symptom of many disorders in which there is increased peristalsis with decreased transit time through the GI tract. Reduced reabsorption of water and watery stools result. The diarrhea may be *functional* (from irritation or stress), *organic* (from intestinal lesion), *osmotic* (from gluten or fat or lactose intolerances), or *secretory* (from bacteria, viruses, bile acids, laxatives, or hormones). Secretory is more serious.

Objectives

1. Determine causation and treatment.
2. Prevent or alleviate dehydration, electrolyte imbalances, anemia, weight loss, and hypoglycemia.
3. Alter stool consistency and quantity. Up to 200 g stool/day is normal.
4. Restore normal bowel motility. Alimentary tract feeding maintains gut integrity, bowel rest (TPN) results in atrophy.
5. Avoid extremes in temperatures, which stimulate colonic activity.
6. Correct intolerances for CHO and protein. Ensure adequate fat intake.

Dietary Recommendations

1. NPO for 12 hours with IV fluids and electrolytes, start oral fluids as soon as allowed. Use TPN only for intractable diarrhea. Osmotic diarrhea abates with NPO.
2. As stools are formed, gradually reintroduce small amounts of food. Temporarily omit lactose, test tolerance. Some fiber or pectins may help. Potassium should be replenished.

    Adults. Start with broth, tea, and toast. Gradually add foods in a normal diet as tolerance progresses. 3–4 small meals may be better tolerated.

    Infants. Use 50% strength formula (low in fat and CHO). Or use Nutramigen. A mixture of 5–10% apple powder, banana flakes, or pectin-sugar can be added to the formula. Or use Pedialyte if allowed. Breast-feeding may continue, or return to lactose-containing formula when feasible.
3. If a tube feeding is being used, check tube placement. A jejunal placement may be too far for some patients.

Profile

Ht	IBW/HBW	K^+, Na^+
Cl^-	Temp	N balance
BP	Stool consistency	Transferrin
Stool culture	Biopsy	H & H
Wt	Alb	Lactose tolerance or
I & O	Cu	H-breath test
Wt changes		

Side Effects of Common Drugs Used

1. *Anti-diarrheal drugs* are used to slow peristalsis or thicken stools. Kaolin (Kaopectate) has no major side effects. Lomotil should be taken with food. Lomotil may cause bloating, constipation, drug mouth, swollen gums, dizziness, nausea, and vomiting.
2. *Antibiotics* are used if the problem is caused by shigellae or amoebae. Some antibiotics can stimulate diarrhea if used for a long period of time.
3. *Cholestyramine* may be used for bile acid diarrhea.
4. *Opiates* can decrease propulsive diarrhea action.
5. *Multivitamin/mineral supplements* may be needed to replace vitamins A and C, zinc, iron and other nutrients.

Patient Education

1. Describe the effects of pectin as a thickening agent (in apples and bananas).
2. Avoid carbonated beverages. Electrolyte content is low, osmolality is high.
3. Avoid alcoholic beverages when using Lomotil.
4. Caffeine can aggravate diarrhea; omit until the problem clears.
5. Once diarrhea improves, gradually return to milk if tolerated.
6. Omit apple juice until tolerance is established.

Comments

In severe PCM, diarrhea and other infections are common. Weight loss can be caused by diarrhea. Hypoglycemia is a potentially fatal complication of infectious diarrhea in children.

Table 7–4.

WHO Oral Rehydration Formula*

1/3–2/3 t. table salt
3/4 t. sodium bicarbonate
1/3 t. potassium chloride
3-1/3 T. sugar
1 liter boiled or sterile water

---

* World Health Organization.

DYSENTERY OR TRAVELER'S DIARRHEA

Usual Hospital Stay

3–4 days.

Notation

Dysentery, inflammation of the bowel, results from poor sanitation (causes range from contact with feces to contamination by house flies). *Traveler's diarrhea*, a GI bacterial infection, is caused by contaminated food or water, usually from *E. coli* or *Shigella*. Symptoms include diarrhea, often with blood and mucus, cramps, fever, and pus in stools.

Objectives

1. Reduce irritation and inflammation of the GI tract.
2. Gradually refeed to prevent dehydration and to restore bowel motility.

Dietary Recommendations

1. Clear liquids (broth, tea, thin gruel) should be taken during the acute condition.
2. Gradually add nonirritating, low fiber foods. Water-soluble fiber, from apples or oatmeal, may be helpful.
3. Products like Enrich have fiber added, for use in TF or supplements.

Profile

Ht	Wt	IBW/HBW
Wt loss	Cl	Alb
K^+, Na^+	I & O	H & H
No. of stools, consistency	Stool exam	Gluc

Side Effects of Common Drugs Used

1. Tetracycline, chloramphenicol or co-trimoxazole may be used.
2. Lomotil may be used.

1. Use only cooked foods and bottled water, juices, and beer.
2. Instruct the patient to brush teeth with bottled water only.
3. Instruct the patient concerning the possible danger of fresh foods, which may have been washed in contaminated water, and foods prepared with unheated water (e.g., jello), and ice cubes added to beverages.

FAT MALABSORPTION SYNDROME

Usual Hospital Stay

3–4 days.

Notation

Fat malabsorption is caused by functional or organic causes (e.g., celiac disease, cystic fibrosis, pancreatitis, or carbohydrate intolerances). Symptoms and signs include fatigue, weight changes, altered bowel movements, lab abnormalities.

Objectives

1. Alleviate steatorrhea and reduce intake of fat sources that are not tolerated.
2. Use medium-chain triglycerides in the diet when possible. The causes of malabsorption are various and include the following:
   GI tract. Postgastrectomy, blind loop syndrome, small bowel resection.
   Pancreas. Cystic fibrosis, chronic pancreatitis.
   Biliary. Biliary atresia.
   Other causes. Gluten enteropathy, beta-lipoprotein deficiency, diabetic steatorrhea.

Dietary Recommendations

1. *Initial treatment* should consist of parenteral solutions or liquid formula emulsions (carbohydrates, 45%; protein, 15%; medium-chain triglycerides, 40%) such as Portagen. Medium-chain triglycerides alleviate steatorrhea in some cases; start with 20 to 60 g and increase gradually.
2. For moderate to severe cases, tube feed if necessary (50 ml/hr full strength initially; advance gradually).
3. For mild cases, oral feeding is preferred since it stimulates brush border activity.
4. Dietary fat may be limited to one egg and 4 to 6 oz of meat, poultry, or fish. Gradually check tolerance for LCTs and work up to 30–40 g.
5. Increase intake of protein, which may be in the form of skim milk, egg white, cereals, or legumes.

6. Complex carbohydrates may be better tolerated than simple sugars. Lactose may not be tolerated.
7. A multivitamin supplement may be necessary to offset fecal losses of nutrients, vitamins, and water in patients with malabsorption syndromes—especially zinc, folate, vitamin B_{12}, calcium, magnesium, iron, and fat-soluble vitamins.
8. Monitor oxalate intake to prevent stones; decrease dietary sources as needed.

Profile

Ht	Wt	Serum carotene, vit. A
IBW/HBW	Alb, prealbumin	Labelled carbon
Fecal Ca^{++}	Chol	breath test
Trig	H & H, serum Fe	Sudan stain test
Fecal fat study results	Na^+	D-Xylose test
K^+	Mg^{++}	Serum Ca^{++}
PO_4	Tryptophan Load Test for B_6	Schilling Test for B_{12}

Side Effects of Common Drugs Used

1. *Medium-chain triglycerides* have an 8- to 10-carbon source of fat when longer-chain fats (16 to 18 carbons) cannot be efficiently digested or absorbed. Medium-chain triglycerides have concentrated calories made from coconut oil for adjunct therapy. Portal rather than lymphatic system transport (as albumin-free fatty acids) and absorption (using less lipase and bile) occur.

   Medium-chain triglyceride oil has 230 kcal per 30 ml (6 to 7 kcal/g). Use instead of vegetable oil in recipes.

   One cup of Portagen powder has 240 kcal (medium-chain triglycerides, 10 g; protein, vitamins, and minerals, 8.4 g). One tablespoon of the powder (14 g) has 116 kcal.

   Many other supplements now contain medium-chain triglycerides as the fat source. Osmolite and Isocal can be used for tube feedings.
2. *Antibiotics* are used for bacterial overgrowth.
3. *Pancreatic enzymes* may be needed for pancreatic insufficiencies.
4. *Cholestyramine* may be needed for bile-salt diarrhea. Fat-soluble vitamins can be depleted.
5. *Antidiarrheals* may be used, such as Kaolin (Kaopectate).

Patient Education

1. Caution patient about rapid consumption of medium chain triglycerides; if they are consumed too rapidly, hyperosmolar diarrhea may result.
2. Remember that a source of essential fatty acids may be needed if medium chain triglycerides are used with a low-fat diet.

3. Abdominal discomfort, flatulence, diarrhea or steatorrhea may indicate continued malabsorption; the physician should be contacted.

Comments

Table 7–5.

Altered Stool/Nutrients Involved

Characteristic	Disorder
Yellow or silver color	Fat malabsorption
Pale, foamy, mushy or floating	Panmalabsorption
Formed in AM, diarrhea in PM	Bile salt malabsorption

Table 7–6.

Fecal Fat Study*

100 g LCT × 3 days should be consumed.
Fat absorption is tested by quantitative measurement of total fat in the stool.
Normal excretion = 3.5 g (5% of a 609–100 g intake).
Mild malabsorption = under 25 g (defects in micelle formation)
Moderate malabsorption = 25–30 g (intestinal mucosal disease)
Severe malabsorption = over 40 g (massive ileal resection or pancreatic disease)

---

* Hermann-Zaidins, M.: *JADA* 86:1171, 1986.

NOTES

CELIAC DISEASE (GLUTEN-INDUCED ENTEROPATHY, IDIOPATHIC STEATORRHEA, NONTROPICAL SPRUE)

Usual Hospital Stay

5 days.

Notation

It is thought that celiac disease is caused either by an inborn error of metabolism or immunologic sensitivity to gliadin by the small intestines. Villi are decreased in number, with less absorptive surface and fewer enzymes in the damaged cells. Symptoms and signs include frequent, foul-smelling stools that are pale and foamy; irritability; a distended abdomen; easy fatigue, pallor; weight loss; vomiting; and anemia. Diagnosis can occur at any age (infancy through old age), often following stress, pregnancy, or viral infections. Pica and growth failure often precede it.

Objectives

1. Remove the offending protein (gliadin fraction) from the diet. Glutenin is harmless. Improvement is noted within 4–5 days.
2. Improve the patient's nutritional status.
3. Replace nutrients (magnesium, calcium, and vitamins A, D, E, and K) lost from diarrhea and steatorrhea.
4. Overcome anorexia with pleasant meals.
5. Reverse bone demineralization. Patient may need calcium supplements.

Dietary Recommendations

1. For infants with diarrhea, provide fluids, electrolytes, and a low fat formula.
2. The diet should provide 1 to 2 g protein/kg body weight (adult intake, 120 g) from lean meat, whole milk, etc.
3. The diet should provide 125 to 200 kcal/kg body weight. Infants may tolerate banana powder; adults may use simple carbohydrates, gelatin, fruit juice, peanut butter, simple cornstarch pudding, bananas.
4. Medium-chain triglycerides are often used with good results, especially in adults.
5. A *gliadin-free/gluten-restricted diet* excludes wheat, buckwheat, oats, rye, and barley. Corn, rice, tapioca, potato, arrowroot, cassava, and gluten-free bread can be used.
6. Initially the diet should include low amounts of fiber because of flattening of the mucosal villi. Intake can be increased as tolerated.
7. Watch lactose intolerances which are temporary or permanent.
8. Supplements to the diet should include water-miscible vitamins A, D, E, and K; iron; calcium; folic acid; and vitamin B_{12}, thiamine and other B-complex vitamins.

Profile

Ht	Wt	Transferrin, TIBC
IBW or growth pattern/	H & H	Cu (dec.)
HBW	Ca^{++}	Intestinal biopsy
Alb	Fecal fat study	LDH (inc.)
Serum carotene	PO_4 ($\downarrow$)	Xylose absorption

Side Effects of Common Drugs Used

1. *Gluten-free laxatives* include psyllium seed laxatives (Metamucil, Naturacil), docusate sodium (Surfak), and bisacodyl (Dulcolax).
2. Check all labels for gluten-containing ingredients.

Patient Education

1. Instruct the patient to read food labels for cereal, starch, flour, thickening agents, emulsifiers, gluten, stabilizers, hydrolyzed vegetable proteins, etc. Wheat starch is acceptable because the gluten has been removed. Caramel coloring and MSG may not be tolerated.
2. Check the ingredients of all recipes.
3. Strict lifelong adherence is essential with permanent damage.

Comments

If the defect is permanent, the diet will also be permanent. It may be helpful to add new foods to the diet; if this is done, the patient's responses should be closely watched.

Foods not well tolerated include cream soups, creamed vegetables, ice cream (labels should be checked for thickening agents), oatmeal (tolerated by some people—check with the physician before using), cakes, cookies, breads (unless made with rice, corn, or potato flours), wheat starch, mixed infant dinners and junior dinners that contain flour thickeners, spaghetti, macaroni, and other pastas.

For More Information

American Celiac Society (ACS)
45 Gifford Avenue
Jersey City, NJ 07304
(201) 432-1207

National Celiac-Sprue Society
5 Jeffrey Road
Wayland, MA 01778
(617) 358-5150 or 651-3230

Gluten Intolerance Group
PO Box 23053
Seattle, WA 98102-0353
(206) 854-8606

CSA-USA
2313 Rocklyn Drive, #1
Des Moines, IA 50322
(515) 270-9609

NOTES

TROPICAL SPRUE

Usual Hospital Stay

3–4 days.

Notation

Villi of the small intestinal mucosa become blunted or obliterated in tropical sprue. A reduced absorptive area and malabsorption occur.

Objectives

1. Improve nutrient absorption with gradual addition of foods.
2. Differentiate between tropical and nontropical sprue.

Dietary Recommendations

1. Use a regular diet with supplements of vitamin B_{12} and folic acid. The diet should provide sufficient amounts of calories, protein, iron, and vitamins.
2. In its early phase, the diet should include a high intake of protein and low intake of carbohydrates and fat until absorption improves. Acceptable carbohydrates would include simple sugars and nonstarchy vegetables; fats would include medium-chain triglycerides.
3. No gluten restriction applies.
4. Good sources of folacin include liver, kidney, yeast, leafy greens, lean beef, and eggs. Good sources of vitamin B_{12} include meat, poultry, fish, dairy products, and eggs.

Profile

Ht	Wt
IBW/HBW	Malabsorption
Gluc	Alb
H & H	Serum B_{12} and folate

Patient Education

Explain to the patient which foods are good sources of folic acid and vitamin B_{12}.

NOTES

LACTOSE MALABSORPTION (LACTASE DEFICIENCY)

Usual Hospital Stay

3–4 days.

Notation

Lactose is a disaccharide (glucose and galactose) found in milk. If lactase is missing, lactose is drawn into the intestinal lumen, causing bloating and cramping. Unabsorbed lactose passes into the colon, where bacteria flourish and draw more water, resulting in diarrhea. Types of lactose malabsorption are *congenital* (rare, present at birth), *primary* or *genetic* (low incidence in children), and *secondary* or *acquired* (from GI disease, food allergy, antibiotics, or intestinal trauma). Lactase "non-persistence" is common in people of African or Asian descent (70-95%), less common in Caucasians (6-10%) and in Hispanics.

Objectives

1. Omit or control lactose intake. Lactose comprises 10% of the carbohydrate found in the American diet.
2. Check for actual tolerance by monitoring intake. Most people can tolerate 1/2 cup milk (6 g lactose) with a meal, eventually if not immediately.
3. Offer calcium and riboflavin from other foods and sources.

Dietary Recommendations

1. Read the labels of foods. Watch for fillers in drugs; milk; whey solids; and milk solids. Casein ("curds") is acceptable.
2. Lactose-hydrolyzed milk may be tolerated.

3. Persons on a *lactose-free diet* can use lactate, lactalbumin, and calcium. *Lact-Aid* (produced by the Sugar-Lo Co., P.O. Box 1017, Atlantic City, NJ 08404) can be used in such a diet.
4. If tolerated, fermented products (buttermilk, natural or aged cheese, yogurt with active cultures, cottage cheese, or sour cream) can be used.
5. For infants with the condition, try Nutramigen, ProSoBee, Isomil, MBF; gradually introduce foods that contain milk or lactose.
6. Beware of processed cheese or cheese foods that have nonfat dry milk solids.
7. Carnation Instant Breakfast with Lact-Aid milk can be a potential supplement or tube feeding.

Profile

Ht	BUN	Lactose challenge test
IBW/HBW	Ca^{++} (better	K^+, Na^+
Alb	absorption can	Hydrogen breath test
Wt	occur over time)	
Mg^{++}	H & H	

Patient Education

1. Pregnant women should receive a calcium supplement.
2. Home-cooked meals and recipes may be useful. Heating milk does *not* change lactose.
3. Kosher foods are often acceptable, if they are pareve (non-milk, non-meat).
4. Indicate what foods are sources of lactose-free products.
5. Recipes are available for use of lactose-free formulas in products like meatloaf.
6. Discuss how to use Lact-Aid drops to allow the enzyme to hydrolyze the lactose.
7. Drink milk with meals rather than alone, to decrease symptoms.
8. *Acidophilus milk* provides no specific relief of symptoms.
9. Dairy foods contain about 1–8% lactose by weight (milk, 4–5%; yogurt, 4%; ice cream, 3–4%; milk chocolate, 8%; cottage cheese, 1–2%).

NOTES

CONSTIPATION

Usual Hospital Stay

3–4 days.

Notation

Constipation occurs when the fecal mass remains in the colon longer than the normal 24 to 72 hours after meal ingestion, or when the patient strains to defecate. For chronic problems, bowel retraining may be necessary.

Objectives

Atonic Constipation ("Lazy Bowel"). Stimulate peristalsis, provide bulk, retain water in the feces.

Spastic Constipation. For the increased narrowing of the colon with small, ribbon-like stools caused by obstruction, nervousness, or anxiety, undue distention and stimulation of the bowel should be prevented during exacerbations. Once well, fiber should be increased.

Dietary Recommendations

Atonic Constipation. The diet should be high in fiber, with liberal use of whole grains, fruits, and vegetables. Adding a carrot and some bran to the diet can be an easy solution. Use adequate fluid, 8–10 cups daily.

Spastic Constipation. The diet should be decreased in fiber during painful episodes. Then increase use of prune juice, dried fruits, bran, raw fruits and vegetables, nuts, and whole grains.

Profile

Ht	Wt	Blood guaiac
IBW/HBW	I & O	BP
Alb	H & H	Gluc
BUN	Recent wt changes	
Bowel habits	Stool color	

Side Effects of Common Drugs Used

1. Medicines containing iron, aluminum, or calcium often cause problems with constipation.
2. *Suppositories, enemas, and laxatives* are used to relieve constipation. Beware of using mineral oil as a laxative, because decreased absorption of calcium and fat-soluble vitamins will occur. Some products may contain excessive amounts of sodium—Sal Hepatica contains 1 g of sodium per dose! Long-term use can alter fluid and electrolyte balance.

Avoid using bisacodyl (Dulcolax) with dairy products; take with a high fiber diet.

3. *Psyllium*, a plant fiber sold as Metamucil, Syllact, etc., must be taken with plenty of water or juice (8 oz per teaspoonful). Results may require 1 to 4 teaspoons of the product. Taste, as well as the cost of the product, must be considered.

Patient Education

1. Explain that proper diet can produce relief, but cannot cure the condition.
2. Explain that a normal bowel routine is needed, but that daily fecal evacuation is not needed for everyone.
3. Identify specifically foods that have a laxative effect for the patient. Explain that fiber may be increased on a gradual basis only, and that prune juice may help. For every gram of cereal fiber, stool weight increases by 3–9 g.
4. Have the patient drink 8–10 glasses of water daily, as permitted.
5. Exercise may be beneficial in maintaining regularity.
6. Discuss overuse of laxatives and cathartics.
7. Discuss foods that have caused constipation, flatus, and GI distress in the past. Offer relevant suggestions.
8. Discuss need for medical assistance for diarrhea, bleeding, infection, and change in bowel habits.

NOTES

MEGACOLON, ACQUIRED

Usual Hospital Stay

3–4 days.

Notation

Megacolon, enlarged bowel, results from an abnormal colonic dilatation. It is often present in elderly persons who have a long history of elimination problems created by laxative abuse or constipation. The colonic dilatation may reach 8–10 cm in diameter. Persons with diabetes, hypothyroidism, sclero-derma, multiple sclerosis, electrolyte imbalances and other conditions may be affected. Obstruction could be caused by tumor, stricture, etc.

Note that the colon provides reabsorption of water and electrolytes as well as elimination of waste and regulation of bacterial homeostasis. Motility is crucial in these roles. Normal urges to defecate are affected by physical activity, neurological status, chemical/drug use, and bowel condition. Normal reflexes are needed for muscular and sphincter control.

Signs and symptoms of megacolon involve abdominal distention, flatus, absence of stool, smearing or diarrheal incontinence; nausea, anorexia, fa-tigue, and headache.

Objectives

1. Prevent complications such as long atelactasis from distention; sepsis, ulceration with hemorrhage or perforation, or sigmoid volvulus.
2. Evaluate bowel pattern by history and at present, including drug use and abuse (laxatives, etc.).
3. Identify and correct any nutrient deficiencies, electrolyte imbalances, or PCM.
4. Normalize bowel function as far as possible.
5. Position patient in whatever way is most comfortable.

Dietary Recommendations

1. Use adequate fluid and fiber, pending status and other conditions (such as CHF). Prune juice added to hot cereal may help normalize bowel function.
2. Raw fruits and vegetables should be used only as tolerated; progress over time.
3. Avoid excesses of refined foods and concentrated sweets to the exclu-sion of desirable foods.

Profile

Ht/wt/IBW or HBW	I & O	BP
Endoscopy	Barium X-rays	Na^+, K^+, Cl^-
BUN, creat	Thyroid function	Stool consistency
Abdominal girth	Stool pattern	Blood guaiac

Side Effects of Common Drugs Used

1. *Anticholinergics, opiates* and *antidepressants* may increase or aggravate constipation. Watch use carefully.
2. *Suppositories* and *stool softeners* may be used, or may have been used excessively. Monitor specific medications accordingly.

Patient Education

1. Discuss the role of exercise in maintaining normal bowel function.
2. Observe closely if colonic irrigations are used (Harris Flush—800 cc warm water slowly introduced into the rectum to relieve flatus).
3. Discuss role of fluid and fiber in bowel regularity.

NOTES

IRRITABLE COLON (SPASTIC COLITIS)

Usual Hospital Stay

3–4 days.

Notation

Spastic colitis, the most common form of inflammation of the colon, can result from anxiety, stress, or lack of adequate fiber in the diet. Signs and symptoms include belching, flatulence, heartburn, mucus in the stools, cramplike pain, constipation (sometimes alternating with diarrhea), and nausea. It is also known as irritable bowel syndrome.

Objectives

1. Encourage regular eating patterns, regular bowel hygiene, adequate rest, and relaxation.
2. Avoid constipation.
3. Use adequate fluid intake.
4. Monitor for lactose intolerance, food allergies, and gluten intolerance.
5. Alleviate pain, symptoms, and flatulence.

Dietary Recommendations

1. Provide an elemental diet for persons with irritable colon in its acute form.
2. As treatment progresses, use bland or soft foods; ensure that fluid intake is high. Gradually introduce fiber.

3. If the patient is at home, use a high fiber diet and bulking agents to avoid constipation.
4. Omit milk or gluten if not tolerated. Add calcium in other forms.
5. Omit gas-forming oligosaccharides (beans, barley, Brussels sprouts, cabbage, nuts, and soybeans) if not tolerated.

Profile

Ht	Wt	Ca^{++}, Mg^{++}
IBW/HBW	Alb	Hydrogen breath test
H & H	Gluc	Na^+, K^+, Cl^-

Side Effects of Common Drugs Used

1. *Methylcellulose.* Bulking agents must always be taken with large amounts of water.
2. *Antispasmodic drugs* can be used to alleviate abdominal pains.

Patient Education

1. Slowly increase dietary fiber to prevent discomfort.
2. Explain that regular times for bowel evacuation should be planned.
3. Ensure that the patient has adequate food intake.
4. Help the patient devise adequate methods for coping with stress.
5. A food diary may help to identify any food sensitivities.
6. Regular exercise may also be important.

NOTES

DIVERTICULAR DISEASES

Usual Hospital Stay

3–4 days.

Notation

Diverticulitis results from inflammation of small pouches (diverticula) formed in the colon wall and lining due to chronic constipation. Inflammation develops when bacteria or other irritants are trapped in pouches, causing spasm and pain in the lower left side of the abdomen, as well as distention, nausea, vomiting, constipation or diarrhea, chills, and fever. Diverticular diseases are rare in societies where a high fiber diet is consumed. Bowel cancer is a risk.

Objectives

Diverticulosis

1. Increase stool caliber and volume.
2. Distend the bowel wall to prevent development of high pressure segments.
3. Relieve intraluminal pressure.
4. Prevent inflammation.

Diverticulitis

1. Allow complete bowel rest to prevent perforation.
2. Avoid the laxative effect of excess fiber.
3. Eliminate food particles that accumulate in sacs. These food particles are capable of causing bacterial contamination.
4. Prevent peritonitis and abscess.

Dietary Recommendations

Diverticulosis (Convalescent State)

1. The diet should include a high intake of fluid.
2. The diet should be high in fiber. Begin with 1 teaspoon bran daily, working up to 2 tablespoons. Whole grains, stewed or dried fruits, potato skins, raw carrots, or celery may be used. Increase fiber *gradually*.

Diverticulitis (Inflamed State)

1. An elemental diet should be used if patient is acutely ill. Progress to clear liquids.
2. As treatment progresses, a bland diet (no excess spices or fiber) may be used. Avoid nuts, seeds, and fibrous vegetables.

Profile

Ht	Wt
IBW/HBW	Stool number, frequency
H & H	Alb
Transferrin, TIBC	BP
Sigmoidoscopy	Barium enema
ESR (inc.)	WBCs (may be inc.)

Side Effects of Common Drugs Used

1. *Bulk-forming agents* (methylcellulose) may be used to initiate normal colonic function and bowel action.
2. *Anticholinergics, stool softeners*, and *antibiotics* may be used. Monitor accordingly.

Patient Education

1. Instruct the patient concerning dietary fiber. Some ingested plant material is not digested by GI enzymes, including cellulose, pectin, lignin, and hemicelluloses. Some dietary fibers (whole grains) resist intestinal disintegration, whereas others (fruits and vegetables) are more or less disintegrated. Increased stool volume and decreased intracolonic pressure alter transit time.
2. High fiber foods are not synonymous with foods high in residue.
3. Have the patient chew slowly.
4. Instruct the patient to avoid constipation and straining.
5. Fluid intake should be adequate.

NOTES

PERITONITIS

Usual Hospital Stay

3–4 days.

Notation

Inflammation of the peritoneal cavity due to infiltration of intestinal contents occurs in peritonitis. Contents from such conditions as ruptured appendix, gastric or intestinal perforation, trauma, fistula, anastomotic leaks, or failure in peritoneal dialysis may initiate the problem.

Objectives

1. Provide bowel rest and recovery.
2. Improve anorectic state; correct ileus if present.

3. Correct dehydration and fluid/electrolyte imbalances where present.
4. Improve nutritional status, especially if patient has been malnourished over a period of time.

Dietary Recommendations

1. Patient is generally NPO with IV feedings for at least 24 hours, or until bowel sounds return.
2. Progress to an increased liquid diet as tolerated, such as a diet including Ensure Plus HN, or other supplemental feeding.
3. Progress as tolerated to a soft or general diet, appropriate for condition which caused the peritonitis originally.
4. Increase protein intake to correct catabolic state. Increase calories since BMR is generally elevated 10–17%.

Profile

Ht, wt	BP	Alb
Temp	BUN, creat	Na^+
H & H	Laparotomy	TLC
X-rays	I & O	Other parameters
WBCs	Gluc	
IBW/HBW	K^+	

Side Effects of Common Drugs Used

Antibiotics are used for bacterial peritonitis.

Patient Education

1. With patients on CAPD, the diet may need to be limited to 1.2–1.5 g protein/kg + 35 kcal/kg as is typical for renal patients.
2. Discuss diet appropriate for the illness of origin (such as diabetes, hypertension, toxemia, or nephritis).

NOTES

CARCINOID SYNDROME

Usual Hospital Stay

3–4 days.

Notation

A rare growth that develops in the wall of the intestine, carcinoid syndrome is usually discovered in x-rays performed for other reasons. The growth can become so large as to cause intestinal obstruction. Diversion of tryptophan to 5HT synthesis occurs, resulting in less tryptophan for protein and nicotinamide synthesis. 10% metastasize to the liver, producing hormone-producing tumors that have signs that include flushing of the head and neck (usually triggered by alcohol or exercise). The symptoms can last for several hours. In addition, the patient may have swollen and watery eyes, explosive diarrhea and abdominal cramps, wheezing like asthma, breathlessness, and symptoms similar to heart failure; 35% will get heart disease from fibrosis of the endocardium. Survival is 3–20 years.

Objectives

1. Ease symptoms and reduce any pain.
2. Control secretory diarrhea and wheezing.
3. Slow progression of the disease, which is not curable through surgery.
4. Control side effects of medications.
5. Replenish electrolyte and fluid losses.
6. Correct pellagra-like rash.

Dietary Recommendations

1. Decrease fiber intake during acute stages of diarrhea. Add pectin and ensure adequate fluid intake during those periods.
2. Use a diet controlled in protein and carbohydrate with use of bronchodilators.
3. Avoid alcoholic beverages. Limit caffeine intake to a controlled amount.

Profile

Ht, Wt	IBW/HBW	H & H
X-rays, GI tract	Biopsy of growth	Endoscopy
Alb	K^+	Na^+
Transferrin	TLC	No. of stools,
5HIAA		consistency

Side Effects of Common Drugs Used

1. Some *vasconstricting drugs* may be used to control flushing.
2. *Kaolin* (Kaopectate) and other medications may be used to control diarrhea.
3. *Bronchodilators* may be used to control wheezing. Check specific type of drug to evaluate potential side effects.
4. *Cytotoxic drugs* may be used in severe cases.
5. *Prednisone* helps to reduce flushing.

Patient Education

1. Discuss measures specifically designed for the patient's status and tolerance levels.
2. Suggest ways to make meals more appetizing if appetite is poor.

Comment

5-Hydroxyindole acetic acid (5HIAA) testing requires several days of a diet free from intake of avocados, pineapple, bananas, kiwi fruit, plums, eggplant, walnuts, hickory nuts, and pecans (*JAMA* 9/16/88).

CROHN'S DISEASE (REGIONAL ENTERITIS)

Usual Hospital Stay

8 days.

Notation

Crohn's disease is a chronic inflammatory granulomatous bowel disease (usually of the terminal ileum and cecum, less often of the colon) of unknown etiology, with onset generally between 15 and 35 years of age. The intestinal lumen decreases; peristalsis from food intake causes cramping pain, especially in the right lower quadrant. Other symptoms include fever, weight loss, debility, bowel narrowing, nausea, vomiting, abdominal pain, intestinal bleeding and sporadic flare-ups. Chronic diarrhea results from edema and ulcers. Children may present with growth failure. It differs from ulcerative colitis by affecting the GI tract from oral cavity to rectum. Only 25% of cases go into remission; an increased risk of colon CA or obstruction exists. Anorectal fistulas and abscesses may occur.

Objectives

1. Replace fluid and electrolytes lost through diarrhea and vomiting.
2. Lessen mechanical irritation and promote rest, especially with diarrhea.
3. Replenish nutrient reserves; correct malabsorption or anemia.
4. Monitor intolerances (lactose, gluten, etc.).

5. Promote healing; rest during an attack.
6. Prevent peritonitis or obstruction.
7. Promote weight gain or prevent losses from ↑ BMR, exudates, etc.
8. Prepare for surgery if necessary (perhaps from failed medical management, obstruction, fistula, or peritonitis). A total colostomy may be done.
9. In a child, promote growth.
10. When controlled, a higher fiber intake may reduce severity of symptoms (Klunfeld: *JADA 87*:1172, 1987).

Dietary Recommendations

1. With strictures or fistulas, use a low residue (elemental) or low fiber/bland diet that is high in calories with a protein content of 1–1.5 g/kg (especially high in HBV proteins). Use TPN if needed, usually 2 weeks or longer. BEE × 1.5 may be calculated.
2. Limit fat intake if steatorrhea is present. Medium-chain triglycerides may be better tolerated.
3. Reduce lactose intake if not tolerated. Check for wheat and gluten tolerances.
4. Supplement diet with adequate amounts of vitamins C and B_{12}, iron, zinc, vitamin B_6, copper, calcium, potassium, folate, vitamin D, and magnesium. Vitamins A, E, and K should be given every other day.
5. Monitor progress carefully. Patients are finicky eaters.
6. Small, frequent meals may be better tolerated.

Profile

Ht	Transferrin, TIBC	BP
IBW/HBW	N balance	H & H
Fe	Wt	TLC
K^+	Schilling test	Serum Cu
Alb, RBP	Ca^{++}	WBCs, ESR (inc.)
X-rays, endoscopy	Serum B_{12}	No. of bowel
Barium enema, barium	TP	movements,
swallow	BUN, creat	frequency
Fecal fat analysis	Serum carotene	Breath hydrogen test

Side Effects of Common Drugs Used

1. *Corticosteroids.* The use of corticosteroids commonly causes electrolyte imbalance. The patient may then need a diet that provides 2 g of sodium daily, with extra calcium and potassium from losses. Corticosteroids are more effective for colon involvement.
2. *Antidiarrheal agents.* The diet should include 2 L of water daily. Sulfasalazine (Azulfidine) decreases folate levels; the patient may need

folate supplements. Fever, hair loss, and nephrotoxicity can occur. Metronidazole may be used with anal involvement.
3. *Antacids, analgesics,* and *antispasmodics* may be used.
4. *Psyllium laxatives* (Metamucil) can help with constipation, diarrhea. Long-term use alters electrolytes. Flatulence or steatorrhea may occur.
5. *Antibiotics* work well for fistulas; vitamin K may be needed.

Patient Education

1. Encourage the patient to eat. Alleviate fears associated with mealtimes.
2. Tell the patient to avoid seasonings if they are poorly tolerated.
3. Ensure that during periods of diarrhea sources of potassium are increased.
4. Help the patient to evaluate tolerance of chilled foods. Have him or her chew foods well and avoid swallowing air.
5. Discuss the roles of fiber, supplements, and fluid intake.
6. Highlight calcium and vitamin D in their roles in bone mineralization; discuss alternate sources when milk cannot be used.
7. Periodic assistance or re-evaluation by a dietitian may be helpful regarding dietary intake.
8. No definite role for sugar or food processing has been documented.

For More Information

Crohn's and Colitis Foundation of America, Inc. (CCFA): (800) 343-3637

NOTES

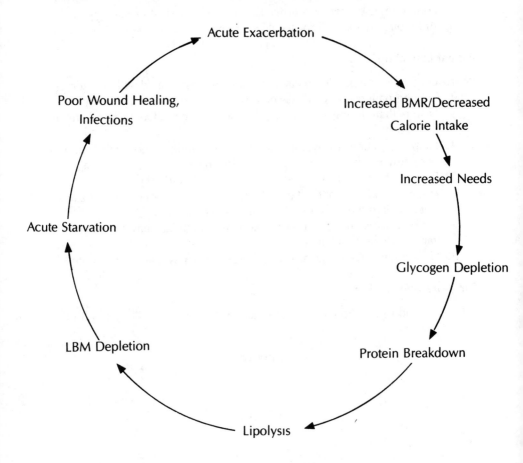

Fig. 7–2. Nutritional Depletion in Inflammatory Bowel Disease.

Adapted from Newman, McCorkle, and Turner: In *Nutritional Support in Critical Care* (C. Lang, ed.), Rockville, MD: Aspen Publishers, 1987.

INTESTINAL FISTULA

Usual Hospital Stay

4 days.

Notation

An intestinal fistula is an unwanted pathway from intestines to other organs, e.g., the bladder. External fistulas are between the SI and the outside (skin, for example). Internal fistulas are between two internal organs. They may occur from Crohn's disease, CA, or following surgery. Weight loss and hypoalbuminemia will affect mortality.

Objectives

1. Promote rest and healing; minimize drainage.
2. Monitor type of dietary regimen according to location of fistula and surgical or medical treatment. Surgery may be done to drain infection or to establish a stoma, or to remove the fistula if possible.
3. Replace fluid and electrolyte losses.
4. Replace malnutrition and infections.
5. Prevent organ damage and death.

Dietary Recommendations

1. Use TPN or elemental diet at first, especially TPN for jejunal fistulas. A jejunostomy may help a duodenal fistula.
2. Progress to a low-residue, soft/bland, and normal diet as tolerated. Or use Vivonex or Vivonex TEN for an extended period of time. Reabilan may also be beneficial.

Profile

Ht	Wt	K^+, Na^+
IBW/HBW	Alb	I & O
H & H	BUN	Transferrin
N balance	Wt. loss	RBP

Patient Education

1. Instruct the patient in the fiber content of foods.
2. Defined formula diets can help support spontaneous closure in about 4–6 weeks. If closure has not occurred, surgery is aided by a better nutritional status.

ULCERATIVE COLITIS

Usual Hospital Stay

10 days.

Notation

An ulceration of the mucosa with passage of pus and blood in the stools, *ulcerative colitis* causes crampy abdominal pain, fever, diarrhea, anemia, pyoderma, endocarditis, cirrhosis, splenomegaly, and stomatitis. Children may have growth failure. The condition is usually one relentless, continuous lesion of the colon with some involvement of the terminal ileum. It may be acute, mild or chronic. There are four theories of its cause: autoimmunity, bacteria, allergy or milk intolerance. Onset is usually between ages 15–35, often in women. Surgery is potentially curative here. The ileocecal valve should be preserved, if possible. Increased risk of colonic CA exists, especially with 10 + years duration.

Objectives

1. Correct fluid and electrolyte imbalance.
2. Replenish depleted stores and correct poor nutritional status, anemia, etc.
3. Avoid further irritation and inflammation of the bowel by decreasing fiber—large fecal volume distends the bowel. Be careful about obstructions.
4. Correct for diarrhea, steatorrhea, obstruction, and anemia.
5. In acute stages, allow bowel to rest and heal.

Dietary Recommendations

1. To treat the condition of its acute state, an elemental diet is needed to minimize fecal volume. TPN should be used if needed, often for 2 weeks in the acute stage.
2. As the patient progresses, a bland, high protein (1–1.5 g/kg), high calorie diet, given in six small feedings, should be used. The diet should

exclude nuts, seeds, legumes, whole grains, and fresh fruits and vegetables.

3. If needed, a low residue diet should be used. Intake of fiber and milk should be controlled. Persons with this condition often have lactose, wheat or gluten intolerance. Ensure or other products may be helpful.
4. Supplement the diet with multivitamins and minerals, especially thiamine, folacin, zinc, calcium and iron.
5. MCTs may be helpful.

Profile

Ht	IBW/HBW	Gluc
Bilirubin	PT	Fecal fat study
Chol	Trig	Stool sample
K^+	Cl^-	Breath hydrogen test
BUN, creat	Transferrin, TIBC	Alk phos
Wt	N balance	CBC, Sed. rate
Alb, RBP	Biopsy	WBCs
H & H	Sigmoidoscopy	Folate
Ca, P, Mg	Schilling Test (B_{12})	Ferritin, Serum iron

Side Effects of Common Drugs Used

1. *Sulfasalazine* (Azulfidine) requires the patient to drink 8 to 10 cups of fluid daily.
2. *Corticosteroids* may require restriction of sodium intake. ACTH is usually more effective than hydrocortisone sodium succinate (Solucortef). Negative nitrogen balance may result. Monitor need for extra vitamins.
3. *Antispasmodics* or *antidiarrheals* are often used.
4. With *antibiotic* therapy, diarrhea can be aggravated and vitamin K may be lost.

Patient Education

1. Ensure that the patient avoids foods that are known to cause diarrhea. Avoid extremes in food or beverage temperatures.
2. Explain that pleasant mealtimes are an important part of treatment.
3. Indicate that frequent small meals may increase the patient's total nutritional intake.
4. Avoid iced or carbonated beverages, which stimulate peristalsis.
5. Instruct the patient to eat slowly and chew foods well.
6. Discuss fears related to eating.
7. Frequent counseling by a dietitian may be helpful.
8. Stop eating 2–3 hours before bedtime.

Comments

Colectomy and Ileostomy

Preoperative Diet. A low residue diet is recommended, to be followed by intake of clear liquids.

Postoperative Diet. IV feeding should continue for 2 days. When bowel sounds return, clear liquids may be taken. The diet should progress slowly to full liquids and then a low fiber, high protein regimen with high calories (carbohydrates especially). The diet should also provide a high intake of vitamins and minerals. The patient will need vitamin B_{12} injections, as well as adequate intake of sodium and potassium and fluids. TPN may be ordered.

In a liberalized diet, foods (those least likely to cause problems) are added one at a time. Avoid gas-forming or acidic foods (the latter may cause increased peristalsis).

ILEOSTOMY

Usual Hospital Stay

10 days.

Notation

Used to treat intractable cases of ulcerative disease, Crohn's disease, polyposis, and colonic CA, ileostomy is a surgical procedure (stoma/opening formation) that brings the ileum through the abdominal wall. This procedure causes a decrease in fat, bile acid and vitamin B_{12} absorption, as well as greater losses of sodium and potassium. Patients will be incontinent of gas and stool. Ideally, ileocecal valve can be kept to decrease bacterial influx into the small intestine. Of these patients, 50–70% will have recurrent disease.

Objectives

1. Modify the diet to counteract malabsorption of nutrients secondary to diarrhea, protein and fluid losses from an ulcerated colon, a negative nitrogen balance from nutrient loss, and anorexia.
2. Correct anemia caused by inadequate intake of blood losses.
3. Counteract weakness and muscle cramping from potassium losses.
4. Counteract increased basal metabolic needs in presence of fever and infection.
5. Replenish calcium to reverse arthritic joint involvement due to steatorrhea and the side effects of steroid therapy.
6. Prevent gallstones, renal oxalate stones, bacterial overgrowth, and fatty acid malabsorption. Note that unabsorbed bile acids act as cathartics in the colon.

Dietary Recommendations

1. If needed, provide a high calorie, high protein diet that is *low* in excess fiber. Pectin in apples guar gum in oatmeal may actually be beneficial.
2. Use dairy products cautiously in preoperative patients as some may have lactose intolerances. Be careful of nuts, legumes, whole grains, and leafy greens in the preoperative patient because of their high residue content with resultant bowel stimulation.
3. The diet should provide an adequate amount of fluids, especially in hot weather.
4. Postoperatively, spinach and parsley may be used as an intestinal deodorizer. Beware of excesses of oxalate-rich foods.
5. The patient needs an adequate intake of protein (provided by low fat sources such as lean meats and egg white), vitamin B_{12} (provided by liver, fish, and eggs), folacin, calcium, magnesium, iron, sodium, vitamin C, and potassium. Add salt as needed to the diet.

Profile

Ht	Alb
IBW/HBW	Transferrin
H & H	TIBC
BUN, Creat	Gluc
Stool (occult blood)	WBC
K^+	BP
Na^+	Ca^{++}
Mg^{++}	Serum B_{12}, Schilling test if needed
Wt	

Side Effects of Common Drugs Used

1. *Prednisone.* Restrict excessive sodium intake.
2. *Lomotil.* This drug is a stool thickener and deodorizer. Plenty of fluids should be used.
3. *Psyllium laxatives* (Metamucil) are used as bulk-forming agents.

Patient Education

1. Explain which foods are common sources of the needed nutrients in a diet, or suggest supplementation with multivitamins.
2. Monitor individual tolerance to offending foods, such as gas-forming or fried foods, highly seasoned foods, nuts, raisins, and pineapple.
3. An enterostomal therapist may be of assistance.
4. Discuss the role of fluid and sodium during hot weather.
5. The patient should avoid obesity.
6. Eating before bedtime should be avoided.

Comment

Alternative involves *ileal reservoir after proctocolectomy*. The colon is the primary site for sodium, potassium, and water absorption and for formation and absorption of vitamin K. This procedure allows fairly normal resumption of colonic functions. No problems with vitamins B_{12} or K or bile salt absorption have been noted. A high fiber diet is recommended to normalize elimination. Fluids may be given between meals, with consideration for sodium and potassium needs. Caffeine should be controlled to decrease diarrhea; concentrated sweets should be avoided in order to prevent osmotic diarrhea, and specific intolerances should be omitted.

COLOSTOMY

Usual Hospital Stay

10 days, medical; 3–4 days surgical.

Notation

A colostomy is an artificial outlet for intestinal wastes created surgically by bringing a portion of the colon through the abdominal wall. Normal fluid reabsorption occurs in the colon. Colostomy output is more formed than ileostomy output. Colostomy can be permanent or temporary. It may be indicated for cancer, diverticulitis, perforated bowel, radiation enteritis, obstruction, and Hirschsprung's disease.

Objectives

1. Speed wound healing and recovery.
2. Prevent weight loss. Correct malnutrition from GI blood loss, anemia, protein malabsorption, and steatorrhea.
3. Prevent blockage.
4. Prevent watery or unscheduled bowel movements. Correct or prevent dehydration.
5. Individualize the diet: eat regularly, avoid odor-causing foods, monitor food preferences.
6. Normalize the patient's lifestyle as much as possible.
7. Avoid infection and skin irritants.

Dietary Recommendations

1. Initially, after the operation, use clear liquids. As patient progresses, use a bland/low residue diet to reduce stoma discharge and irritation. To speed healing, the diet should also be high in protein and calories. Gradually introduce new foods; if done slowly, offending foods can be identified and obstruction can be controlled or prevented.

2. The diet should provide normal or increased salt intake. One to two quarts of fluid, taken between meals, should be ingested daily.
3. Beware of highly spiced foods and excessive raw fruits and vegetables, if these foods cause diarrhea. Prune juice may also be a problem for some patients.
4. Odor-causing foods include alcohol (beer), beans, onions, green peppers, cabbage, turnips, beets, Brussels sprouts, radishes, cucumbers, fish, eggs and garlic.
5. Gas-forming vegetables like corn, broccoli and cauliflower may cause discomfort; omit if necessary.
6. Regular mealtimes and "constipating foods" like boiled milk, rice or peanut butter can help to normalize evacuation times.
7. Progress to a high fiber diet. Short-fibered foods are best—no whole-kernel corn, celery, nuts, pineapple, popcorn, coleslaw, apple skins, seeds, or coconut.

Profile

Ht	Wt	Transferrin, TIBC
IBW/HBW	Alb	Serum B_{12}, Fe, folacin
H & H	Ca^{++}	PT
K^+, Na^+	I & O	Hydration status
Gluc	Chol	
Trig		

Patient Education

1. The use of a commercial deodorant in the colostomy bag is preferred to eliminating highly flavored foods or nutrient-dense foods.
2. Tell the patient to eat slowly, chew foods well, and avoid swallowing air.
3. Irrigations should not be done when there is vomiting or diarrhea.
4. Regular mealtimes should be encouraged.
5. Enterostomal therapy can be very helpful.
6. Reassurance is needed, without misleading the patient.

Comments

If diarrhea results from the colostomy, use strained bananas, applesauce, boiled rice, boiled milk, and peanut butter.

If calcium oxalate stones develop after the colostomy, the diet should provide a high fluid intake. Restrict intake of oxalates from spinach, rhubarb, wild greens, coffee and tea, and chocolate.

Approximately 6 weeks are required to acclimate the bowel to new procedures of irrigation. Enemas are used to wash the bowel up to the ileocecal valve (with 1000 cc tap water). Constipation can occur with dehydration; therefore, adequate intake of fluid and fiber is important.

NOTES

INTESTINAL LYMPHANGIECTASIA

Usual Hospital Stay

3–4 days.

Notation

Intestinal lymphangiectasia is a generalized disorder of intestinal lymphatics which results in a protein-losing enteropathy. Increased intestinal lymphatic pressure with vessel dilatation occurs, discharging fluid into the bowel lumen. The fluid is then digested by intestinal enzymes and is reabsorbed. Only marginal loss of protein stores occurs in most cases.

Objectives

1. Decrease symptoms and promote recovery.
2. Decrease ingested fat since it stimulates lymphatic flow into the gut.
3. Meet all nutritional needs for age and sex.
4. Monitor absorption of fat-soluble vitamins; ensure adequacy from dietary or supplemental sources.

Dietary Recommendations

1. A diet using MCT oil may be necessary.
2. Adequate protein and calories are needed, appropriate to the individual's needs.
3. Fat-soluble vitamins may be required in water-miscible form for adequate absorption.

240

Profile

Ht, wt	IBW/HBW	H & H
Steatorrhea	Alb (dec.)	Transferrin (dec.)
RBP	Chol, trig	TLC
BUN, creat	TSF, MAC, MAMC	Gluc

Patient Education

1. Discuss the role of fat in digestion, with the need for MCT oils in the daily diet.
2. Discuss fat-soluble vitamins and their sources in the diet.

NOTES

SHORT-BOWEL SYNDROME

Usual Hospital Stay

8–14 days.

Notation

Short bowel syndrome (SBS) usually involves surgical resection of a portion of the small bowel, compromising the absorptive surface and resulting in malabsorption (especially if over 50% of the small intestine has been removed). Malnutrition and steatorrhea may result. SBS may also result from Crohn's disease, CA, scleroderma, or fistula. If only 30% of the SI remains in an adult (or less than 30 cm in infants), the resulting malabsorption may be life-threatening. An attempt should be made to keep the ileocecal valve to prevent contamination of the SI.

Symptoms and signs include dehydration, electrolyte losses, hypokalemia; deficiencies of calcium, magnesium, and zinc; carbohydrate and lactose malabsorption; protein malabsorption; oxalate stone formation; cholesterol biliary stones; gastric acid hypersecretion; vitamin B_{12} or iron deficiency; fat-soluble vitamin deficiency; and diarrhea. SBS generally leaves less than 150 cm small intestine; 100 cm is necessary to completely absorb bile salts.

Objectives

1. Prevent and correct fluid and electrolyte imbalances and dehydration.
2. Utilize remaining bowel surface and maximum efficacy.
3. Correct symptoms of deficiency and malabsorption, where possible, for trace minerals and for vitamins B_{12}, A, D, E, and K.
4. Decrease weight loss (approximately 10 lbs monthly until adaptation occurs).
5. Omit lactose if not tolerated; provide adequate calcium replacements.
6. Decrease oxalate from the diet to reduce stone formation.
7. Control or prevent gallstone formation, anemia, and protein-losing enteropathy.
8. Allow remaining intestine to compensate over time by hypertrophy of villi and increased diameter. Less than 100 cm yields more severe problems; less than 60 cm remaining intestine may require long-term parenteral nutrition.
9. Provide nutrient replacements, dependent on area of resection (proximal jejunum—calcium, iron, magnesium, protein, CHO and fat absorbed here; terminal ileum—bile acids and IF-bound vitamin B_{12} absorbed here).
10. For care of colostomy or ileostomy, see those entries.

Dietary Recommendations

1. IVs or TPN may be appropriate immediately before and after surgery to allow rest before feeding. Determine if patient has problems with bloating, etc. TPN should continue until adaptive processes are complete, if and when that occurs. Glutamine-enriched solutions may be beneficial against intestinal atrophy during TPN.
2. When patient is ready (stable fluid and electrolyte balance, return of bowel sounds, less than 2 L daily of diarrhea), elemental diet may be tried. Monitor osmotic diarrhea, which can result.
3. Frequent, small feedings (5–6 times daily) may be needed to utilize the diet as ingested. Reabilan may be beneficial.
4. Increased calories (35–45 kcal/kg); 40–50 g fat + MCT oil; high protein (1.5–2 g/kg) may be needed.
5. Adequate zinc, potassium, magnesium, calcium, manganese, iron, glucose, vitamin C, selenium, B-complex (especially folic acid) and other nutrients may be needed as supplements—determine needs based on site of resection and signs of malnutrition.
6. Lactose-restricted and oxalate-restricted diets may be needed for an extended period of time. Rhubarb, spinach, beets, chocolate and peanuts are high oxalate foods.
7. Water-miscible forms of the fat-soluble vitamins may be useful.
8. Omit alcoholic beverages and caffeine unless physician permits small quantities.

9. Taking fluids between instead of with meals may be helpful in reducing dumping.
10. With osmotic diarrhea, a reduction in simple carbohydrates and an increase in complex carbohydrates may be needed.

Profile

Ht, wt	IBW/HBW	Wt changes
H & H	Ca^{++}	Mg^{++}
Transferrin	Na^+	K^+
Serum Fe	Fecal nitrogen	N balance
Bile acid breath test	Fecal fat test	Serum oxalate
Lactose tolerance test	GTT, Gluc	Alb
D-Xylose absorption	RBP	Prealbumin
Serum gastrin (↑)	I & O	Serum amylase, lipase

Side Effects of Common Drugs Used

1. *Cholestyramine* may be used for choleraic diarrhea when less than 100 cm is resected; prevent excessive use.
2. *Pancrelipase* improves fat and protein absorption after jejunal resection.
3. *Cimetidine* and *antacids* may be needed to decrease gastric hypersecretion.
4. *Oral calcium supplements* (OsCal) are often used to bind oxalate excesses.
5. *Anti-diarrheals* may be needed, as will *antibiotics* (especially with blind loop).

Patient Education

1. Importance of adequate nutrition and supplementation must be discussed to prevent or correct malnutrition and malabsorption.
2. A supportive attitude from family and caregivers will be essential.
3. Recipes and food preparation tips will be needed to support the specific dietary regimen and to evaluate tolerances over time.
4. Progression in diet is allowed when the SI hypertrophies over several weeks or months.
5. Discuss the need for free water.

Comments

Loss of Colon. Oxalate absorption occurs here; fewer malabsorption problems will occur.

Loss of Ileum. This is more serious than loss of jejunum because vitamin B_{12} and bile salts will be poorly reabsorbed as a result. The ileocecal valve keeps colonic bacteria out of the small intestine and regulates chyme flow.

In SBS, short-chain triglycerides have a precursor in pectin; they increase O_2 uptake in the colon, therefore maintaining gut integrity. Mucosal growth is stimulated by early refeeding (free fatty acids, sugars, proteins). Hyperphagia can increase enterocyte production.

NOTES

HEMORRHOIDS AND HEMORRHOIDECTOMY

Usual Hospital Stay

6 days.

Notation

Chronic constipation is thought to be the main cause of hemorrhoids. The disorder is common in Americans (1/2 over age 50 will have suffered at least once, especially if obese). Pregnancy or labor and jobs with excessive standing may also cause the problem.

Hemorrhoids can also be caused by excessive straining for bowel evacuation. *Internal* hemorrhoids are normal anatomical structures and are rarely painful (they may only bleed). *External* hemorrhoids are usually from excessive diarrhea or from constipation; they are tender, painful, bluish localized swellings of varicose veins at the anal margin. Bleeding is common.

Objectives

Hemorrhoids

1. Provide comfort. Prevent prolapse and thrombosis.
2. Avoid constipation, infection, and anemia.
3. Reduce possible irritation from too much roughage.
4. Avoid irritants such as laxatives.

Hemorrhoidectomy

1. Reduce irritation while patient heals.
2. Promote rapid healing. Prevent future recurrence.

Dietary Recommendations

Hemorrhoids

1. The diet should be low in fiber only when a patient is in pain. Otherwise, a high fiber diet should be used.
2. Fluids should be increased to eight to ten glasses daily.
3. Exclude highly seasoned foods or relishes.

Hemorrhoidectomy

1. Begin with clear liquids and progress to full liquids.
2. A low fiber/soft diet should be used until full recovery occurs.
3. Eventually, adequate to high fiber (up to 20 g) should be taken.
4. Omit lactose only if necessary.

Profile

Ht	Wt	Proctoscopy
IBW/HBW	Fe	PT
H & H	BUN	Alb
Stool (occult blood)	Transferrin, TIBC	Hx diarrhea or
I & O	BP	constipation

Drugs Commonly Used

1. *Laxatives* and *enemas* may have caused faulty bowel function. Avoid use unless prescribed by the doctor.
2. *Preparation H* contains vitamin A from shark oil, as well as yeast derivatives. No shrinkage is actually verifiable (*Consumer Reports* 9/86).

Patient Education

1. Ensure that the patient adequately exercises, rests, and maintains regular bowel habits.
2. Teach the patient about the role of fiber in the diet.
3. Persistent or recurrent bleeding requires medical attention, especially to monitor vitamin K, iron and B-complex levels, and to prevent additional losses.
4. Keeping the anal skin area dry will be important.
5. Over-the-counter products like Lanacane may aggravate an allergic response.

NOTES

INTESTINAL LIPODYSTROPHY (WHIPPLE'S DISEASE)

Usual Hospital Stay

5 days.

Notation

An uncommon systemic disease, Whipple's disease involves infiltration of the SI with glycoprotein-laden macrophages and some rod-shaped bacilli in varying body tissues. It normally occurs in males, with insidious onset.

Signs and symptoms include malabsorption, fever, hypoproteinemia, anemia, arthritis, endocarditis, CNS involvement, lymphadenopathy, edema, gray to brown skin pigmentation. The disease is usually fatal.

Objectives

1. Reduce fever and inflammatory processes.
2. Correct malnutrition and malabsorption.
3. Prevent or correct weight loss.
4. Correct anemia and hypoproteinemia.
5. Prevent or correct dehydration and electrolyte imbalances.

Dietary Recommendations

1. Use a high protein/high calorie diet appropriate for age and sex.
2. Supplement diet with a multivitamin/mineral preparation, especially for vitamin D and calcium when steatorrhea is a problem. Vitamin A may also be needed.
3. Ensure adequate intake of a diet rich in HBV proteins, iron, B-complex vitamins and other nutrients for blood-building.
4. Provide adequate fluid intake to reduce fever and replenish tissues.
5. If edema is a problem, control of sodium to 4–6 grams daily may be helpful.

Profile

Ht, wt	IBW/HBW	H & H (dec.)
Serum Ca^{++}	Mg^{++}	K^+
Na^+	Transferrin	Temp
I & O	Alb (dec.)	RBP

Side Effects of Common Drugs Used

1. *Tetracycline*—do not take with calcium antacids or with dairy products.
2. *Penicillin* may also be used to reduce bacterial overgrowth.

246

Patient Education

1. Discuss inclusion of high quality proteins in the diet. Frequent snacks may be beneficial if large meals are not tolerated.
2. Provide lists for nutrient-dense foods rich in specific and needed nutrients (iron, calcium, etc.).

Section 8
Pancreatic, Hepatic, and Biliary Disorders

Chief Assessment Factors

pain, abdominal or radiating

hepatomegaly

diarrhea, steatorrhea

vomiting, nausea

anorexia, malaise

fatigue

diabetes, hyperglycemia, hyopglycemia

jaundice

abnormal liver function tests

altered pancreatic enzyme levels

altered bleeding/clotting times

Table 8–1.
Liver, Gallbladder, and Pancreatic Functions
LIVER   The largest single organ of the body; it is the central biochemical organ of the body. Functions include:

1. Converts galactose and fructose to glucose; makes glycogen; degrades glycogen upon demand.
2. Converts proteins into glucose; synthesizes albumin, globulin, fibrinogen, prothrombin, transferrin; removes nitrogenous wastes (ammo-

nia); provides transamination; synthesizes purines and pyrimidines; forms amines by decarboxylation.
3. Synthesizes triglycerides; forms VLDLs; oxidizes fatty acids for energy and ketones; synthesizes cholesterol from acetate; makes HDLs.
4. Stores vitamins A, D, E and K and some vitamin B_{12} and vitamin C; hydroxylates vitamin D for renal activation.
5. Stores minerals (iron, copper, zinc, magnesium).
6. Detoxifies drugs.
7. Produces bile.

GALLBLADDER
Stores bile, which helps counteract stomach acidity and aids in fat digestion through emulsification.

PANCREAS
1. The pancreas produces pancreatic juice when stimulated by secretin. Pancreatic juice contains bicarbonate, which helps to neutralize acid chyme.
2. The pancreas also secretes insulin and glucagon hormones.
3. The pancreas secretes digestive enzymes (trypsin, lipase and amylase) into the collecting duct as stimulated by cholecystokinin (also called pancreozymin), produced by the duodenum.
4. The pancreas secretes metabolic/digestive enzymes involved in protein, carbohydrate and fat metabolism. Pancreatic secretion has gastric, cephalic, and intestinal phases. The *islets* secrete insulin (beta) and glucagon (alpha). The *acini* secrete lipase, amylase, trypsin, chymotrypsin, ribonuclease, and carboxypolypeptidase.

For More Information

American Liver Foundation
Cedar Grove, NJ 07009
(800) 223-0179

NOTES

PANCREATITIS

Usual Hospital Stay

6 days.

Notation

Pancreatitis involves inflammation with edema, fat necrosis, and cellular exudate.

Acute pancreatitis is an acute inflammatory disease in which autodigestion occurs owing to obstruction of the pancreatic duct (perhaps from chronic alcoholism, biliary tract disease or gallstones, trauma, certain hyperlipidemias, and pancreatic CA).

Chronic pancreatitis is a fibrotic, necrotic disease state with decreased enzymatic processes. Both types cause abdominal pain, nausea, vomiting, and distention.

Objectives

1. Inhibit activity and secretion of pancreatic enzymes to promote rest and to reduce pain.
2. Avoid pancreatic irritants, especially alcohol and caffeine.
3. Correct fluid and electrolyte imbalances and malnutrition; avoid overfeeding.
4. In *acute* cases, allow the pancreas to rest; reduce fever; prevent shock.
5. In *chronic* cases, alleviate steatorrhea and prevent or control secondary tetany, hyperglycemia, PCM, maldigestion, and diarrhea.
6. Avoid or control complications (cardiovascular, pulmonary, hematological, renal, neurological, or metabolic); prevent multiple organ failure.
7. Feed intravenously if necessary to reduce morbidity.

Dietary Recommendations

1. For the patient with *acute pancreatitis*, start NPO with IV feedings, 24–48 hours. By the 3rd day, check glucose tolerance and progress to clear or full liquids. Eventually add amino acids and predigested fats; medium chain triglycerides may be well tolerated as well. Progress to a light, moderate fat diet given in six daily feedings. Use TPN for excessively slow progression such as ileus. Transition to jejunostomy can then be considered.
2. For the patient with *chronic pancreatitis*, use a low to moderate fat, moderate protein, high carbohydrate diet. It should be low fiber and it

should be taken in the form of six small meals a day. Alcoholic beverages are prohibited; adequate calcium and fat-soluble vitamin supplementation should be provided. In addition, caffeine or gastric stimulants should be prohibited. The diet should include adequate amounts of vitamin C, vitamin B complex, and folic acid for water-soluble vitamin needs, and zinc as well.

3. For the patients with severe *steatorrhea*, the diet should include an increase of MCTs. Mild cases are not usually a problem.
4. Needle catheter jejunostomy may be useful.

Profile

Ht	Chol (LDL up, or total	Steatorrhea
IBW/HBW	decreased)	Alb, RBP
BEE	Trig (inc.)	Pco_2, Po_2
K^+, Na^+	Mg^{++} (dec.)	BUN
PT	LDH (over 700)	H & H
Bilirubin	SGOT (over 250)	Serum folate
Wt	Temp	LUQ abd. pain
Ca^{++} (altered)	WBCs (over 200)	Alk phos
Gluc (inc.)	Chvostek's sign	CT scan
Lipase (inc.)	Amylase (over 200)	Vomiting

Side Effects of Common Drugs Used

1. *Pancreatic enzymes (Pancreatin)* may be needed to reduce steatorrhea to less than 20 g/day. Enteric coating is necessary to prevent destruction by enzymes. Capsules or tablets should be swallowed whole. Take enteric-coated enzymes with cimetidine, food, or antacids.
2. *Antibiotics, antispasmodics,* and *anticholinergics* may be used.
3. *Acetazolamide* may be needed.
4. *Antacids* may be helpful; beware of extended use.
5. *Steroids* can cause sodium retention, potassium and calcium depletion, negative nitrogen balance.
6. *Insulin* may be necessary.
7. *Bile salts* or water-miscible forms of fat-soluble vitamins may be needed.

Patient Education

1. Instruct the patient to watch for signs and symptoms of diabetes and tetany.
2. Discuss omission of alcohol from the typical diet.
3. Discuss what should be done about nausea and vomiting.
4. Coffee, tea, and gas-forming foods may need to be omitted.

NOTES

PANCREATIC INSUFFICIENCY

Usual Hospital Stay

6 days.

Notation

Pancreatic insufficiency is caused by decreased secretion of lipase, often from cystic fibrosis, PCM, congenital problems, pancreatic cancer, or pancreatitis. Lipase is the key enzyme for breaking down triglycerides.

Objectives

1. Correct states of maldigestion, diarrhea, and steatorrhea.
2. Provide adequate caloric intake while lowering intake of fats.
3. Provide missing fat-soluble vitamins, if needed, from malabsorption.
4. Prevent iron overloading.
5. Correct steatorrhea; maintain below 20 g/day.

Dietary Recommendations

1. Use a moderate to low fat diet; 3 to 4 teaspoons of fat daily are allowed. Medium-chain triglycerides may also be tolerated because they do not require lipase. They may be taken with simple sugars, jelly, and jams in mixed dishes.
2. Use tender meats and low-fiber fruits and vegetables.
3. Alcoholic beverages are prohibited.
4. Zinc may be needed in supplemental form or from an elemental diet.
5. Tube feed in severe cases.

Profile

Ht	Bicarbonate	Lipase
IBW/HBW	Wt	H & H
K^+	Gluc	Amylase ($\downarrow$)
Ca^{++}	Na^+	I & O
Trig	Chol	Steatorrhea
PT	Alk phos	Serum Carotene

Side Effects of Common Drugs Used

1. *Pancreatic enzymes [pancreatin or pancrelipase (Cotazym)]* should be taken with food. Take enteric-coated tablets with cimetidine or antacids.
2. Fat-soluble vitamins should be taken in water-miscible form.

Patient Education

1. Instruct the patient in the role of the pancreas in digestion.
2. Discuss appropriate measures for recovery, control.

ZOLLINGER-ELLISON SYNDROME

Usual Hospital Stay

6 days.

Notation

The Zollinger-Ellison syndrome is a severe form of peptic ulcer disease with ulceratogenic tumor (gastrinoma) of the delta cells of the pancreatic islets of Langerhans. It results in hypersecretion of gastric acid and fulminating ulceration of the esophagus, stomach, duodenum, and jejunum. It is frequently accompanied by secretory diarrhea. Of all cases, 60% occur in males; 2/3 are malignant. D-cell adenoma may be malignant or benign. Insulin is often increased by the beta cells, interestingly.

Objectives

1. Overcome malabsorption.
2. Decrease steatorrhea with losses of nitrogen, fat, sodium, and potassium.
3. Lessen diarrhea.
4. Eliminate gastric acid secretion, usually with medications or, less often, surgery (gastrectomy).
5. Where existing, lessen problems with dysphagia and reflux.

Dietary Recommendations

1. The diet should provide low to moderate fat (50–70 g).
2. According to the patient's stool losses, modify calories, fat, protein, and electrolytes as needed.
3. Modify fiber, seasonings, and textures as necessary.
4. Alter feeding modality to TF or TPN if needed.

Profile

Ht	Wt	Serum insulin
IBW/HBW	Alb	Serum gastrin > 1000
N balance	H & H	pg/ml
Na$^+$	K$^+$ (dec.)	Stool volume
Ca^{++} (may be	Mg^{++}	BP
elevated)	BUN	Trig, Chol
Steatorrhea	CT scan	Gluc
		Gastrin
		radioimmunoassay

Drugs Commonly Used

1. *Histamine H$_2$ receptor antagonists* (ranitidine or cimetidine) can reduce hypergastric acid secretion.
2. *Omeprazole* can also inhibit gastric acid secretion.
3. *Pancreatic enzymes* may be needed if steatorrhea is excessive.

Patient Education

1. Explain which modifications of fiber in the diet are appropriate.
2. Explain how malabsorption compromises nutritional status.

GALLBLADDER DISEASE

Usual Hospital Stay

Medical, 4 days; surgical*, 12 days.

Notation

Cholecystitis is inflammation of the gallbladder. Its acute form is almost always caused by stones; its chronic form may be caused by bacteria, chemical irritants, or stones. Symptoms and signs include abdominal pain, radiating to back; vomiting; nausea, and fever.

Cholelithiasis is defined as the presence of gallstones. Of the general population, 10% (especially women), and of American Indian women over 30, 70%, have gallstones. Incidence is greater with aging. Some gallbladders can concentrate bile normally, but cannot acidify it. The result is that calcium may be less soluble in bile, and precipitates out.

There are two forms of stones—cholesterol or pigment stones. Cholesterol precipitates as gallstones whenever cholesterol is greater than bile acids and phospholipids.

Extracorporeal lithotripsy breaks up gallstones with shock waves, thus reducing the hospital length of stay. Some can be done on an outpatient basis.

Objectives

1. Lose excess weight if needed. Avoid *rapid* weight loss, which can lead to gallstones.
2. Limit foods that cause pain or flatulence.
3. For the patient with *cholelithiasis,* overcome fat malabsorption caused by obstruction and prevent stagnation in a sluggish gallbladder, which may be caused by decreased bile secretion, bile stasis, bacteria, hormones, or fungi. Bacterial overgrowth alters bile acids so they no longer can emulsify fats.
4. Prevent biliary obstruction, cancer, and pancreatitis.
5. Provide fat-soluble vitamins if needed.

Dietary Recommendations

1. Provide a calorie-controlled, balanced diet. Use NPO during an acute attack.
2. For the patient with *acute cholecystitis,* use a fat-free diet. Progress to a diet with fewer condiments and gas-forming vegetables, which cause distention, increased peristalsis, and irritation.
3. For the patient with *chronic cholecystitis,* use a fat/calorie controlled diet to promote drainage of the gallbladder without excessive pain. The patient should consume adequate amounts of carbohydrates, especially fiber (such as pectin, which binds excess bile acids.)
4. For the patient with *cholelithiasis,* encourage a diet that is high in fiber and, when needed, low in calories.
5. Fat-soluble vitamins may need to be replaced in water-miscible forms.

Profile

Ht	Wt	Na^+
IBW/HBW	SGOT	Lipase (often ↑)
WBCs	Temp	Amylase
Jaundice	PT	Ca^{++}
Alb	H & H	Alk phos
Bilirubin (inc.)	Chol	GGT (↑)
Trig	K^+	

Side Effects of Common Drugs Used

1. *Chenodeoxycholic acid and lithium* may be used to dissolve small stones and prevent new formation if consumed daily for at least 6 months. Chenodiol (Chenix) may cause nausea, vomiting, or diarrhea; take with food or milk.
2. *Bile salts (Festal)* are used to facilitate fat metabolism. They contain protease, lipase, hemicellulose, amylase, and bile constituents.

3. *Antibiotics* may be used to counteract any infection.
4. *Oral contraceptives* and *estrogens* may increase risk for gallbladder diseases, especially after years of use.

Patient Education

1. After a *cholecystectomy*, fat intake should be limited for several months to allow the liver to compensate for the gallbladder's absence. Fats should be introduced gradually; excessive amounts of fat or bulky foods at one meal should be avoided.
2. Recommend weight control because stone formation can occur even after cholecystectomy.
3. Avoid fasting and rapid weight loss schemes.

Comments

Table 8–2.
Hypotheses for Risk Factors in GBD
Advanced Age
Sex (female)
Obesity with high fat intake
Hormonal imbalance (estrogen, progestin, insulin)
Drugs (OCs, clofibrate, cholestyramine)
Enzyme defects
Starchy foods (*Arch. Int. Med. 150*:1409, 1990)

JAUNDICE

Usual Hospital Stay

1–3 days.

Notation

A yellowish discoloration of the skin, mucous membranes, and some body fluids, jaundice results from accumulation of bile or bilirubin. It is a sign, not a disease itself. Causes include excessive RBC destruction, liver cell infection, and bile obstruction from gallstones, tumors or parasites.

Objectives

1. Coordinate efforts to lose or maintain ideal body weight.
2. Correct inadequate fat absorption.
3. Prevent osteopenia.

Dietary Recommendations

1. Use a high calorie, high protein diet with low fat intake, unless hepatic failure is imminent.
2. Supplement the diet with iron, calcium, vitamin K, and other nutrients. Check the need for vitamin D.
3. Exclude alcoholic beverages from the diet.
4. Monitor protein intake according to clinical status.

Profile

Ht	Chol (inc. if obstructive)	Trig
IBW/HBW		Alk phos
SGPT	SGOT	Ca^{++}
Serum ammonia	BUN	H & H
Alb	Bilirubin	Carotenoids (inc./dec.)
Serum lipase	Globulin	Gluc
Wt	Amylase	GGT

Side Effects of Common Drugs Used

1. *Bile salts (Festal)* may be used to correct faulty fat absorption if that is causative.
2. Avoid excesses of vitamins A and D.

Patient Education

1. Show the patient how to make appetizing meals that are low in fat.
2. Discuss the role of organs in digestion and absorption.

For More Information

American Liver Foundation
998 Pompton Ave.
Cedar Grove, NJ 07009

NOTES

HEPATITIS

Usual Hospital Stay

4 days.

Notation

Hepatitis is defined as liver inflammation resulting from infectious mononucleosis or cirrhosis, toxic materials (carbon tetrachloride), or viral infection (transmitted in food, liquids, or blood transfusions). It causes nausea, fever, liver tenderness and enlargement, jaundice, pale stools, and anorexia. Infectious (type A) has a rapid onset; Serum (type B) has a slow onset.

Objectives

1. Promote liver regeneration. Prevent further injury. Promote rest.
2. Prevent or correct weight loss, which often results from a poor appetite and nausea.
3. Replenish glycogen stores and correct hypoglycemia.
4. Prevent or alleviate hepatic coma, which may be a risk due to transient liver damage and therapy with a diet of normal to high protein intake.
5. Spare protein by providing a diet high in carbohydrates.
6. Force fluids to prevent dehydration, unless contraindicated.

Dietary Recommendations

1. For patients with acute hepatitis, provide nutrients with a 5% to 10% glucose solution with IV amino acids. BCAAs are acceptable.
2. As the patient progresses, use a liquid diet, and then a diet of small, frequent feedings of regular or soft foods. TPN only if necessary.
3. The diet should be high in calories (3000–4000 kcal). Intake of carbohydrates should be between 300–400 g, and intake of protein should be 90–100 g, or 1.5–2 g/kg body weight. Fat intake should be moderate to liberal (150 g), depending on tolerance.
4. Supplement the diet with vitamin B complex (especially thiamine and vitamin B_{12}), vitamin K (to normalize bleeding tendency), vitamin C, and zinc for impoverished appetite.
5. Extra fluid should be encouraged, unless contraindicated.

Profile

Ht	Wt	Gluc
IBW/HBW	Alb	Transferrin (inc. in
Globulin	BUN	acute stage)
Bilirubin (inc.)	Serum ammonia	H & H
SGOT (inc.)	SGPT	I & O

Alk phos (inc.)	Lipase	WBCs
Chol	Amylase ($\downarrow$)	GGT
LDH (inc.)	PT	

Side Effects of Common Drugs Used

1. *Analgesics* are used for pain.
2. *Steroids* may cause side effects (sodium retention, nitrogen depletion, or hyperglycemia).
3. *Antiemetics.*
4. Avoid excessive fat-soluble vitamin intake (vitamins A and D).

Patient Education

1. Ensure that the patient abstains from alcohol for at least 4–6 months.
2. Help the patient make attractive and appetizing meals, especially frequent small meals.
3. With anorexia and nausea, breakfast may be the largest meal.
4. Teach safe personal hygiene in regard to handwashing and disinfectants.

Comments

A and B types are viral (B from needle punctures, blood transfusions, etc.) Of persons with type B, 10% develop some form of chronic liver disease.

Non-A/non-B hepatitis involves contact with infected blood; symptoms are less evident—interferon may help.

With *chronic active hepatitis*, inflamed liver cells continue for years. It is usually an autoimmune response following type B or non-A/non-B hepatitis. Steroids may be needed in this form.

BILIARY CIRRHOSIS

Usual Hospital Stay

6 days.

Notation

Cholangiolitic hepatitis (obstructive jaundice) is caused by excessive storage of copper in the liver, spleen, and kidney. It causes progressive destruction of intrahepatic bile ducts. Symptoms include pruritus, jaundice, and portal HPN. Primary biliary cirrhosis is progressive, etiology unknown, perhaps an autoimmune response.

Objectives

1. Decrease copper stores; support effective cupresis.
2. Correct diarrhea, steatorrhea, malnutrition, and osteomalacia.
3. Limit or control other complications.

Dietary Recommendations

1. The diet can be limited in copper (approximately 2 g daily). It should limit nuts, shellfish, tea, cocoa, wheat germ, bran, chocolate, broccoli, and dried beans.
2. Increase vitamin D and calcium intake if osteopenia occurs.
3. Increase water-miscible sources of vitamins A, D, E, and K in steatorrhea.
4. Reduce cholesterol and saturated fats in hpercholesterolemia.

Profile

Ht	Transferrin	Ca^{++}
IBW/HBW	Globulin	Chol (inc.)
Alb	Jaundice	Ceruloplasmin
Serum Cu	Bilirubin (inc.)	Xanthomas
PT (dec.)	Gluc	SGOT/SGPT
Wt	Alk phos (inc.)	GGT

Side Effects of Common Drugs Used

1. *D-penicillamine* may be used to reduce circulating immune complexes.
2. *Cyclosporine* can be nephrotoxic over a long time.
3. *Cholestyramine* may be used to decrease bile acids.
4. *Colchicine* may cause diarrhea.

Patient Education

1. Instruct the patient about which foods are sources of copper in a diet.
2. Discuss the role of bile salts in fat and fat-soluble vitamin absorption.

NOTES

ALCOHOLIC LIVER DISEASE

Usual Hospital Stay

7–8 days.

Notation

Alcohol is a hepatotoxin. It is also ulcerogenic, usually to the esophagus. Nicotine-adenine dinucleotide (NAD) is the rate-limiting factor in the metabolism of alcohol. Metabolism of alcohol is slower during the deprivation of calories. Alcohol decreases absorption of fats, fat-soluble vitamins, thiamine, folic acid, and vitamin B_{12}. Alcohol dehydrogenase is made from zinc.

Detoxification takes 5–7 days; rehabilitation 2–3 weeks; convalescence 6–12 months. Symptoms and signs include restlessness, agitation, spider angiomas on face, insomnia, anorexia, weight loss, GI cramps, malnutrition, delirium tremens, and hand tremors. Counselors must understand addiction.

Objectives

1. Allow the disabled liver to function more effectively while protecting it from metabolic stress.
2. Prevent hypoglycemia from blocked gluconeogenesis. Correct alternate states of hyperglycemia, especially with hypertriglyceridemia.
3. Repair hepatic damage from fatty liver.
4. Repair neural damage from malnutrition.
5. Help liver tissue regenerate and replenish plasma proteins.
6. Correct fluid and electrolyte imbalances, nutritional deficits (anemia from chronic blood loss in varices, ulcers, etc.), and vomiting.
7. *Avoid alcohol.*
8. Be honest in approach; avoid playing games.

Dietary Recommendations

1. The diet should provide high amounts of protein (2 g/kg body weight), as well as adequate amounts of carbohydrates and fat to spare protein. Monitor CHO intake carefully in hyperglycemia and type IV HLP; monitor fat/cholesterol as well.
2. The diet should provide adequate intake of potassium.
3. Supplement the diet with B-complex. Synthetic folacin is also needed because the patient cannot use what is provided by the diet. The diet should provide adequate amounts of vitamins A, D, E, and K, as well as zinc and calcium.
4. Make the meals appetizing to stimulate appetite.
5. Use no alcohol in any form.

Profile

Ht	Trig (inc.)	H & H (dec.)
IBW/HBW	PT	Uric acid (inc.)
Gluc (inc. or dec.)	WBCs	Globulin
Serum ammonia	Serum B_{12}	Alk phos (inc.)
Chol	Serum folate	Transferrin

BP	I & O	TIBC
Wt	SGPT	Mg^{++} (dec.)
Ascites	SGOT (inc.)	Ca^{++}
BUN (may be low)	Bilirubin	Phosphorus (dec.)
Alb	K^+	

Side Effects of Common Drugs Used

1. *Antabuse (Disulfiram)* is given with the patient's consent. It causes the patient to vomit after ingesting alcohol and can be dangerous. Avoid alcohol in vinegar, sauces, and cough syrup.
2. *Insulin* may be necessary. Do not mix with alcohol.
3. Avoid excesses of vitamins A and D.
4. *Methylprednisolone* may be used in alcoholic hepatitis, with improved ability to produce albumin and to normalize PT and bilirubin levels.

Patient Education

1. Help the patient in the preparation of appetizing, nutrient-dense meals.
2. Instruct the patient in the sources of necessary nutrients in the diet, as well as the use of the prescribed multivitamins.
3. Explain that alcohol is the preferred fuel by the liver but cannot be used for muscular activity.
4. Zinc supplementation may improve a poor appetite.
5. Discuss the fact that chemical addiction is a disease. Self-help programs and follow-up reduce dependency.

Comments

Table 8–3.
Stages of Alcoholism—Related Effects
I. Obesity, HLP, HPN, diabetes
II. Hepatomegaly, hypertriglyceridemia, hypoalbuminemia
III. Chronic hepatitis, pancreatitis
IV. Cirrhosis
V. Encephalopathy
VI. Coma and death if untreated

For More Information

National Council on Alcoholism
733 Third Ave.
New York, NY 10017

Contact the local Alcoholics Anonymous, Al-Anon, or Ala-Teen

NOTES

ASCITES

Usual Hospital Stay

3–4 days.

Notation

Ascites is defined as fluid in the peritoneal cavity due to portal hypertension, low serum proteins, or sodium retention. It is seen in patients with hepatic cirrhosis, cardiac failure, or renal insufficiency, and may result from fluid loss from cells because of osmolar or nutrient imbalances. A distended abdomen results.

Objectives

1. Reduce fluid retention, usually by paracentesis.
2. Prevent potassium and electrolyte imbalances.
3. Prevent further distress, dyspnea, fatigue, loss of LBM, and anorexia.
4. Correct hepatorenal syndrome.
5. Individualize diet as needs change.

Dietary Recommendations

1. The diet should be high in potassium if serum levels so indicate.
2. Restrict the patient's intake of sodium (usually to 500–1000 mg). Increase the intake of sodium as retention subsides.
3. Fluid restriction may also be necessary (1–1.5 L/day); 2/3 with meals and 1/3 for thirst/medicines.
4. BEE is often 1.5, protein 1.25–1.75 g/kg IBW after paracentesis.
5. If TF or TPN is needed, a nutrient-dense formula may help.
6. Ensure RDAs for vitamins and minerals are adequate. Check signs of malnutrition.

Profile

Ht	Wt	TLC (dec.)
IBW/HBW	BP	I & O
Alb (dec.)	Globulin	Temp

K⁺	Na⁺	Chol, trig
BUN, creat	SGOT	Abd girth
SGPT	Transferrin	TSF, MAC
H & H	Gluc	

Side Effects of Common Drugs Used

1. *Diuretics.* Check whether the specific drug retains or spares potassium; if furosemide (Lasix) is used, added potassium is needed.
2. *Albumin replacement* may help maintain oncotic pressure.

Patient Education

1. Instruct the patient concerning good sources of potassium.
2. Ensure that the patient follows a low sodium diet. Explain which foods have hidden sources of sodium.
3. Salt substitutes (KCl, for example) can lower the pH of the ileum, making vitamin B_{12} absorption less effective. Discuss controlled intake.

Comments

Chylous ascites results from increased hydrostatic pressure and lymphatic blockade, with accumulation of LCT-dense chyle in the peritoneum; often from CA, trauma, or fistula. MCT is the preferred fat source, with the addition of EFAs. Adequate protein and calories are needed. PN is best, with extra zinc, vitamin C, and fat-soluble vitamins.

HEPATIC CIRRHOSIS

Usual Hospital Stay

7–8 days.

Notation

Hepatic cirrhosis is caused by chronic degeneration of the liver cells and thickening of the surrounding tissue. Symptoms and signs include fatigue, weight loss, lowered resistance, vomiting of blood, jaundice, and GI disturbances. It may result from severe malnutrition (seen in alcoholic patients), viral hepatitis, or other diseases. *Alcoholic cirrhosis,* also called Laennec's cirrhosis, is the 4th leading cause of death over age 40.

Objectives

1. Support residual liver function.
2. Provide supportive treatment for ascites, renal failure, esophageal varices, and portal hypertension.

3. Promote liver regeneration and healing. Correct fibrosis.
4. Prevent fat stasis and steatorrhea.
5. Correct nutritional deficiencies.
6. Prevent or correct protein intolerances. Drowsiness and disorientation are potential signs.
7. Provide adequate glucose for brain metabolism, but beware of glucose intolerance (common in 50–80% of patients), especially in alcoholic cirrhosis.
8. Prevent bone disease, hypokalemia, and anemia.
9. Prevent or correct decubitus ulcers.

Dietary Recommendations

1. The diet should be high in calories, with 1–2 g protein/kg body weight (a high percentage should be HBV proteins). It should also provide adequate carbohydrates to spare protein. Intake of methionine and choline should be high. 40–50% NP calories should be from fat.
2. Ensure that fat intake is moderate. Monitor use of medium-chain triglycerides; they may cause diarrhea and acidosis. Ensure adequate EFA intake.
3. Supplement diet with vitamin B-complex, vitamin C, vitamin K, zinc, magnesium-rich foods or supplements. Monitor need for vitamins A and D.
4. Encourage the use of vegetable proteins and BCAAs (pasta, vegetables, rice, fruits, and lima beans). Decrease BCAAs when patient is well.
5. If there is an *impending coma,* restrict the patient's intake of glycine, serine, threonine, glutamine, lysine, asparagine, and histidine. No mayonnaise, bleu or Cheddar cheese, margarine, French dressing, onions, relish, catsup, salami, or wine.
6. Avoid alcoholic beverages.
7. With steatorrhea, decrease LCTs.

Profile

Ht	PT (prolonged)	Mg^{++}
IBW/HBW	SGPT	Alk phos (inc.)
BUN	BP	WBCs
TSF	Na^+	Trig (inc.)
Wt; Wt. loss	Ca^{++}	Chol
Alb	Transferrin	Cu (inc.)
Globulin	H & H (dec.)	LDH (inc.)
TP	Ammonia	RBP, Prealbumin
Bowel changes	SGOT (inc.)	Free fatty acids (inc.)
UA	Bilirubin (inc.)	Ceruloplasmin (inc.)
Gluc (inc. or dec.)	K^+	Folate
		GGT

Side Effects of Common Drugs Used

1. *Albumin replacement* may be used. Check tolerance and encephalopathic status.
2. *Insulin* may be needed.
3. *Colchicine* has been demonstrated to improve survival of many patients with cirrhosis. More studies are being completed at this time.
4. Other drugs are used for patient-specific symptoms.

Patient Education

1. A better appetite at breakfast seems common. Encourage the patient to make breakfast the biggest meal of the day.
2. Dietary intake must be adjusted according to the changing status of the patient.
3. Large meals increase portal pressure. Ensure that the patient eats smaller meals.
4. Avoid skipping of meals. Discuss proper menu planning.
5. Avoid high doses of vitamin A, which can lead eventually to cirrhosis.

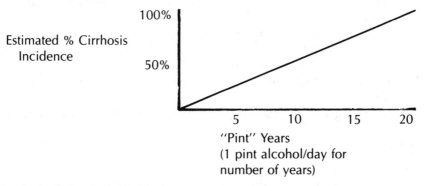

Fig. 8–1. Role of Alcohol in Creating Cirrhosis. (Lelbach)

PORTACAVAL-SPLENORENAL SHUNT FOR PORTAL HYPERTENSION

Usual Hospital Stay

21 days, surgical; 4–5 days hypertensive encephalopathy.

Notation

Portacaval blood flow is diverted from the liver by anastomosing portal vein to inferior vena cava. The shunt is performed for intrahepatic obstruction. Splenorenal shunting is done when flow is diverted from the liver by anastomosis of the splenic vein to the renal vein (done when the portal vein is obstructed). Portal hypertension contributes to esophageal varices, the most serious complication of cirrhosis.

Objectives

1. Support preoperative and postoperative medical care. The liver fares better when adequate glycogen stores are available.
2. Correct inadequate intake, which is a common problem.
3. Correct malabsorption and fatty liver.
4. Avoid excess fiber when esophageal varices are present.
5. Avoid encephalopathy and coma.
6. Normalize amino acid patterns.

Dietary Recommendations

1. Provide TPN or TF when needed; increased BCAAs seem to be beneficial.
2. Control fluid intake—prevent dehydration and overhydration.
3. No alcoholic beverages should be consumed.
4. If needed, an IV with Freamine can be added to other therapeutic approaches.
5. Progress as tolerated to a regulated protein, adequate to high carbohydrate, controlled sodium (lower with ascites), adequate calorie diet.
6. Provide a multivitamin/mineral supplement if needed, especially ensuring that fat-soluble vitamins A, D, E and K are available in an appropriate form.
7. Generally, 1–1.5 g protein/kg if patient is not comatose can be tolerated.

Profile

Ht, Wt	IBW, HBW	Gluc
PT	Alb	H & H
Nausea, vomiting	Jaundice	Globulin
Ammonia (inc.)	BUN, Creat	Urea
I & O	GGT	Tarry stools
Na^+, K^+		Ca^{++}, Mg^{++}
SGOT, SGPT		

Side Effects of Common Drugs Used

Antibiotics may be needed for bacterial infections. Extensive use may deplete vitamin K levels.

Patient Education

1. The importance of dietary regulation should be addressed extensively.
2. The patient should be advised to omit alcoholic beverages from the diet, probably permanently.
3. The patient should eat slowly and chew well.

NOTES

LIVER TRANSPLANTATION

Usual Hospital Stay

17–18 days.

Notation

Liver transplantation is now a viable alternative for patients with end-stage hepatic failure, usually from cirrhosis, hepatitis, chronic active liver disease, α_1 antitrypsin deficiency, cholangiocarcinoma, primary biliary cirrhosis. Patients are carefully screened for other underlying conditions; many will not be suitable for transplantation.

Symptoms and signs generally leading to the need for transplant include ascites, jaundice, edema, CNS dysfunction, and cachexia.

Objectives

1. Enhance liver cell function to correct malnutrition, lessen edema, and prevent rejection.
2. Prevent or correct catabolic wasting of muscle mass with increased hormonal levels (insulin, glucagon, epinephrine and cortisol may be elevated).
3. Reduce fluid and electrolyte imbalances.
4. Provide nutritional support in an appropriate mode of feeding (considering nausea, vomiting, etc.) to provide a normalized nitrogen balance and other normalized lab values.
5. Promote normalized protein synthesis in the liver (i.e., albumin, globulins, clotting factors, etc.).
6. Prevent or correct hyperglycemia, fasting hypoglycemia, abnormal glucagon storage.

7. Correct any fat malabsorption, with or without steatorrhea or diarrhea.
8. Correct abnormal amino acid metabolism and neural accumulation of amino acids that are precursors for dopamine, serotonin, and norepinephrine. Normalize serum ammonia.
9. Postoperatively, support wound healing.

Dietary Recommendations

1. Protein requirements may be 1.3–2.0 g/kg dry weight, unless in encephalopathy.
2. Adequate calories are needed—35–45 kcal/kg est. dry weight, or 1.5–1.75 × BEE.
3. Decrease long chain fatty acids; increase MCTs. 25–40% of total calories as fat may be needed. Decrease simple sugars if glucose is elevated.
4. Increase BCAAs and decrease aromatic amino acids (tyrosine, phenylalanine, tryptophan). Parenteral Hepatamine may be useful. Hepatic Aid or Travasorb Hepatic may be beneficial with enteral feedings. In patients with encephalopathy, decreasing methionine may also be necessary.
5. Mineral supplementation may be helpful (calcium, magnesium, zinc) if muscle cramps or altered taste acuity are noted.
6. Adequate vitamin intake will be essential to maintain immunity, and to support wound healing. Beware of excesses because of liver functioning.
7. Alter sodium and potassium intakes according to profile. Usually sodium is maintained at a maximum of 2–4 g. Hyperkalemia can be a problem with cyclosporine.
8. If TF, use a low volume, diluting concentration as needed. TPN if needed.

Profile

Ht, Wt, Present Wt	IBW/HBW	H & H
BUN, Creat	Bilirubin	Transferrin
Alb, Prealbumin	Serum ammonia	Urea
N Balance	Edema	BP
I & O	CSF	Chol, Trig.
Amino acid profiles	Mg^{++}, Ca^{++}	Carotenoids
Na^+, K^+	Nausea, vomiting	SGOT, SGPT, GGT
		Gluc

Side Effects of Common Drugs Used

1. *Cyclosporine*—as indicated, hyperkalemia may be a concern. Monitor carefully. HPN may also occur, or HLP, ↓ Mg^{++}, nausea or vomiting as well.

2. *Steroids* can decrease nitrogen balance and potassium, calcium, and magnesium while increasing sodium retention. Decrease caffeine intake if needed because of GI distress.
3. *Insulin* may be necessary during periods of hyperglycemia.
4. *Furosemide* (Lasix) and other diuretics may be needed with edema. Assess each medication's effects.
5. *Lactulose* and neomycin are often used. See other Hepatic entries.
6. Monitor effects of *bile acid sequestrants*.
7. Other *immunosuppressants*, such as *azathioprine*, can cause mouth sores, nausea, vomiting, stomach pain, etc. *Muromonab-CD³* can cause nausea, vomiting, diarrhea, and anorexia.

Patient Education

1. Snacks such as brownies or custards can be made which contain BCAAs and other supplemental nutrients.
2. Discuss the role of diet in wound healing, graft retention, and improvement in health status.
3. Recipes for no-added-salt and sugar-free foods may be needed; provide to patient or family as appropriate.
4. Discuss sources of HBV foods, calcium and magnesium foods, etc. Individualize to patient preferences and needs.
5. Discuss the need for such services as alcohol rehabilitation, family counseling and other available services. ETOH abuse affects such key nutrients as niacin, folate, vitamin B_{12}, zinc, phosphorus, and magnesium.
6. Obesity can occur unless fat and CHO intakes are controlled.

NOTES

HEPATIC ENCEPHALOPATHY, FAILURE, OR COMA

Usual Hospital Stay

4 days.

Notation

Hepatic failure is common in critical illnesses. Decreased dopamine and elevated serotonin can occur, as well as decreased BCAAs and increased aromatic AAs.

Coma is a potentially serious complication of advanced liver disease. The following are signs of an impending coma:

1. Irritability, change in mentation.
2. Disorientation to time and place.
3. Asterixis, or metabolic flap (involuntary jerky movements, especially of hands).
4. Constructional apraxia (inability to draw simple diagrams).
5. Difficulty in writing.
6. Ascites, edema, fetor hepaticas (sweet, musty odor of the breath).
7. Bleeding.

Objectives

1. Limit protein concentration in the intestines to decrease ammonia and toxin production. Normalize amino acid patterns.
2. Avoid hypoglycemia. Provide adequate O_2 and glucose and brain functions.
3. Avoid tissue catabolism from altered catabolic hormone levels.
4. Promote regeneration of liver tissue.
5. Support other systems (respiratory, neurological, GI, circulatory) while liver regenerates.
6. Correct anemia or nutritional deficits.
7. Prevent hypokalemia, sepsis, starvation, and acute crises.
8. Reduce circulating amines and lessen shunting of blood around the liver.
9. Control hemorrhage and blood loss into the gut.

Dietary Recommendations

1. For the patient with *coma*, use tube feeding or parenteral nutrition. Control protein intake; ensure higher intake of BCAAs. It may be helpful to use Hepatic Aid II or similar products. Freamine, Aminosol and Hepatamine* are for PN.
2. For the patient who is not comatose, the diet should provide moderate restrictions of protein (in the form of HBV proteins). If severe, restrict protein intake further and advance by increments of 10–20 g as the patient's condition improves. BCAAs can be added to PN or EN solutions by the pharmacist. Generally, 0.6–0.8 g/kg is acceptable.

---

*35% BCAAs—leucine is most essential.

3. To minimize muscle catabolism, the diet should provide 1800 kcal/day or more. Adequate intake of carbohydrates and fats is needed; 30 kcal/kg IBW is common.
4. Ensure adequate intake of fluids and electrolytes as monitoring determines. Often, sodium is limited to aid diuresis.
5. Use more milk, pasta, and vegetables; less meat.
6. Restrict fluid only with dilutional hyponatremia; usually 1000–1500 cc.
7. Vitamin-mineral supplements may be needed (vitamins A, D, E, and K, niacin, thiamine, phosphate, and zinc). Calcium or magnesium may be supplemented as needed. Monitor fat-soluble vitamin use with damaged liver.

Profile

Ht	Alb (dec.)	Gluc (dec.)
IBW/HBW	Wt	Globulin (dec.)
BUN (dec.)	SGOT (inc.)	Plasma AAs
Bilirubin (inc.)	PT	(isoleucine,
Alk phos (inc.)	Ca^{++}	leucine,
SGPT, GGT	Na^+	valine,
Mg^{++}	BP	tryptophan,
H & H (dec.)	Transferrin	phenylalanine
K^+	Prealbumin, RBP	tyrosine)
Chol, Trig	N balance	Serum insulin,
UA	I & O	epinephrine
Ammonia		adrenocorticol
		steroids,
		thyroxine

Side Effects of Common Drugs Used

1. *Neomycin*. Used to destroy intestinal bacteria, neomycin treatment is started before protein restriction begins. This drug alters the absorption of most nutrients, and can cause nausea, vomiting, diarrhea, sore mouth, elevated BUN/creatinine.
2. *Lactulose* (Cephulac, Chronulac) is used to decrease ammonia and aromatic AA formation and to improve protein tolerance. Constipation, nausea, and diarrhea may occur.
3. *Levodopa* is used to relieve psychiatric symptoms. It may also be necessary to restrict protein intake with this drug, and to watch the vitamin B_6 content of the diet.

Patient Education

1. Milk and eggs produce less ammonia than meats do.
2. Explain that guidelines for hepatic cirrhosis also apply.

Comments

Table 8–4.

Nutrient Relationships in Hepatic Failure and Hepatic Encephalopathy

Decreased protein—swollen belly (ascites) from decreased albumin production

Decreased niacin—memory loss

Decreased folacin—degeneration of spinal cord

Decreased B-complex, iron and protein—glossitis, anemias

Decreased vitamins C and K—hemorrhage, scurvy

Decreased zinc—poor taste acuity, impaired wound healing

Decreased magnesium, niacin, thiamine—hallucinations, delirium, beriberi, pellagra

Increased Na^+ and fluid—fluid retention

Decreased thiamine—amnesia, confabulation, Korsakoff's psychosis

Decreased vitamin A—increased respiratory infections

Decreased vitamin K—muscle weakness

Decreased protein and fat with malabsorption—somnolence, euphoria, asterixis, coma

Decreased magnesium—marked anxiety, hyperirritability, confusion, seizures, tremor

---

CHOLESTATIC LIVER DISEASE

Usual Hospital Stay

4 days.

Notation

Cholestasis interferes with excretion of the bile salts required for emulsification and absorption of dietary fat. A deficiency of fat-soluble vitamins may occur. Of particular concern is vitamin E, which tends to be low in this condition for reasons not well established. Vitamin E circulates in the blood almost exclusively attached to the lipoprotein fractions.

In cholestatic liver disease, biliary obstruction can occur, with hyperlipidemia and accumulation of copper resulting.

Symptoms and signs can include glossitis from B-complex deficiency, protein and iron deficiency, hemorrhagic tendencies due to vitamins C or K inadequacy, and flatulence.

Objectives

1. Promote return of normal liver function and bile flow.
2. Correct fat malabsorption and deficiency of any nutrients.
3. Correct steatorrhea if present.

Dietary Recommendations

1. A low fat diet may be beneficial during acute stages or pain.
2. Water-miscible forms of fat-soluble vitamins A, D, E, and K may be needed. Vitamin E may be given intramuscularly if malabsorption is severe.
3. Some research suggests the need for adequate taurine, especially if the patient is fed by tube feeding or TPN.
4. Carnitine may be beneficial for some patients.
5. Small, frequent feedings and snacks may be better tolerated than large meals.

Profile

Ht, Wt	Bilirubin (inc.)	Serum carotene (inc.
Chol, Trig (inc.)	Alk phos (inc.)	or dec.)
PT (prolonged)	RBP	Transferrin
SGOT/SGPT (inc.)	Bun, Creat	Globulin
Serum Fe	H & H	Serum cholic acid
IBW/HBW	Alb	GGT
		Amylase, lipase

Side Effects of Common Drugs Used

Bile salts may be needed with extensive malabsorption.

Patient Education

1. Discuss the role of fat in normal metabolic processes; simplify the explanation in correlation to absorption of the fat-soluble vitamins and other nutrients affected by the liver.
2. Discuss ways to increase satiety from the diet with appetizing recipes.

Section 9
Endocrine Disorders

Chief Assessment Factors

fatigue

numbness

tingling, paresthesias

bone pain

headache

seizures

syncope

anorexia, nausea

abdominal pain

weight changes

shortness of breath

hoarseness

decreased libido

dysuria

frequent infections

pruritus

altered consciousness

hormone imbalances

Table 9–1.
Endocrine Gland Functions

Gland	Functions	Hormones
Pituitary (Anterior)	growth, lactation, control of other endocrine glands	(ACTH, growth hormone, (corticotropin) gonadotropins (FSH, LH)
Pituitary (Posterior)— Hypothalamus	body temperature regulation, sleep, behavior, appetite, emotional response	oxytocin, vasopressin, corticotropin-releasing factor, pitocin
Thyroid	growth and development, metabolism	thyroxine, triiodothyronine
Pancreas	control of many metabolic functions, blood glucose control	glucagon (A cells), insulin (B cells), gastrin (D cells)
Pineal Gland	skin blanching	melatonin
Thymus	immunity/T cells/ lymphocytes	thymosin
Gonads	reproduction	estrogen, progesterone, androgens
Andrenal glands	control of many hormones (28 total)	mineralocorticoids, glucocorticoids, androgens (adrenal cortex) epinephrine/ norepinephrine (adrenal medulla)
Parathyroids	regulation of calcium/ phosphorus	parathormone, calcitonin

Anabolic Hormones
   growth hormone, androgens, sex hormones

Catabolic Hormones
   stress hormones (causing gluconeogenesis from protein) such as catecholamines (epinephrine, norepinephrine), glucocorticoids (cortisone, cortisol), and glucagon.

For More Information of Diabetes

American Diabetes Association
1660 Duke St.
Alexandria, VA 22314
800-ADA-DISC (232-3472)

National Institutes of Diabetes and Digestive and Kidney Diseases
   (NIDDKD)
National Institutes of Health
Bethesda, MD 20892

National Diabetes Information Clearinghouse
Westwood Bldg., Room 603
Bethesda, MD 20205

TYPE I, INSULIN-DEPENDENT DIABETES MELLITUS (IDDM)

Usual Hospital Stay

4–5 days.

Notation

Diabetes mellitus is the No. 3 killer in the U.S., usually related to CHD or stroke. It is the chief cause of blindness, renal failure and amputations. In the third world nations, type I diabetes results from decreased protein/high CHO diets; insulin is often not available there.

Resulting from a defect in the pancreatic beta cells (the islets of Langerhans), insulin-dependent diabetes mellitus may be related to the adrenal cortex, thyroid, anterior pituitary gland, etc. Onset often follows viral infection such as mumps. IDDM accounts for 10% of all cases of DM. Old names included "juvenile," "brittle," or "ketosis-prone" diabetes.

Objectives

1. Encourage regular mealtimes plus interval feedings. If necessary, make two plans—one for weekdays, one for weekends.
2. Achieve and maintain IBW according to age. Assess whether insulin has caused weight gain, making loss difficult. Children need 75–90 kcal/kg IBW.
3. Determine the patient's meal pattern according to the type of insulin and the frequency of injection. If more than 45 units are used, the patient is probably insulin-resistant; multiple doses and meal regulation may be needed.
4. Prevent or minimize complications:

Acute (See NIDDM entry). The *Somogyi effect* is defined as hormonal rebounding effects of insulin/blood sugar levels. Hypoglycemia or fasting hyperglycemia occurs, with potentially dangerous results. Check 3 AM BS.

Intermediate. Children's growth and development are impaired. Add 300–500 kcal for pregnancy and lactation, plus extra iron, calcium, protein, and folic acid.

Chronic. Achieve and maintain normal blood glucose and lipids. Common complications include CHD, osteoporosis, retinopathy, neuropathy, nephropathy, anorexia nervosa or bulimia.

Dietary Recommendations

1. Serve three meals daily plus scheduled snacks: 50–60% CHO, 15–20% protein*, 20–25% fat.
2. Teach the basic four food categories, use of exchanges, and calorie content of foods. Children benefit from unmeasured, sugar-controlled diets.
3. Severely limit or omit simple sugars. Increase intake of complex carbohydrates (fiber) as with high CHO/high fiber diets (25 gms/1000-kcal) from rice, beans, vegetables, barley, and oat bran. Pectin and guar gum are beneficial.
4. Include adequate chromium and potassium.
5. Prevent ketosis by including at least 40–45% carbohydrates daily.
6. Encourage control of reduction in total sodium, cholesterol, and saturated fat intake. Cut down or eliminate fried, creamed, and scalloped foods.
7. Assess dietary history, physical exercise and activity patterns. Discuss use of artificial sweeteners, alcohol, and food diaries. Alcohol calories = 0.8 × proof × No. oz.
8. Determine appropriate calorie level for age, with pregnancy or growth receiving more. Sedentary = 15–20 kcal/kg; normal = 30 kcal/kg; undernourished or active = 45–50 kcal/kg. For *children*, average is 1500 kcal at age 6, 2000 kcal at 11; 2400–2700 kcal teen girls, and 3100–3600 kcal teen boys. Reassess as activity changes.
9. Glucose and vitamin C compete for uptake. Vitamin C and B-complex are needed for cases of infection, polyuria, ketoacidosis.
10. Fish, garlic and amylose are suggested in research for control of blood lipids and glucose. More studies are needed. Studies are also needed for glycemic index results with a mixed diet.
11. Include adequate vitamin A since carotene is poorly converted.
12. Vitamin E may be protective against angiopathy.

Profile

Ht	Fasting glucose
IBW/HBW	Hgb A_1c (normal, less than 7%)
GTT results	Chol—HDL/LDL
BUN	Urine glucose
Trig	BP
Urinary ketones	CA^{++}, Mg^{++}
K^+, Na^+	PO_4
Wt	

---

*There is some evidence that controlled *protein* intake (e.g. 40 g HBV) will slow down progression of nephropathy and increase HDL—cholesterol. There is no final conclusion. Children under 3 need 2.5 g protein/kg; adults need 0.8–1 g protein/kg. More protein is needed in ketogenesis states.

Side Effects of Drugs Used

1. Insulin/diet correlation is essential to avoid nausea or anorexia. *Insulin is affected by timing of meals:*
   a. Long-acting—PZI or ultralente—onset 4–8 hrs., peak 10–30 hrs., duration 36 hrs.
   b. Intermediate—NPH or lente—onset 1–2.5 hrs., peak 7–15 hrs., duration 24 hrs.
   c. Short-acting—Regular—onset 1/2–1 hr., peak 2–5 hrs., duration 6–8 hrs.
      Continuous subcutaneous insulin infusion (CSII) may be good for triglyceride levels. A pump is used; meal schedules are not as strict but should not be abused.
2. Vitamin C in high doses can give false-positive urinary glucose results. Check use of supplements.
3. Check drugs for content of sugars and alcohol.

Patient Education

1. Teach the patient the symptoms of ketosis, since insulin-dependent patients are prone to it.
2. Teach the patient the importance of self-care and optimal functioning; what to do during illness or stress; how to dine away from home; how to read labels; when to use sweeteners, fructose, sorbitol; and the role of exercise in dietary control.
3. Teach the patient about potassium in the production of insulin.
4. Encourage regular mealtimes and snacks; same size/total quantity.
5. In fever, decrease intake by about 20% because of stress hyperglycemia. However, be careful to avoid ketosis.
6. Discuss typical downfalls—restaurants, food offers from others.
7. Discuss dietary compliance (i.e., careful adherence to dietary pattern with rare indiscretions).
8. Key factors in success include self-discipline, emotional stability, positive influence from others, work and social events under control, and economics.
9. Discuss visual assessment of portions. Practice with scales if necessary.
10. Frequent follow-up visits are helpful (at least every 2 weeks for the first 2 months, then monthly for the rest of the year).
11. *Glycemic Index* (GI) yields white bread @ 100, cornflakes @ 119, apples @ 53, instant potatoes @ 116, sucrose @ 86, milk @ 49, soybeans @ 22. A mixed diet yields varying results on blood glucose levels. The index is very controversial.

Comments

Table 9–2.

Sugar and Sweeteners: Some Facts

Sugar (sucrose)	16 kcal/t. (4 g CHO)
Saccharin	300–400 × sweeter than sugar
Fructose	11 kcal/t. (3 g CHO))
Sorbitol	50% as sweet as sucrose; it is a sugar alcohol
Xylitol	16 kcal/t. (4 g CHO)
Aspartame	180 times sweeter than sugar; 4 kcal/g
Acesulfame-K (Sunette)	200 times sweeter than sugar and suited for baking

---

TYPE II, NON-INSULIN-DEPENDENT DIABETES MELLITUS (NIDDM)

Usual Hospital Stay

7 days.

Notation

Patients with non-insulin-dependent diabetes mellitus have beta-cell dysfunction and insulin resistance in peripheral tissues (muscle, liver, fat). Hyperinsulinism decreases insulin receptors (down regulation).

NIDDM accounts for 90% of all DM and affects 10,000,000 Americans. The majority (80%) are overweight. Risk factors include genetics, obesity and age. Rates of NIDDM are high among American Indians, blacks, and Mexican Americans. Tailoring of their diets will be important.

Old names of NIDDM include "Adult-Onset," "Maturity-Onset," "Ketosis-Resistant" diabetes.

Objectives

1. Achieve and maintain IBW. The patient's caloric needs are determined by multiplying the IBW by ten for the basal value, and then adding three times the IBW for sedentary, five times IBW for moderately active, and ten times IBW for very active patients. If the patient needs to gain weight add 500 or more kcal to the normal diet; if the patient needs to lose weight subtract a minimum of 500 kcal per day. These dietary changes will yield a gain or loss of 1 lb per week, respectively.
2. The diet should be nutritionally adequate: three meals per day, small bedtime snack. Maintain the diet through behavior modification, a structured diet, and planned activities.
3. Improve beta-cell functioning.

4. Prevent or minimize complications:

Acute. For patients with *hyperglycemia* (nocturia, polydipsia, polyuria), values under 130 mg/dl two-thirds of the time are preferred.* For patients with *glucosuria*, 80% negative urines are desired.* *Hypoglycemia* can cause confusion, sweating, tremors, hunger, dizziness, irritability, weakness, and nightmares. Keep simple sugars on hand.

Chronic. Complications include hypertension, hyperlipidemia, retinopathy, nephropathy, neuropathy, and coronary heart disease.

Dietary Recommendations

1. Three meals a day—if patient requests a snack, give a small snack at bedtime. 50–60% CHO, 15–20% protein, 25–30% fat should be maintained.
2. Teach the basic four food categories, proper caloric intake, and the concept of energy metabolism. Teach food exchanges only at the patient's request.
3. Simple sugars are limited.[†] Use more complex carbohydrates—like the high CHO/high fiber diets, (25 g fiber/1000 kcal)—rice, beans, vegetables, oat bran, legumes, barley, produce with skins, apples. Soluble fiber should be high.
4. Limit intake of cholesterol to less than 300 mg daily. Ensure that only 10% of total fat intake is saturated.
5. As a preventive measure, limit intake of sodium to 3–4 g per day.
6. Ensure that the patient has an adequate intake of chromium, potassium, vitamins A, C, and E.
7. To prevent ketosis, ensure that intake of carbohydrate is at least 80 to 100 g. Fasting diets (e.g. 400–600 kcal) should only be done in a hospital setting.
8. Assess dietary history, physical exercise, and activity patterns. Discuss use of artificial sweeteners, alcohol and food diaries.

Profile

Ht, Wt	Body mass index, waist-to-hip
IBW/HBW	ratio (WHR)[‡]
GTT results	Hgb A_1c
BUN, Creatinine	Chol (usually low HDL/high
Trig (inc.)	LDL)
Urinary ketones	Urinary gluc
K^+, Nat$^+$	BP (inc.)

---

*Albert Einstein School of Medicine, Diabetes Research and Training Center.

[†]Limit simple sugars to no more than 5% total in lean patients and in persons without type IV HLP.

[‡]Upper body (android) obesity is more strongly associated with NIDDM than lower body (gynoid) obesity. (NIH Consensus Development Conference, Dec. 1986).

Fasting gluc
SGOT, SGPT
LDH, Alk Phos

Ca^+, Mg^{++}
PO_4

Side Effects of Drugs Commonly Used

1. *Sulfonylureas*: tolazamide (Tolinase), tolbutamide (Orinase), and chlorpropamide (Diabinese). Avoid alcohol, which can cause an Antabuse-like reaction. Diarrhea, GI distress, nausea, vomiting, and metallic taste may also occur.
2. Large dose of *vitamin C* can cause false positive urinary glucose levels.
3. *Insulin* may be needed for stress, infection, or pregnancy.
4. Other *oral hypoglycemia agents* (OHAs) may be used—glyburide (Diabeta and Micronase), and glipizide (Glucotrol). Nausea, GI distress, diarrhea, and heartburn may occur.
5. *Steroids, beta-blockers,* and *diuretics* may cause hyperglycemia.

Patient Education

1. Emphasize the importance of regular mealtimes and the types of allowed snacking.
2. Emphasize the importance of self-care and optimal functioning. Include instructions on how to handle illness, stress, dining out, exercise, label reading, and how to use sucrose or fructose and sugar alcohols.
3. Differentiate between "dietetic" and "diabetic" in food labeling.
4. Discuss handling parties and food offers from others.
5. Encourage group support, behavior modification and nutritional counseling for overweight persons.
6. Small-step changes lead to greater self-esteem than continued failures at change. Sequential rather than simultaneous dietary manipulations work better for most people.
7. Purified fiber supplements should not be recommended.

Comments

1. *Hypertension* is common (2.5 million people have both hypertension and diabetes). Maintain IBW; prevent hypokalemia, which can blunt insulin release; control glucose; use 10–15% protein, 25–30% fat, 50–55% CHO; omit alcohol and smoking; add exercise.
2. For *Diabetic Nephropathy*, liberalize CHO intake and restrict protein to 0.5–-0.8 g/kg IBW (75% HBV, 25% LBV). Control insulin levels accordingly. Prevent hypoalbuminemia and loss of lean body mass. Slow the progression of ESRD. Diagnosis involves persistently positive urinary albumin over 0.3 g/dl in the absence of other renal disease. Control of HPN is also necessary. Diabetes is now the leading cause of ESRD, especially among blacks, Mexican Americans, and American Indians. The onset of ESRD is 5.7 years after noted renal damage.

NOTES

DIABETIC GASTROPARESIS

Usual Hospital Stay

4 days.

Notation

Gastroparesis occurs in 20–30% of all diabetics, with delayed gastric emptying (heartburn, nausea, abdominal pain, vomiting, early satiety, and weight loss for some persons). The condition occurs as a result of vagal autonomic neuropathy. The problems occur more in IDDM than in NIDDM.

Objectives

1. Reduce or control pain, diarrhea, and constipation.
2. Ensure adequate intake of diabetic diet as prescribed to prevent weight loss.
3. Prevent further symptoms and problems.
4. Prevent ketoacidosis, which can aggravate the condition.
5. Prevent bezoar formation.

Dietary Recommendations

1. Monitor intake carefully to replace CHO with tolerated foods. Blood sugar delays its return to normal in hypoglycemia with gastroparesis.
2. Six small meals may be better tolerated than large meals.
3. Alter fiber intake according to needs (diarrhea, constipation, etc.).
4. If patient complains of dry mouth, add extra fluids and moisten foods with broth or allowed sauces or gravies.
5. In severe problems, a jejunostomy tube feeding may be indicated.
6. Soft to liquid diet and low fat (40 g) may be useful to prevent delay in gastric emptying.

Profile

Ht, Wt	IBW/HBW	Gluc
Hgb A_1c	H & H	Alb
Abd pain	Gastrin	Chol, trig

Side Effects of Common Drugs Used

1. *Metoclopramide* (Reglan) may be given 30 minutes before meals to increase gastric contractions and to relax pyloric sphincter. Dry mouth or nausea can be side effects.
2. *Insulin* should be matched with meals to monitor delayed absorption and glucose changes.

Patient Education

1. Discuss the source of pain and problems.
2. Discuss the role of diet in maintaining weight and controlling pain. Emphasize nutrient-dense foods if intake has been poor.
3. Bezoar formation is common with oranges, coconuts, and green beans, apples, figs, potato skins, Brussels sprouts, and sauerkraut.

NOTES

DIABETIC KETOACIDOSIS OR DIABETIC COMA

Usual Hospital Stay

6 days.

Notation

Diabetic Ketoacidosis (DKA) is a medical emergency, with mortality from 5–15%. Alkaline reserves may be depleted by infection, too little insulin, fever, pregnancy, stress, trauma, insulin resistance, less activity, or too much food. Preceding coma, symptoms and signs include intense thirst, nausea and vomiting, dim vision, labored breath, and sweet acetone breath, pruritus, polyuria, and hot and dry flushed skin. Hyperketonemia from DKA results in classic metabolic acidosis.

Objectives

1. Allow hyperglycemia and glucosuria to subside. Provide insulin.*
2. Replace depleted electrolytes and fluids.
3. Promote return to wellness, since patient has most likely been in poor health for several days preceding acidosis.
4. Control precipitating factors, such as surgery, MI, or trauma.
5. Prevent complications, such as shock.

Dietary Recommendations

1. If the patient is in a coma, intravenous insulin, electrolytes, and fluids are used.
2. As treatment progresses, a 5% glucose solution is usually given as glucosuria and hyperglycemia subside. If glucosuria and hyperglycemia do not decrease, try tea and salty broth. Later, fruit juices and liquids high in potassium may be given.
3. Eventually, return to usual diet. Monitor closely.

Profile

Ht	Gluc (350–750 mg/dl)	Temp
IBW/HBW	Pco_2 (dec.)	HCO_3
Blood pH	Acetone (inc.)	Phosphate (dec.)
BUN, creat	BP	Chol (inc.)
K^+, Na^+ Cl^- (dec.)	Uric acid (inc.)	I & O
Hgb, A_1c	Trig	Mg^{++}
Wt	SGOT (dec.)	pH below 7.3
Amylase (inc.)	SGPT, LDH, CK ($\uparrow$)	bicarbonate < 15 mmol/L

Patient Education

1. Explain the role of food and insulin during illness and infection.
2. Explain the role of exercise in lowering blood glucose levels.
3. Ensure that there is adequate fiber in the patient's diet.
4. Beware of the Somogyi effect; discuss.

NOTES

*Frequent monitoring is necessary. For IDDM, the physician must be contacted if glucose levels do not return to normal. For NIDDM, the physician may suggest increase in use of regular insulin during this times.

HYPEROSMOLAR HYPERGLYCEMIC NONKETOTIC DEHYDRATION OR COMA

Usual Hospital Stay

6 days.

Notation

HHNK dehydration involves a metabolic disorder that compromises osmosis, leading to increased serum osmolality. Blood glucose is extremely elevated but ketosis does not exist. The condition is common in elderly patients with NIDDM.

Symptoms and signs include polydipsia, polyuria, nausea and vomiting, diarrhea, fever, hypertension, respirations that are normal to rapid, profound dehydration, lethargy, confusion, grand mal seizures, tachycardia, hypotension, oliguria.

Predisposing factors include pancreatic disease, sepsis, surgery, extensive burns, infections, renal or cardiovascular disease, cortisol steroid use, diuretics, TPN, dialysis, and excessive tube feeding.

Objectives

1. Prevent or correct dehydrated state, shock, cardiac arrhythmias, and death.
2. Monitor fluid status (deficits may be 10–20% of total body weight).
3. Reduce elevated blood glucose levels, generally with isotonic saline and then hypotonic saline.
4. Prevent future crises by appropriate patient/caretaker education.

Dietary Recommendations

1. Patient is likely to be NPO during a crisis, or perhaps tube fed during comatose state.
2. As appropriate, the intake may be progressed gradually to a balanced diet, controlling calories as needed.
3. Offer fluids as ordered, 1–2 liters in 24 hours.
4. Potassium may be needed; check serum levels.

Profile

Ht, Wt	Wt. changes	Alb
IBW/HBW	BUN, creat	H & H
K^+	Na^+	I & O
Bicarbonate	BP	Ketones
Hyperosmolality (us. over 350–475)	Gluc (under 600 mg/dl)	PO_4

Side Effects of Common Drugs Used

Insulin may be needed to normalize blood glucose levels.

Patient Education

1. Discuss, where possible, predisposing factors, how to avoid future incidents, etc.
2. Calorie-controlled diets may be beneficial if the patient can comprehend. Family intervention may be required.

NOTES

HYPOGLYCEMIA

Usual Hospital Stay

4–5 days.

Notation

True low blood sugar (40 mg% or lower) releases hormones, such as the catecholamines, that produce hunger, trembling, headache, dizziness, weakness and palpitations. Many different causes can stimulate hypoglycemia, and treatments through dietary means will differ accordingly.

The body makes great effort to supply glucose for the central nervous system and for the red blood cells.

Fasting hypoglycemia—glandular problem that has many potential causes. It may be related to an islet cell tumor, or may occur with fasting.

Postprandial hypoglycemia—reactive hypoglycemia that occurs 1.5–5 hrs after meals, especially carbohydrate-rich meals.

Objectives

1. Minimize length of time between times of eating.
2. Prevent seizures and coma in true hypoglycemia (i.e., neuroglycopenia with confusion, light-headaches, aberrant behavior, seizures and frank coma.)
3. Normalize blood glucose levels.

4. Stabilize blood glucose levels through normal mealtimes and meal consistency.

Dietary Recommendations

1. *Fasting Hypoglycemia.* Use a normal diet with adequate to high levels of carbohydrates. Have the patient ingest fruit juice or carry candy as needed. Fat is not as effective in normalizing blood glucose. Frequent feedings may be beneficial.
2. *Postprandial/Reactive Hypoglycemia.* Because the response may occur in response to a high carbohydrate load, use a balanced diet with a reduction in concentrated sweets. If necessary, limit CHO to 100 g daily and increase protein intake accordingly. Use more soluble fibers (fruits, vegetables), but avoid concentrated sugar in dried fruits. Try 3 meals + 3 snacks daily.
3. *Leucine-Induced Hypoglycemia.* The diet should be limited in leucine (i.e., 150–230 mg leucine/kg body weight). Restrict intake of milk and eggs until tolerance levels are established. Avoid simple sugars, but have the patient consume 10g CHO 30–40 minutes after meals to counteract the diminished BS.

Profile

Ht	Wt	IBW/HBW
Serum gluc	Acetone	Chol
GTT results using	BP	Trig
1g gluc/kg	Na^+	Ca^{++}
Serum insulin	K^+	I & O

Side Effects of Common Drugs Used

1. *Insulin* and other glucose-lowering medications must be carefully prescribed and monitored.
2. *Chemotherapy* for insulinoma (streptozocin, 5-fluorouracil) can be nephrotoxic.

Patient Education

1. Explain which foods are appropriate for between-meal snacks. Beware of the use of "dietetic" items when blood sugar levels need to be controlled more carefully.
2. Explain the role of exercise in reducing blood sugar levels. Discuss appropriate snacking patterns.
3. Discuss observations that require medical attention.
4. Promote regular meal times, meal spacing and exercise levels.

5. Examples of fast-acting CHO are to be used or avoided for the individual person, such as (10 g fast-acting CHO each):

   4 oz orange or apple juice
   2 oz grape juice
   3 oz cola
   4 oz ginger ale
   2 teaspoons corn syrup
   2 1/2 teaspoons sugar
   5–6 lifesavers

Table 9–3.
Signs and Symptoms of Hyperglycemia and Hypoglycemia
Hyperglycemia

Polyphagia, polydipsia, polyuria, dehydration, weight loss, weakness, muscle wasting, recurrent or persistent infections, hypovolemia, ketonuria, glycosuria, blurred or changed vision, fatigue, and muscle cramps.

Hypoglycemia

Fatigue, confusion, diplopia, personality changes, hunger, weakness, headache, psychosis, rapid and shallow breathing, numbness of mouth or lips or tongue, pulse normal or abnormal, convulsions, lack of coordination, coma, dizziness, staggering gait, pallor, slurred speech, tingling, diaphoresis, and nausea.

NOTES

HYPERINSULINISM (FUNCTIONAL HYPOGLYCEMIA)

Usual Hospital Stay

4–5 days.

Notation

Excessive amounts of insulin are secreted in response to carbohydrate-rich foods. Symptoms resemble those of the dumping syndrome: weakness and agitation 2 to 4 hours after meals, perspiration, nervousness, mental confusion. If the cause is a beta-cell tumor, surgery may be needed.

Objectives

1. Reduce concentrated sweets intake to a level that does not overstimulate the pancreas to secrete inappropriately large amounts of insulin, which may cause blood sugar to drop to 40 mg/dl or lower.
2. Monitor the patient carefully since this condition can precede diabetes or can be related to mild overt diabetes.
3. If required, ensure that the patient loses weight.
4. Prevent seizures or coma.

Dietary Recommendations

1. Limit carbohydrate intake to 100–125 g daily. Use more soluble-fiber foods, like fruits and vegetables. Reduce excess starches. Simple sugars and dried fruits are allowed in limited amounts.
2. Limit milk to 2 cups daily to reduce insulin-triggering effect of lactose. Alcohol and caffeine are prohibited.
3. Increase protein intake to 1–1.5 g/kg daily. Fat furnishes the remainder of the calories.
4. The diet should include three meals and two or three snacks daily, or should at least provide a well-balanced diet.

Profile

Ht	Wt	Ca^{++}, Mg^{++}
IBW/HBW	GTT results	BP
Gluc (dec.)	K^+, Na^+	Acetone
Chol	Trig	PO_4

Patient Education

1. Explain that children with hyperinsulinism need calcium supplementation.
2. Explain that alcohol blocks gluconeogenesis and should be avoided.
3. Ensure that the patient keeps available high protein snacks such as cheese and crackers.
4. Emphasize that meals should not be skipped, and that large meals should not be taken. Meals should be eaten on time.
5. Excessive insulin must be avoided.
6. Avoid any one meal that is unbalanced or especially high in CHO.
7. Control caffeine intake since it alters glucose levels.

NOTES

ADRENOCORTICAL INSUFFICIENCY, CHRONIC, AND ADDISON'S DISEASE

Usual Hospital Stay

4–5 days.

Notation

The adrenal cortex atrophies with loss of hormones (aldosterone, cortisol, and androgens). The condition often results from tuberculosis, cancer, or surgery for hypertension. Of patients with adrenocortical insufficiency, 33% also have diabetes. Addison's disease is a strict insufficiency state. Signs and symptoms include abdominal pain, vomiting, weakness, fatigue, weight loss, dehydration, nausea, diarrhea, hyperpigmented (tan or bronze) skin, and hypotension.

Objectives

1. Replace lost hormones with synthetic hormones.
2. Prevent hypoglycemia; avoid fasting.
3. Prevent weight loss. Improve appetite and strength.
4. Modify sodium according to drug therapy. Prevent hyponatremia, especially in warm weather.
5. Prevent dehydration and shock.
6. Correct diarrhea, hyperkalemia, nausea, and drug overdosage.

Dietary Recommendations

1. Use a high protein, moderate carbohydrate diet. Snacks may be needed.
2. Ensure that intake of sodium is high, unless drugs are used to retain sodium.
3. Restrict simple sugars to prevent overstimulation of insulin (with resulting hypoglycemia).
4. Supplement diet with B complex and vitamin C for increased metabolic requirements.
5. Beware of foods high in potassium, unless drugs are used to control the potassium.
6. Force fluids—up to 3 L if allowed.

Profile

Ht	Na$^+$ (dec.)	BUN (inc.)
IBW/HBW	Ca^{++} (inc.)	Cortisol (dec.)
Gluc (dec.)	BP (dec.)	Alb
K$^+$ (inc.)	Cl$^-$ (dec.)	Mg^{++} (inc.)
N balance	WBCs (dec.)	I & O
Wt	ACTH (inc.)	

Side Effects of Common Drugs Used

1. *Cortisone* (20–30 mg common). Extra dietary salt may be needed.
2. *Fludrocortisone*. A sodium-retaining hormone, fludrocortisone does not demand an increase in dietary sodium. Be wary about overdosing. Side effects include HPN, and ankle edema, or postural hypotension with a low dose.

Patient Education

1. Help the patient individualize the diet according to symptoms.
2. To decrease gastric irritation, ensure that patient takes the hormone with milk or antacid.
3. Ensure that the patient does not skip meals. Tell patient to carry a cheese or cracker snack to prevent hypoglycemia.
4. Discuss the simple meal preparation to lessen fatigue.

Comments

Aldosterone functions to conserve sodium and excrete potassium. When aldosterone is no longer secreted normally, the following events occur:

1. Excretion of sodium takes place.
2. The body's store of water decreases, leading to dehydration, hypotension, and decreased cardiac output.
3. The heart becomes slower due to reduced work load.
4. Increased serum potassium can lead to arrhythmias, arrest, even death.

Other Comments

Acute adrenal insufficiency involves low blood pressure, low serum sodium, high serum potassium, and low corticosteroid levels. It may be temporary or may become a chronic insufficiency.

Addisonian crisis can be precipitated by acute infection, trauma, surgery or excessive body salt loss.

Adrenalectomy may require steroid therapy and a 2 g Na$^+$ diet. Hyperglycemia may result.

ACROMEGALY

Usual Hospital Stay

4–5 days.

Notation

This disease is caused by overproduction of growth hormone (GH).

Symptoms and signs may include disproportionate growth (facial features, tongue, hands and feet); increased, coarse body hair; coarse and leathery skin; excessive diaphoresis and oiliness; visual impairment; headache; moderate weight gain; heart failure; and diabetes in 25–30%.

Surgical removal of the pituitary gland may help.

Objectives

1. Control weight and metabolic rate, which may be increased.
2. Control diabetes and heart disease where involved.
3. Alter phosphorus intake where needed (as tubular reabsorption of phosphate may be increased).
4. Prevent osteoporosis with calcium balance (often negative in acromegaly).

Dietary Recommendations

1. A diet controlled in calories (higher or lower) may be needed to control weight.
2. Extra fluid intake may be needed, often 2–3 liters daily.
3. Adequate Ca:P ratio is needed, with at least a ratio of 1:1.

Profile

Ht, wt	IBW/HBW	GTT
BP (inc.)	Urine sugar	K^+
N Balance	Gluc	I & O
P (inc.)	Ca^{++}	H & H
BUN	Alb	
Serum creat (inc.)	Growth hormone	

Side Effects of Common Drugs Used

Insulin may be needed with diabetes.

Patient Education

1. Discuss body changes and self-image alterations.
2. Teach the patient about control of diabetes, where present.

HYPERALDOSTERONISM

Usual Hospital Stay

4–5 days.

Notation

An increased production of aldosterone by the adrenal cortex, *hyperaldosteronism* may be primary (usually from adenoma) or secondary (cancer, CHF, hyperplasia, malignant hypertension, pregnancy, estrogen use, or cirrhosis). *Conn's syndrome* is a benign tumor in one adrenal gland that can cause this condition.

Signs and symptoms include hypertension, headache, cardiomegaly, retinopathy, hypokalemia, paresthesia, polyuria, polydipsia, azotemia, muscle spasms in hand and feet, and tetany.

Objectives

1. Hydrate adequately.
2. Alter diet as needed for testing (sodium, potassium).
3. Correct hypokalemia and other altered electrolytes.
4. Prepare for surgery if a tumor is involved.

Dietary Recommendations

1. Provide adequate fluid intake (unless contraindicated for other reasons).
2. Use a high or low sodium intake for testing (6 g Na^+ load is common).
3. A high potassium intake may be required.
4. Small, frequent feedings may be needed.

Profile

Ht, wt	IBW/HBW	K^+
Urine sugar	Plasma renin	Na^+
BP	Aldosterone levels	H & H

Side Effects of Common Drugs Used

1. *Antihypertensives* may be used; monitor side effects specifically for these medications.
2. *Digitalis* is often used.
3. *Spironolactone* may be used if surgery is not indicated.

Patient Education

1. Explain altered sodium and potassium requirements, as appropriate.
2. Have the patient avoid fasting, skipping meals, fad dieting.
3. Provide recipe suggestions.

NOTES

HYPOPITUITARISM

Usual Hospital Stay

4–5 days.

Notation

A deficiency in production of pituitary hormones, hypopituitarism may be caused by tumor, aneurysm, infarction or surgery. The condition is relatively rare. In children, short stature results (10% of all dwarfism). Skinfold thickness over 50% for age shows greater subcutaneous fat deposition with decreased muscle mass.

Symptoms and signs include sexual dysfunction, weakness, easy fatigue, and lack of resistance to cold and stress.

Objectives

1. Replenish stores.
2. Prevent dehydration and hypoglycemia.
3. Improve lean muscle mass stores.
4. Monitor serum levels of cholesterol and triglycerides; prevent side effects of elevated levels.

Dietary Recommendations

1. High calorie/high protein diet with a moderate to high salt intake may be needed. A low fat and cholesterol intake should be assured.
2. Six small feedings may be better tolerated.
3. Increase fluids unless contraindicated.
4. Ensure adequate intake of all vitamins and minerals.

Profile

Ht, wt	T_4 (dec.)	Na^+
Chol & trig	Osm	GTT, Serum gluc
Alb, transferrin	PBI uptake (dec.)	FSH, LH, TSH (dec.)
IBW/HBW	T_3	Uric acid
CBC	BP	

Side Effects of Common Drugs Used

1. *Corticosteroids* [hydrocortisone (Cortef), cortisol] are often used and can alter glucose, calcium, and phosphate tolerance. One needs to increase K^+ and folacin and to decrease sodium.
2. *Thyroid preparations* may be needed.
3. *Growth hormone*, when given, requires no specific dietary interventions.
4. *Other hormonal replacements* may be needed.

Patient Education

1. Have the patient avoid fasting and stress.
2. Discuss the need to use small frequent meals instead of large meals.

NOTES

PHEOCHROMOCYTOMA

Usual Hospital Stay

4–5 days, surgical.

Notation

Pheochromocytoma is a rare tumor of the sympathoadrenal system resulting in increased secretion of the hormones epinephrine and norepinephrine.

Symptoms and signs include very high blood pressure, headache, excessive diaphoresis, palpitations, syncope, blanching or blushing of skin, hyperglycemia, nausea and vomiting, anorexia, polyuria, tetany, blurred vision, nervousness, heart failure, and hypermetabolism with normal T_4.

Objectives

1. Avoid overstimulation (even slight exercise, cold stress, or emotional upsets).
2. Correct nausea, vomiting, anorexia and CHO intolerance.
3. Prepare for surgery to remove tumor, if feasible.
4. Prevent crisis (which could cause sudden blindness or CVAs).

Dietary Recommendations

1. Increase fluids, but not with caffeinated beverages.
2. Six small feedings may be better tolerated than large meals.
3. For testing, a VMA diet may be required for lab results (i.e., omit chocolate, vanilla extract, and citrus). Check with the diagnostic personnel.
4. Increase protein and calories if patient will have surgery. Post-operatively, provide adequate vitamins and minerals for wound healing.

Profile

Ht, wt	T_3, T_4	H & H
Epinephrine levels (inc.)	IBW/HBW	VMA in urine (inc.)
Gluc (inc.)	Norepinephrine (inc.)	Glycosuria
CT scan	Urinary cate-	Alb
	cholamines	

Patient Education

1. Discuss avoidance of caffeinated foods and beverages (coffee, tea, and chocolate).
2. Maintain a calm atmosphere for the patient; prevent undue stress.

NOTES

HYPERTHYROIDISM

Usual Hospital Stay

4–5 days.

Notation

Hyperthyroidism results from oversecretion of thyroxine and/or triiodothyronine, which causes an elevated metabolic rate, tissue wasting, diaphoresis, tremor, tachycardia, heat intolerance, cold insensitivity, tremor, nervousness, increased appetite, exopthalmos and loss of glycogen stores. *Thyrotoxicosis* and *Graves' disease* (toxic goiter) are the more severe forms. Hyperthyroidism is 8 times more common in women.

Objectives

1. Prevent or treat the complications accompanying the high metabolic rate, including bone demineralization.
2. Replenish glycogen stores. Correct anorexia. Replace lost weight (usually 10–20 lbs).
3. Correct negative nitrogen balance.
4. Replace fluid losses from diarrhea, diaphoresis, and increased respirations.
5. Monitor fat intolerance, steatorrhea.

Dietary Recommendations

1. Use a high calorie diet (3500–4000 kcal). The patient's caloric needs are increased by 50–60% in this condition (or 10–30% in mild cases). Ensure high intake of carbohydrates, and protein in the range of 1–2 g/kg body weight.
2. Fluid intake should be 3–4 L per day, unless contraindicated by renal or cardiac problems.
3. The diet should include 1 quart of milk daily to supply adequate calcium, phosphorus, and vitamin D.
4. Use less seasoned, fibrous foods. Caffeine stimulants should be excluded from the diet.
5. Supplement the diet with vitamins A and C, as well as the B-complex, especially thiamine, riboflavin, B_6 and B_{12}.
6. Be cautions in regard to the use of natural goitrogens (cabbage, Brussels sprouts, kale, cauliflower, etc.) concomitant with anti-thyroid medications.

Profile

Ht	Na$^+$	Phosphorus
IBW/HBW	Wt	Thyroid scan
Triiodothyronine (T$_3$)	Thyroxine (T$_4$)	Temp
Gluc (inc.)	PBI	N balance
Alb	H & H	Alk phos (inc.)
Ca^{++}	Chol, Trig (dec.)	BP
K$^+$	Mg^{++} (dec.)	I & O

Side Effects of Common Drugs Used

1. *Anti-thyroid drugs* [methimazole (Tapazole)] can cause vomiting and GI distress; take with food. Watch the use of natural goitrogens with these drugs, which can increase the effects of the drug.
2. Radioactive iodine can cause temporary burning sensation in the throat.

Patient Education

1. Encourage quiet, pleasant mealtimes.
2. Exclude the use of alcohol, which may cause a hypoglycemic state.
3. To avoid obesity, adjust the patient's diet as the condition corrects itself.
4. Beware of hyperglycemia after carbohydrate-rich meals.
5. Frequent snacks may be needed.

Comment

1. *Exophthalmos*, which is caused by increased accumulation of extracellular fluid in the eyes, may require fluid and salt restriction. Thyroidectomy may be needed.
2. Fifty percent of persons suffering from *Graves' disease* have had relatives with altered thyroid functioning. Some underlying hereditary condition may exist.
3. With *thyroidectomy*, often subtotal, the patient may require a high-calorie, high protein diet preoperatively. Evaluate needs postoperatively with the doctor's care plan.

NOTES

HYPOTHYROIDISM

Usual Hospital Stay

4–5 days.

Notation

Hypothyroidism, the underfunctioning of the thyroid gland (from surgery, hypofunctioning of the pituitary or hypothalamus gland) may show with such signs and symptoms as dry skin, hand and face puffiness, weight gain, slow speech, mental apathy, constipation, hearing loss, memory impairment, decreased perspiration, cold intolerance, and brittle nails. *Endemic goiter*, the enlargement of the thyroid gland with swelling in front of the neck, results from iodine deficiency due to inadequate dietary intake or drug effects.

Objectives

1. Control the weight gain that results from a 15–40% slower metabolic rate. Measure weight frequently to detect losses or fluid retention.
2. Correct the reasons for imbalance, which can be due to inadequate intake of iodine, increased intake of goitrogens, or congenital imbalance.
3. Correct vitamin B_{12} or iron deficiency anemias if present.

Dietary Recommendations

1. Use a calorie-controlled diet adjusted for age, sex, and height.
2. Ensure an adequate supply of fiber and laxative foods.
3. In diets for pregnant women or children, check to make sure that adequate amounts of iodine are provided.
4. Foods that are natural goitrogens must be limited. Such foods are from the Brassica family: cabbage, Brussels sprouts, kale, and cauliflower. Asparagus, broccoli, soybeans, lettuce, peas, spinach, turnip greens and watercress have also been implicated.

Profile

Ht	Wt	Na^+ (dec.)
IBW/HBW	T_3 (dec.)	Serum B_{12}
T_4 (dec.)	PBI	CPK
Chol, Trig (inc.)	Gluc	Thyrotropin
Ca^{++}	Temp	Uric acid (inc.)
H & H (dec.-less O_2 needed)	Alk phos (dec.)	Mg^{++} (inc.)
	Cu (dec.)	Carotenoids (inc.)
		K^+ (dec.)

Side Effects of Common Drugs Used

Thyroid Hormones (Liotrix, Sodium Levothyroxine or Synthroid). Monitor diabetics carefully. Use caution with long-term use of soy protein products and the Brassica family. Changes in appetite and decreased weight can occur. Thyroid hormones elevate glucose and decrease cholesterol.

Patient Education

1. Provide a list of the foods that contain progoitrin, an anti-thyroid agent. Cooking destroys goitrin. Urge cooking of vegetables.
2. Encourage the use of iodized salt, as permitted.
3. Encourage adequate fluid intake.
4. Be careful not to self-medicate with iodine.

Comments

1. T_3 and T_4 are elevated with pregnancy and OC and estrogen use.
2. Simple and nodular goiters are unrelated to presence of iodine.
3. *Cretinism* is endemic goiter in a child, with dwarfism or short stature, deafness, retardation, and large tongue. It is rare at birth.
4. *Myxedema* is an endemic goiter in an adult. In myxedema coma, severe unconsciousness can occur with sedative use or cold weather. Vitamin A may be poorly converted from carotene. Calcium may be retained.

NOTES

DIABETES INSIPIDUS

Usual Hospital Stay

4–5 days.

Notation

Diabetes insipidus results from primary (inherited) or secondary (resulting from trauma, tumor, or infection) deficiency of the pituitary gland hormone (vasopressin or ADH), and is marked by excessive thirst and urination, dry skin, and weakness. Urine output may be 5–10 L/24 hours. The disease is more common in the young, especially in males.

Nephrogenic diabetes insipidus can be an inherited disorder of defective kidney tubules or it can be acquired.

Objectives

1. Prevent dehydration and hypovolemic shock from the excretion of large amounts of very dilute urine.
2. Check the patient's weight three times weekly to determine fluid retention and the effectiveness of drug therapy.

Dietary Recommendations

1. Ensure increased fluid intake to compensate for losses. Up to 20 L may be needed!
2. Ensure that potassium intake is high or use supplements.
3. If patient has the *nephrogenic* form, limit protein intake to 1–2 g/kg body weight, and liberalize the regimen as the patient (usually a child) learns to satisfy fluid needs.

Profile

Ht	IBW/HBW	Alb
BP	I & O	Urinary specific
K^+	BUN	gravity (dec.)
Wt	Na^+ (inc.)	Uric acid
		(inc. in adults)

Side Effects of Common Drugs Used

Vasopressin (Pitressin) tannate or *benzothiazine diuretics* will reduce volume by 50% for this type of pituitary disorder. Supplements of K^+ may be needed. Angina or intestinal cramping can occur. Vasopressin is not effective for the nephrogenic type.

Patient Education

1. Caution patient not to limit fluid intake in an effort to lessen urine output. Cold water may be preferred.
2. Select low calorie beverages to prevent excessive weight gain.
3. Avoid stimulant/diuretic-type beverages (coffee, tea, alcohol).

NOTES

SYNDROME OF INAPPROPRIATE ANTIDIURETIC HORMONE (SIADH)

Usual Hospital Stay

4–5 days.

Notation

SIADH involves water intoxication with hypernatremia and hyperosmolarity of urine and serum. Normal renal and adrenal functioning with abnormal elevation of plasma vasopressin occur (inappropriate for serum osmolality). The condition may occur as a result of oat cell bronchial cancer, pulmonary tuberculosis, acute MI, myxedema, CNS disorders, acute leukemia, stroke, meningitis, or craniotomy.

Symptoms and signs include irritability, lethargy, seizures or confusion.

Objectives

1. Restrict water intake.
2. Replace electrolytes as appropriate.
3. Normalize ADH secretion.

Dietary Recommendations

1. Restrict fluid intake.
2. Alter dietary sodium and potassium, as deemed appropriate for the condition.

Profile

Ht, wt & dry wt	IBW/HBW	Na^+ ($\downarrow$)
I & O	ADH levels	Osmolality (dec.)
BUN	Creatinine	K^+

Side Effects of Common Drugs Used

1. *Lithium carbonate* may be used.
2. *Demeclocycline (Declomycin) may be used with side effects like those of tetracycline.*

Patient Education

1. Provide counseling regarding water restrictions and fluid intake, as ordered.
2. Discuss any underlying conditions which may have caused the syndrome; highlight needed dietary alterations.

CUSHING'S SYNDROME

Usual Hospital Stay

4–5 days.

Notation

Cushing's syndrome is a rare disorder, mainly of women, characterized by virilism, obesity, hyperglycemia, glucosuria, hypertension, moon face, emotional lability, buffalo hump, purple striae over obese areas, and pitting ankle edema. It can be caused by extrinsic and excessive hormonal stimulation of the adrenal cortex by tumor of the anterior pituitary gland, adrenal hyperplasia, or exogenous cortisol use. Excess ACTH is secreted.

Objectives

1. Control symptoms of elevated blood glucose.
2. Promote weight loss if needed. Control patient's weight, while increasing lean body mass.
3. Control symptoms of hypertension. Prevent vertebral collapse and other side effects, such as CHF, bone demineralization, osteoporosis, and hypokalemia.
4. Control side effects of corticosteroid therapy.

Dietary Recommendations

1. Restrict sodium if steroids are used.
2. Use a calorie-controlled diet if needed. Calculate diet according to the patient's IBW. Control glucose levels if required.
3. Ensure adequate intake of calcium and potassium.
4. Ensure adequate intake of protein if losses are excessive. For example, 1 g protein/kg, or more.

Profile

Ht	Chol
IBW/HBW	K^+ (dec.)
Urinary gluc (inc.)	N balance

Urinary Ca^{++}	Na^+ (inc.)
BP (inc.)	P_{CO_2} (inc.)
Alb	CT Scan
Edema	WBC, TLC (dec.)
Wt	Urinary and plasma cortisol
Gluc (inc.)	(inc.)
Serum Ca^{++}	GTT

Side Effects of Common Drugs Used

1. *Glucocorticoid therapy.* Osteoporosis and hypercalciuria are common side effects of these drugs.
2. *Vitamin D* may be necessary (e.g., 50,000 IU twice weekly).

Patient Education

1. Help the patient control weight as needed.
2. Explain which foods are good sources of calcium in the diet.
3. Explain how to control elevated blood sugars through balanced dietary intake.

NOTES

PARATHYROID DISORDERS AND ALTERED CALCIUM METABOLISM

Usual Hospital Stay

4–5 days.

Notation

Hypoparathyroidism/hypocalcemia is one of the most common results of damage to parathyroid glands during surgery. Other causes include magnesium deficiency, neonatal immaturity, and defects. In states of permanent hypoparathyroidism, requirements are large for calcium (1–2 g) and vitamin D (25,000–200,000 IU/day) to maintain normal calcium.

Hyperparathyroidism/hypercalcemia may be caused by elevated levels of parathyroid hormone or (rarely) dietary excesses of vitamin D. Hyperparathyroidism may also result from renal failure. Increased serum Ca^{++}, decreased serum P and dehydration are common.

The Ca:P ratio is 1.2:1 in cow's milk, 2:1 in breast milk.

Parathormone is regulated by serum Ca^{++} levels. *Calcitonin* from the thyroid has an action opposite that of PTH. PTH affects calcium, phosphorus, and vitamin D metabolism by removing calcium from bone to raise serum levels; it hydroxylates vitamin D to 1,25 $(OH)_2$-D.

Objectives

Hyperparathyroidism/hypercalcemia

1. Lower elevated serum calcium and urinary calcium.
2. Normalize serum and urinary phosphate; 80% of phosphorus is usually absorbed from the diet. *Parathyroidectomy* may be necessary.

Hypoparathyroidism/hypocalcemia

Normalize serum and urinary levels of calcium, phosphorus, and vitamin D.

Dietary Recommendations

Hypercalcemia/hyperparathyroidism

Use a low calcium diet. Use fewer dairy products, nuts, salmon, peanut butter, green leafy vegetables. Use more jelly. Compleat-B, which is low in calcium and high in phosphorus, can be used.

Hypocalcemia/hypoparathyroidism

Use a high calcium diet. Increase dairy products, nuts, salmon, peanut butter, green leafy vegetables. Reduce excess use of meats, phytates (whole grains) and oxalic acid (spinach, chard, etc.). If tolerated, lactose should be included in the diet. Intake of vitamin D and protein should be adequate. Meritene and Sustacal are high in calcium. Calcium carbonate may be needed.

Profile

Ht	PTH	Alk phos
IBW/HBW	Wt	Chvostek's sign (+
Mg^{++}	Ca^{++}	to tapping of
Urinary Ca^{++}	P	facial muscles)

Side Effects of Common Drugs Used

1. Overuse of *steroids* may cause hypocalcemia, with resulting severe muscle spasms, and convulsions.
2. Beware of hypervitaminosis A or D—either may aggravate or cause

hypercalcemia (e.g., 10,000 of vitamin A or 50,000 of vitamin D). It takes 12–36 hours to show changes in serum Ca^{++} levels.

3. Use of antacids and excessive amounts of iron lower phosphorus absorption. Be careful!
4. *Calcium lactate* (8–12 g) may be used in hypoparathyroidism.
5. *Ergocalciferol, (Calciferol),* and *calcitriol (Rocaltrol)* are calcium supplements that may be used for hypocalcemia.

Comments

1. *Hyperparathyroidism* results from adenoma, renal failure, increased growth of the parathyroid gland or from a hypocalcemic state. Signs and symptoms include weakness, fatigue, anorexia, constipation, weight loss, hypercalcemia and hypercalciuria and elevated PTH. See also—Paget's disease.
2. *Hypoparathyroidism* results from a deficiency of PTH from biologically ineffective hormones, damage or accidental removal of the glands, impaired skeletal or renal response. Vitamin D may be deficient. Signs and symptoms include tetany, thinning hair, coarse skin, cataracts, dental hypoplasia, chronic cutaneous moniliasis, hypocalcemia, hyperphosphatemia and low PTH.

Patient Education

1. Indicate which foods are sources of calcium, phosphorus and vitamin D.
2. Indicate which foods are sources of phytates and oxalates.
3. Discuss sunlight's role in vitamin D formation.

NOTES

GESTATIONAL DIABETES

Usual Hospital Stay

3 days.

Notation

Gestational diabetes (GDM) occurs in 1–3% of all pregnancies, with hyperglycemia (over 130 mg/dl) and glycosuria first recognized during pregnancy. The condition may indicate diabetes for the mother postnatally as well (20–30%). This condition yields an abnormally high risk for perinatal complications. In general, these mothers may be older or may have been obese prenatally.

Symptoms and signs include a large weight gain, hypoglycemia, diabetic ketoacidosis, pregnancy-induced hypertension, and anxiety. Infants may be born with macrosomatia (LGA), hypoglycemia, respiratory distress, hypocalcemia, hyperbilirubinemia.

Objectives

1. Minimize morbidity and prevent death of mother and infant.
2. Prevent complications of diabetes or fetal problems. Avoid infections.
3. Control blood pressure.
4. Control blood sugars (BS under 90–100 mg/dl would be needed). Avoid glucosuria. Maintain normoglycemia.
5. Prevent hypoglycemic episodes; urinary tract infections; candidiasis.
6. Prevent weight loss, but avoid excessive weight gain patterns also.
7. Achieve an approximate total weight gain of 20–30 lbs.

Dietary Recommendations

1. The diet should match age needs, weight gain or control measures. The typical diet may include 30–35 kcal/kg; 20–25% total calories as protein (1.3–2.0 g/kg), 50–60% CHO (especially complex sources), and 20–25% fat.
2. Ensure intake of prenatal vitamin-mineral supplement (especially for folic acid, 30–60 mg iron, adequate calcium). Monitor adequate chromium intake.
3. Avoid concentrated sweets, where possible.
4. A minimum of 150–200 grams CHO may be needed to prevent hypoglycemia.
5. Carefully spaced meals and snacks, especially before bedtime, are needed. Four to six small meals may be helpful, and a snack upon arising may be important to prevent hypoglycemia. Some physicians use the rule of 18's (2/18, 1/18, 5/18, 2/18, 5/18, 2/18 and 1/18 during the day).
6. No meals can be skipped.

Profile

Ht/Wt/IBW, HBW	BP
GTT (if possible)	Na^+, K^+

EDC   BUN
Ketones   Prenatal wt
H & H   Glycosuria
Hgb A_1c Edema
Weight gain pattern   Alb
Serum gluc (often over Ca^{++}
    105 mg % fasting)

Side Effects of Common Drugs Used

Insulin may be required to control blood glucose. Careful physician monitoring will be needed.

Patient Education

1. The importance of meal spacing and timing, adequacy; not skipping meals.
2. Careful instructions on what to eat/what to avoid will be important.
3. Carrying a snack at all times is helpful (e.g., fruit, thermos of milk, crackers).
4. Exercise after meals may be beneficial in controlling blood sugar; walking is generally recommended.
5. Counseling regarding future pregnancies may be needed.
6. Encourage breast-feeding.

Comments

Pregnancy is a metabolic stress test for all women. Some women fail the test and become diabetic. Women at risk for GDM may be obese, hyperglycemic and insulin-resistant; others may be thin and insulin-deficient. Pregnancy-induced diabetes in either group is called gestational diabetes. Women with IDDM and NIDDM who are in poor control at conception and during the first two months of pregnancy are at greater risk for bearing infants with congenital malformations.

In *any pregnancy*, increased insulin resistance occurs because gestational hormones counteract insulin action. Glycosuria can occur in the presence of normal blood sugars from decreased renal glucose thresholds. During the first half of pregnancy, transfer of maternal glucose to fetus occurs; during second half of pregnancy, diabetogenic action of placental hormones outweighs glucose transfer (average insulin requirement increases by 67%).

Monitor starvation ketosis (glucose needed) versus diabetic acidosis (where insulin and potassium are needed).

PREGNANCY-INDUCED HYPERTENSION

Usual Hospital Stay

3 days.

Notation

Pregnancy-induced hypertension (PIH), also called EPH-gestosis, pree-clampsia and other terms, is a syndrome of hypertension, edema and protein-uria that occurs during the second half of pregnancy (usually after week 20), more often in primigravidas and women over the age of 35. The condition occurs in approximately 6–7% of all pregnancies.

Signs and symptoms include increased blood pressure, proteinuria, facial edema, pretibial pitting edema, irritability, nausea and vomiting, nervousness, severe headache, altered states of consciousness, epigastric pain, and oliguria. This state of edema-proteinuria-hypertension (140/90 or greater) can lead to convulsions (eclampsia).

Objectives

1. Prevent eclamptic seizures and death.
2. Prevent, if possible, chronic hypertension after delivery.
3. Normalize abnormal blood pressures.
4. Lessen any edema that is present.
5. Correct any underlying protein-calorie malnutrition.
6. Monitor any sudden weight gains (over 1 kg/week), unexplained by food intake.

Dietary Recommendations

1. Maintain diet as ordered for age and pregnancy stage (generally 300 kcal above prepregnancy diet).
2. A multivitamin-mineral supplement may be needed, since inadequate intakes of vitamins C and B_6 have been implicated by some studies.
3. Adequate calcium, protein, calories and potassium will be necessary.
4. Sodium intake can be controlled to 1–2 g/day; present body weight may determine needs.
5. Linoleic and arachidonic acids have been used to serve as vasodilators in some cases. This should be done under careful medical supervision.

Profile

Ht/WT/IBW, HBW
GFR
Ca^{++}
Alb
Proteinuria
(over 0.3 g/L/day
mild; over 5 g/L/day
may be severe)
H & H
Gluc

Mg^{++} (↑)
BP (severe over 160/110)
Wt. gain pattern
K^+, Na^+
Uric Acid (↑)
LDH, CPK
SGOT, SGPT
Edema
BUN

Side Effects of Common Drugs Used

Thiazide diuretics can cause electrolyte imbalances, hyperglycemia, hyperuricemia, and pancreatitis. They are not usually beneficial in treatment and may harm the fetus. They are used only in rare cases of congestive heart failure and severe chronic hypertension during pregnancy.

Patient Education

1. Rest is essential during this time.
2. Meal-skipping should be avoided at all costs.

Section 10
Weight Control and Malnutrition

Chief Assessment Factors

height

weight—history, present, ideal/healthy wt

% IBW, recent changes, goal weight

Lab values—glucose, BUN, albumin, H & H, chol/trig.

Table 10–1.
Important Weight Calculations and Conversions

$$\% \text{ IBW} = \frac{\text{actual wt}}{\text{IBW}} \times 100$$

$$\% \text{ usual body wt} = \frac{\text{actual wt}}{\text{usual wt}} \times 100$$

$$\% \text{ wt change} = \frac{\text{usual wt less actual wt}}{\text{usual wt}} \times 100$$

Table 10–2.
Ideal Body Weight/Healthy Body Weight. Acceptable Weights for Men and Women*

Height (Without Shoes)	Weight in Pounds (Without Clothes)	
	19 to 34 Years	35 Years and Over
5'0"	97–128	108–138
5'1"	101–132	111–143
5'2"	104–137	115–148
5'3"	107–141	119–152
5'4"	111–146	122–157
5'5"	114–150	126–162
5'6"	118–155	130–167
5'7"	121–160	134–172
5'8"	125–164	138–178
5'9"	129–169	142–183
5'10"	132–174	146–188
5'11"	136–179	151–194
6'0"	140–184	155–199
6'1"	144–189	159–205
6'2"	148–195	164–210

* Report of the Dietary Guidelines Advisory Committee for Americans, USDA, 1990.

Conversion Factors

1 foot = 30.48 cm
1 inch = 2.54 cm (1 cm = 0.39 inches)
1 m = 39.37 inches
1 fluid oz = 29.57 cc^3
1 oz = 28 g
1 pound = .453 kg
1 kg = 2.2 pounds

Table 10–3.
Malnutrition

Undernutrition
    Primary—from insufficient intake
    Secondary—from impaired utilization
Overnutrition—excessive calorie intake

OBESITY

Usual Hospital Stay

4–5 days.

Notation

Overweight is defined as body weight 10–19% above IBW for sex and age. *Obesity* is defined as body weight 20% or more above the IBW (or by triceps skinfold thickness equal to or greater than 18–19 mm in adult men, 25–26 mm or more in women). Obesity is diabetogenic, especially with longer duration. Evaluate cause (i.e., emotional, acquired from family, or metabolic.) Approximately 1/4–1/3 of adults are obese; obesity is the most common form of disturbed nutrition in the United States. Some patients may suffer from undernutrition for some nutrients. Risks increase for CAD, diabetes, HLP, liver and gallbladder disease, EPH-gestosis in pregnancy, DJD, surgery, accidents, some CA, and respiratory problems.

Objectives

1. Determine the category of obesity: *hypertrophic obesity* results from an increased lipid content of adipocytes. It is the more common type and is usually seen in adults. *Hyperplastic-hypertrophic obesity* results from increased fat cell number and lipid content of fat cells. It most often occurs in patients whose obesity began in their early years. Juvenile obesity is hyperplastic.
2. Decrease the patient's calorie intake to induce a weight loss of 1–2 lbs weekly. Ensure loss of fat, not LBM. Create an energy deficit.
3. Provide a nutritionally balanced, individualized diet pattern.
4. Maintain a normal or slightly higher protein intake to maintain nitrogen balance.
5. Alleviate associated risk factors such as elevated lipids, blood pressure, uric acid, and glucose levels. For patients 100–300 lbs. above IBW, surgery may be indicated.
6. Weigh weekly on same scale with same clothing.

Dietary Recommendations

1. Schedule six to eight small meals at frequent intervals to prevent cheating and overeating. Breakfast is crucial.
2. The diet should provide adequate fluid intake to excrete metabolic wastes. Beverages with meals increase fullness.
3. Decrease salt intake if fluid retention exists.
4. Intake of protein should follow RDAs appropriate to the patient's age, or slightly higher to maintain satiety while fat is being decreased.
5. If an anorexiant has been prescribed, avoid using caffeine in the diet.

6. Have patient set his or her own goal: a weight loss of 1/2–1 per week. Each pound of body fat contains approximately 3500 kcal.
7. With type IV HLP, decrease concentrated sweets and sugars, fats.
8. Increase fiber content; it takes longer to chew, is low in kcal and increases satiety. High fiber cereal at breakfast seems to curb appetite at lunch slightly.
9. Teach the patient to splurge by plan, not by impulse.
10. For a modified fast, a physician may prescribe *Optifast*. (*Optifast* program gives 420 kcal, 70 g egg-white and milk protein, EFAs, small % CHO, 100% USRDA of vitamins and minerals. Product is available from Sandoz or through a physician. Physical and psychological screenings are needed. Phase I—Optifast; Phase II—Optifast plus one meal; Phase III—Maintenance.) Very low calorie diets (VCLDs) may cause reduced REE by 20%. Moderation is better.

Profile

Ht	Trig	Wt changes
IBW/HBW	Gluc	Wt
BP	Skinfold thicknesses	Hypoxemia
Uric Acid	Waist: Hip Ratio =	Chol
T_3, T_4	(<1:1 men)	
BMI*	(<0.8:1 women)	

Side Effects of Common Drugs Used

1. *Appetite suppressants* may cause excitability, GI distress, and other problems. This is especially true of drugs containing amphetamine.
2. *Fenfluramine HCl* (Pendimin) or *Phentermine HCl* (Adipex-P) may be used. Side effects are common.
3. *Dexedrine* causes elevated glucose levels, dry mouth, unpleasant taste, dizziness, diarrhea, anorexia, extreme weight losses, GI disturbances, and drowsiness. It can cause growth disturbances in children.

Patient Education

1. Instruct the patient on how to maintain a proper diet; use of menus, recipes; tips on restaurant dining; portion control; eating at parties; low calorie snacking; and food preparation methods.
2. Behavior therapy may be helpful in self-monitoring (food diaries, weights, activity). Teach stimulus control of cues, family intervention, slowing down of eating. Be wary of eating in groups, parties, breaks. Avoid eating most calories late at night.

---

* $BMI = \dfrac{\text{wt in kg}}{(\text{ht in meters})^2}$

3. One lb requires 1 extra mile of capillary blood vessels for additional circulation.
4. Promote aerobic exercises, especially 1–3 hours after meals.
5. Avoid yo-yo syndrome dieting, which ↓ BMR, ↓ LBM, ↑ fat.
6. Make meals last 20 minutes +.
7. Eat slowly; chew well. Sugarless gums can help.
8. Avoid bizarre, fad dieting; skipping meals; emphasis on any one dietary component.
9. Obesity *can* be successfully treated.
10. Soup before a meal and fructose-sweetened beverages can retard appetite.

Comments

1. Be careful! Do not provide too *low* a calorie level. Caloric intake less than 1200 kcal for women and 1500 kcal for men requires an additional multivitamin supplement.
2. A patient with *Pickwickian syndrome* is obese and hypersomnolent. Cor pulmonale, polycythemia, nocturnal enuresis, and personality changes may also occur.
3. *Sleep apnea* is common in morbidly obese males (20%). Generally, they have 12× the mortality rate of their normal weight peers.
4. *Smoking cessation* can aggravate obesity because of increased caloric consumption as well as changes in activity levels. Moderate to heavy smokers may need to reduce intake by 100–200 kcal, just to maintain weight. Fruit helps relieve the craving for sweets.
5. Upper body fat, especially in stomach, increases risk for heart disease.
6. *Premenstrual weight gain* may include 2–5 lbs of fluid. Otherwise, only 5% of all obesity is related to endocrine or pathologic disorders.
7. There is no such tissue as cellulite.
8. Various theories (such as brown fat for thermogenesis) are being evaluated. There *are* neuroendocrine stimulants for food intake; mediating peptides may be found.
9. Obesity is primarily related to fat calories more than carbohydrate or protein. 1% of the population is morbidly obese.
10. Overweight is more common in black women than in white women.
11. Weight loss in morbid obesity leads to enhanced lipoprotein lipase activity and greater lipid storage (*NEJM* 1990).

UNDERWEIGHT OR GENERAL DEBILITY

Usual Hospital Stay

4–5 days.

Notation

Being underweight is defined as having weight at least 10% below IBW standards. Body fat is 80% of total fuel storage; body storage of glycogen is about 1100 calories; body storage of protein equals 40,000 kcal of muscle tissue (loss of 30–50% is incompatible with survival.) Death in starvation is often from decreased respiratory muscle function and terminal pneumonia. 8–9% of the population is underweight.

Objectives

1. Increase body weight gradually.
2. Encourage weight gain of approximately 1 lb. weekly.
3. In the case of *general debility,* provide diet as tolerated to improve nutritional status. Progress slowly—it may take several days to stimulate the patient's appetite. If confusion exists, dehydration may be a factor.

Dietary Recommendations

1. Calculate the patient's IBW:
   Women: 100 lbs for the first 5 feet plus 5 lbs for each inch, ±10%.
   Men: 106 lbs for the first 5 feet plus 6 lbs for each inch, ±10%.
2. Calculate the patient's metabolic rate, which is determined in the non-stressed patient by multiplying the ideal weight by ten.
3. Each lb of fat requires 3500 kcal; therefore, the diet should be increased by 500 kcal daily to promote a weight gain of 1 lb per week.
4. Use a high protein/high calorie diet with frequent feedings. Tube feed if needed. See Decision Tree, Section 17.
5. The diet should provide adequate amounts of Zn to stimulate appetite; plus a general vitamin-mineral supplement if needed.

Profile

Ht	Wt	N balance
IBW/HBW	Usual wt	TSF, MAC, MAMC
Recent changes	Alb	Alk phos
H & H	Chol	I & O
Trig	BUN, Creat	Ca^{++}, Mg^{++}
Na^+	K^+	TLC

Patient Education

Help the patient make meals in a simple manner, using attractive foods.

NOTES

PROTEIN-CALORIE MALNUTRITION (KWASHIORKOR, MARASMUS, MIXED, PCM)

Usual Hospital Stay

4–5 days.

Notation

Of patients admitted to hospitals, 25–50% are malnourished on admission; 25–30% more become malnourished during the stay. About 50% of hospitalized patients are malnourished to some degree.

Kwashiorkor. Patient appears well-nourished or even over-nourished, but has had recent stress with protein intake insufficient to maintain visceral stores. Albumin and transferrin levels are depressed. Depressed cellular immunity also exists. TLC, BUN and creatinine are low.

Marasmus. Patient appears to be chronically starved. Decreased anthropometric values (MAMC, TSF, etc.) are produced by chronically inadequate diets and a moderate catabolic illness. The patient may have normal albumin and transferrin levels. Even muscle mass may be WNL.

Mixed Marasmic Kwashiorkor. Patient is depleted of somatic and visceral protein stores and consequently is less able to withstand added metabolic stress and catabolic illness. Anthropometric measures, muscle mass and serum values are low.

Moderate PCM. Patient's wt. is 60–80% of healthy body weight. Lymphocytopenia, energy, and anemia exist. Edema is generally not present. PCM is common in GI patients, especially IBD.

Objectives

1. Prevent weight loss, weakness, apathy, infections, poor wound healing.
   Kwashiorkor. Correct protein deficiency, edema, fatty liver.
   Marasmus. Provide energy immediately. Correct complications, which can include dehydration, electrolyte imbalances, infections, and vitamin-mineral deficiencies.
2. Prevent complications (sepsis, overfeeding with HHNK or hyperglycemia, CHF).
3. Avoid hazards of refeeding (hypophosphatemia, low Mg^{++}, low K^+.)

Dietary Recommendations

1. Vitamin-mineral supplementation is needed to treat *both conditions*.
2. *Kwashiorkor.* Begin initial treatment with small amounts of skim milk, perhaps lactose-treated. After a week, gradually add a mixed diet.
   Start treatment with 2.5–5 g protein/kg body weight, 0.8–1.0 × BEE at first.
   The diet should provide adequate carbohydrate and caloric intake to spare protein and correct weight loss. Use TF or TPN if appropriate (see Section 17). Add thiamine if needed.
3. *Marasmus.* Start treatment with intravenous or oral glucose. Gradually add lactose-treated skim milk to the diet, adding solids later.
   Provide HBV proteins and calories adequate to utilize N effectively. TF or TPN if appropriate. Avoid overfeeding. Add a vitamin-mineral supplement if necessary, including thiamine.

Profile

Ht or arm length/knee length	Transferrin	BUN (dec.)
	TSF	TLC, WBCs (dec.)
Recent wt	MAMC, MAC	Na^+, K^+, Cl^-
IBW/HBW	Usual wt, present wt	TIBC (<250 ug/dl)
Alb*	Changes in wt	Serum B_{12}, and
BP	Gluc (inc. or dec.)	folacin
Chol, trig (dec.)	H & H	Ca^{++}, Mg^{++}
Serum Fe	Urine acetone	Edema
Alk phos (dec.)	T_3, T_4	Muscle wasting
PO_4	Mg^{++}	Serum Cu (dec.)

---

* Albumin shifts intravascularly in marasmus, extravascularly in kwashiorkor.

Patient Education

1. Emphasize the importance of gradual refeeding.
2. Unless nutritional therapy is aggressive, infection is a major risk. Surgery becomes life-threatening and sepsis is more likely.
3. PCM can increase fistula formation, lessen recovery and wound healing after surgery, lead to pneumonia or poor drug tolerance.

Comments

1. Patients with *hypoalbuminemia* are at greater risk for complications resulting from medical/surgical interventions. *Malnutrition* decreases cardiac output, BP, O_2 consumption, TLC, T cells, and GFR; increases infection rate, fatty infiltration, anergy, emphysema and pneumonia, anemia, GI tract atrophy, bacterial overgrowth, hepatic mass losses. (See Bibliography—Cerra, p. 6).
2. *Tissue catabolism* usually begins with lowered albumin and plasma proteins, RBCs, and leukocytes; later wasting of organs, skeletal muscle, bone skin, subcutaneous tissue. CNS is the last tissue to be catabolized.

Table 10–4.
Complicating Effects of Chronic Malnutrition
(Protein-Calorie Deprivation)*

Progressive weight loss

Progressive weakness and apathy

Decreased activity with delayed physical rehabilitation

Decubitus ulcers at pressure points

Depressed cell-mediated immunity with increased infection, particularly gram negative sepsis

Depressed ventilatory response to hypoxia

Impaired wound healing, wound infections, wound disruption, and bowel fistula

Increased incidence of pneumonitis and urinary tract infection

Endocrine changes

Decreased response to chemotherapy for infection and cancer control

Delayed reponse in the completion of radiotherapy

Increased difficulty with fluid, electrolyte, and acid-base management

Increased and prolonged use of critical care facilities with expensive drugs and excessive requirements for hospital support services

Delayed discharge and delayed ability to work.

Protein Measurements

Somatic (CHI, renal function)

Visceral (albumin, transferrin)

General (nitrogen balance)

* From Gastineau, C. (Ed.): Malnutrition in the Hospital. *Dialogues Nutr. 2(2):3*, 1977.

Section 11
Musculoskeletal, Arthritic, and Collagen Disorders

Chief Assessment Factors

pain, edema in muscles, joints, bones

extremity weakness

movement problems

weight loss, anorexia

insomnia

easy fatigue

height loss

unsteady gait

contractures

ANKYLOSING SPONDYLITIS

Usual Hospital Stay

4–5 days.

Notation

Spondylitis is inflammation of the joints linking the vertebrae. In ankylosing spondylitis, inflammation recedes but leaves hardened and damaged joints that fuse together the bones of the spinal column; etiology is unknown. The

325

sacroiliac joints are generally affected first. The condition is most common in men 20–40 years of age, and may run in families.

Symptoms and signs include lower back pain and stiffness, vague chest pains, tender heels, weight loss, anorexia, slight fever and chest pain, and reddened eyes.

Objectives

1. Reduce pain.
2. Improve appetite and intake.
3. Control weight loss.
4. Correct anorexia, nausea and febrile state.

Dietary Recommendations

1. A normal diet is generally useful, with weight loss/calorie control if needed to normalize weight.
2. Food preferences can be offered to stimulate appetite.

Profile

Ht, Wt	IBW/HBW	Wt changes
Ca^{++}	P	Back pain
HL-A-B_{27} Test	Anorexia	Leg pain
Alk. phos.	Temp	SGOT/SGPT
BUN, creat	H & H	

Side Effects of Common Drugs Used

1. *Anti-inflammatory drugs* may be used, such as indomethacin (Indocin) or phenylbutazone. Many side effects can result, such as hyperglycemia, hyperkalemia or anemia. Nausea, dizziness and headache can also result.
2. *Fenoprofen* (Nalfon) can cause constipation, nausea, and vomiting.

Patient Education

1. Exercise is crucial, especially swimming, to relieve back pain.
2. The patient should practice deep breathing exercises.
3. The patient should be sleeping on a hard bed, supine.
4. Discuss the role of calories in weight control.

IMMOBILIZATION, EXTENDED

Usual Hospital Stay

20 days or longer.

Notation

Patients with orthopedic injuries may lose 15 to 20 lbs from stress, immobilization, trauma, and bed rest. *Immobilization hypercalcemia* involves nausea, vomiting, abdominal cramps, constipation, headache, and lethargy.

Objectives

1. Correct negative nitrogen balance from nitrogen losses (perhaps up to 2–3 g nitrogen/day). Prevent decubitus ulcers and infections.
2. Prevent deossification and osteoporosis of bones. Prevent hypercalcemia from low serum levels of albumin (which normally binds calcium).
3. Prevent kidney and bladder stones from hypercalcemia.
4. Provide adequate fluid intake to aid excretion of calcium.
5. Prevent constipation, impactions, and obstruction.
6. Prevent anemias that result from inadequate nitrogen balance.

Dietary Recommendations

1. The diet should provide a high intake of HBV proteins in order to correct nitrogen balance. An intake of 1.2 g protein/kg body weight is recommended. Provide adequate CHO, plus 1–2% total kcal as EFAs.
2. Increased intake of phosphorus during the first few weeks may be useful.
3. Encourage adequate (but not excessive) intake of calcium. A high protein diet raises the body's calcium requirements.
4. The diet should provide a high fluid intake.
5. Intake of vitamin C and zinc should be adequate to protect against skin breakdown.
6. The diet should provide adequate amounts of fiber to prevent constipation. Avoid overuse of bulk with impaction.

Profile

Ht or arm length/knee length	Wt
IBW/HBW	Ca^{++} (inc.)
P	N balance
H & H	RBCs
Alb	BUN, creat
Prealbumin, RBP	

Side Effects of Common Drugs Used

Diuretics may be used to prevent urinary stasis.

Patient Education

1. Explain to the patient that early ambulation is the best treatment possible.
2. Explain that calcium intake will have to be monitored for patients on tube feeding or liquid diet for a long time.

NOTES

GOUT

Usual Hospital Stay

4–5 days.

Notation

Gout is the abnormal metabolism of purines, which causes a form of acute arthritis, with inflamed joints (usually the knees and feet). Hyperuricemia results, with deposition of urate crystals and sometimes sodium. The disease tends to affect men, especially older men, and is sometimes hereditary. More then 1 million people in the United States are afflicted with gout.

Objectives

1. Have patient lose weight if obese, gradually to prevent increased purine release.
2. Increase excretion of urates.
3. Force fluid intake to prevent uric acid kidney stones.
4. Correct any existing hyperlipidemia.
5. Prevent complications such as renal disease, hypertension, and stroke.

Dietary Recommendations

1. A high carbohydrate diet increases excretion, as does a low fat intake. Increase carbohydrate ingestion and decrease fat ingestion.
2. If patient's condition is acute, avoid excessive intake of purines by limiting ingestion of anchovies, smoked meat, sardines, liver, kidney, brain, heart, caviar, herring and gravies.

3. The diet should exclude alcoholic beverages.
4. Use a calorie-controlled diet if weight loss is necessary.
5. Ensure a high fluid intake.
6. If needed, use a type IV hyperlipidemia diet.

Profile

Ht	Wt	SGOT
IBW/HBW	Uric acid (inc.)	SGPT
Na$^+$	Chol	
Trig (inc.)	Alb	
Urate crystals in urine	BUN (inc.)	
Use of alcoholic beverages	Gluc	

Side Effects of Common Drugs Used

1. *Analgesics* (e.g., *colchicine*) may cause vomiting. Avoid using them with uricosuric drugs. Take with adequate fluids.
2. *Uricosuric drugs.* Probenecid (Benemid) and sulfinpyrasone (Anturane) block renal absorption of urates. Adequate intake of fluid is needed. Anorexia, nausea, vomiting, and sore gums may result.
3. *Allopurinol* (Zyloprim) blocks uric acid formation. Adequate intake of fluid is needed. Mild GI upset can occur; take after meals.
4. *Indocin or ACTH.* Used to reduce fever and inflammation, Indocin or ACTH may require a restricted sodium intake. Beware of elevated glucose levels.

Patient Education

1. Advise the patient that alcohol may precipitate a gouty attack.
2. Have the patient avoid fasting.
3. Stress may precipitate an acute attack. Encourage relaxation and pleasant activities.
4. Inflammatory response may be suppressed by an increase in omega-3 fatty acids, as found in fatty fish (mackerel, herring, and salmon).

Comment

Table 11–1

Phases of Gout

1. Asymptomatic hyperuricemia
2. Acute gouty attack
3. Interval phase
4. Chronic arthritis

MUSCULAR DYSTROPHY

Usual Hospital Stay

4 days.

Notation

Actually a group of disorders, *muscular dystrophy* involves a hereditary condition with progressive degenerative changes in the muscle fibers, leading to weakness and atrophy.

In the Duchenne type of muscular dystrophy, the facial muscles are involved, and the patient cannot suck, close lips, bite, chew, or swallow. Aggressive forms appear gradually in males ages 1–15, with frequent falls and difficulty in climbing.

Objectives

1. No specific treatment exists. Encourage the patient to lead an active life. Exercise programs can help prevent contractures.
2. Prevent obesity, which may result from inactivity. Obesity complicates therapy.
3. Avoid constipation because fecal impaction is frequent.
4. Encourage other activities besides eating to prevent dependency on food as a source of pleasure.

Dietary Recommendations

1. Use a low calorie diet to control or lessen obesity. Check the patient's IBW according to age.
2. Use foods that are easy to chew and swallow for Duchenne type.
3. Use pureed or blenderized foods where needed.
4. Provide adequate fiber (prune juice, bran, etc.) if constipation becomes a problem. Beware of excesses as well.

Profile

| Ht | Wt | Hand-to-mouth |
| IBW/HBW | Ability to chew | coordination |

Ability to swallow	Creatinine (often	Alb
N balance	decreased)	Gluc
H & H	CPK (inc.)	BUN
LDH (inc.)		

Patient Education

1. Provide low calorie snacks.
2. Help the patient modify food textures to meet needs.
3. Discuss problems related to inactivity or weight gain.

For More Information

Muscular Dystrophy Association
810 Seventh Ave.
New York, NY 10019

NOTES

OSTEOARTHRITIS AND DEGENERATIVE JOINT DISEASE

Usual Hospital Stay

4–5 days.

Notation

Osteoarthritis may be primary (more common in the elderly) or may follow an injury or disease involving the articular surfaces of synovial joints; it is technically "Osteoarthrosis." Symptoms and signs include pain, swelling, synovial joint stiffness. *Spondylosis* is osteoarthritis of the spine (see entry).

Objectives

1. If patient is obese, lessen pressure on weight-bearing joints.
2. Encourage patient (especially if elderly) to consume adequate amounts of protein and calcium. Fat and carbohydrate intake should be limited if these prevail in the diet.
3. Evaluate any food allergies.
4. Joint replacement may be necessary; prepare accordingly.

Dietary Recommendations

1. Use a calorie-controlled diet if obesity is present.
2. Dry skim milk can be used as a lower-calorie, less expensive source of calcium than fluid whole milk.
3. Increase use of fish and fish oils in the diet. Ensure adequate intake of zinc and vitamins C and E.

Profile

Ht	ASO titer	LE prep
IBW/HBW	Wt	X-rays
Antinuclear bodies	Sedimentation rate	Uric acid
Rheumatoid factor	C-reactive protein	K^+, Na^+
BUN, creat	Gluc	

Side Effects of Common Drugs Used

1. *Aspirin* can be taken with meals to reduce gastric distress. Prolonged use can cause GI bleeding. Intake of vitamin C and folate should be increased.
2. *Steroids* may cause sodium retention; calcium, nitrogen, and potassium depletion; truncal obesity; and hyperglycemia.
3. *Non-steroidal anti-inflammatory agents* indomethacin (Indocin), sulindac (Clinoril) may cause nausea or RF or diarrhea. Ibuprofen (Advil/Motrin) may cause nausea and vomiting, take with food. Anorexia, flatulence, and GI distress may also occur.

Patient Education

1. Encourage the patient to avoid fad diets for "arthritis cure."
2. Ensure that the patient's diet is balanced and includes all nutrients.
3. DJD is seldom a serious problem and has no life-threatening risks.
4. "Rest frequently, and sleep on a firm bed" is wise advice.
5. Do not allow muscles around the joints to become weak through disuse.

For More Information

Arthritis Foundation
1314 Spring St., NW
Atlanta, GA 30309
(800) 523-1429/2210

Arthritis Medical Center: (800) 327-3027

OSTEOMYELITIS, ACUTE

Usual Hospital Stay

4–5 days.

Notation

The acute form of osteomyelitis may be due to localized infection of the long bones or bone trauma. Infectious agents may include *E. coli, Staphylococcus aureus, Streptococcus pyogenes*.

Symptoms and signs include sudden, acute pain in the joint nearest the site of infection, fever, chills, tachycardia, diaphoresis, nausea and vomiting, dehydration, electrolyte imbalance, contractures in affected extremities, and pressure sores.

Objectives

1. Decrease febrile state.
2. Correct nausea and vomiting.
3. Prevent further infection, dehydration and other complications.
4. Promote recovery and healing.

Dietary Recommendations

1. Encourage adequate fluid intake.
2. Maintain a normal to high calorie and protein intake, with adequate amounts of vitamins and minerals included (e.g., vitamin C).

Profile

Ht, Wt	IBW/HBW	WBCs (inc.)
ESR (inc.)	I & O	Temp
K^+	Na^+	BP
Other symptoms	Ca^{++}	Gluc

Side Effects of Common Drugs Used

Antibiotics may be needed to correct any infections that are present.

Patient Education

1. Discuss the role of nutrition in wound healing, immunity and other conditions related to this disorder.
2. Discuss signs that may indicate reversal in status or recovery.

OSTEOMALACIA

Usual Hospital Stay

4 days.

Notation

Deossification of the bone (osteomalacia, or adult rickets) results from deficiency of vitamin D, calcium, or phosphorus. Bones become softened and deformed. Other symptoms include muscular weakness, listlessness, aching and bowing of bones. Osteomalacia may occur in conjunction with bone loss and hip fractures, but more generally with vitamin D deficiency. Risk factors include Crohn's disease with colonic resection, CRF, CF, and celiac disease.

Objectives

1. Provide the correct amount of calcium, phosphorus, or vitamin D.
2. Prevent or reverse (if possible) bone density loss resulting from Ca loss in the bone matrix.
3. Monitor long-term use of TPN; check contents of calcium and vitamin D.

Dietary Recommendations

1. Encourage use of milk, especially vitamin-D-fortified milk. The diet should be high in calcium; adults need 1000 mg or more.
2. If the patient is lactose-intolerant, try Lact-aid or other forms of lactose-free milk.

Profile

Ht	Serum Ca^{++} (dec.)	X-ray ("washed out"
IBW/HBW	Bone pain	bones)
Serum P (dec.)	Bone biopsy	Alk phos (inc.)
Wt		

Side Effects of Common Drugs Used

1. Treatment with *calcium salts* should be monitored frequently to prevent hypercalcemia.
2. TPN solutions may need to exclude excess vitamin D, which may be one cause of this problem.
3. *Anticonvulsant therapy* may deplete vitamin D and calcium.
4. Tranquilizers, sedatives, muscle relaxants, and oral diabetic agents may also deplete vitamin D.

5. Phosphate binders with aluminum may precipitate the disorder. Calcium carbonate may be an effective substitute; do not take with whole grains, bran, high oxalate foods, or with iron or vitamin D supplements.
6. Drugs that inhibit calcium absorption include furosemide (Lasix), neomycin, thyroid hormone, triameterene, heparin, steroids, or cholestyramine.

Patient Education

1. Explain which foods are good sources of calcium, phosphorus, and vitamin D. Encourage the patient to spend time in the sun!
2. Explain that fortified margarine and milk are good sources of vitamin D.
3. Vegetarians who avoid animal products may be at risk.

NOTES

OSTEOPOROSIS

Usual Hospital Stay

4–5 days.

Notation

Osteoporosis is defined as porousness and brittleness of bones. Type I is *postmenopausal,* occurring in women 18–20 years after menopause, with pain in the vertebrae, rounding of shoulders, height loss, and proneness to fractures. Type II is *senile* osteoporosis. Of the population aged more than 85 years, 4% sustain a serious fracture related to osteoporosis each year. Symptoms and signs range from asymptomatic conditions to severe backache. Ten percent of women over 50 have some form of it; lactase deficiency is common. Type I responds best to estrogen replacement. Type II may respond to calcium increases.

Objectives

1. Help the obese patient lose weight.
2. Normalize the Ca:P ratio to reverse the decline in bone density; 1:1 is suggested.

3. Lessen the risk of spontaneous fractures.
4. Decrease precipitating factors: anticonvulsants, corticosteroids, lactase deficiency, low milk intake, general low intake of calcium or calcium malabsorption, and sedentary lifestyle.
5. Provide adequate time for improvement, which takes 6–9 months.

Dietary Recommendations

1. The diet should be high in calcium, at least 800–1000 mg daily before menopause, 1.5 g daily after menopause. To fulfill the requirement, 1 quart of milk daily can be prescribed, or calcium supplements can be used if dairy products are not tolerated.
2. If the patient is obese, use a calorie-controlled diet.
3. In the early stages of treatment, try controlling the phosphorus from dietary sources; a 1:1 ratio is needed.
4. Dry skim milk powder can be added to many foods. Cheese is also a good calcium source, especially aged cheese. Live-culture yogurt is beneficial.
5. Check that the water is fluoridated in the area.
6. 1–2× normal RDA of vitamin D may be needed.
7. Adequate manganese (meat sources, for example) is beneficial.
8. Beware excesses of fiber, phytates, magnesium, cellulose, and protein.

Profile

Ht	Wt	Back pain
IBW/HBW	Ca^{++}, serum	Ca^{++}, urine
P (dec.)	PTH	Mg^{++}
Bone densitometry	Alk phos	

Side Effects of Common Drugs Used

1. *Os-Cal,* a calcium supplement, can cause hypercalcemia. Its use should be carefully watched. Beware of excess vitamin D, which can cause vitamin D calcinosis.
2. *Estrogen* increases the risk of cancer of the endometrium. Ensure adequate calcium intake.
3. *Calcium carbonate* (Tums, Titralac) temporarily decreases gastric acidity, which is needed for calcium absorption. Dietary calcium is better absorbed.
4. Elemental calcium varies in supplements (calcium carbonate 40%; calcium chloride 36%; bone meal, which may include contaminants, 33%; calcium citrate 21%; calcium gluconate 9%).
5. *Sodium fluoride* can cause changes in bone quality and may actually increase fractures.
6. *Etidronate plus phosphorus* may be used to increase bone mass, if approved by the FDA.

Patient Education

1. Encourage the patient to stand upright, rather than sit or recline, as often as feasible.
2. Explain that the efficiency of calcium absorption declines with age.
3. Use fluids liberally to prevent formation of calcium stones or hypercalcemia.
4. Describe the use of milk and other alternate calcium sources in the diet.
5. Change a sedentary lifestyle. Walking is a beneficial exercise.
6. Decrease use of alcohol, cigarettes and caffeine.
7. Encourage adequate exposure to sunlight.
8. Beware of vegetarian diets that are low in absorbable manganese, a factor in bone reformation/maintenance.
9. Beware of excessive weight-bearing exercise, which can cause amenorrhea when a low-calorie diet is consumed.

Comments

Table 11–2.
Osteoporosis Risk Factors
Premature menopause
Family history of osteoporosis
Slender frame
Smoking and alcohol use
Low dietary calcium availability (poor diet, excess fiber)

For More Information

National Osteoporosis Foundation
1625 I (Eye) St., NW, Suite 1011
Washington, DC 20006
(202) 223-2226

NOTES

PAGET'S DISEASE (OSTEITIS DEFORMANS)

Usual Hospital Stay

6 days.

Notation

Paget's disease is a nonmetabolic bone disease of unknown etiology, with excessive bone destruction and repairing. There is a strong familial occurrence, usually after the age of 40. Of all persons over age 50, 3% have an isolated lesion; the actual clinical disease is much less common. Prognosis is good in mild cases; unfavorable in severe cases.

Symptoms and signs include deep "bone pain," skull enlargement, headaches, thickening of long bones, heart failure (especially in severe form), spontaneous fractures, anemia or bone sarcoma.

Objectives

1. Prevent complications, especially related to the nervous system (e.g., blindness, fractures, vertebral collapse, and deafness).
2. Prevent side effects of drug therapy.
3. Promote full recovery where possible.
4. Differentiate from other conditions with bone lesions.

Dietary Recommendations

1. A high protein diet may be useful, with adequate calories to spare protein.
2. Adequate levels of calcium and vitamin C may be needed.
3. To correct anemia, monitor serum levels of iron and vitamin B_{12} to determine need for an altered diet.

Profile

Ht, Wt	P	Urinary Ca^{++}
Ca^{++}	PTH (abnormal)	(altered)
X-rays (denser, expanded bones)	UA (often elevated)	H & H
	Transferrin	Serum B_{12}
Alb	Alk phos	
IBW/HBW	Bone scans	

Side Effects of Common Drugs Used

1. *Thyrocalcitonin* or synthetic salmon *calcitonin* may be used; often parenteral as Calcimar. Monitor for nausea or vomiting.
2. *Aspirin* is often used to relieve bone pain; monitor GI effects.
3. *Vitamin D* may be used (e.g., 50,000 IUs 3 × weekly).
4. *Mithramycin* may be used.
5. *Estrogen* or *testosterone* may be given if osteoporosis co-exists.

Patient Education

1. Discuss appropriate dietary alterations for patient's condition.
2. Discuss side effects for the specific drugs ordered.

NOTES

POLYARTERITIS NODOSA

Usual Hospital Stay

4–5 days.

Notation

In this condition, medium and small arteries become inflamed in several organs, causing damage (often in brain, heart, liver and renal tissues). The condition is rare, 3× more common in men.

Symptoms and signs include chest pains (heart); shortness of breath (lungs); abdominal pain (liver and intestines); weakness and numbness (nerves); edema; and hematuria (kidneys). Fatigue, aches and pains, persistent fever, anorexia, weight loss and tachycardia may result.

Objectives

1. Treat as soon as possible to decrease heart and renal damage.
2. Improve appetite and intake.
3. Prevent weight loss.
4. Increase calorie intake to counteract fever.
5. Reduce edema, anorexia.

Dietary Recommendations

1. Adequate to high calorie intake may be beneficial in case of weight loss.
2. A normal to high protein intake is generally required.
3. Fluid or sodium intake may be limited with excessive edema, or with steroid use.

Profile

Ht, Wt	IBW/HBW	Edema
Hematuria	I & O	Temp
K$^+$	Na$^+$	BP
Alb	Transferrin	H & H

Side Effects of Common Drugs Used

1. *Steroids,* such as prednisone, may be used. Side effects of long-term use include negative nitrogen and potassium balances; decreased calcium and zinc levels; CHO intolerance; excessive sodium retention.
2. *Pain relievers* may be needed; monitor individually.

Patient Education

1. Discuss alternate dietary guidelines as appropriate for medications and side effects of the disease.
2. Discuss sources of nutrients as appropriate for the ordered diet.

RHEUMATOID ARTHRITIS

Usual Hospital Stay

5 days.

Notation

A chronic polyarthritis mainly affecting the smaller peripheral joints, rheumatoid arthritis is accompanied by general ill health and crippling deformities. Its cause is unknown, although autoimmunity has been suggested. Inflammation of synovial tissues is the dominant manifestation. Of all cases, 75% are in women.

Objectives

1. Maintain satisfactory nutritional status; malnutrition is common in this condition. Monitor weight changes.
2. Suggest ways of simplifying meal preparation.
3. Restrict sodium intake if needed.
4. Modify the patient's diet if hyperlipidemia is present (usually Type IV).
5. Avoid or correct constipation.

Dietary Recommendations

1. Use a high protein/high calorie diet if patient is malnourished.
2. Restrict saturated fats and sodium if other problems exist.
3. Provide bland meals if the drugs being used cause gastric irritation.

4. Ensure that the diet provides adequate intake of protein and calcium in the diet.
5. Adequate fluid, fiber, vitamins and minerals are important.
6. With dysphagia, tube feed or use soft/thick pureed foods as needed.

Profile

Ht	Wt	Temp
IBW/HBW	Sedimentation rate	Ceruloplasmin (inc.)
RBCs	(ESR)	H & H
C-reactive protein	Antinuclear bodies	Cu
(CRP)	Rheumatoid factor (RF)	TP
LE prep	Antistreptococcal	Alb
Creatinine (often dec.)	antibody titer	Gluc

Side Effects of Common Drugs Used

1. *ACTH.* Restrict sodium if needed.
2. *Salicylate/Aspirin.* Prolonged use can cause GI bleeding. Intake of vitamin C and folate should be increased.
3. *Phenylbutazone* (Butazolidin) can cause peptic ulceration.
4. *Indomethacin* (Indocin) can also cause GI ulceration, renal failure, hyperkalemia.
5. *Gold salts* may be used when conservative management fails.
6. *Fenoprofen* (Nalfon), *ibuprofen* (Motrin), and *naproxen* (Naprosyn) can cause headaches or nausea.
7. *Methotrexate* can cause anemia, nausea, vomiting, and stomatitis.

Patient Education

1. Instruct the patient about simplified planning and preparation tips.
2. No nutrients can replace needed blood transfusions for anemia.
3. Discourage quackery and substitute sound health practices. The "Dong" diet is farcical, for example.
4. Carbohydrate tolerance must reflect individual needs; sometimes carbohydrate intolerance occurs because of chronic inflammation.
5. Inflammatory responses may be affected by use of omega–3 fatty acids, from herring, salmon, and mackerel.

Comments

1. *Juvenile RA* can occur in children or adults. Salicylates, gold salts or glucocorticoids may be used.
2. *Sjögren syndrome* is a variant form of RA, with insufficient production of lacrimal and salivary secretions. Artificial tears, artificial saliva and glucocorticoids may be needed.

3. *Felty syndrome* is a triad of RA, granulocytopenia and splenomegaly. Infections, leg ulcers and anemia can also complicate the condition. Sometimes splenectomy is indicated. Drug therapy may be helpful to others.
4. *Rheumatoid vasculitis* can be life-threatening. Fatigue, weight loss, fever and peripheral neuropathy can occur. D-penicillamine and prednisone are generally used.

NOTES

RUPTURE OF INTERVERTEBRAL DISC

Usual Hospital Stay

5 days, medical back problems.

Notation

Slipping or prolapse of a cervical or lumbar disc can occur, with neck/shoulder pain or low back pain accordingly. With lumbar disc involvement, ambulation may be painful and limping can occur. Muscular weakness may also result.

Percutaneous automated discectomy (PAD) surgery can be performed in some cases; this surgery breaks up the disc and removes fragments.

Objectives

1. Maintain adequate rest and activity levels, as assigned by the physician.
2. Prevent weight gain from decreased activity.
3. Encourage adequate hydration.
4. Prevent constipation and straining.
5. Feed if patient is in traction.

Dietary Recommendations

1. A regular diet to control calories and weight gain is generally sufficient. For some, a more strict regimen may be beneficial.
2. Increased fluid and fiber intake can be helpful to reduce constipation. Fresh fruits and vegetables, bran and other foods may be needed.

Profile

Ht, Wt	Myelogram	Alb
I & O	Constipation	Ca^{++}
BP	X-rays	Alk. phos.
H & H	Edema	Gluc
IBW, HBW	Na^+, K^+	

Side Effects of Common Drugs Used

1. *Anti-inflammatory drugs* may be used.
2. *Analgesics* may be helpful to relieve pain.
3. *Muscle relaxants* may be ordered.

Patient Education

1. Instruct patient on effective methods of relieving constipation.
2. Discuss the role of nutrition and exercise in health maintenance.

SCLERODERMA

Usual Hospital Stay

5 days.

Notation

In scleroderma, also known as progressive systemic sclerosis (PSS), pathological deposition of fibrous connective tissue in the skin and visceral organs occurs. The GI tract is affected, and Raynaud's syndrome (ischemia of fingers) is common. There is no known cure, and the disease can be fatal.

Symptoms and signs include dysphagia, heartburn, fibrosis of salivary and lacrimal glands, abdominal pains, flatulence, weight loss, nausea and vomiting, diarrhea, and constipation.

Objectives

1. Prevent or correct PCM and nutrient deficiencies.
2. Correct xerostomia from Sjögren's syndrome (decreased saliva with dysphagia and difficulty in chewing as a result).
3. Monitor dysphagia with esophageal involvement; alter mode of feeding as needed.
4. Counteract vitamin B_{12} and fat maldigestion and absorption.
5. Monitor hypomotility of the GI tract, with altered fiber intake as appropriate.

Dietary Recommendations

1. A soft diet with moistened foods and extra fluids may be useful. Add fiber if constipation is a problem (e.g., adding crushed bran to hot cereal).
2. Tube feed if patient is dysphagic; use TPN if the condition is extreme.
3. Reduce lactose if lactose intolerance occurs.
4. Small, frequent feedings may be needed.
5. Reduce fiber in case of obstruction; low residue or tube feeding may be needed.
6. Give fat- and water-soluble vitamins in supplemental form if needed; extra calcium may be needed if lactose is not tolerated orally.
7. Calories (30–40 kcal/kg); high protein (NPN:kcal ratio of 150:1); low fat (less than 40 g daily) and reduced sodium may be useful.

Profile

Ht, Wt	B_{12}	Other parameters as
Serum folate	I & O	needed
IBW/HBW	Gluc	Skinfold
H & H	PT	measurements
Fecal fat test	Alb	
Hydrogen breath test	Temp	

Side Effects of Common Drugs Used

1. *Bethanecol* may be given to augment LES pressure.
2. *Antacids* may be used to reduce gastric hyperacidity.
3. *Antibiotics* may be necessary to decrease intestinal bacteria overgrowth.
4. Monthly *vitamin B_{12}* shots are beneficial to some patients, as required.
5. *Anti-inflammatory agents* are often used.

Patient Education

1. Artificial saliva (Xerolube) may be useful.
2. If eating orally, adequate chewing time will be required.
3. For heartburn, keep head elevated after meals; decrease or limit intake of chocolate, caffeine, fatty foods, alcohol, citrus, and tomatoes.

For More Information

United Scleroderma Foundation, Inc.
P.O. Box 350
Watsonville, CA 95077-0350

NOTES

SYSTEMIC LUPUS ERYTHEMATOSUS

Usual Hospital Stay

5 days.

Notation

A collagen disorder of unknown etiology, systemic lupus erythematosus (SLE) involves areas of erythema of the skin, pyrexia, toxemia, malaise, butterfly rash on cheeks, hepatosplenomegaly, weight loss, diarrhea, pleurisy, pericarditis, and renal damage. Women of child-bearing age are most affected.

Objectives

1. Counteract steroid therapy.
2. Replenish potassium reserves.
3. Reduce fever and replace nutrient losses, and weight loss.
4. Control disease manifestations. Cure is not yet possible.

Dietary Recommendations

1. Use a high potassium diet, unless potassium replacements are provided.
2. If needed, mildly restrict sodium intake.
3. The diet should be high in protein and kcal to compensate for nitrogen losses during fever. If renal damage is excessive, the diet can be adjusted.

Profile

Ht	Wt	Serum Cu (inc.)
IBW/HBW	K^+	TP (dec.)
BP	Na^+	WBCs (dec.)
Alb	H & H (dec.)	Gluc (inc.)
Transferrin	Serum Fe	Specific gravity, urine
LE prep	Antinuclear bodies	($\downarrow$)
Sedimentation rate	(inc.)	Chol (inc.)

Side Effects of Common Drugs Used

1. *Steroid therapy* may cause sodium retention, hyperglycemia, potassium and calcium depletion, negative nitrogen balance.
2. PABA lotions are needed to screen the sun's rays.

Patient Education

1. Ensure that the patient has an adequate intake of fluids during febrile periods.
2. Explain which foods are sources of sodium and potassium in the diet.
3. Adequate rest is needed during flare-ups.

For More Information

Lupus Foundation of America
1717 Mass. Ave. SW, Suite 203
Washington, DC 20036

Section 12
Hematology: Anemias and Blood Disorders

Chief Assessment Factors

concurrent illness, diseases (CVD, MI, asthma, hemorrhage, CA, renal disease)

surgery, especially gastric or hepatic or renal

infections, sepsis

family hx (leukemias, CA, anemias, immune disorders, allergies)

alcohol and nicotine use

dietary habits (heme vs. nonheme iron, etc.)

occupation

decreased protein intake

medications (prescriptions, OTC)

anorexia, fatigue

beefy, red tongue; other signs of deficiencies

Table 12–1.
Nutritional Factors in Blood Formation

Iron
Vitamin B_{12}
Folic acid
Vitamin B_6
Vitamin C
Protein
Vitamin E

Notation

Erythrocyte life span—120 days.
Microcytic anemias—usually iron deficiency causes or results.
Macrocytic anemias—folic acid or vitamin B_{12} insufficiency.
Normocytic anemias—from inhibition of marrow by infection or chronic disease.

Anemias can be encountered in generalized or in specific nutritional deficiencies.

"Nutritional anemias . . . caused by lack, corrected by provision."

—Dr. Victor Herbert

NOTES

HEMOCHROMATOSIS (IRON OVERLOADING)

Usual Hospital Stay

4–5 days.

Notation

Hemochromatosis is a condition in which iron stores are deposited in excess, often from excess intake or liver/pancreatic diseases, from renal dialysis, or frequent and long-term transfusions. Iron accumulation can occur as an inherited condition or can be from conditions listed above. The problem is ten times more common in males than in females.

Symptoms and signs include bronzing of the skin, cirrhosis, cardiomegaly with congestive failure, and diabetes mellitus.

Objectives

1. Remove excess iron from the body (usually with phlebotomies of 500 ml weekly).
2. If excess iron intake is a problem, discontinue its use.
3. Teach principles of nutrition and menu planning to incorporate adequate intake of other nutrients that may be depleted with excessive phlebotomies.

Dietary Recommendations

1. Provide a normal diet, unless renal or hepatic function are altered.
2. Ensure adequate protein intake, and provide calories to meet needs and activity.
3. Check food labels for iron fortification; discuss alternatives.

Profile

Ht, Wt	HBW, HBW	Serum Fe
Transferrin (inc.)	TIBC	H & H
I & O	Alb	Gluc
Serum Cu (inc.)	Ferritin (inc.)	

Patient Education

1. Discuss nutrient sources as appropriate for the individual.
2. Highlight iron fortification and review food labeling issues.

For More Information

Hemochromatosis Research Foundation
P.O. Box 8569
Albany, NY 12208

Iron Overload Disease Association (IOD)
224 Datura St., Suite 912
West Palm Beach, Florida 33401
(305) 659-5616

NOTES

APLASTIC ANEMIA

Usual Hospital Stay

4–5 days.

Notation

This anemia is a normocytic, normochromic anemia where normal marrow is replaced with fat. It may be caused by exposure to drugs, chemicals, diseases or radiation.

Symptoms and signs include fatigue, slow thought processes, headache, dizziness, irritability, waxlike pallor, petechiae, ecchymosis; hemorrhagic diathesis (gums, nose, GI tract, urinary tract, vagina); tachycardia, tachypnea, dyspnea, upper respiratory infections; hemosiderosis with resulting cirrhosis, diabetes, heart failure, and bronzing of skin.

Objectives

1. Prevent infections or sepsis.
2. Reduce bleeding tendencies and hemorrhages.
3. Prepare for splenectomy or bone marrow transplantation.
4. Reduce febrile status.
5. Prevent further complications and decline in cardiovascular and hepatic functions.

Dietary Recommendations

1. Replenish nutrient stores.
2. Provide a balanced diet with six small feedings.
3. Provide extra fluid unless contraindicated (e.g., 3 liters daily).
4. If patient has mouth lesions, avoid excesses in hot or cold foods, spicy or acidic foods, or rough textures.
5. If steroids are used, limiting sodium intake may be beneficial.

Profile

Ht, Wt	IBW/HBW	H & H
RBC count (dec.)	Granulocytes (dec.)	Platelets (dec.)
PT	BP	WBCs (under 1500)
Serum Fe	TIBC	Alb
Gluc	Transferrin	Other parameters

Side Effects of Common Drugs Used

1. *Corticosteroids* may be used. Watch side effects of chronic use, such as elevated serum sodium levels, decreased potassium and calcium levels, negative nitrogen balance.
2. *Aspirin* must be avoided.
3. *Antibiotics* may be required when infections are present.
4. Other drugs which may aggravate the condition include *chloramphenicol, phenylbutazone, sulfa drugs,* and *ibuprofen.*

Patient Education

1. Discuss the needs of the patient that are specific for signs and symptoms and for side effects of any medications.
2. Discuss meal planning that is simplified but nutritious.

NOTES

ANEMIA, FOLIC ACID DEFICIENCY

Usual Hospital Stay

4–5 days.

Notation

Folic acid is needed for the synthesis of DNA and maturation of red blood cells. Folic acid deficiency is generally caused by inadequate diet, intestinal malabsorption, alcoholism, or pregnancy. It is a hyperchromic/macrocytic/nonmegaloblastic anemia with signs and symptoms of weight loss, anorexia, malnutrition, smooth and red tongue, and cold extremities.

Objectives

1. Increase folic acid in the diet to allevaite anemia.
2. Improve the diet to provide nutrients needed to make red blood cells.
3. Instruct the patient to correct faulty diet habits, if they are the cause of the anemia.
4. Check for other malabsorption syndromes, and correct these as well.

Dietary Recommendations

1. Provide a diet that is high in folic acid, protein, copper, iron, vitamin C and vitamin B_{12}.
2. Ingestion of one fresh fruit or vegetable would provide sufficient folic acid, but other sources include fish, legumes, whole grains, leafy greens, broccoli, grapefruit, and meats. Avoid overcooking.
3. Diets that provide bland, liquid, or soft foods may be needed for sore mouth. 6–8 small meals may be helpful.

Profile

Ht	Wt	Serum Fe (inc.)
IBW/HBW	H & H	MCV
Serum folate (under 5 mg/dl)	CBC (macrocytic cells)	Leukopenia, WBCs
	Transferrin	Forminoglutamic acid (FIGLU)
Low RBCs		

Side Effects of Common Drugs Used

1. Supplements of *folic acid* are better than diet alone to alleviate the anemia. A common dose is 1–5 mg folic acid. *Leucovorin* is an active reduced form.
2. *Anticonvulsants* (primidone, phenytoin, phenobarbitol) interfere with the body's use of the folic acid.
3. *Folic acid antagonists* (cancer treatments) affect the body's use of folic acid. Methotrexate, for example, is especially depleting; it is common to administer leucovorin as a "folinic acid rescue."
4. *Oral contraceptives* decrease the body's ability to use folic acid.
5. *Multivitamin preparations* may not contain folic acid because folacin masks a vitamin B_{12} deficiency. Check the labels. Vitamin B_{12} helps folate travel into cells via transport form (5-methyl tetrahydrofolate).

Patient Education

1. Vitamin C promotes absorption of folic acid from foods.
2. Pregnant women should receive appropriate counseling; 30% may have a folate deficiency. Daily needs increase by about 400 micrograms.
3. Large intakes of folate (1 mg + /day, etc.) can cure the anemia but may mask a correlated vitamin B_{12} anemia; monitor carefully.
4. Attractive meals may help the appetite.
5. Fad and restrictive diets should be avoided.
6. Alcoholic beverages interfere with folate metabolism and absorption.

NOTES

ANEMIA, IRON DEFICIENCY

Usual Hospital Stay

4–5 days.

Notation

The most commonly deficient nutrient in the world is iron. This anemia results from inadequate intake or impaired absorption of iron, blood loss, or repeated pregnancies. When caused by an inadequate diet, it may take years to produce symptoms when there are adequate iron stores. Iron is the basic nutritional component of heme.

About 90% of the body's store of iron is reused. The diet replaces iron lost through sweat, feces, and urine. Menstruation increases iron losses by 30 mg per month. Infants, preschoolers, and teenagers are also at risk.

Pica is seen in approximately 50% of patients with this condition. Symptoms and signs include weakness, fatigue, vertigo, headache, irritability, heartburn, dysphagia, flatulence, vague abdominal pains, anorexia, glossitis, stomatitis, pale skin, ankle edema, tingling extremities, and palpitations.

Objectives

1. Provide adequate oral iron to replace losses or deficits, especially heme sources.
2. Provide an acid medium to favor better absorption.
3. Monitor and correct geophagia (clay-eating), ice-eating, and other forms of food pica. Excessive consumption of life savers, ice, lettuce, celery, snack chips, and chocolate are commonly seen forms of pica.
4. Alleviate the anemia and associated anorexia. Correct causation.
5. Avoid constipation.

Dietary Recommendations

1. Use a diet with adequate iron in addition to medications. Sources of iron include liver, eggs, kidney, beef, dried fruits, whole-grain cereals, molasses. Heme iron is readily found in beef, pork, and lamb; consume with fruit or fruit juice.
2. Use liberal amounts of HBV proteins (needed for production of red blood cells and Hgb). Foods with HBV proteins include meat, cheese and eggs.
3. Increase intake of vitamin C (oranges, grapefruit, tomatoes, broccoli, cabbage, baked potatoes, strawberries), *especially* when the patient is taking an iron pill, to increase the acid medium. Sugars also enhance iron absorption.
4. Detect pica and discuss with the patient. Foods chosen are often crunchy or brittle. After cure of the anemia, the craving often becomes a revulsion.

Profile

Ht

IBW/HBW

H & H (Hgb more sensitive)

MCH, MCHC (dec.)

CBC

Transferrin

*% Transferrin Saturation = Serum Fe/TIBC × 100 (normal = 35 + 15%)

*Free Erythrocyte Protoporphyrin (FEP) (normal 30 μg%)

Wt

*Ferritin (dec. stores in liver, spleen, bone marrow)

MCV (below 80)

RBCs (small, microcytic, hypochromic)

WBC/differential (inc.)

TIBC (inc. over 350)

Pallor, diarrhea

Brittle fingernails, spoon-shaped

Serum Cu

---

* Best Tests.

Side Effects of Common Drugs Used

1. *Ferrous salts* are better utilized for iron therapy than other forms; 10–100 mg × 4 daily after meals, for example.
2. *Iron tablets* should not be taken simultaneously with tetracycline since they decrease the effectiveness of the antibiotic. Gastric irritation is common with iron medications; increase their use slowly. *Feostat, Fergon, Feosol* are commonly used brands.
3. Coffee and tea with meals may reduce iron absorption.
4. *Imferon* can be given intramuscularly if oral iron is not tolerated. Pain and skin discoloration may result.
5. *Enteric-coated or sustained-release remedies* are more expensive and often carry the iron past maximal absorption site in the upper intestine.
6. *Aspirin* or *corticosteroids* can increase GI bleeding or cause peptic ulceration.

Patient Education

1. Hemoglobin is made from protein, iron, and copper. Red blood cells are made from vitamin B_{12}, folacin, and amino acids.
2. Explain food pica—ice, clay, starch, plaster, paint chips, etc.
3. Explain which foods are good sources of iron, protein, vitamin C, and related nutrients.
4. Changes in stool color (green or tarry and black) are common, with supplements.
5. Beware of excessive phytates, phosphates, oxalates, fiber, alkalis, antacids, tannins, calcium phosphates. Discuss food sources.
6. To avoid side-effects of supplements, take them with meals or milk. "Food iron" has fewer side effects.
7. The average American diet contains 10–20 mg iron daily, roughly 10% of which is absorbed.

8. Overdosing (200 mg iron or more daily) with supplements does no good. The body can only synthesize 5–10 mg hemoglobin per day. The process cannot be expedited.
9. Local or systemic infections interfere with iron absorption and transport.

Comment

Upper SI is where iron is best absorbed. Damage or surgery here can greatly inhibit total iron absorption, thus leading to greater risk of deficiency.

NOTES

ANEMIA, PERNICIOUS AND B_{12} DEFICIENCY

Usual Hospital Stay

6 days.

Notation

Pernicious anemia is a conditioned vitamin B_{12} deficiency with defective RBC production caused by a lack of intrinsic factor of the stomach. If there is no intrinsic factor, extrinsic factor (vitamin B_{12}) is not absorbed. This is rare before age 35. Vitamin B_{12} is needed for maturation of the red blood cells.

With poor intake of extrinsic factor (vitamin B_{12}) the *megaloblastic anemia* is corrected by use of oral cyanocobalamin once weekly for a month. Vitamin B_{12} deficiency may take 5–6 years to appear. It is rare, and occurs mostly in vegetarians.

Symptoms of either type of anemia may include fatigue, flatulence, nausea and vomiting, diarrhea, constipation, anorexia, weight loss, pale waxy skin, tachycardia, cardiomegaly, achlorhydria, and glossitis. Lemon-yellow pallor of skin often occurs in pernicious anemia.

Objectives

1. Alleviate the anemia and causation, where possible.
2. Provide foods that won't hurt a sore mouth. Glossitis (a beefy, red tongue) decreases the desire to eat.
3. Correct the patient's anorexia.

Dietary Recommendations

The following suggestions are supportive measures for the *required* B_{12} injections in pernicious anemia:

1. The diet should make liberal use of HBV proteins.
2. If the patient has a sore mouth, use a soft or liquid diet, of bland foods especially.
3. Supplement the diet with iron, vitamin C and other B-vitamins (folic acid), and copper.
4. Good sources of vitamin B_{12} include liver. Daily average intake is 2–30 micrograms.

Profile

Ht	CBC	Beefy red tongue
HBW/HBW	Schilling test (dec.)	TIBC
RBCs	Transferrin	Urinary
Macrocytic/nucleated	Gastrin (inc.)	methylmalonic acid
cells	Serum B_{12}	for B_{12} status
LDH (may be inc.)	MCV, MCHC, MCH	
Wt	(inc.)	

Side Effects of Common Drugs Used

1. *Vitamin B_{12} injections* must be given daily until remission of pernicious anemia, after which six to eight injections yearly will suffice. Usual dose is 100 micrograms/dose. Avoid megadoses.
2. *Trinsicon* contains vitamin B_{12}, ferrous fumarate, vitamin C, folacin and intrinsic factor. Avoid taking it with dairy products.
3. *Crystimin* or *Rubramin PC* are cyanocobalamin drugs for vitamin B_{12} deficiency.

Patient Education

1. Beware of vegetarian diets since vitamin B_{12} is found only in animal foods. Avoid fad diets as well.
2. Pernicious anemia develops after total gastrectomy unless vitamin B_{12} is administered. The problem can occur in patients with only partial gastrectomy, or with patients who have had gastrojejunostomies.
3. Avoidance of fatigue is essential.
4. *Megalobastic B_{12} anemia* may be common in the elderly; careful food choices are essential.
5. For *pernicious anemia,* lifelong injections are necessary.

ANEMIA, PROTEIN DEFICIENCY

Usual Hospital Stay

4–5 days.

Notation

Protein is required for production of hemoglobin and red blood cells. When intake is deficient, the body frees protein from red blood cells for other uses.

Protein-deficiency anemia usually occurs in combination with other deficiencies. It may occur in patients with nephrosis.

Objectives

1. Gradually reintroduce the patient to a high protein diet if the patient has had deficient protein intake for a long time.
2. Correct concurrent deficiencies of other nutrients.
3. Supply adequate amounts of calories and carbohydrates so that amino acids can be used for erythropoiesis.

Dietary Recommendations

1. Use a normal, well-balanced diet with emphasis on HBV proteins.
2. Ensure that the diet supplies adequate amounts of iron, vitamin B_{12}, and folic acid to support red blood cell formation. Pyridoxine should also be adequate.
3. Ensure that the diet includes 1.5–3 g protein/kg body weight (approximately 100–150 g for adults).
4. Ensure that the diet is high in carbohydrates and calories.

Profile

Ht	Wt	Serum B_{12}
IBW/HBW	H & H	Serum folacin
Alb, prealbumin	CBC	Serum pyridoxine
Transferrin	Fe	Serum copper
RBP	WBCs	Total protein

Patient Education

1. Protein deficiency leads to nutritional edema, which may mask signs of poor nutrition.
2. Indicate which foods are low cost sources of protein (e.g., textured vegetable protein, peanut butter). Two tablespoons of peanut butter contain 8 g of protein and 0.6 mg of iron.
3. Explain that less expensive cuts of meat contain as much protein as expensive ones.

ANEMIA, COPPER DEFICIENCY

Usual Hospital Stay

4–5 days.

Notation

Copper is needed in minute amounts for the formation of hemoglobin. People with poor diets who have a high intake of milk may become deficient in copper. The copper-deficient anemias may actually be related to iron and protein deficiencies.

Objectives

1. Correct the anemia.
2. Instruct the patient about good sources of protein, iron and copper to prevent recurrences.

Dietary Recommendations

1. Good sources of copper include oysters, liver, nuts, dried legumes, and raisins.
2. Protein should be at least 1 g/kg; iron intake adequate for age and sex.

Profile

Ht	Serum copper	RBP
IBW/HBW	H & H	Hypochromic anemia
CBC	Ceruloplasmin	
Alb, prealbumin	Transferrin	
Wt	Serum Fe	

Patient Education

1. Indicate which foods are good sources of copper, iron and protein.
2. Have the patient avoid fad diets. Monitor vegetarian (nonheme iron) diets carefully.

NOTES

ANEMIA FROM PARASITIC INFESTATION

Usual Hospital Stay

4–5 days.

Notation

Infestation of the GI tract by parasitic worms that feed on blood (hookworm) or on nutrients (tapeworm) may occur. Anemia can result as a side effect of blood loss, deficiencies in iron or vitamin B_{12} or folic acid.

Symptoms include anemia, fatigue, abdominal discomfort, nausea, vomiting, fever and irritability.

See also the Ascariasis and Trichinosis entries in Section 15.

Objectives

1. Correct the anemia from blood losses; eliminate the parasitic infestation.
2. Prevent GI tract perforation or obstruction, where likely to exist.
3. Improve nutritional status and appetite.

Dietary Recommendations

1. A diet high in protein, B-complex vitamins and iron may be appropriate.
2. Provide adequate calories to meet individual needs for anabolism, if needed.
3. Heme iron sources and vitamin C should be included in foods chosen.
4. Iron inhibitors should be excluded from the diet as far as possible until recovery is complete.

Profile

Ht, Wt	IBW/HBW	H & H
Serum B_{12}	Serum Fe	Transferrin
TIBC	Serum folic acid	Gluc
Alb	Other parameters	Serum Cu

Side Effects of Common Drugs Used

If needed, oral or parenteral iron may be given to correct the anemia more rapidly. Beware of excessive use of oral supplements because of their potential side effects with iron overloading; monitor all sources (including iron-enriched foods).

Patient Education

1. Discuss ways to prevent further parasitic infestations, as with small children playing in soil.

2. Discuss ways to prepare foods high in necessary nutrients, and methods to increase bioavailability (e.g., combining orange juice at breakfast with an iron-fortified cereal, etc.)

NOTES

ANEMIA, HEMOLYTIC FROM VITAMIN E DEFICIENCY

Usual Hospital Stay

4–5 days.

Notation

In hemolytic anemia caused by a vitamin E deficiency, the red blood cells have an abnormal membrane, which results in hemolysis.

This condition often occurs in infants who receive PUFAs without adequate vitamin E.

Symptoms and signs include edema, anemia, noisy breathing, puffy eyelids. In severe cases, encephalomalacia can result (in infancy.)

Objectives

1. Correct vitamin E deficit.
2. Prevent further complications.
3. Correct the anemia.

Dietary Recommendations

1. Decrease excessive PUFA intake, which depletes vitamin E.
2. Provide diet as usual for age and sex.
3. Avoid excesses of iron.
4. Ensure adequate intake of zinc, which may become deficient.

Profile

Ht, wt or growth %	TIBC	Transferrin
Serum a-tocopherol	Bilirubin	Gluc
levels	IBW/HBW	SGOT (inc.)

Side Effects of Common Drugs Used

Water-soluble vitamin E (alpha tocopherol) is likely to be given daily. Avoid taking with an iron supplement, which could interfere with utilization.

Patient Education

1. Discuss, in layman's terms, the role of vitamin E in lipid oxidation and utilization. Discuss sources of polyunsaturated fats and why excesses should be controlled.
2. Discuss sources of vitamin E in the diet.

NOTES

ANEMIA, SIDEROBLASTIC/SIDEROTIC

Usual Hospital Stay

4–5 days.

Notation

Sideroblastic anemia is a microcytic, hypochromic anemia similar to that caused by iron deficiency, except that serum iron is normal or elevated. In some cases, a vitamin B_6 deficiency impairs hemoglobin synthesis.

The disorder may also have nonnutritional causes, such as from CA, isoniazid (INH) use (nonsupplemented), collagen disorders, and chronic alcoholism.

Signs and symptoms are the same as those found in iron-deficiency anemia.

Objectives

1. Correct problems and symptoms.
2. Identify causes and solutions.
3. Correct any suppression of bone marrow, iron-loading, etc.

Dietary Recommendations

1. A diet high in vitamin B_6 may be beneficial (often drugs are used).
2. Protein and carbohydrate intake should be adequate; calories as well.

3. Folic acid may also be needed.
4. Alcohol intake should be severely limited.
5. Balanced meals and snacks as necessary may be appropriate.

Profile

Ht, Wt	IBW/HBW	B_6 levels
Transferrin saturation	Serum folic acid	Serum Cu
(often elevated)	WBCs	
RBC count	Serum Fe	

Side Effects of Common Drugs Used

1. 50–200 mg vitamin B_6 may be ordered (age-dependent doses).
2. Chloramphenicol may cause drug-induced bone marrow suppression, resulting in sideroblastic anemia.
3. Isoniazid (INH) and cycloserine can cause abnormal vitamin B_6 metabolism.

Patient Education

1. Discuss adequate sources of all needed nutrients, such as vitamin B_6—especially if the deficiency was causative.
2. Discuss attractive menu planning and balancing of meals.

NOTES

HEMORRHAGE, ACUTE OR CHRONIC

Usual Hospital Stay

Varies.

Notation

A hemorrhage is defined as the escape of blood from a ruptured vessel. The bleeding (bright red and in spurts from an artery; dark red and in a steady flow from a vein) can be external, internal, or into skin or other tissue. When massive, a hemorrhage can cause such symptoms as rapid, shallow breathing;

cold, clammy skin; thirst; visual disturbances; and extreme weakness. Loss of over 20% of blood volume causes hypotension and tachycardia.

Objectives

1. Medical management is designed to control bleeding, take care of the underlying cause of the bleeding, and replace lost blood. Transfusions may be given.
2. Less severe hemorrhages may require iron, vitamin B_{12}, and folic acid to help replace red blood cells.
3. Support erythropoiesis.
4. Control intestinal effects from GI bleeding, which can cause a protein overload.

Dietary Recommendations

1. Ensure that the diet is rich in proteins, iron, folic acid, vitamin B_{12}, and copper.
2. Check for the need for vitamin K.

Profile

Ht	BUN, creat	Serum Fe
HBW/HBW	Wt	Serum B_{12}
Transferrin	Occult blood	Serum folate
RBCs	CBC	PT
Alb	H & H	TIBC (inc.)

Patient Education

1. Blood donors should be alerted to the need to replace daily iron intake by 0.7 mg for a year. Every pint is equivalent to 250 mg of iron lost.
2. Discuss adequate dietary replacement for lost nutrients.

Comment

Blood clots when its fibrinogen is converted to fibrin by action of thrombin. Factors involving nutrition include:

I Fibrinogen
II Prothrombin
III Thromboplastin
IV Calcium

SICKLE CELL ANEMIA

Usual Hospital Stay

4–5 days.

Notation

Sickle cell anemia is a hereditary hemolytic anemia. Cells are crescent-shaped. It is most common in black populations and is usually detected within the first year of life. Bone marrow functions at $6 \times$ normal rate.

Objectives

1. Supplement treatment with missing nutrients. Correct any malnutrition.
2. Reduce the oxygen debt. Improve the patient's ability to participate in the activities of daily life.
3. Reduce painful cramps, liver dysfunction, cholelithiasis, jaundice, and hepatitis.
4. Lessen decubiti, infections, renal failure.
5. Promote normal growth and development, which could be stunted in children.

Dietary Recommendations

1. Use vitamin B_6 and folic acid supplements and adequate diet.
2. The diet should include HBV proteins, adequate vitamin B_{12}.
3. The diet should provide adequate intake of vitamin C, zinc, riboflavin, vitamin E, vitamin A, and calories. Avoid excesses of vitamin C and iron.
4. Nightly tube feeding can help to improve nutritional status.

Profile

Ht	Wt	MCV, Serum ferritin
IBW/HBW	H & H	TLC
Serum Fe (inc. from hemolysis)	% Transferrin sat.	Po, Pco_2
	Urinary zinc	Serum folacin
Alb (normal)	N balance	TSF
RBP (dec.)	Chol, trig (dec.)	Uric acid (inc.)

Patient Education

Indicate which foods are good sources of folic acid, HBV proteins, vitamin C, zinc, riboflavin, and vitamins A, E, and B_6.

Comments

1. Iron deficiency, through reduction of MCHC, may actually be beneficial for longer RBC survival and O_2 affinity. Studies are not conclusive.
2. Be careful about iron overloading, especially after transfusions.

For More Information

National Association for Sickle Cell Disease, Inc.
3460 Wilshire Blvd.
Los Angeles, CA 90010

NOTES

POLYCYTHEMIA VERA (OSLER'S DISEASE)

Usual Hospital Stay

4–5 days.

Notation

This condition is a chronic, progressive disease in which increased blood volume and increased erythrocyte levels occur.

Signs and symptoms may include: belching, fullness, thirst, flatulence, constipation, headache, vertigo, lassitude, tinnitus, blurred vision, diplopia, dyspnea on exertion, chest pain, paresthesias, pruritus, dusky reddish skin on face and hands, thrombosis (which could lead to MI or CVA), gout, hemorrhagic tendency, hypertension, enlarged spleen, seizures, confusion, slurred speech, peptic ulcer, or CHF.

Objectives

1. Prepare patient for phlebotomy by ensuring adequate nutrient stores.
2. Prepare, as needed, for chemotherapy or radiation therapy, which may be provided.
3. Correct or control the condition.

Dietary Recommendations

1. A diet of preferred foods and balanced meals should be offered.
2. Extra fluids will be helpful, as with 3–4 liters daily (unless contraindicated, as with CHF).
3. Changes in dietary texture or content may be needed if radiation or chemotherapy alter nutrient or dietary needs.

Profile

Ht, Wt	IBW/HBW	I & O
H & H (elevated)	RBCs (7–12 million)	Alb
Gluc	BP	

Side Effects of Common Drugs Used

Chemotherapeutic agents (busulfan, chlorambucil, cyclophosphamide) may be used. Nausea and vomiting are some of the common side effects.

Patient Education

Discuss the need to maintain a healthy lifestyle and to eat adequate protein and calories because of the frequent phlebotomies (where completed).

NOTES

THROMBOCYTOPENIC PURPURA

Usual Hospital Stay

4–5 days.

Notation

Idiopathic (ITP) is caused by platelet destruction by antibodies, causing bleeding disorders. Mild to excessive bleeding occurs in skin, gingiva, nose, and internally.

Thrombotic (TTP) is a platelet disorder manifested by vascular lesions. Headache, slurred speech, numbness and weakness of extremities, increased temperature, and bleeding (as in ITP) occur.

Objectives

1. Avoid infections, especially upper respiratory infections and flu to prevent coughing, which increases intracranial pressure.
2. Rest adequately.
3. Prepare patient for splenectomy, if indicated. Ensure adequate nutrient stores.
4. Reduce bleeding tendency and complicating results.

Dietary Recommendations

1. Maintain diet of preference or as ordered. Use small, frequent feedings if patient has nausea or vomiting.
2. Adequate folic acid will be needed.
3. Increase fluids (e.g., to 3 liters daily) unless contraindicated.
4. After splenectomy, a patient will need adequate protein, calories, zinc, vitamin A, and vitamin C for wound healing.
5. Vitamin K in the diet may need to be monitored.

Profile

Ht, Wt	N Balance	Ca^{++}
Proteinuria	PT	K^+, Na^+
Alb	H & H (dec.)	
IBW/HBW	Casts in urine	

Side Effects of Common Drugs Used

Corticosteroids may be used to control bleeding. Side effects are numerous, and may affect nutritional status—e.g., decreased serum Ca^{++}, K^+ and nitrogen; increased serum Na^+; glucose intolerance.

Patient Education

Discuss altering nutrients as needed, dependent upon medications ordered and their use over time; surgery if required; and ability to eat adequately.

NOTES

THALASSEMIA (COOLEY'S ANEMIA)

Usual Hospital Stay

4–5 days.

Notation

Thalassemia is a hereditary disease with an increased rate of destruction of red blood cells. It is most common in persons with Mediterranean ancestry. The red blood cells are fragile and contain abnormal hemoglobin.

Signs and symptoms include anemia, bone abnormalities, jaundice, enlarged spleen, and leg ulcers.

The most common form, beta-thalassemia, may allow a normal lifespan; some other forms may be fatal.

Objectives

1. Offer temporary relief with blood transfusions.
2. Improve hematological status with oxygen availability.
3. Correct failure to thrive and GI problems, which complicate the condition in infants.
4. Reduce or correct infections.
5. Promote healing of any ulcerations.

Dietary Recommendations

1. A diet high in quality protein, calories, B-complex vitamins (especially folic acid), zinc and vitamin C will be beneficial.
2. Provide adequate fluid intake.

Profile

Ht, Wt	IBW/HBW	H & H
Alk phos	RBCs	Serum Fe
Transferrin	CBC	Alb
Gluc	I & O	Jaundice

Patient Education

1. Discuss ways to improve nutritional intake, where deficient.
2. Discuss the importance of diet in the maintenance of hematological health.

NOTES

Section 13
Leukemias, Lymphomas, and Cancer

Chief Assessment Factors

weight changes

anorexia, nausea, vomiting, dysphagia

7 warning signs:

—change in bowel/bladder habits

—sore that dose not heal

—unusual bleeding or discharge

—thickening or lump in breast or elsewhere

—indigestion or dysphagia

—obvious change in wart or mole

—nagging cough or hoarseness

Table 13–1.
Categories of Nutritional Care in Cancer
  a. Preventive care
  b. Maintenance care in therapy
  c. Palliative care in terminal patients

Table 13-2.

Nutritional Implications of Cancer Treatments*

Surgery

Oropharynx	Tube dependency from decreased access to GI tract
Esophagus	Fat malabsorption, loss of normal swallowing, decreased motility, obstruction
Stomach	Dumping syndrome, delayed emptying, anemia, malabsorption
Pancreas	Exocrine or endocrine insufficiency
Small intestines	Bile acid depletion, steatorrhea, fat malabsorption, B_{12} deficiency and anemia, short-gut syndrome
Colon	Loss of electrolytes and water

Chemotherapy

Alkylating agents	Nausea, vomiting
Antibiotics	Anorexia, diarrhea, nausea and vomiting, stomatitis
Antimetabolites	Diarrhea, nausea, vomiting, stomatitis
Corticosteroids	Sodium and fluid retention
Sex hormones	Anorexia, nausea, vomiting, sodium and fluid retention
Vinca alkaloids	Nausea and vomiting

Radiation

Head-neck	Anorexia
Oropharyngeal	Nausea, vomiting, dysphagia, dry mouth, mouth blindness, altered taste sensations, weight loss
Abdominal, Intestinal, Pelvic	Early: enteritis, diarrhea, distention, abdominal pain, nausea and vomiting
	Late: intestinal stenosis, edema, fluid and electrolyte loss, weight loss

* Adapted from *A Guide to Nutritional Care.* Evansville, IN, Mead Johnson Nutritional Division, 1980.

Table 13-3.

Protective/Preventive Nutritional Factors in Cancer*

Conservative Recommendations—Protective Nutrients

12,500 IU vitamin A (β-carotene)	1000 mg vitamin C
200–800 IU vitamin E	50–200 µg selenium
omega-3 fatty acids	vitamin B_6
vitamin D_3	folacin, thiamine, niacin, riboflavin

Other preventive suggestions: (note—80–90% of cancers are environmental/preventable)

1. Reduce frying, grilling, and use of smoked and salt-cured foods.
2. Decrease use of alcoholic beverages. Monitor additives.
3. Increase use of cruciferous vegetables, fiber, fish, and garlic (allicin).
4. Control weight, avoid obesity.
5. Decrease fat (saturated or unsaturated) intake to 30% total kcal.

* *JADA* 86:505, 1986

Table 13–4.

Potentially High Risk Nutrients and Factors

Oral CA—alcohol, tobacco. low beta-carotene and vitamin E

Breast and Prostate CA—high fat (especially PUFA because of EFAs), high calories, low omega-3s (Wistar Institute), and alcohol

Respiratory Tract CA—smoking, alcohol, low vitamin E and C

Liver CA—aflatoxins

GI Tract CA—nitrosamines, alcohol, amino acid pyrosalates in broiled meat and fish, low carotenoids and low vitamins C and E

Cervical CA—low vitamin C, E, and beta-carotene

Ovarian CA—fried foods and eggs (*JAMA* 7/19/85)

Colorectal CA—high red meat and protein, alcohol, high calories, low vitamins C and D, low calcium, sedentary lifestyle, low intake of carotenoids and vegetables

Melanoma—low vitamin B_6 and carotenoids (AICR)

Natural carcinogens: UV radiation, dyes, environmental chemicals, (smoke, mines), viruses, nitrosamines, aflatoxins, saffrole

For More Information

American Cancer Society
777 Third Ave.
New York, NY 10017
AMC Cancer Hotline: (800) 525-3777

Cancer Information Service
1825 Connecticut Ave., NW
Washington, DC 20009

National Cancer Institute
Bldg. 31, Room 10A18
Bethesda, MD 20205

American Institute for Cancer Research (AICR)
1759 R St. NW
Washington, DC 20009
(202) 328-7244

NOTES

CANCER

Usual Hospital Stay

Average, 4–5 days: radiation. 6–7 days; chemotherapy, 2–3 days.

Notation

There are 100 + variations. Cancer is the No. 2 killer in the U.S., with 20% of all fatalities.

Cancer. Abnormal, uncontrolled growth of a lump or mass that also destroys normal tissue.

Oncology. Scientific study of tumors.

Leukemia. Patients have abnormally high white blood cell counts with frequent hemorrhages and mouth ulcers.

Lymphoma. A tumor of lymphatic tissue.

Carcinoma. A form of cancer involving epithelial tissue and coverings of internal and external surfaces. Breast, stomach, uterus, skin, and tongue cancers are included in this group: 80–90% of all cancers.

Metastasis. A transfer of disease from one organ to another that is not directly connected to it, especially the spread of carcinoma.

Multiple myeloma. A malignant disease of bone marrow, causing persistent bone pain, weight loss, and infections.

Oat cell carcinoma. A rapidly spreading, highly fatal cancer of the bronchus.

Epithelioma. Carcinoma consisting of many epithelial cells.

Sarcoma. Cancer arising from connective tissue (bone, kidney, liver, etc.)

Objectives

1. Overcome the side effects of treatment. Diminish the toxicity of treatment. Coordinate total care plan with MD, RN, etc.
2. Correct cachexia from weakness, anorexia, redistribution of host nutrients, and nutritional depletion. Control the cancer and complications, such as anemia or MOSF.
3. Prevent weight loss from increased basal metabolic rate* (usual increase is 15%). Greatest losses occur from protein stores and body fat. Early nutritional status is a good prognostic indicator.
4. Prevent further depletion of humoral and cellular immunity from malnutrition.
5. Prevent infection or sepsis; further morbidity, and death from starvation or infections.
6. Provide appropriate micronutrients.
7. Control glucose intolerance (NIDDM is common).

---

* Some patients may be hypometabolic; others hypermetabolic by 10–30% above normal rates.

Dietary Recommendations

1. In general, intake of protein should be high (1–1.5 g/kg body weight to maintain; 1.5–2 g/kg body weight to replete weight losses). Intake of calories should be high* (25–35 kcal/kg body weight to maintain; 40–50 kcal/kg body weight to replete body stores). Add calories if patient is febrile or septic. Fat should be 30–50% NPC.
2. Schedule a large meal earlier in the day. If needed, schedule five to six small meals daily, tube feeding, or IV feeding. If the gut works, use it. Use TPN with weight loss over 20% and with a good prognosis. Routine TPN parenteral therapy should not be used with chemotherapy.
3. Provide adequate supplementation: vitamin B-complex (vitamin B_6, pantothenic acid, folic acid, etc.), vitamins A and C.
4. Nutritional treatment for specific cancers: see specific entries.
5. Force-feed *only* if tumor is treatable. Review each case individually.
6. Leucine and methionine may be needed. Increases in BCAAs have been suggested; data are not conclusive. After surgery or abdominal radiation, glutamine may be useful.
7. Alter dietary therapy as needed; each person's needs vary before and after treatments.
8. Control simple sugars with CHO intolerance.

Profile

Temp	Type of cells	I & O
Trig, Chol	Tumor grade (growth	Wt
N Balance, RBP	rate)	Wt changes
Alk phos	Constipation	Alb (risk inc. below
PO_4	Edema	3.5 mg; 2.1 may
Mg^{++}	Ceruloplasmin (inc.)	increase sepsis)
N, V, diarrhea	Ca^{++}	K^+
Taste changes	Ht	Cl
Food aversion	IBW/HBW	BUN (often dec.)
Ascites	H & H	MCV
WBCs, ESR	Na+	Platelets
SGPT, GGT	Pco_2, Po_2	TLC (not reliable here)
Dysphagia	Fe, ferritin	Urinary acetone
Sore mouth	Transferrin, TIBC	Creatinine
Chewing problems	WBCs	Ca^{++} (inc. with bone
Choking	SGOT, SGPT	resorption)
MRI or CT scan	Lactate (inc. 5×),	Uric acid
Tumor stage	from lactic acid	
	Gluc (inc.)	

---

* Some patients may be hypometabolic; others hypermetabolic by 10–30% above normal rates.

Side Effects of Common Drugs Used

1. *Methotrexate.* Folate preparations can alter drug response. Folate, lactose, vitamin B_{12} and fat are less well absorbed. Mouth sores are common.
2. Other *antineoplastic agents.* Side effects include nausea, anorexia, stomatitis, diarrhea, taste alterations, some vomiting, sloughing of colonic mucosa. Hyperuricemia, N and V are common with *alkylating agents.*
3. *Immunotherapy.* Side effects include nausea, vomiting, abdominal pain, fatigue, and anorexia. Interleukin and interferon are used.
4. *Antibiotics* and *steroids* also alter nutritional status.

Patient Education

1. The patient's improved nutritional status may allow neoplastic cells to become more susceptible to treatment. This may make patients more suitable for treatments previously denied them. An improved nutritional status also reduces side effects, promotes better rehabilitation, and improves the quality of life while perhaps increasing survival rates. Malnutrition can potentiate the toxicity of anti-neoplastic agents.
2. Malnutrition does not have to be accepted in the case of the cancer patient. Try all treatment modes. Start "where the patient is."
3. Have patient avoid unscientific treatments, such as Laetrile, herbal teas, and megavitamins.

Comments: Side Effects of Treatment

1. *Loss of teeth* makes the patient's mouth more sensitive to cold, heat, and sweets. Food should be served at room temperature.
2. *Xerostomia,* dry mouth from atrophy of mucous membranes, causes difficulty in eating and swallowing. Use salivary substitutes, lip balm, sugarless gum and candies, gravies and sauces. Increase fluids, and use of softened, moist foods (custard, stews, soups). Sip beverages with each bite of food. Cut food into small pieces. Ice chips and popsicles can also help. Pureed or baby foods are often useful.
3. For the patient with *poor dentition and caries,* avoid sweets and use sodium fluoride three times daily. Mouth care should be provided several times daily.
4. *Thick saliva* can produce more caries. Use less bread, milk gelatin, and oily foods. Blenderize foods such as fruits and vegetables.
5. *Sore mouth and throat* (stomatitis, mucositis or esophagitis) result from local bleeding and lesions. Pain and inflammation are common. Modify the texture and consistency of the foods as needed. Use a bland diet with fewer spices and seasonings in the food. Have the patient rinse mouth with water and $NaHCO_3$. Avoid acidic juices, salty foods or soups, grainy breads and cereals. Grind meats. Have the patient swish

his mouth with lidocaine before meals. Use the "mechanical soft diet" as needed. Offer fluids frequently, and by straw—cold or tepid. Popsicles and cold liquid foods may help. Smaller meals are useful.

6. *Mouth blindness* (dysgeusia) is defined as disinterest and aversion to foods. Emphasize the aroma and colors of foods. Provide a variety of foods and use garnishes. Acidic foods (e.g., lemonade) may help stimulate the patient's ability to taste foods. Use highly flavored foods and sauces. Try milk shakes that are coffee or mint flavored. Fresh vegetables, special breads, highly flavored snacks, olives, and pickles may be well received by patient. Add sauces to meats.

7. *Anorexia* may be caused by mental depression, altered sensory experiences, or tumors. The condition aggravates cachexia. Use small, frequent feedings and supplements. Teach ways to increase calories and protein. Fortify foods where possible.

8. *Weight loss* can be treated by adding fats to foods, dry milk to mashed potatoes and shakes, extra sugar to coffee and cereals. Use small, frequent feedings and the patient's favorite foods. Use 40–50 kcal/kg for repletion.

9. To treat *diarrhea*, alter fiber in the diet. Beware of lactose intolerance secondary to disease process or drug/radiation therapies. Decrease fatty foods; increase fluids and potassium. Use cold or room temperature foods.

10. *Constipation* requires fiber and fluids to be added to the diet. Milk may also be beneficial if tolerated. Fruits, vegetables and bran may help.

11. *Aversion to tastes.* In some patients a lower threshold for urea causes aversion to meat; these patients may say that the meat "smells rotten." Substitute milk, eggs, peanut butter, legumes, poultry, fish, and cheese. In addition, the patient may have a decreased ability to taste salt and sugar. Add other seasonings, sauces, more salt or sugar as desired by the patient; however, do not allow sweet foods to replace nourishing foods. Ensure adequate zinc intake.

12. *Preference for cold foods.* Cold foods are often better accepted than hot foods. Use cold, clear fluids; carbonated beverages; ices; gelatin; watermelons; grapes and peeled cucumbers; cold meat platters; ice cream; and salted nuts.

13. *Nausea* can be treated by deep breathing, ice chips, or sips of carbonated beverages. Try a dry diet also (liquids between meals). Try relaxation measures. Antivert may be helpful. Eat small meals; rest afterward. Keep crackers handy. Cut down on fatty foods.

14. If meals are interrupted by *treatment*, the evening may be the best time to catch up on food intake. Keep the kitchen well stocked.

15. To treat *pain*, give pain medications before meals, or have the patient eat when pain is lowest. Encourage trying foods again after time lapse. Try biofeedback or muscle relaxation.

16. *Loneliness* may affect eating habits. Social eating may improve food intake. Visitors should be encouraged to come and bring gifts of food.
17. Meals may be prepared in quantity when the patient is less tired. To prevent further *fatigue* foods may be used that require less chewing. Provide frequent rest periods, especially before meals.
18. In the case of *malabsorption*, elemental diets can only be used if the patient has an intact duodenum and jejunum. Total parenteral nutrition can only be used in some cases, considering risks of infection.
19. If the patient has *difficult in swallowing* (dysphagia), use moist foods. Add gravies and sauces to foods. Some patients tolerate semisolid foods better than liquids. The patient should sip fluids throughout the meal. To prevent aspiration, the patient should try placing liquid under the tongue. Some patients may also find that tilting their heads will be useful.
20. For *anemias*, a balanced diet with HBV proteins, B-complex vitamins, iron and vitamin C may be helpful. Ensure use of heme sources, if possible, to increase iron bioavailability.
21. *Early satiety* can be a problem. Never give plain water; always use a calorie-containing beverage. Take liquids between meals. Avoid fatty, greasy foods. Use small meals and frequent snacks, "nibbling."
22. During periods of *vomiting*, use sips of clear liquids every 10–15 min. "Flat" carbonated beverages are useful. Call doctor if abdominal pains persist.
23. With *chemotherapy*, alter sodium, potassium and fluid intake as necessary. Avoid drinking or eating 2 hours after treatment to prevent N or V. Cardiotoxicity, nephrotoxicity and pulmonary toxicity may occur.
24. *Radiotherapy* can cause N or V. Avoid eating immediately before or after therapy. Diarrhea may occur in radiation enteritis.
25. Following *curative surgery*, direct efforts at restoring nutritional health to pre-illness status.

Comment

TPN should not be used to prolong life in patients at the end stage of their disease. TPN can be used for patients with controllable CA, when enteral and oral feedings are poorly tolerated. The patient must be included in this ethical decision.

Studies indicate that increased body iron stores are associated with increased risk for cancer in men (*NEJM* 10/20/88). Further investigation is warranted.

NOTES

LEUKEMIA, ACUTE

Usual Hospital Stay

7–8 days.

Notation

Leukemia involves uncontrolled proliferation of leukocytes and their pre-cursors in blood-forming organs, with infiltration into other organs. Various types exist:

1. *Acute Lymphocytic (Lymphoblastic) Leukemia,* also called ALL, pri-marily affects bone marrow and lymph nodes. This condition affects mainly children, and represents approximately 90% of all childhood leukemias. Prognosis is 2–3 years.
2. *Acute Nonlymphocytic Leukemia* represents 10% of childhood leuke-mias. Together, this leukemia and ALL comprise 30% of all childhood cancers.
3. *Acute Myelogenous Leukemia* (AML) consists of proliferation of mye-loblasts, which are immature polynuclear leukocytes; more common in adults. Prognosis is 10–12 months.

Symptoms and signs of leukemias include easy fatigue, malaise, irritability, fever, pallor, petechiae, ecchymosis, purpura, hemorrhage, palpitations, short-ness of breath, slight weight loss, bone or joint pain, cough, sternal tenderness, splenomegaly, hepatomegaly, anemia, headache, nausea and vomiting, and mouth ulcers.

Blood has a grayish-white appearance.

Objectives

1. Prevent hemorrhage and infections.
2. Promote recovery and stabilization prior to bone marrow transplanta-tion.
3. Prevent constipation; correct anorexia and nausea or vomiting.
4. Prevent complications and further morbidity.
5. Prevent weight loss; correct as needed.

Dietary Recommendations

1. Attractive meals should be served at proper temperatures; avoid extremes.
2. Small meals may be better tolerated to avoid overwhelming the patient.
3. In some cases, cold or iced foods may be preferred.
4. A high protein/high calorie/high vitamin-mineral intake should be offered; use tube feeding or TPN if necessary.
5. Extra fluids will be important during febrile states.

Profile

Ht, Wt	H & H	Temp (101°F. or
WBCs (↑)	Platelets	greater)
Alb	LDH (elevated)	Uric acid (inc.)
N Balance	Zinc (dec.)	Transferrin
Serum copper (inc.)	IBW/HBW	Ferritin (inc.)
Gluc	TLC (reliability varies)	Other problems
Wt changes		

Side Effects of Common Drugs Used

1. *Chemotherapy* is generally used—methotrexate and daunorubicin may cause stomatitis, nausea or vomiting. Coadministration with glucose may help. Adequate fluid intake is important.
2. In some cases, *interferon* may be used.
3. *Prednisone* may be used, with side effects related to steroids with chronic use. Alter diet and intake accordingly.
4. If *L-asparaginase* (Elspar) is used, hepatitis or pancreatitis may result. Watch carefully. This drug is often used with ALL.

Patient Education

1. A well-balanced diet is essential; discuss ways to improve or increase intake. See general entry for Cancer regarding side effects of the disease or therapy.
2. Adequate fluid intake is important.

NOTES

LEUKEMIA, CHRONIC

Usual Hospital Stay

7–8 days.

Notation

Chronic lymphocytic leukemia involves a crowding out of normal leukocytes in lymph glands, interfering with the body's ability to produce other blood cells. *Chronic granulocytic leukemia* has similar overproduction of WBCs in the bone marrow, often thought to be developed through an abnormal acquired chromosome (Philadelphia, Ph_1) perhaps as a result of ionizing radiation.

Chronic lymphocytic leukemia is more common in people over age 50 and in males.

Symptoms and signs include anemia, increased infections, bleeding, enlarged lymph nodes (in lymphatic form), night sweats, fever, weight loss and anorexia. Prognosis is 3–5 years.

Objectives

1. Prevent hemorrhage, infections, further complications and morbidity.
2. Promote recovery and stabilization prior to bone marrow transplantation, if required.
3. Prevent or correct constipation, nausea, vomiting, and anorexia.
4. Alter diet according to medications and therapies, such as chemotherapy.
5. Correct weight loss if possible.

Dietary Recommendations

1. Serve attractive meals at temperatures that are tolerated. In some cases, cold foods are preferred.
2. Small, frequent meals are generally more desired than large meals.
3. Tube feed or use TPN if appropriate or necessary, but avoid sepsis.
4. Extra fluids will be important to reduce a febrile state.

Profile

Ht, wt	IBW/HBW	WT changes
PT	BP	Platelets
WBCs	TLC (varied results)	H & H
Transferrin	N Balance	Alb
Serum ferritin (inc.)	Uric acid (inc.)	

Side Effects of Common Drugs Used

Chemotherapeutic agents may be used, with varying side effects. Chlorambucil (Leukeran) and busulfan are common. Nausea, vomiting, glossitis and cheilosis may result. Avoidance of hot, spicy, or acidic foods may be beneficial.

Patient Education

1. Discuss alternative ways to make meals more attractive and appealing.
2. For side effects of the disease and therapies, see the general entry for cancer.

NOTES

BONE MARROW TRANSPLANTATION

Usual Hospital Stay

15 days.

Notation

This procedure involves intravenous replacement of medically destroyed bone marrow with histocompatible donor bone marrow to establish a graft and reinstate production of normal cellular blood components. The transplantation is often necessary in leukemia or in aplastic anemia. It is also undergoing trials with other diseases.

Objectives

1. Prepare preoperatively by providing adequate nutrient stores (glucose, calories, vitamins and minerals as well as protein).
2. Individualize needs; promote engraftment of marrow.
3. Reduce nausea, vomiting and diarrhea, where present.
4. Improve weight status; promote anabolism.
5. Correct anorexia, stomatitis, xerostomia, depression—all of which reduce total intake.

6. Avoid or prevent "graft vs. host disease" (GVHD), with rash, erythroderma, hair loss, jaundice, abdominal pain, emaciation, pneumonitis, infections, and GI tract problems.
7. Prevent oral infections, gastroenteritis, pneumocystitis.
8. Postoperatively, replenish nutrient stores and promote wound healing.

Dietary Recommendations

1. TPN may be needed to prepare the patient preoperatively, and to initiate recovery postoperatively. Tube feeding is less frequently used because of nausea, vomiting and risk of infections.
2. In some cases, the use of a "low bacteria" (neutropenic) diet may be useful for several months before and after transplantation. Protective isolation may be needed, and products may require special preparation (as with a laminar flow hood).
3. Provide 35–40 kcal/kg and 1.5–2 g protein/kg of weight; fat 1–2.5 g/kg.
4. Keep foods at a temperature that is safe to prevent food infection. Microwave hot foods immediately prior to service.
5. Sterile water may be used to keep hydration at an adequate level to prevent renal problems.
6. If needed, a low lactose/low fiber/low fat/bland diet may be needed by the patient. Progress, as tolerated, to a normal diet over time.
7. To increase bowel flora, use of live-culture yogurt may be beneficial; *Lactobacillus acidophilus* therapy can also be helpful.

Profile

Ht, Wt	CBC	Trig
H & H	Na^+, K^+	TLC (varied reliability)
Bilirubin	Alb	I & O
Gluc	Uric acid	Ferritin
IBW/HBW	Weight changes	Transferrin
Mg^{++}		BUN, creat

Side Effects of Common Drugs Used

1. *Total body irradiation* (TBI) may be done in some cases. Side effects vary for each individual.
2. *Chemotherapy drugs* may be used, such as busulfan (to destroy marrow stem cells) or cyclophosphamide (Cytoxan) (which can cause nausea, vomiting, diarrhea, anorexia).
3. *Antibiotics* may be used to fight infections.
4. *Clotrimazole* may be used for bowel preparation.
5. *Cyclosporine* (CSA) and *Prednisone* are often given to prevent GVHD for 1 to several months postoperatively. Numerous side effects can result

(e.g., nausea and vomiting, skin rashes, hemorrhagic cystitis, altered potassium metabolism).
6. Analgesics, antihistamines, and antidepressants may be used; monitor side effects.

Patient Education

1. Discuss needed protection against environmental infections (safe food handling and preparation, keeping foods below 40° or above 140°F, use of sterile water, etc.)
2. The "low bacteria" (also called neutropenic) diet used in some cases may include careful use of raw fruits and vegetables, milk, and shell-fish—all of which may be easily contaminated with bacteria. Results with this diet are not always conclusive.
3. Small, frequent meals of bland, cold consistency may be well tolerated.

NOTES

BRAIN TUMOR

Usual Hospital Stay

7–8 days.

Notation

A neoplasm arising from intracranial cells, a brain tumor may be benign if it is unlikely to spread or malignant if it is likely to spread. In children, brain tumors are most common in girls ages 5–9.

Constituting 50% of brain tumors, a *glioma* is a tumor of neurological origin. A *neuroma*, a tumor composed of nerve cells, may occur along any nerve and is not necessarily associated with a brain tumor. A *glioblastoma multiforme* is a CNS neoplasm, especially related to the cerebrum.

Symptoms and signs include headache, vertigo, altered consciousness or convulsions, inability to follow commands, mental or personality changes, unequal pupil response, hemianopsia, blurred or decreased vision, ptosis, tinnitus, altered gait, dysphagia, vomiting with or without nausea, aphasia, obesity, elevated blood pressure, and loss of sense of smell.

Objectives

1. Provide adequate calories without excess.
2. Avoid constipation and straining.
3. Prevent upper respiratory infections with coughing, which can increase intracranial pressure.
4. Counteract side effects of therapy—radiation, surgery, etc.
5. Correct hypoalbuminemia.

Dietary Recommendations

1. Maintain diet as ordered, with extra fluid unless contraindicated.
2. Provide adequate fiber in the diet.
3. Alter texture and liquids if necessary for dysphagia. If necessary, tube feed or offer TPN.
4. Limit sodium to 4–6 grams daily to correct cerebral edema.

Profile

Ht, wt	EEG	Wt changes
Gluc (elevated)	Alb	CT scan
CSF-elevated protein	Temp	Transferrin
Skull x-ray	TLC, WBCs (altered)	BP
Aphasia	WBCs in CSF (NL or	Cerebral edema
IBW/HBW	inc.)	SGPT ($\uparrow$)

Side Effects of Common Drugs Used

1. *Steroid therapy* may be used. Decrease sodium and increase potassium as appropriate. Negative nitrogen balance may result over time.
2. *Anticonvulsants* are often used. Side effects may include a decrease in serum folacin levels and other nutrients; monitor individually.
3. *Analgesics* are generally used to relieve pain.

Patient Education

1. The importance of attractive meals should be stressed to help appetite if fair or poor. Keep in mind that the sense of smell may have declined recently.
2. Discuss the importance of a balanced diet.

NOTES

BRONCHIAL CARCINOMA

Usual Hospital Stay

7–8 days.

Notation

There are several kinds of lung cancer, but only bronchial cancer is common. It is almost always caused by smoking. Cancer cells of the lung often spread to the brain, bone, liver and skin.

This cancer is the most common type of cancer in the Western world. It generally affects men more than women, but is increasing in women.

Heavy smokers are 25 × more susceptible to this cancer, with oat cell carcinoma common. Oat cell CA is a rapidly spreading, highly fatal lung CA.

Objectives

1. The patient must be encouraged to stop smoking.
2. Prepare the patient for therapy—surgery, radiation, chemotherapy.
3. Meet calorie needs (with BMR elevated by about 30%).
4. Counteract side effects, such as cachexia.
5. Prevent or correct other side effects, such as weight loss and anorexia.

Dietary Recommendations

1. Increase calories and protein, CHO, and fluids.
2. Alter diet as appropriate for side effects (See general entry for Cancer).
3. Small, frequent meals may be beneficial.
4. Adequate vitamin/mineral provision will be needed. Vitamins A & C are especially important.

Profile

Ht, Wt	IBW/HBW	Chest x-ray
Bronchoscopy	Biopsy	P_{CO_2}, P_{O_2}
Alb	Ca^{++}	K^+
Na^+	Na^+	I & O
Gluc	TLC (varies)	SGPT ($\uparrow$)

Side Effects of Drugs Commonly Used

Cytotoxic drugs (vincristine, which can cause severe constipation); (methotrexate, N & V common); doxorubicin (Adriamycin) causes stomatitis, anorexia and diarrhea. Coadministration with glucose may alleviate toxic GI effects.

384

Patient Education

1. Discuss alternate methods of eating if meals are not consumed as usual.
2. Discuss side effects of drugs that are being used.

NOTES

CHORIOCARCINOMA

Usual Hospital Stay

3 days.

Notation

This condition involves a highly malignant neoplasm from the chorionic epithelium; it may develop after a hydatidiform mole, a miscarriage, or a full-term delivery. Rarely, it may occur in males (testes).

Symptoms and signs include profuse or intermittent vaginal bleeding, discharge between menses, cough, hemoptysis, headache, nausea and vomiting, hypertension, tachypnea, vaginal or vulvar lesion, anemia, sepsis, weight loss and cachexia.

Objectives

1. Prepare the patient for surgery, should that be necessary. Often, a TAH is done.
2. Correct weight loss and cachexia.
3. Correct side effects of chemotherapy if used.
4. Treat and correct all other side effects of therapy and the disease state.

Dietary Recommendations

1. Modify diet to patient preferences.
2. Increase liquids as needed.
3. Provide adequate protein, B-complex vitamins, iron, calories, and other nutrients for wound healing, as appropriate.
4. Alter texture of diet if patient is fatigued at mealtimes, or if stomatitis exists with chemotherapy.

Profile

Ht, wt	IBW, HBW	Temp
Alb	H & H	I & O
Transferrin	Nausea, vomiting	K^+
BP	Ca^{++}, Mg^{++}	Na^+
Gluc	TLC (varies)	SGPT ($\uparrow$)

Side Effects of Common Drugs Used

1. *Methotrexate* may be used; nausea and vomiting are common side effects. Administer with glucose to reduce toxicity.
2. *Vincristine* or *dactinomycin* may also be used.

Patient Education

The appropriate suggestions should be offered according to the specific needs of the individual—e.g., nausea or vomiting may require small, frequent feedings and control of fluid intake at mealtimes. See the general entry for Cancer for more suggestions.

NOTES

ESOPHAGEAL CANCER

Usual Hospital Stay

4–5 days.

Notation

This type of cancer develops in the middle or lower third of the esophagus. Formerly fatal because the condition is often advanced before symptoms appear, resection may now be beneficial.

Symptoms and signs include dysphagia, painful swallowing, substernal pain, feeling of fullness, weight loss, malaise, malnutrition, dehydration, anemia, regurgitation after eating, electrolyte imbalance, hiccups, foul breath, aspiration, increased salivation, hoarseness and coughing, hepatomegaly.

This condition is more common in elderly persons (especially males), and is generally found only in 5–7/100,000 persons.

Objectives

1. Prevent sepsis, further weight loss, malnutrition, cachexia.
2. Hydrate adequately.
3. Feed adequately if resection is needed; some fat malabsorption may occur.
4. Omit alcoholic beverages, especially if ETOH abuse has occurred by history.
5. Promote positive nitrogen balance and prevent loss of LBM.
6. Meet increased glucose needs for gluconeogenesis.
7. Prepare for treatments (usually surgery, but sometimes radiation as well).
8. Correct anemia.

Dietary Recommendations

1. Patient is generally NPO, with parenteral (PPN or TPN) or gastrostomy feedings.
2. If swallowing is possible, provide a diet high in calories & protein with bland or pureed foods as required. Adjust individually to meet patient needs.
3. Increase fluid intake as tolerated, with up to 3.5 L daily unless contraindicated.
4. MCT may be beneficial if fat malabsorption exists, especially with steatorrhea.
5. Increase intake of vitamin A, zinc, and other nutrients that may be low or at risk.
6. If *esophagectomy* has been performed, fat malabsorption is common, as well as gastric stasis, diarrhea due to vagotomy, hypochlorhydria. MCT are especially important in this case.
7. Calorie requirements may equal 1.5 REE (70% CHO and 30% fat for NP kcal); 1.5–2 g protein/kg.

Profile

Ht, Wt	IBW/HBW	Gluc
BP	Temp	Endoscopy
TLC (varies)	Barium swallow	T_3, T_4, TSH
I & O	Transferrin	
Alb	H & H	

Side Effects of Drugs Commonly Used

1. *Cisplatin* can cause nausea and vomiting.
2. *Bleomycin* and *methotrexate* can also aggravate N & V. Coadminister with glucose.

Patient Education

1. If the patient can eat orally, encourage him or her to chew slowly.
2. If gastrostomy feeding is required, teach the patient/family/caretaker how to prepare feedings and how to produce the item in a sterile environment.
3. Encourage help from Speech Therapy.
4. Hypothyroid status can cause dysphagia; counsel accordingly.

NOTES

GASTRIC CARCINOMA

Usual Hospital Stay

4–5 days.

Notation

This carcinoma most commonly occurs in the pyloric segment and along the lesser curvature. Often, no early definitive signs are evident.

Symptoms and signs include a feeling of fullness, indigestion, dysphagia, anorexia, weight loss, anemia, pallor, vertigo, nausea & vomiting, malnutrition, melena, occult blood, and dehydration. Gastric CA often follows long-term pernicious anemia, Menetrier's disease or chronic gastritis. It is generally found in males ages 50–70.

Objectives

1. Prevent weight loss and further malnutrition.
2. Force fluids.
3. Counteract side effects of chemotherapy or radiation, or gastrectomy. If gastrectomy is performed, dumping syndrome or hypochlorhydria may result.
4. Correct protein-losing enteropathy.

Dietary Recommendations

1. Parenteral therapy or TPN may be used, especially before surgery.
2. If oral intake is allowed, try light meals that are nutrient-dense and well-balanced. A high protein/high calorie diet will be needed.
3. 2–3 liters of fluid are generally required, unless contraindicated for other reasons.
4. Postgastrectomy, beware of dumping syndrome (see that entry). Small, frequent feedings may be better tolerated and concentrated CHO may need to be limited.
5. Jejunostomy at resection may be helpful.
6. Be sure that the dietary intake (or supplementation) includes selenium and other key nutrients for wound healing and correction of anemia.

Profile

Ht, Wt	IBW/HBW	Transferrin
Alb	Gluc	Barium swallow
Na$^+$, K$^+$	Occult blood	Temp
Endoscopy	BP	Anorexia
I & O	N or V	SGPT ($\uparrow$)
TLC (varies)	H & H	

Side Effects of Drugs Commonly Used

Cytotoxic drugs. Mitomycin C (fever, N, V, anorexia, stomatitis can result); 5 Fluorouracil (anorexia and nausea are common). Sore mouth, taste changes and vomiting may also result. For some cases, added thiamine is needed with 5–fluorouracil treatment.

Patient Education

1. Encourage patient to chew slowly and well, when and if oral intake is possible.
2. Feeding tubes may be useful in the home setting (e.g., jejunostomy).

HEPATIC CARCINOMA

Usual Hospital Stay

6–7 days.

Notation

Malignant hepatic tumors are commonly due to metastatic lesions from other organs. Primary tumors are common with alcohol abuse.

Symptoms and signs include slow onset, anorexia, weakness, progressive weight loss, N and/or V, increased flatulence, steatorrhea, diarrhea, abdominal fullness, low-grade fever, dehydration, anemia, malnutrition, abnormal LFT, decreased albumin levels, portal hypertension, dyspnea, jaundice, ascites, hepatic coma.

Objectives

1. Reduce fluid retention, ascites.
2. Correct serum protein levels and production.
3. Prevent further N & V, weight loss, anorexia, malnutrition.
4. Counteract side effects of therapy (surgery, chemotherapy, radiation).
5. Improve overall nutritional and hematological status.
6. Improve prognosis as long as possible.

Dietary Recommendations

1. Patient may be NPO with parenteral/TPN as needed.
2. Progress, if and when tolerated, to high calorie/high protein diet with an increased CHO intake. If hepatic coma occurs, decreased protein with supplemented amino acids will be needed. See entry for hepatic encephalopathy/coma (Section 8).
3. Reduce sodium if ascites and edema are significant.
4. Monitor serum levels of other values to determine other restrictions or needed alterations.
5. Supplemental vitamin A, D, K, and B-complex may be beneficial. Be careful of toxic levels because of poor hepatic clearance.
6. With surgery, monitor nutrients needed for adequate wound healing, recovery.

Profile

Ht, Wt	IBW/HBW	Alb & RBP
PT (prolonged)	Sed. rate (inc.)	Gluc (dec.)
GI bleeding	Melena	Fever, Temp
H & H	Hepatomegaly	Alk phos
I & O	Na$^+$	K$^+$
Transferrin	Therapy—OR, etc.	TLC (varies)
SGOT, SGPT	Ammonia	

Side Effects of Drugs Commonly Used

1. *Antiemetics* may be used for vomiting.
2. *Diuretics* are commonly used; monitor side effects carefully.

Patient Education

1. Teach the patient about signs of deficiency of vitamins K and C, such as bleeding gums.
2. Discuss signs of hepatic coma that require dietary alterations.

Comments

With hepatic resection, decreased albumin and serum glucose levels are the major problems. Adjust intake accordingly.

NOTES

INTESTINAL CARCINOMA

Usual Hospital Stay

4–5 days.

Notations

Colorectal cancer is the 3rd most common type of CA. Maintaining the ileocecal valve is crucial if surgery is needed. In CA of the *small intestine*, malignancy is generally found in the lower duodenum and lower ileum, with a high rate of mortality and few early symptoms; it presents in about 5% of cases. In the *large intestine*, slow-growing malignancies are usually found in the cecum, lower ascending and sigmoid colon; prognosis is optimistic but few early symptoms are found. *Rectal* CA is more common in men than in women and often occurs after middle age, with bleeding, pain and irregular bowel habits.

Symptoms and signs include: weakness, weight loss, anorexia, anemia, dehydration, electrolyte imbalance, intestinal obstruction, bowel abscess, fistula, metastases to other organs (lungs, kidneys, bone). For SI cancer, symptoms include N & V, anorexia, upper abdominal pain, weight loss, anemia. In the LI, symptoms include altered bowel habits, rectal bleeding, abdominal cramping, pain and distention.

It may be of interest to note that the diet may have been high in fat and low in fiber over a long time before symptoms appear.

Objectives

1. Decrease residue, especially with obstruction, until fiber is better tolerated.
2. Prevent further weight loss, correct anemia and dehydration.
3. Counteract side effects of therapies; resection is common (see the short

gut syndrome entry in Section 7). Chemotherapy or radiation are also used in some cases.

4. Provide nutrients in a tolerable form—oral, parenteral or enteral.

Dietary Recommendations

1. Administer parenteral fluids with adequate electrolytes, vitamins C and K, selenium (if used over a long time). Vitamin D, calcium, iron, and fat intakes should also be monitored for adequacy.
2. TPN may be needed for an extended period of time; or tube feeding.
3. Ostomy diets may be provided (see the ileostomy and colostomy entries in Section 7).
4. Increase calories; ensure adequate protein.
5. Decrease residue; eventually increase (if tolerated) wheat bran, cereal and vegetable fibers (insoluble).

Profile

Ht, wt	X-rays	WBCs, ESR (inc.)
H & H (dec.)	IBW/HBW	Alb, RBP
Na^+, K^+, (K^+ often dec.)	Transferrin	Ca^{++}
	Chol, trig	Melena
Proctoscopy, colonoscopy	Serum Fe	Other parameters
	TLC (varies)	

Side Effects of Drugs Commonly Used

1. *Steroid* therapy may be administered.
2. *Chemotherapy* may be used; monitor side effects accordingly. Monitor side effects.
3. *Fluorouracil* plus *levamisole* are commonly used. Diarrhea, nausea, vomiting, low WBCs, and mouth sores can occur.

Patient Education

1. Discuss the appropriate dietary regimen for the specific problems generated by the therapy.
2. Encourage family participation in all levels of care.

Comments

1. *Ileal resection*—vitamin B_{12} deficiency can occur; bile salts may be lost in diarrhea; hyperoxaluria and renal oxalate stones can be a problem. Massive bowel resection—malabsorption, malnutrition, metabolic acidosis, and gastric hypersecretion may result.
   Ileostomy and Colostomy—salt and water balance are a problem.

2. Right side of colon (ascending) absorbs fluids & salts; CA spreads upward here; obstruction is rare.
Left side of colon stores feces; CA here tends to encircle the bowel and cause obstructions. This portion is the descending colon.
3. High risk for intestinal CA exists among ulcerative colitis patients with over 8 years' duration. A similar risk with Crohn's disease exists.

NOTES

LYMPHOMA, HODGKIN'S DISEASE

Usual Hospital Stay

7–8 days.

Notation

A malignant tumor of lymphoid tissue, Hodgkin's disease usually presents with enlarged lymph nodes that are firm and rubbery; pruritus, generalized and severe; night sweats; fatigue and malaise; weight loss; slight fever; alcohol-induced pain; cough; dyspnea; chest pain.

Patients who present with weight loss initially have a worse prognosis than those without such loss.

Objectives

1. Prevent infections, such as candidiasis.
2. Counteract side effects of chemotherapy and radiation.
3. Prevent or correct weight loss, fever, and malaise.

Dietary Recommendations

1. A diet as tolerated is acceptable. Bland foods may be better accepted for a while. Increase protein, kcal, fluids.
2. Six small feedings are generally better tolerated than 3 large meals.
3. Arachidonic acid metabolites may play a role; monitor appropriate fat intake.

Profile

Ht, wt	IBW/HBW	H & H
TLC (varies)	Ceruloplasmin (inc.)	Bilirubin (inc.)
Uric acid (inc.)	Bone marrow bx	Lymphangiogram
TP (inc.)	Sed. rate	Alk phos (often inc.)
Diarrhea	Temp	I & O
Gluc	Serum Cu (inc.)	Ferritin (inc.)
		SGPT (↑)

Side Effects of Drugs Commonly Used

1. *Chemotherapy*—(Nitrogen mustard can cause N, V, anorexia, diarrhea or weakness); vincristine or mechlorethamine can also cause problems, such as constipation and mouth sores.
2. *Corticosteroids* can aggravate electrolyte status and will decrease potassium and nitrogen balance over time.

Patient Education

1. Discuss methods of improving appetite by use of attractive meals.
2. Encourage rest periods before and after meals to reduce fatigue.

NOTES

LYMPHOMAS, NON-HODGKIN'S

Usual Hospital Stay

7–8 days.

Notation

These are malignant tumors of lymphoid tissue other than Hodgkin's disease. They are generally due to invasion of the lymph nodes and other tissues by lymphocytes.

Symptoms and signs are similar to those of Hodgkin's disease and to those of enlarged tonsils and adenoids. It is possible as well to develop chylous ascites or chyloperitoneum.

Objectives

1. Correct dysphagia, nausea and vomiting, and anorexia.
2. Prevent infections, candidiasis, etc.
3. Prevent or counteract weight loss.
4. Control protein-losing enteropathy, chylous ascites and other side effects.
5. Modify diet according to side effects of therapy (radiation, chemotherapy).

Dietary Recommendations

1. A normal diet is allowed as tolerated. Bland foods may be preferred at least temporarily.
2. Six small feedings are often better tolerated.
3. Increase protein and calories as appropriate to maintain or gain weight.
4. MCT and decreased LCT may be appropriate in chylous ascites.

Profile

Ht, wt	IBW/HBW	LDH (inc.)
Abnormal lymphocytes	Ca^{++} (inc.)	Uric acid (inc.)
Lymphangiogram	+ Antiglobulin test	Gamma globulin (inc.)
Bilirubin (inc.)	(Coombs' test)	RBP
Ceruloplasmin (inc.)	Chol, trig	Temp
Na^+, K^+	I & O	SGPT ($\uparrow$)
Gluc	Serum Cu (inc.)	
	Alb	

Side Effects of Drugs Commonly Used

1. *Procarbazine* (Matulane) can cause N, V, stomatitis, diarrhea, constipation. It is also an MAO inhibitor. Avoid foods high in tyramine, such as aged cheese.
2. *Nitrosoureas* (carmustine, lomustine)—N & V are common, and abnormal renal or hepatic function can occur.
3. *Vinblastine* (Velban) may cause constipation; *stool softeners* may be helpful. Nausea, vomiting, anorexia, and stomatitis are also common.

Patient Education

1. Discuss any specific side effects of chemotherapy or radiation.
2. Highlight methods for making meals more attractive.
3. Discuss fiber as an alternative to stool softeners where appropriate.

NOTES

MYELOMA

Usual Hospital Stay

7–8 days.

Notation

Myeloma is a malignant disorder of the hematopoietic system in which plasma cells proliferate, invade the bone marrow, and produce abnormal immunoglobulin. Rare, the condition affects only 4/100,000 persons. Males are affected more often than females, and the disorder usually strikes after age 50.

Multiple myeloma affects several areas of bone marrow.

Symptoms and signs include bone pain, weight loss, infections, pathological fractures, shortened stature, paraplegia, fatigue, weakness, apathy, sudden confusion, renal disorders, bleeding tendency (especially gums), N & V, anorexia, URIs and UTIs.

Objectives

1. Avoid fasting. Space meals and snacks adequately.
2. Counteract episodes of fatigue and weakness.
3. Prevent narcotic addiction from excessive pain medication.
4. Counteract side effects of antineoplastic therapy, steroid therapy, and radiotherapy.
5. Avoid infections and febrile states.
6. Prevent spontaneous fractures, as far as possible.
7. Correct anorexia, N & V, and weight loss.

Dietary Recommendations

1. Provide the diet as usual, with six small feedings rather than large meals.
2. A higher protein intake may be useful to counteract losses.
3. Provide adequate calories to meet needs of weight control, preventing unnecessary losses.
4. Avoid dehydration by including adequate fluid intake (e.g., 3 liters daily).

Profile

Ht, wt	IBW/HBW	Proteinuria
Ca^+ (inc.)	BP	Sed. rate (inc.)
Skeletal survey	Hypercalciuria	Uric acid (inc.)
TP	Alb (often ↑)	RBP
PTH (inc.)	Transferrin	Hx bleeding
I & O	N, V, anorexia	SGPT (↑)
TLC (varies)	H & H	

Side Effects of Drugs Commonly Used

1. *Melphalan* (Alkeran) or *nitrosoureas* are commonly used. Monitor side effects, such as anorexia, anemia, nausea, vomiting, and stomatitis.
2. *Prednisone*—if used chronically, can increase nitrogen losses, potassium and magnesium depletion, and can cause hyperglycemia and sodium retention.

Patient Education

1. Discuss the rationale for spacing meals throughout the day to avoid fatigue.
2. Offer recipes and meal plans that provide nutrients required to improve status and immunological competence.

NOTES

ORAL CANCER

Usual Hospital Stay

5 days.

Notation

Oral cancer occurs more often in unclean mouths, or in those persons with poorly fitted dentures. A goal includes elimination of irritation and infections. The disorder is rare under the age of 40. The risk of metastasis is great.

Objectives

1. Abstain from smoking, alcohol and irritants to the mouth such as chewing tobacco and snuff at this time.
2. Prevent abscesses and infection; provide good mouth care.
3. Monitor dysphagia and difficulty with chewing.
4. Correct for chemotherapy and radiation or surgical procedures with their side effects (mucositis, xerostomia, fibrosis).
5. Prevent weight loss and malnutrition.

Dietary Recommendations

1. Decrease use of condiments if they are irritating (e.g., black pepper, chili powder) and decrease use of acidic fruits or juices, such as orange, grapefruit and tomatoes.
2. Tolerance will vary for hot and cold foods and drinks. Monitor and alter intake accordingly.
3. TPN or gastrostomy feeding may be needed at least temporarily, or for an extended period of time.
4. A dysphagia diet (thick pureed foods, decrease in thin liquids) may be needed if swallowing is difficult.

Profile

Ht, Wt	IBW/HBW	Wt changes
Biopsy	Dysphagia	H & H
Albumin, RBP	BP	TLC (varies)
Transferrin	Na^+, K^+	Gluc
		SGPT ($\uparrow$)

Side Effects of Drugs Commonly Used

1. *Steroids* may be used to reduce inflammation; sodium retention, potassium depletion and negative nitrogen balance can result. Hyperglycemia can also occur.
2. Chemotherapy medications may be used. Monitor according to the medication utilized.

Patient Education

1. Relaxation therapy or biofeedback can be very beneficial.
2. Discuss a diet rationale that is appropriate for the patient's condition.

Comments

Rarely do mouth ulcers from stress or trauma indicate any major sign of a health problem. Ulcers that fail to heal after 10 days or those that recur should be seen by a physician. Leukoplakia, thickened white patches, should be biopsied if they exist for a prolonged time.

NOTES

OSTEOSARCOMA

Usual Hospital Stay

6–7 days.

Notation

Osteosarcoma involves rapidly growing malignant bone tumor(s) of unknown origin, occurring most often in the long bones of young people (generally males between 10–25 years old).

Symptoms and signs include pain over one affected extremity, weight loss, limited use of the extremity, fatigue, warmth in a local area, fever, and cough. This type of cancer often spreads to the lung.

Objectives

1. Prevent dehydration; correct fever (often 103–104°F).
2. Relieve pain; prolong life.
3. Counteract effects of surgery (perhaps amputation), radiation and cobalt therapy.
4. Meet needs related to growth and elevated BMR.

Dietary Recommendations

1. A balanced diet (high in calories and protein) will be needed.
2. Extra fluids (3 liters, for example) are used, unless contraindicated.
3. Supplement with foods or nutrients that are low in the patient's intake.
4. Small, frequent feedings may be better tolerated than large meals.
5. A diet rich in zinc, vitamins A & C, and other key nutrients will help with wound healing after surgery.

Profile

Ht, wt	IBW/HBW	Wt changes
Temp	Alk phos (inc.)	Na^+, K^+
Ca^{++} (inc.)	I & O	Alb, RBP
H & H	Gluc	TLC (varies)
		SGPT ($\uparrow$)

Side Effects of Drugs Commonly Used

1. *Hormone therapy* may be given, usually with temporary results.
2. *Doxorubicin* may be used, with side effects affecting intake.

Patient Education

1. Discuss ways to make meals more attractive and appetizing.
2. Discuss with patient and family how to adjust diet for the therapies given (see general entry for cancer).

NOTES

PANCREATIC CARCINOMA

Usual Hospital Stay

6–7 days.

Notation

Malignancy in the pancreas has a high mortality rate, owing to lack of early symptoms, symptoms that mimic other conditions, and rapid metastasis to other organs. 50–70% have CA in the head of the pancreas; 50% in the body and tail. Pancreatic CA is the 5th most common cause of death from CA.

Symptoms and signs include midepigastric pain, signs of biliary obstruction, rapid weight loss, anorexia, hyperglycemia, steatorrhea, N & V, fatigue, ascites, thrombophlebitis, hepatomegaly. A fistula may also occur. Jaundice occurs in about 50%.

There is a slight correlation between cigarette smoking and pancreatic CA.

Objectives

1. Reduce nausea and vomiting; control future episodes.
2. Prevent or correct weight loss.
3. Restore LBM.
4. Control side effects of therapy and the disease, such as diabetes.
5. Counteract therapies—surgery, chemotherapy, radiation.
6. Provide foods or supplements that include all necessary nutrients to prolong life and health.
7. Augment nutritional status; correct anemia.

Dietary Recommendations

1. TPN may be beneficial for short term or long term, altering nutrients according to serum values.
2. Small, frequent meals may be better tolerated when and if the patient can eat orally.
3. Increased calories and protein should be provided to restore weight, unless patient is hyperglycemic or has extensive liver impairment.
4. Eventually, a calorie-controlled diabetic diet may be needed.
5. MCT and fat-soluble vitamins (water-miscible form) may be added to the diet. EFAs should also be included.
6. Selenium may be needed for some patients, especially with TPN solutions.

Profile

Ht, wt	Temp	Alb
Alk, phos (inc.)	X-rays	Chol, trig
IBW/HBW	Transferrin	BP
PT (inc.)	Serum insulin	Serum amylase (inc.)
Gluc (↑)	TLC (varies)	H & H
Serum lipase (inc.)	Bilirubin (inc.)	CT scan
Secretin	Cholecystokinin	SGOT, SGPT (↑)

Side Effects of Drugs Commonly Used

1. *Pancreatic enzymes** (pancrelipase and pancreatin) are given only if serum levels of nutrients are inadequate.
2. Insulin may be needed if the patient is hyperglycemic. In islet cell tumors, hypoglycemia may occur instead. Monitor accordingly.
3. *Vitamin B_{12}* supplements may be required with total pancreatectomy, especially with steatorrhea.
4. *Antiemetics* may be needed.

---

* NOTE: All enzymes are digested when taken as an oral supplement. Enteric coating aids in maintaining integrity of the enzymes until they reach the small intestine.

5. *Bile salts* may also be needed, especially with extensive diarrhea and steatorrhea.
6. *Streptozocin* can cause or aggravate nausea.

Patient Education

1. Discuss specific dietary recommendations appropriate for the patient's condition and therapies.
2. With *pancreatectomy*, a diabetic diet may be absolutely essential. Discuss the rationale with the patient.
3. Explain how the diet affects malabsorption in regard to fat, protein, vitamins and minerals.

Comment

Whipple's procedure (pancreatoduodenectomy) involves many operations where the entire duodenum, pancreas, spleen, and gallbladder may all be removed.

NOTES

RADIATION COLITIS AND ENTERITIS

Usual Hospital Stay

4–5 days.

Notations

Serious injury to the intestinal epithelium and arterioles of the small or large intestines results in cell death, fibrosis and obstruction after radiation therapy. 7000 rads usually causes damage, especially to the small intestine (enteritis). If the radiation must be given chronically, resection may be needed. The ability of the intestines to become hyperplastic and to increase absorptive capacity is thus prevented. Radiotherapy may involve high-energy radiation from x-rays, cobalt-60, radium, etc.

Symptoms and signs include nausea, vomiting, mucoid diarrhea, abdominal pain, bleeding. (Later—colic, decrease in stool caliber, progressive obstipation with stricture and fibrosis).

Of patients who are given abdominal or pelvic radiotherapy, 5–40% will develop radiation enteritis or colitis. Of these persons, many will require home TPN or chronic PN because of the effects on the intestinal tract. Radiation to the ileum is especially devastating.

Objectives

1. Correct malnutrition and malabsorption from diarrhea, bacterial overgrowth, protein exudative losses, CHO loss from decreased enzymes, and steatorrhea from ileal damage.
2. Prevent or correct intestinal ischemia.
3. Prepare the patient for surgery if needed, to relieve obstruction.
4. Meet hypermetabolic needs from infection and complications.
5. Prevent gallstones, renal stones and other effects following radiation.
6. Replace folic acid and vitamin B_{12} if ileal damage has occurred.
7. Ensure adequate electrolyte and fluid intake.

Dietary Recommendations

1. An elemental diet may be best tolerated, especially if obstruction or constipation has occurred. If taken orally, products like Vivonex or Vivonex TEN should be sipped slowly to avoid a dumping effect. Encourage patient to consider it a medication.
2. TPN may also be appropriate for the patient, before or after surgery.
3. If oral intake is possible, 6–8 small feedings may be better tolerated. Low residue, low fat, milk and gluten-free diet may be necessary.
4. Gradually add foods back to the diet as tolerance increases.
5. Fluid and electrolyte balance and intake should be carefully maintained.

Profile

Ht, wt	Gluc	Wt changes
Alb, Transferrin, RBP	IBW/HBW	Na^+, K^+
H breath test	Ca^{++}, Mg^{++}	Schilling test
Intestinal bx if needed	Fecal fat test	I & O
	H & H	SGPT

Side Effects of Drugs Commonly Used

1. *Sedatives* may be used as needed.
2. *Antispasmodics* may be used if intestinal colic persists.
3. *Corticosteroids* may cause or aggravate sodium or potassium depletion, negative nitrogen balance, hyperglycemia and other problems.
4. *Sulfasalazine* has side effects that should be carefully monitored.

Patient Education

1. Home TPN may be needed for a short-term or long-term use.
2. Discuss ways to make meals appetizing and palatable, and how to decrease nausea (see general entry for cancer).

NOTES

WILMS' TUMOR (EMBRYOMA OF THE KIDNEY)

Usual Hospital Stay

3–4 days.

Notation

Wilms' tumor, also called nephroblastoma or embryoma of the kidney, is a highly malignant tumor occurring almost exclusively in young children (under age 6); 62% are aged 1–4 years. Metastasis to lungs, liver and brain can occur.

Symptoms and signs include weight loss, anorexia, enlarged kidney, hypertension, fever, anemia, and abdominal pain.

A cure may be possible if metastases have not occurred before nephrectomy.

Objectives

1. Prepare the patient for surgery (nephrectomy) and for postsurgical wound healing.
2. Control side effects of radiotherapy and chemotherapy.
3. Promote normal growth and development, as far as possible.
4. Control hypertension; correct anemia.

Dietary Recommendations

1. Provide adequate calories and protein according to age. If needed, include a safety measure for weight loss that has occurred.
2. Ensure adequate intake of foods high in HBV proteins, iron and B-complex vitamins to help prevent anemia from worsening.
3. Restrict excessive sodium if patient is hypertensive. Monitor calcium and magnesium levels as well; supplement if necessary.
4. Monitor protein tolerance; increase as tolerated.

Profile

Ht, wt, growth %	Wt changes	X-ray
BP (inc.)	Mg^{++}	I & O
Ca^{++}	Gluc	Transferrin
Alb	TLC (varies)	Abd. CT scan
Creatinine	BUN	Liver function tests
IBW/HBW	H & H	SGPT

Side Effects of Drugs Commonly Used

1. *Dactinomycin* or *vincristine* may cause nausea and other side effects. Monitor accordingly.
2. *Doxorubicin* may also be used.

Patient Education

1. Discuss side effects that the patient is experiencing in light of therapies used (e.g., radiation, chemotherapy, and surgery).
2. Discuss normal growth and desirable weight for the patient.
3. Highlight meals that are attractive so that the patient eats as well as possible.

Comment

Tumor Staging

Stage I	limited to kidneys (can be excised)
Stage II	extension into peri-renal tissue occurs; excision may still be possible
Stage III	tumor is not completely resectable
Stage IV	metastasis occurs
Stage V	bilateral renal involvement occurs

WOMEN'S MAMMARY CARCINOMA (BREAST CANCER)

Usual Hospital Stay

6 days; 3–4 days without complications.

Notation

The breast is the most common site of CA in women. In early stages, a single nontender, firm, or hard mass with poorly-defined margins may exist. Later, skin or nipple retraction, axillary lymphadenopathy, breast enlargement, redness, edema and pain may occur. In late stages, ulceration, edema, and metastases to bone, liver or brain are common.

The incidence is higher in women who are nulliparous, who have a family history of breast CA, or a personal history of breast CA or dysplasia. 1/9 of all women develop some form of mammary carcinoma. It is more common after age 30, but is not limited to one specific decade of life in onset. A Boston University study suggests that OC use over 10 years will increase risk.

Lactation is not now viewed as protective, as was once believed. Fertility and ovarian function probably play a role. Tumors are frequently found in the upper/outer quadrant of the breast (45%), nipple area (25%), with 30% identified in the other breast areas.

Objectives

1. Control side effects of therapy and treatments (radiotherapy, local or extensive mastectomy, chemotherapy).
2. Promote good nutritional status in order to reduce future incidents and recurrence.
3. Encourage regular breast self-examinations.
4. Promote weight control (lose if obese, but be careful not to lose LBM).
5. Increase likelihood of survival and wellness.
6. For mastectomy patients, promote wound healing and decrease infection.

Dietary Recommendations

1. A normal diet with control of excessive calories and fat may be helpful. Some theories suggest that obesity may promote the original tumor growth, and calories seem to play the greatest role.
2. No other specific alternate foods are required.
3. Alcoholic beverages should be strongly discouraged, since there is some possible etiological role.

Profile

Ht, wt	H & H	Chol, trig
Anorexia, nausea	Sed rate (for mets)	IBW/HBW
Mammography	Gluc	Serum estrogen
TLC (varies)	Any wt changes	Alb
Ca^{++}	Alk phos	Temp
Biopsy	CBC	
I & O	Prolactin	

Side Effects of Drugs Commonly Used

1. *Hormonal therapy* may be given—estrogens, androgens, corticosteroids are commonly used.
2. *Chemotherapy* may also be used. Taste alterations are common for beef, chicken, coffee, and cake.

3. *Megestrol acetate* (a hormonal antineoplastic drug) can reverse anorexia and weight loss in some women.

Patient Education

1. Breast cancer detection projects are available throughout the United States. Check with the local chapter of the National Cancer Institute (NCI) and the American Cancer Society (ACS). Early detection of new tumors is crucial.
2. Discuss ways to make meals more appetizing, especially if appetite is poor.

Comments

1. Breast CA in men is uncommon and is generally preceded by gynecomastia.
2. Staging of breast CA
   Stage I   rarely metastasizing/noninvasive
   Stage II   rarely metastasizing/invasive
   Stage III   moderately metastasizing/invasive
   Stage IV   highly metastasizing/invasive
3. Studies are now including genetic predictors, such as the HER-2 gene and the NM23 gene.
4. The natural protein *mammastatin* is present in the circulation in normal cells. Some women have more than others, as in the end stages of pregnancy. Studies are underway.

For More Information

Y-Me Breast Cancer Support Program: (800) 221-2141

Section 14
Surgical Disorders

Chief Assessment Factors

presurgical illness—acute or chronic (diabetes, CVD, etc.)

recent weight changes, especially loss

serum albumin, transferrin, RBP

skinfold measures

hydration status

electrolyte status

blood pressure, abnormal

anemia

nausea, vomiting

surgical procedure (GI versus non-GI involvement)

obesity

infections

Table 14–1.
Postsurgical Phases
1. 3–7 days—Marked catabolic response.
2. 2–5 weeks—Turning point and anabolic phase where spontaneous improvement begins.
3. 6 weeks or longer—Fat gain phase, where vigorous nutritional support could promote excessive fat stores.

Table 14–2.

Elective Versus Major Surgery*

Elective Surgery—minimal increases in nitrogen loss and 10–15% increase in carlorie needs.

Major surgery—greater intensity and duration will increase catabolic effects. Preoperative hyperalimentation may be needed for up to one month, if possible.

---

* Cerra, F: *Pocket Manual of Surgical Nutrition.* St. Louis: C. V. Mosby, 1984.

For More Information

Second Surgical Opinion Hotline: (800) 638-6833

Table 14–3.
Extent of Body Reserves of Nutrients*

Nutrient	Time Required to Deplete Reserves in Well-Nourished Individual
Amino acids	several hours
Carbohydrate	13 hours
Sodium	2–3 days
Water	4 days
Fat	20–40 days
Thiamine	30–60 days
Vitamin C	60–120 days
Niacin	60–180 days
Riboflavin	60–180 days
Vitamin A	90–365 days
Iron	125 days (women); 750 days (men)
Iodine	1000 days
Calcium	2500 days

* Guthrie, H.: *Introducing Nutrition,* 2nd ed. St. Louis: C. V. Mosby, 1986.

SURGERY, GENERAL

Usual Hospital Stay

Preoperative procedures, 1 day; postoperative stay varies by procedure, complications.

Notation

Metabolic effects after surgery may be related to the extent of the surgery, the prior nutritional state of the patient, and the effect of surgery on the patient's ability to digest and absorb nutrients. After surgery or injury, plasma cortisol generally increases rapidly with an acceleration in the breakdown of fat to fatty acids and glycerol.

Increased excretion of nitrogen and sodium retention occurs, but is reversed in approximately 5–7 days (or as late as 12–14 days in the elderly); this may be prolonged after severe burns. Increased excretion of potassium occurs but begins to reverse itself 1–2 days after surgery. An increased excretion of calcium is seen after skeletal trauma or during immobilization. Major surgery or stress to the soft tissue is followed by increased calcium excretion in children and adults, and decreased calcium excretion in the elderly. Vitamin C may be destroyed by extensive inflammation in the postoperative condition.

A fever causes increased nutritional needs; for every 1°F increase, there is an increased caloric need of 7% to 8%. With wounds, burns, and hemorrhage there is an increased protein need; major wounds and burns can cause a loss of up to 50 g protein/day. With hemorrhage or major blood loss, or even when much blood is drawn for laboratory tests, loss of iron and plasma protein may be great (1L blood is equivalent to 150 Hb [500 mg iron] and 50 g plasma protein.) Fluids should also be increased.

Nutritional intervention should occur if treatment has been NPO for 3 days and the patient will not be eating for another 7 days. Remember that D_5W has only 170 kcal/L.

Objectives

Preoperative

1. Prepare reserves. Proper nourishment should be emphasized in order for the patient to prepare for stress, wound healing, hemorrhage, and potential dehydration. Some authors suggest glucose/potassium IV loading in nondiabetic/nonrespiratory patients for preoperative preparation.
2. Monitor patients who are grossly overweight. Fatty tissues are not resistant to infections; they are hard to suture. Dehiscence may occur. Controlled weight loss should be instituted before surgery whenever possible.

Postoperative

1. Replace protein and glycogen stores.
2. Correct electrolyte and fluid imbalances (water, sodium, potassium).
3. Shorten the time needed for wound healing. The wound has priority for first 5–10 days; tensile strength peaks at 40–50 days.
4. Restore lost protein and iron from hemorrhage/bleeding.
5. Replace important nutrients (vitamin C, 100–200% RDA; vitamin k; zinc, vitamin A. Arginine has been shown to speed wound healing (Rutgers U.)
6. Minimize weight loss, which is not obligatory. Prevent or correct PCM.
7. Attend to special needs, such as fever, trauma, pregnancy, infancy or childhood.
8. Prevent infection, which can occur in over 10% of surgical cases.

Dietary Recommendations

Preoperative

1. Use a high protein/high calorie diet. TF or TPN if needed.
2. If patient is obese, use a low calorie diet that includes CHOs adequate for glycogen stores.
3. Ensure that intake of vitamin C and vitamin K is adequate.
4. Gradually restrict diet to clear liquids, and then NPO.

Postoperative

1. Immediately after surgery use IV glucose and electrolytes as needed.
2. As treatment progresses, clear liquids may be followed by full liquids; diet may be changed as tolerated.
3. If oral feeding is not possible, use tube feeding or parenteral nutrition.
4. The patient's increased appetite requires a high calorie intake, HBV proteins and increased fluid, zinc, vitamins C & A. 40–45 kcal/kg; 1.5 g protein/kg (16% total kcal) and a 1:150 N:kcal ratio are needed.
5. Increase BCAAs for stress greater than usual.
6. Alter care plans by degree of net catabolism (losses of 5–15 g of nitrogen daily may be common). Alter calories accordingly.
7. With infection, use care with zinc and iron, which are bacterial nutrients.

Profile

Ht	Na^+	I & O
IBW/HBW	PT	P
Alb	Wt	TLC
BUN	Gluc	Ca^{++}, Mg^{++}
K^+	H & H	3-methyl histidine
N balance	RBP	Wt changes
Transferrin	N, V	Other parameters

Side Effects of Drugs/Anesthesia

1. *Anesthetics* delay peristalsis. Nausea is common. Have the patient eat ice chips or sip carbonated beverages until the nausea subsides.
2. *Pain medications* should be taken sufficiently in advance of meals to allow a pleasant, pain-free mealtime.
3. Treatment with *warfarin* (Coumadin), a blood thinner used to prevent emboli, requires that the patient reduce excessive intake of vitamin K foods (cabbage, kale, and spinach) to control levels. The vegetarian should be watched in particular. *Heparin* has no dietary consequences.
4. *Metoclopramide* (Reglan) may help with postoperative ileus. Dry mouth or nausea can result after prolonged use.

Patient Education

1. Immobilization of the patient can produce unwanted side effects. Have the patient drink plenty of fluids and ambulate as soon as possible.
2. Patients tend to lose 0.5 lb daily early in the postoperative period. Weight gain during this time suggests fluid excess.
3. Eat and drink slowly to prevent gas formation from swallowed air.
4. Discuss the role of surgery as planned trauma, allowing adequate time for a return to homeostasis.
5. Discuss wound healing priority, tensile strength, role of nutrients (zinc, vitamin C, vitamin A, and amino acids). Substrate failure can decrease anabolism, decreasing scar tissue formation.
6. Discuss rebound scurvy and controlled intake of vitamin C.
7. During the fat gain stage (3 months to 1 year postoperatively) calories should be controlled.

NOTES

HYPONATREMIA

Usual Hospital Stay

4–5 days.

Notation

Low serum sodium concentration can occur as a result of loss of sodium in excess of osmotically obligated water (*primary salt depletion*), a dehydration where sodium loss is greater than water loss. In this case, contracted extracellular fluid volume is evident and a hypertonic or isotonic saline solution is given (perhaps along with salty broths).

Retention of water in excess of sodium can also cause hyponatremia (with water intoxication, dilutional hyponatremia, SIADH, etc.) In *dilutional hyponatremia*, impaired water excretion occurs (as in CHF, cirrhosis, or nephrotic syndrome); sodium is abnormally retained and a low sodium diet with diuretics may be indicated. With *water intoxication*, fluid will be restricted. For *SIADH*, with such conditions as oat cell CA, pulmonary diseases, CVA, brain tumor, thiazides, sulfonalureas, myxedema, etc., see SIADH entry.

Objectives

1. Correct hyponatremic state.
2. Prevent future episodes, as far as possible.

Dietary Recommendations

1. Provide appropriate dietary alterations, as indicated above by causation.
2. Monitor effects on serum sodium levels; prevent further problems.

Profile

Ht, wt	IBW/HBW	Na^+
K^+	Cl^-	Osm
I & O	P_{CO_2}	P_{O_2}
BUN	Underlying problems	Urinary Na^+

Side Effects of Drugs Commonly Used

1. In appropriate cases, a 3 or 5% NaCl solution may be given.
2. D_5W used in excess can cause hyponatremia in water intoxication.
3. Furosemide (Lasix) and vigorous diuretic therapy may cause hyponatremia.

Patient Education

1. Inform the patient about good sources of necessary electrolytes.
2. Advise against self-medication with unusual diets or supplements—discuss the need to adhere carefully to medical suggestions.

HYPERNATREMIA

Usual Hospital Stay

4–5 days.

Notation

Hypernatremia usually occurs in persons who cannot obtain sufficient water to replace losses (CV, etc.) Some people may have damage to the thirst center while undergoing surgery for aneurysms. *Sodium intoxication* may result from excess intake of NaCl or sodium bicarbonate. Steroids can also cause hypernatremia.

Objectives

1. Correct dehydration.
2. Monitor thirst, the first sign of water loss.

3. Flushing, fever, loss of sweating, dry tongue and mucous membranes may result from hypernatremia. Tachycardia, hallucinations or coma can result if the condition is not corrected.

Dietary Recommendations

1. Monitor use of all tube feedings carefully; high protein formulas can cause simple dehydration.
2. Nonketotic hyperosmolar coma or diabetes insipidus can also cause water loss; replace water appropriately—orally or parenterally.

Profile

Ht, wt	Underlying	Na^+
Pco_2	conditions	K^+
I & O	Po_2	Osm
IBW/HBW	Skin turgor	

Side Effects of Common Drugs Used

Excessive *steroid* use can cause hypernatremia; monitor carefully.

Patient Education

Discuss the appropriate fluid intake for age and underlying condition(s).

HYPOKALEMIA

Usual Hospital Stay

4–5 days.

Notation

Hypokalemia results from inadequate intake, excessive GI losses from diarrhea or vomiting or fistulas; from urinary losses of adrenal or renal origin. Diuretic therapy is a key cause. Aspirin and penicillin may also cause problems when used chronically.

Symptoms and signs include severe muscle weakness, ECG changes and arrhythmias, lethargy, fatigue, anorexia, constipation, confusion and impaired CHO tolerance.

Chloride depletion usually accompanies hypokalemia. Alkalosis also is common.

Objectives

1. Replace potassium (generally with KCl except in renal tubular acidosis).
2. Prevent future episodes of hypokalemia, wherever possible.

Dietary Recommendations

1. A potassium-rich diet includes bananas, oranges, grapefruit, potatoes and most other fruits and vegetables. In addition, most salt substitutes contain potassium (read labels). Avoid overuse.
2. Monitor sodium intake to prevent underdoses and overdoses.
3. Discuss fiber sources if constipation is a problem.
4. Fluid intake should be adequate.

Profile

Ht, Wt	IBW/HBW	I & O
K^+	Na^+	Cl^-
Osm	BUN	Creat

Side Effects of Common Drugs Used

1. *Diuretics* can cause potassium wastage (e.g., furosemide [Lasix]).
2. As indicated, *penicillin* and *aspirin* can cause or aggravate potassium depletion.
3. *Steroids* in combination with diuretics can especially deplete potassium levels.
4. Kaochlor, Kay-Ciel, K-Lor, K-Lyte, K-Tab, Klotrix, Micro-K, and Slow-K are all sources of potassium.

Patient Education

1. Discuss dietary sources of potassium (colas, coffee, tea, etc.).
2. Discuss the importance of following medical advice carefully, and reading labels of all supplements to avoid overdoses of K^+ on the opposite extreme.

NOTES

HYPERKALEMIA

Usual Hospital Stay

4–5 days.

Notation

Because the distal nephron has such a large capacity for secreting potassium, even in advanced renal failure, hyperkalemia occurs only when an additional problem exists (e.g., oliguria, tissue catabolism, K^+ supplementation, use of penicillin G, severe acidosis, excessive spironolactone or triamterene therapy, deficiency of endogenous steroids.

Symptoms and signs include weakness, anxiety, altered ECGs (over 7 mEq/liter, a fatal arrhythmia can occur).

Objectives

1. Treat immediately to prevent arrhythmias.
2. Prevent constipation and fecal impaction.
3. If all else fails, dialyze.

Dietary Recommendations

1. IVs are likely to be used (glucose, insulin, bicarbonate), to shift K^+ intracellularly; Na^+ and Ca^{++} may also be needed as physical antagonists to K^+. Infusions will be given until excess K^+ is permanently removed.
2. When the patient can eat orally, a controlled K^+ intake will be needed to avoid further exacerbation.

Profile

Ht, wt	IBW/HBW	Serum K^+
Na^+	Cl^-	Ca^{++}, Mg^{++}
I & O	BUN, creat	Gluc

Side Effects of Common Drugs Used

Sodium polystyrene sulfonate (Kayexalate) may also be needed (given with sorbitol to prevent constipation).

Patient Education

Discuss potassium sources from the diet, and how medications affect serum levels.

NOTES

HYPOCALCEMIA

Usual Hospital Stay

4–5 days.

Notation

Vitamin D deficiency caused by nutritional deficiency or malabsorption; renal insufficiency, hepatic dysfunction, hypoparathyroidism, hyperphosphatemia, acute pancreatitis, or calcitonin-producing tumors of the thyroid will cause hypocalcemia.

Symptoms and signs include tetany, seizures, and cardiac arrest. In the long term, bone demineralization with bone pain and compression fractures may result.

Objectives

1. Correct symptomatic condition (usually with Ca^{++} gluconate by IV).
2. Be careful when correcting coexisting acidosis with sodium bicarbonate.
3. Provide adequate vitamin D_3 supplementation, as needed.

Dietary Recommendations

1. Once able to eat, offer calcium-rich foods. Discuss with patient.
2. Beware of excesses of caffeine, oxalates, fiber and aluminum-containing antacids.
3. Increase consumption of vitamin D and lactose-containing foods, if tolerated.

Profile

Ht, wt	IBW/HBW	Na^+, K^+
Mg^{++}	T_3, T_4	Osm
I & O	Alk phos	Urinary Ca^{++}
P	Ca^{++}	

Side Effects of Common Drugs Used

1. *Corticosteroids, furosemide, isoniazid* (INH), and *tetracycline* can reduce calcium availability.
2. *Calcium carbonate* (as in Tums) provides 40% elemental calcium.
3. *Aluminum* in antacids can reduce calcium bioavailability.
4. *Citrated blood transfusions* may cause hypocalcemia.

Patient Education

1. Beware of bone meal and dolomite because of their toxic metal content.
2. Calcium is found in milk, cheese, leafy greens, and yogurt. Dry milk can be added to foods.
3. Oxalates in chocolate appear to have no adverse effect on calcium bioavailability in chocolate milk. (*Dairy Council Digest* 60:3, May–June 1989).
4. Spinach should be omitted because of its effect on calcium bioavailability.

NOTES

HYPERCALCEMIA

Usual Hospital Stay

4–5 days.

Notation

Hypercalcemia can be caused by increased parathormone activity, increased vitamin D activity (as in TB or sarcoidosis), enhanced bone resorption from bone tumors, multiple myeloma, immobilization, milkalkali syndrome, adrenal insufficiency, breast-cancer, or head/neck cancer.

Symptoms and signs include drowsiness, lethargy, stupor, muscle weakness, decreased reflexes, nausea and vomiting, anorexia, constipation, ileus, polyuria, renal stones, azotemia, nocturia, hypertension, bradycardia, pruritus, and eye abnormalities. Short-term therapy is generally undertaken in the ICU.

Objectives

1. Correct underlying condition with rehydration (usually with normal saline), and hemodilution.
2. IV organic phosphate can help remove excess calcium. Neutra-Phos or Phospho-Soda may be used. Steroids are an alternative.
3. Prevent recurrence.
4. Correct nausea, vomiting, constipation and other side effects of elevated calcium.

Dietary Recommendations

1. Be careful not to provide excesses of milk, vitamins D or A, calcium supplements or antacids, and lactose until the condition has been normalized.
2. Caffeine, oxalates, fiber and phytates will decrease calcium absorption and help to promote greater excretion.
3. Monitor potassium and magnesium losses with treatment; these are common. Correct diet accordingly.

Profile

Ht, wt	IBW/HBW	Na^+, K^+
Alk phos	I & O	BUN
Mg^{++}	Osm	
P	Ca^{++}	

Side Effects of Common Drugs Used

1. *Furosemide* and *ethacrynic acid* can help increase calcium excretion. Impaired renal function may contraindicate use.
2. *Prednisone* can be used to decrease vitamin D-mediated calcium absorption. Monitor impact on serum glucose, sodium, etc. Nausea and vomiting may result.
3. *Didronel* (IV) can decrease calcium levels. Nausea and vomiting may result.
4. *Antacids* with aluminum can also be used to increase excretion. Be aware of the high calcium levels in Tums (an OTC drug).
5. *Lithium* and *thiazides* may increase serum calcium levels; monitor carefully.

Patient Education

1. Discuss the calcium content of supplements, tube feedings and antacids—highlight the need for the physician to be aware of all products taken.
2. Discuss how to avoid future problems from diet and medications.

Comment

Malignant disease produces hypercalcemia via bone destruction or metastasis with resulting release of calcium into the bloodstream (*Hospital Medicine* 4/89).

HYPOMAGNESEMIA

Usual Hospital Stay

4–5 days.

Notation

Hypomagnesemia is usually seen with diarrhea, PCM, malabsorption or alcoholism. Of patients in tertiary care units 10% may have this condition. Rarely, hypomagnesemia is seen with hyperparathyroidism, diabetic ketoacidosis or hypercalcemia, excessive diuretic therapy, renal tubular disease or acute pancreatitis.

Symptoms and signs include anxiety, hyperirritability, confusion, hallucinations, seizures, tremor, hyperreflexia, tetany, tachycardia, hypertension, arrhythmias, vasomotor changes, profuse sweating, muscle weakness, grimaces of facial muscles, and refractory hypocalcemia.

Objectives

1. Correct low serum magnesium levels.
2. Prevent sudden death.
3. Correct symptoms and side effects of the condition.

Dietary Recommendations

1. No specific foods are exceptionally excellent sources; chocolate, nuts, fruits and green vegetables, beans or potatoes, wheat and corn are considered good sources. Meats, seafood and dairy products are fair to poor.
2. Discuss long-term measures to prevent further episodes. Long-term use of magnesium-free TPN can be one aggravating source of the problem. Monitor intake form all sources—oral, TF or TPN.

Profile

Ht, wt	IBW/HBW	BP
Ca^{++}	Osm	Gluc
I & O	BUN	
PTH	Mg^{++}	

Side Effects of Common Drugs Used

1. Many medications can cause hypomagnesemia—furosemide, ethacrynic acid, thiazides, some antibiotics, cisplatin, cyclosporine.
2. Normal renal function is needed for use of $MgSO_4$.
3. Milk of magnesia can be used for liquid form.

HYPERMAGNESEMIA

Usual Hospital Stay

4–5 days.

Notation

Hypermagnesemia is usually found in patients with renal failure who are treated with such antacids as Maalox or Gelusil, or with cathartics such as milk of magnesia.

Symptoms and signs include lethargy, hyporeflexia, and respiratory depression.

Objectives

1. Reduce or terminate sources of exogenous magnesium.
2. Treat respiratory depression with calcium, gluceptate or other medication.
3. Prevent further morbidity and side effects.

Dietary Recommendations

1. No specific dietary alterations are required, except omission of rich magnesium sources until the condition is corrected.
2. Monitor intake of all magnesium (as with TPN solutions).

Profile

Ht, wt	IBW/HBW	Mg^{++}
Ca^{++}	I & O	Gluc
BP	Na^+, K^+	Osm

Side Effects of Common Drugs Used

1. Calcium-containing medications may be given to help with excretion of excessive magnesium.
2. TPN solutions should be carefully monitored for all electrolytes.

Patient Education

Discuss effects of magnesium on the body, sources from the diet, as well as use of OTC medications and supplements. Discuss prevention of toxic levels.

PHOSPHATE IMBALANCES

Usual Hospital Stay

Varies by cause.

Notation

Phosphorus is a major component of bone and is one of the most abundant constituents of all metabolic processes and tissues. 85% is found in the skeleton. Only about 12% is bound to proteins, so a typical laboratory assessment is of elemental P, with some additional values for HPO_4 and $NaHPO_4$ as well.

Phosphorus levels tend to be higher in children and tend to rise in women after menopause. Ingestion of CHO acutely depresses serum phosphorus levels, probably resulting from cellular uptake and phosphate formation. Lowered plasma phosphorus can occur from alkalosis, hyperparathyroidism, hypovitaminosis D, malabsorption syndrome, starvation or cachexia, chronic alcoholism, renal tubular defects, acid-base disturbances, diabetic ketoacidosis, and genetic hypophosphatemia. *Hypophosphatemia* can also occur as a result of unmonitored total parenteral nutrition. *Hyperphosphatemia* can result from renal insufficiency, hypoparathyroidism, or hypervitaminosis D.

In *hyperphosphatemia*, calcium phosphate may be deposited in abnormal sites. In addition, abnormal renal phosphorus clearance occurs.

In *hypophosphatemia*, anorexia, weakness, bone pain, dizziness, and waddling gait may be observed. In severe cases, elevated CPK levels are seen, with rhabdomyolysis superimposed on myopathy. Congestive heart failure can result if phosphorus is not administered. Additionally, low serum phosphorus levels will result in lowered 2,3-diphospoglyceric acid (2,3-DPG), which facilitates oxyhemoglobin dissociation (leading to tissue hypoxia and low Po_2). Rapid delivery of intravenous glucose, such as with TPN, may accentuate phosphorus depletion syndrome and can lead to convulsions, muscle weakness and hemolytic anemia.

Objectives

1. Normalize serum phosphorus levels.
2. Prevent further abnormalities and complications.
3. Control phosphorus delivery to all tissues.

Dietary Recommendations

1. Appropriate levels of phosphorus should be provided according to age and serum status.
2. Monitor glucose intake, especially from PN or TPN. Check all tube feedings for phosphorus content as well.
3. During treatment, keep a normal Ca:P ratio (ideally, 1:1).
4. Monitor dietary intake of milk, meat and other foods high in P. Observe serum levels regularly, especially in renal patients.

Profile

Ht, wt, IBW/HBW	Gluc	Alb
Po_2, Pco_2	CPK	I & O

| Alk phos | 2,3-DPG levels | H & H |
| Serum P | Serum Ca^{++} | |

Side Effects of Drugs Commonly Used

1. *Antacids* containing aluminum will prevent phosphorus absorption in the intestinal lumen. They are used to correct hyperphosphatemia, as in renal disease, but can aggravate or cause hypophosphatemia in other conditions.
2. *Diuretics* may affect phosphorus to a varying degree, depending on chemical content. Monitor accordingly.
3. *Potassium acid phosphate* (K-Phos Original), an acidifier, can be used to correct hypophosphatemia.

Patient Education

1. The appropriate measures should be provided to the patient according to his or her condition. For example, a low phosphorus diet with high calcium and adequate vitamin D will be needed for patients with renal osteodystrophy. For conditions causing hypophosphatemia (such as Reye's syndrome and other infectious illnesses), adequate dietary phosphorus would be warranted. A balance is required.
2. The patient may be advised that about 50–60% of dietary phosphorus is absorbed (more in depleted persons) from dietary intakes.

NOTES

AMPUTATION

Usual Hospital Stay

10 days; lower limb amputation for endocrine disease, 17–18 days.

Notation

Amputations may result from trauma, PVD, congenital deformity, chronic infections, or tumors. In amputation, the percentage of total body weight lost depends on body part lost: foot, 1.8%; below knee, 6%; above knee, 15%; entire lower extremity, 18.5%; hand, 1%; below elbow, 3%; entire upper extremity, 6.5%.

"A-K" means above knee; "B-K" means below knee.

Objectives

Immediate Postoperative

1. Provide adequate protein and calories for healing.
2. Provide adequate intake of vitamins and minerals (zinc, vitamin C, vitamin K, vitamin A, etc.)

Long-term

1. Patients with an A-K amputation who walk (with/without prosthesis) use 25% more energy than a normal person who walks the same speed. These patients may have difficulty maintaining weight. Otherwise, immobilized patients may tend to gain weight and will need control measures.
2. Other types of amputations will alter care plans accordingly.

Dietary Recommendations

Immediate Postoperative

1. Use a high protein/high calorie diet.
2. Supplement diet with vitamins and minerals, especially zinc, vitamins A, C and K; arginine.

Long-term

1. Provide a low calorie diet if needed.
2. For patients who lose weight, a high calorie diet should be used to compensate for increased energy use.

Profile

Preop Ht, postop ht	Preop wt, present wt
Pre/postop IBW/HBW	% BW of amputated area
Alb	H & H
K^+, Na^+	Gluc
P_{CO_2}, P_{O_2}	BP
I & O	PT
	Transferrin, RBP

Patient Education

1. Describe the role of nutrition in wound healing.
2. Describe the role of activity in the synthesis of protein tissues.
3. Indicate how to control or increase calories in the diet for energy usage.
4. For hand or arm amputations, consider adaptive feeding equipment. OT specialists can help. Discuss meal preparation.

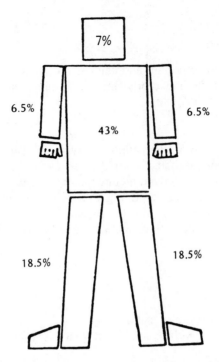

Fig. 14–1. Weight proportions of body segments in % total body weight (from cadavers of young adult men). From Brunnstrom S.: *Clinical Kinesiology*. Philadelphia: F.A. Davis, 1972.

For More Information

National Amputation Foundation
12–45 150th St.
Whitestone, NY 11357

Dietitians in Physical Medicine and Rehabilitation
c/o The American Dietetic Association
Chicago, IL

NOTES

APPENDECTOMY

Usual Hospital Stay

Uncomplicated surgery, 7 days; if complicated, 11 days.

Objectives

1. Reduce any febrile condition that exists.
2. Lower the risks of infection, sepsis.
3. Replace nutrient losses.

Dietary Recommendations

1. Use a high protein/high calorie diet. Ensure that the diet provides adequate amounts of vitamin C, zinc, vitamin K, and vitamin A.
2. Use a soft diet to lessen fiber content.
3. When the patient is able to eat fiber, include foods high in fiber as tolerated.

Profile

Ht	H & H	Gluc
IBW/HBW	Alb	WBCs, ESR (inc. in
Gluc	BP	appendicitis)
K^+, Na^+	I & O	
Wt	PT	

Patient Education

1. Indicate which foods are sources of protein and calories in the diet.
2. Evaluate presurgical intake. A history of poor fiber intake may be evident. A low intake of green vegetables and tomatoes may have altered the bacterial environment of the intestinal tract.

NOTES

BOWEL SURGERY

Usual Hospital Stay

14–15 days.

Objectives

Preoperative

1. Relieve distress.
2. Replenish depleted reserves.

Postoperative

1. Reduce bowel residue while healing occurs.
2. Progress slowly back to a normal diet.
3. Modify diet as needed for the part of the bowel that was affected.

Dietary Recommendations

Preoperative

Regress from soft diet to full then clear liquids. If needed, use an elemental diet, jejunostomy or other enteral/parenteral mode.

Postoperative

1. Use an elemental diet or total parenteral nutrition as needed.
2. Slowly progress from a low residue to normal diet.
3. Good sources of sodium include milk and broth/bouillon.
4. Good sources of potassium include juices, milk, and cocoa.

Profile

Ht	Wt	PT
IBW/HBW	H & H	I & O
Alb	Gluc	BUN, creat
Stoma drainage	Electrolytes	
BP	Temp	

Patient Education

1. Suggest that the patient eat slowly and chew foods well.
2. Excessive intake of roughage should be avoided.
3. Control fluids carefully to include adequate amounts.
4. Long-term nutritional support may be needed.

Comment

Patients who have had a *hemorrhoidectomy* usually tolerate a low residue diet to delay defecation and allow healing at the operative site. After the patient is healed, it is important to have the patient return to a high fiber diet to prevent constipation. See appropriate entry (Section 7).

Patients who have had an *ileostomy* lose a considerable amount of fluid that contains sodium and potassium. Fat and vitamin B_{12} absorption are reduced. Check drainage from ileostomy for electrolytes. Prune juice should be avoided because of its laxative effects. Moderately low fiber foods may be added gradually. Avoid foods high in roughage: nuts, cabbage, prunes, celery, corn, pineapple, beans, onions, etc. Use large amounts of fluids. See appropriate entry (Section 7).

Patients who have had a *colostomy* may follow the same pattern once oral feedings are resumed. See appropriate entry.

In the case of a *jejunoileostomy*, food bypasses 90% of the small intestine. See the jejunoileal bypass surgery entry in Section 7.

See also: *Short-Gut Syndrome* (Section 7).

Comment

Absorptive Role of the Small Intestine

The SI has a large adaptive capacity, with resection of small segments generally not causing nutritional problems. If the terminal ileum is removed, vitamin B_{12} and bile salts will not be reabsorbed.

Diarrhea can be massive if the ileocecal valve is removed with the terminal ileum, with great electrolyte losses and hypovolemia. Cholestyramine may be needed to bind the bile salts. Fat malabsorption with steatorrhea and inadequate vitamins A, D, E and K absorption may also occur. MCT and water-miscible supplements may be necessary. Hyperoxaluria and renal stones may occur. Calcium supplements, altered PUFA intake and aluminum hydroxide binders may be needed.

NOTES

JEJUNOILEAL BYPASS SURGERY

Usual Hospital Stay

7–8 days.

Notation

Formerly used to treat morbid obesity, jejunoileal bypass surgery causes food to bypass 90% of the small intestine. This operation is now seldom done.

Objectives (Postoperative)

1. Improve the reduced absorption of nutrients other than calories.
2. Alleviate electrolyte disturbances.
3. Prevent long-term side effects when possible.

Dietary Recommendations

1. Restrict fluid intake to between meals.
2. Use a high protein, low fat, low carbohydrate, low fiber diet. Intake of lactose should also be low to avoid diarrhea.
3. Schedule six small feedings daily.
4. Replace electrolyte losses, especially potassium.
5. Use a multivitamin supplement to replace malabsorbed nutrients.

Profile

Ht	I & O
IBW/HBW	Postop wt changes
Alb	Gluc
K^+	H & H
Cl^-	Na^+
BUN	Ca^{++}
Mg^{++}	PT
Preop wt	

Patient Education

Adjust diet according to problems and complications seen.

Comments

Complications and Suggestions

1. Diarrhea/vomiting and dehydration. Eliminate spicy, greasy, and fatty foods. Drink tepid water. Eliminate large meals. Avoid fluids for 30 minutes before and after meals.
2. Electrolyte imbalance. Include foods high in calcium (four servings

daily), potassium (four to six servings daily), and magnesium (two or more servings daily).

3. Renal calculi (calcium oxalate stones). Avoid foods high in oxalate, and keep urine volume high by drinking small amounts of tepid water frequently. Aluminum hydroxide binders may be needed.

4. Liver disease. Avoid alcoholic beverages. Do not skip meals—food is essential to the proper functioning of the liver. Increase intake of high quality protein. Cirrhosis occurs in 80–90% of these patients.

5. Insufficient protein absorption. Eat tender, broiled/baked/boiled fish, beef, lamb, or skinless chicken. Use egg white and nonfat milk powder when no lactose intolerance exists.

6. The patient with cholelithiasis or cholecystitis should eat a balanced diet.

7. If the patient has a vitamin deficiency (especially vitamins B_{12}, A, D, and E), a balanced diet and supplements of high potency vitamins should be used.

8. The patient with a lactase deficiency should sip milk slowly. Use non-milk foods that are high in calcium. Have the patient try yogurt.

NOTES

GASTRIC BYPASS OR STAPLING

Usual Hospital Stay

7–8 days.

Notation

Gastric bypass or stapling is a surgical procedure used to bypass a portion of the stomach as a measure of weight loss in the morbidly obese patient. Stretching the pouch postoperatively can defeat the purpose of the gastroplasty.

Objectives

Preoperative

Provide adequate glycogen stores and vitamins C and K for the surgical procedure.

Postoperative

Promote wound healing, restoration of depleted glycogen in the liver. Prevent side effects during weight loss. Prevent complications (alkaline reflux gastritis, esophagitis, perforation, gastric dilation, stomal obstruction, peptic ulcer, staple line disruption, and excessive vomiting).

Dietary Recommendations

Preoperative

Use a balanced diet with adequate calories, protein, vitamins, and minerals. The diet should regress from liquids to NPO.

Postoperative

Over a period of several weeks, progress from clear liquids to full liquids. Until weight loss is achieved, semisolid foods should be added in small amounts. Initial gastric capacity is 30–60 ml; progression is up to 120–150 mls.

Some patients have problems with vomiting if they eat too rapidly, chew improperly, drink fluids right after eating, lie down after eating, or overeat. Recommend eating slowly.

Dehydration or dumping syndrome can also occur.

Profile

Ht	Preop wt	Chol, trig
IBW/HBW	Postop wt	TLC
Alb	H & H	CHI
Gluc	K^+	N balance
Cl^-	BP	PT
Mg	Ca^{++}	Vomiting

Patient Education

1. Indicate the appropriate quantities and qualities of the foods that will be consumed.
2. Help the patient progress to a normalized diet, with the 120–150 ml per meal.
3. Have the patient eat slowly to prevent vomiting, and sip liquids slowly as well. Meat and bread/toast should be taken in very small bites.
4. A multivitamin-mineral preparation is generally needed. Vitamin B_{12}, folacin, iron, potassium and vitamin A are especially at risk.
5. Discuss methods of blenderizing foods.
6. Discuss high protein supplemental beverages.
7. Fasting can cause hypoglycemia; discuss this detail.

Comment

Stapling is the preferred technique, because bypass can cause deficiencies in vitamin B_{12} and iron.

CESAREAN DELIVERY

Usual Hospital Stay

4–5 days, uncomplicated.

Notation

Delivery of a fetus through a uterine incision could have such complications as hemorrhage, infection, fever, drainage, cystitis or pneumonia after the operation. A cesarean delivery is performed for numerous reasons, including maternal diabetes or EPH-gestosis.

Objectives

1. Replenish stores of nutrients from blood and fluid losses.
2. Reduce fever; prevent or correct infections.
3. Promote wound healing.
4. Correct any anemia as a result of the pregnancy or hemorrhage.
5. Encourage mother to breast-feed.

Dietary Recommendations

1. NPO with IVs or clear liquids will be given until nausea subsides.
2. Progress to the usual diet, with increased fiber to soften stools.
3. Increase fluids to 2–3 liters, unless contraindicated.
4. High calorie/high protein intake will be essential to promote adequate wound healing. An iron supplement or vitamin C and vitamin A and zinc in a multiple vitamin-mineral capsule may be beneficial.

Profile

Ht	Pre-PG Wt	Postpartum wt
IBW/HBW (non-PG)	H & H	BP
I & O	Temp	Alb
Chol, trig	Transferrin	Serum Fe
Gluc	Goal wt in 6 months	TIBC

Side Effects of Drugs Commonly Used

1. An *iron supplement* may be given. Ferrous salts are more beneficial and bioavailable than ferric salts.
2. The prenatal supplement can be used for several months postpartum.

Patient Education

1. Discuss importance of nutrition for wound healing, recovery of blood losses, lactation, etc.
2. Stress that the mother should not diet excessively for at least 6 weeks (longer if breast-feeding) to allow healing.

CRANIOTOMY

Usual Hospital Stay

14 days (nontraumatic).

Notation

Craniotomy involves an operative procedure which consists of removing and replacing the bone of the skull to provide access to intracranial structures, usually for a brain tumor.

Symptoms and signs to monitor during or after the procedure involve altered states of consciousness, nausea and vomiting, seizures, paralysis of face or extremities, drainage from the site, shock, aspiration, hyperthermia, dysphagia, thrombophlebitis, diabetes insipidus, or SIADH.

Objectives

1. Prevent aspiration.
2. Limit fluids if necessary.
3. Prevent or correct dysphagia, constipation, UTIs, nausea and vomiting, and diabetes insipidus.
4. Normalize electrolyte levels.

Dietary Recommendations

1. NPO is needed until N & V subside.
2. Progress from clear liquids to soft diet as ordered; patient should be fed while lying on side or with head elevated 30° to prevent aspiration. Check swallowing reflex.
3. Spoon feed as needed.
4. Adequate fiber may be beneficial.
5. If necessary, TF (such as gastrostomy) may be helpful.
6. If steroids are used, reduce sodium intake to 4–6 g daily (or less).

Profile

Ht, wt	IBW/HBW	EEG
H & H	Alb	TLC
CT scan	Consciousness	Gag reflex
BP	WBCs, ESR	CSF
Other parameters		

Side Effects of Drugs Commonly Used

1. *Steroids* may be used, with numerous consequences (such as sodium retention, nitrogen depletion, potassium or calcium losses, hyperglycemia). Alter diet as needed.
2. *Anticonvulsants* may be used (phenytoin [Dilantin], etc.) Monitor specific drugs accordingly.
3. *Analgesics* may be used as pain relief.

Patient Education

1. Discuss the importance of diet in correcting any malnutrition or anemia. As needed, teach family about a diet for dysphagia (e.g., thick, pureed foods with reduced thin liquids).
2. When and if patient can eat, teach him or her to chew slowly and thoroughly.
3. Promote eventual self-feeding.
4. Discuss anxiety related to pain, poor vision, headaches, and seizures. Some patients may be aphasic.

NOTES

CATARACT SURGERY

Usual Hospital Stay

2–3 days.

Notation

A cataract, an opacity of the crystalline lens of the eye, may be congenital, senile, traumatic, or caused by diabetes mellitus. After cataract removal, visual acuity is restored by lens implant, contact lens, or eyeglasses.

Objectives

1. Postoperatively, nutrient losses from bleeding and tissue destruction should be restored.
2. Prevent accidental tearing from excessive facial movement.
3. Improve visual/perceptual field.

Dietary Recommendations

1. The diet should be soft with no stringy meats, pepper, or excessive spices. It should be adequate in protein and calories for healing.
2. Supplement the diet with zinc, vitamin C, vitamin K and vitamin A.

Profile

Ht	Wt	Chol, trig
IBW/HBW	H & H	Serum ascorbate
Alb, RBP	Gluc	PT
K^+, Na^+	BP	

Patient Education

Instruct the patient to eat soft foods, which do not require excessive chewing, until healing is complete.

Comments

1. Some cataracts have been linked to hypercholesterolemia.
2. Ascorbate is especially concentrated in eye tissue. The lens is especially sensitive to O_2 damage, from which vitamin C offers protection. Some persons with cataracts have been found to have low levels of vitamin C. (International Conference on Vitamin C, New York Academy of Sciences, Oct. 8–10, 1986.)
3. Studies at the Human Nutrition Research Center on Aging at Tufts University/Brigham and Women's Hospital in Boston revealed that both vitamins C and A are essential to prevent cataract occurrence.

NOTES

HYSTERECTOMY, ABDOMINAL

Usual Hospital Stay

12 days.

Notation

An abdominal hysterectomy is the surgical removal of the uterus, effected through an abdominal incision. In extensive surgery, 5–10 pints of blood may be lost.

Objectives

1. Promote wound healing and rapid recovery.
2. Replete nutrient reserves and glycogen stores.
3. Replace protein, iron, and vitamin K from heavy blood losses (when they occur).
4. Prevent complications such as urinary tract infections, incisional infections, fever, nausea, and vomiting.

Dietary Recommendations

1. Use a high protein/high calorie diet.
2. Increase fluid intake.
3. Ensure that adequate fiber is provided for alleviation of constipation.
4. Supplement the diet with iron, zinc, vitamin K, vitamin C, and vitamin A.

Profile

Ht	I & O	BP
IBW/HBW	Wt	PT
Alb	H & H	Blood losses
K^+, Na^+	Gluc	Temp

Patient Education

1. Explain that resumption of normal activity may be slow, but exercise improves nutrient repletion and tissue repair.
2. Emphasize the importance of nutrition for wound healing.

Comment

Laser surgery for some women may prevent the need for extensive surgery.

NOTES

PELVIC EXENTERATION

Usual Hospital Stay

12 days.

Notation

This surgery involves removal of all reproductive organs and adjacent tissues in the female patient (i.e., radical hysterectomy, pelvic node dissection, cystectomy and formation of an ileal conduit, vaginectomy, rectal resection with colostomy). The procedure is a major operation.

Objectives

1. Preoperatively, a low residue or elemental diet may be needed, regressing to clear liquids, NPO. Vitamin K may be needed 24–48 hours before the procedure.
2. Prevent hemorrhage, infection, urinary or GI problems, shock, fever, and sepsis.
3. Provide colostomy teaching if needed.
4. Normalize condition as far as possible.
5. Correct anemia or other problems.

Dietary Recommendations

1. Parenteral fluids with electrolytes may be needed (3–4 liters daily unless contraindicated). TPN or tube feeding may also be appropriate.
2. Progress as tolerated to a high protein/high calorie intake with snacks (eggnog, custard, etc.).
3. If nausea is an extensive problem, using fluids between instead of with meals may help.
4. Adequate iron, zinc, vitamins A and C will help with wound healing procedures.

Profile

Ht, wt	IBW/HBW	H & H
Temp, fever	I & O	Alb
PT	BP	Gluc
Transferrin	TLC, WBCs	Other parameters

Side Effects of Drugs Commonly Ordered

1. *Antibiotics* may be useful in correcting bacterial infections.
2. *Iron* in ferrous form may be used.
3. Other drugs may be used to correct UTIs and other complications. Monitor accordingly.

Patient Education

1. Nutrients needed for wound healing must be discussed with the patient and family.
2. The need to take rest with mealtimes and not to become fatigued should be addressed.
3. Recovery may take 6 months or longer.
4. Colostomy teaching should be done as necessary.

NOTES

OPEN HEART SURGERY

Usual Hospital Stay

14–15 days.

Notation

Open heart procedures require the use of a cardio-pulmonary machine. In the case of coronary artery bypass surgery, narrowed or blocked arteries are bypassed. The vein usually comes from the leg. Blood can then flow normally, directly into the heart muscle. CABG usually takes 4–5 hours.

Objectives

Preoperative

Monitor serum levels of electrolytes, albumin, and glucose. Provide a normal diet as ordered by the physician (the diet may be sodium-restricted, calorie-controlled, etc.). Provide ample amounts of glycogen for stores. Use PN support as needed in malnourished cardiac patients (see the CHF and cardiac cachexia entries in Section 6).

Postoperative

Promote wound healing. Restore normal fluid and electrolyte balance. Promote weight control. Wean from ventilator support when possible. Prevent HNKH coma, sepsis, and wound dehiscence.

Dietary Recommendations

1. Control fluid intake by measuring the previous day's output plus 500 ml for insensible losses.
2. Control sodium and potassium intake by monitoring serum levels, controlling edema, and measuring blood pressure. Modify the diet as needed.
3. As treatment progresses, control the intake of cholesterol in the diet (check serum levels and discuss history with patient). Modify sodium intake as needed. The normal amount of sodium needed by adults is 2 g. At home, 2–4 g of sodium is reasonable.
4. Provide adequate protein and calories for wound healing; zinc, vitamins A and C and K as well.
5. The AHA Prudent Heart diet may be utilized.
6. TF or use TPN if severely malnourished. Replete *slowly* and keep head of bed elevated 30° to prevent worsening of CHF. Low sodium TF products would be needed.

Profile

Ht	IBW/HBW	Gluc
BP	H & H	Heart failure
Chol	Edema	RBP
LDH (inc.)	Trig	Transferrin
PTT, PT	CPK	Serum insulin
Na^+	K^+	Acetone
Wt	Ca^{++}	
Alb	I & O	

Side Effects of Drugs Commonly Used

1. *Diuretics* and *digoxin* may deplete potassium.
2. *Insulin* may be needed.
3. *Niacin* and *colestipol* may be used also. Monitor effects.

Patient Education

1. Teach appropriate measures for changes in the daily diet to prevent further problems while the wound is healing.
2. Discuss the need to alter lifestyle (diet, exercise, and stress) to prevent additional problems. Many patients continue to have atherogenic activity after heart surgery.
3. Restriction of simple sugars and alcohol may be needed for patients with diabetes or hypertriglyceridemia.

NOTES

PANCREATIC SURGERY

Usual Hospital Stay

14–15 days (pancreatectomy).

Notation

Surgery of the pancreas may include total pancreatectomy with/without islet cell autotransplant for chronic pancreatitis and cancer; subtotal for islet cell tumor and CA; or pancreatoduodenectomy (Whipple's operation) for carcinoma.

Objectives

1. Monitor any history of ETOH abuse (with resulting malnutrition and malabsorption problems).
2. Encourage nourishing, well-balanced meals if ordered and tolerated.
3. Monitor medications and replacement enzymes or hormones if ordered.
4. Reduce an elevated temperature.

Dietary Recommendations

1. NPO will be needed preoperatively, with PPN or TPN to prepare the patient for a major operation.
2. Postoperatively, TPN or oral intake may progress as tolerated. Clear liquid to soft diet is a general order.
3. A calorie-controlled diabetic diet may be needed.
4. Small, frequent feedings may be helpful.
5. Force fluids unless contraindicated.
6. Alter fat source if malabsorption or steatorrhea occurs.

Profile

Ht, wt	IBW/HBW	Gluc
PT	Alb	Amylase
Acetone	Lipase	Serum insulin

Na$^+$, K$^+$, Cl$^-$ Glucosuria   Temp, fever
Hgb, A$_1$c   I & O
Chol (may be inc.)   H & H

Side Effects of Drugs Commonly Used

1. *Antibiotics* may be used for bacterial infections.
2. *Insulin* may be needed for patients with hyperglycemia.
3. *Vitamin K* can help with clotting.
4. *Pancreatic enzymes* and *bile salts* may be needed.

Patient Education

1. Resources are available to help with diabetes, if the patient becomes a new diabetic.
2. The need for balanced meals will be essential for wound healing and recovery.
3. If the patient has any history of ETOH abuse, discuss how alcohol affects the pancreas.

NOTES

PARATHYROIDECTOMY

Usual Hospital Stay

4–5 days.

Notation

The surgical removal of the parathyroid glands may cause hypoparathyroidism (with tingling, tetany, hoarseness, and seizures).

Objectives

1. Prepare patient preoperatively for surgery.
2. Force fluids unless contraindicated.
3. Alter calcium, vitamin D and phosphorus intake if needed.

Dietary Recommendations

1. Immediately after surgery, IVs or TF may be needed. TPN may not be recommended because of the potential for sepsis in the neck area.
2. 3–4 liters of fluid may be needed.
3. A high calcium/low phosphorus diet may be necessary. Monitor carefully.

Profile

Ht, wt	IBW/HBW	H & H
Ca^{++}	PT	P
Alk phos	Gluc	Alb
TLC	I & O	Temp
BP	Mg^{++}	BUN, creat

Side Effects of Drugs Commonly Used

Vitamin D, calcium chemotherapy and a low phosphorus diet with aluminum hydroxide gel may be ordered for symptoms of hypoparathyroidism.

NOTES

SPINAL SURGERY

Usual Hospital Stay

14 days.

Notation

Spinal surgery is generally performed to relieve pressure on the spinal nerves or cord due to herniated discs, trauma, displaced fractures, osteoporosis, incomplete vertebral dislocation from R.A.

A laminectomy, diskectomy, or spinal fusion may be done.

Objectives

1. Preoperatively, nutrients may be needed for adequate stores (e.g., glucose, protein, vitamins A, C, and K and zinc).

2. Correct nausea and vomiting, if they have been a problem.
3. Avoid weight gain.
4. Prevent calculi, UTIs, and decubitus ulcers.

Dietary Recommendations

1. Parenteral fluids may be given as ordered.
2. A balanced diet, when the patient is ready, with control of total calories to prevent excessive weight gain, may be used.
3. If the patient has been malnourished, a gradual increase in calories may be beneficial.
4. Adequate hydration with 3 liters of fluid will be necessary unless contraindicated. Monitor to prevent overhydration.
5. Increasing fiber intake may be helpful if constipation is a problem. Prune juice, crushed bran and other items may be used if chewing is a problem for the patient. Otherwise, extra fruits and raw vegetables may be used.

Profile

Ht, wt	IBW/HBW	BP
Alb	Gluc	Temp
Na^+, K^+, Cl^-	I & O	CSF
Alk phos	Ca^{++}, Mg^{++}	
BUN, creat	H & H	

Side Effects of Drugs Commonly Used

1. *Antibiotics* may be used with bacterial infections.
2. *Analgesics* and other drugs are used for pain relief.
3. Many *anti-inflammatory drugs* may have been used prior to surgery; monitor time used and side effects accordingly.

Patient Education

1. Discuss the importance of hydration in prevention of UTIs and other problems, such as renal stones.
2. Discuss how fiber can prevent or correct constipation.

NOTES

TOTAL HIP ARTHROPLASTY

Usual Hospital Stay

14 days.

Notation

A total hip arthroplasty is the formation of an artificial hip joint.

Objectives

1. Replenish stores postoperatively.
2. Prevent side effects of immobilization (renal calculi, decubitus, and urinary tract infections.)
3. Promote adequate wound healing.

Dietary Recommendations

1. Use a high protein/high calorie diet.
2. Supplement the diet with zinc, vitamins A, C, and K. Check to see if the patient's iron stores need replenishing after blood loss.
3. If weight loss is needed, provide a balanced, low calorie diet after wound healing is completed.
4. The diet should provide adequate amounts of calcium and phosphorus—calculi should be prevented, but bone tissue adaptation to the new joint should be promoted.

Profile

HT	Ca^{++}	Transferrin
IBW/HBW	Gluc	Wt
I & O	H & H	K^+
BP	BUN	Prealbumin
PT	Alk phos	RBP
Alb	Phosphorus	

Patient Education

1. Ambulation, when possible, will help promote healing and increase strength.
2. Have the patient eat small, frequent meals if nausea is a problem.

NOTES

TONSILLECTOMY AND ADENOIDECTOMY

Usual Hospital Stay

1.5 days.

Objectives

1. Supply adequate nourishment for glycogen stores preoperatively.
2. Postoperatively provide cold liquids that will not produce discomfort and progress to nonirritating foods.
3. Prevent or correct vomiting and nausea.

Dietary Recommendations

1. Postoperatively, give cold liquids (sherbet, ginger ale, nectars, and gelatin). Avoid milk products only if the patient cannot tolerate them. On the second or third day, use soft, smooth foods (pudding, strained cereals, soft cooked eggs).
2. Progress to regular diet as tolerated. A soft diet may be preferred for a few more days.
3. Use supplements of vitamin C if patient cannot tolerate juices.
4. Use adequate fluid intake (adults 3 L, children 2L, for example).

Profile

Ht	Wt
IBW/HBW	H & H
Gluc	Alb
K$^+$	BP
I & O	

Patient Education

1. Help the patient select nonirritating foods for use at home. Avoidance of hot, spicy foods; raw vegetables; toast and crackers; citrus juices; and other related foods until full recovery will be recommended.

446

2. Straws should not be used, temporarily.
3. Taking large swallows of water causes less pain than small swallows.
4. The patient should remain on cool liquids until pain subsides.
5. Some doctors recommend avoidance of red gelatin in case of hemorrhage.

Section 15
Hypermetabolic, Infectious, Traumatic, and Febrile Conditions

Chief Assessment Factors

recent illnesses, surgery

presence of chronic diseases

medications (prescription and OTC)

anemia, anorexia, malnutrition

fever

accidents, other trauma

metabolic rate

edema

infectious processes, sepsis

multiple organ involvement

Table 15–1.

Nutritional and Host Factors in Immunity*

INFECTIOUS DISEASE DETERMINANTS
Host immunity, including nutritional status
Microorganismic virulence
Environmental sanitation
Personal hygiene

HOST-RESISTANCE FACTORS
1. Physical barriers (skin, mucous membranes)
2. Mucus and cilia on epithelial surfaces
3. Phagocytes (leukocytes, macrophages)
4. Complement system
5. Immunoglobulins and antibodies (B cells) from bone marrow
6. Cell-mediated immunity (T cells) from thymus

GROUPS AT GREATEST RISK FOR INFECTIOUS ILLNESSES
Infants
Elderly patients
Malnourished and hospitalized persons

KEY NUTRIENTS IN IMMUNOCOMPETENCE
1. Vitamin A/beta-carotene
2. B-complex, especially, vitamin B_6 and folacin
3. Vitamin C
4. Vitamin E and selenium
5. Iron and zinc (beware of excesses, especially IM or IV)
6. Copper
7. Iodine
8. EFAs are needed, but beware of excess PUFA and obesity

IMMUNE SYSTEM
Bone marrow
Spleen
Lymph nodes
Thymus
Tonsils
Lymphoid tissue (Peyer's patches in gut; Luster patches in bronchioles)

---

* Adapted from Chandra, R.K.: *Nutrition and Immunity—Basic Considerations Contemp. Nut.* 11:11, 1986. Minneapolis, MN: General Mills Co.

Assessment of immunocompetence by currently available methods . . . can identify individuals who are most in need of appropriate nutritional support and thus provide crucial prognostic information in terms of risk of disease, duration of hospitalization and chances of survival.
—Puri, S. and Chandra, R.K.: Nutrition and immunity. *Pediatr. Clin. North Am., 32:*493, 1985.

NOTES

AIDS AND HIV INFECTION

Usual Hospital Stay

4–5 days.

Notation

Acquired Immune Deficiency Syndrome (AIDS) is a viral infection caused by the HIV* virus. A diverse array of problems result, with opportunistic infections (e.g., 60% have *Pneumocystis carinii* pneumonia (PCP); many others develop Kaposi's sarcoma). Persons at risk include homosexual and bisexual males, hemophiliacs, IV drug addicts, Haitian immigrants, and heterosexuals with multiple partners. BF infants of HIV$^+$ mothers are also at risk.

Symptoms and signs include fever, chills, sore throat, headache, tachypnea, anxiety, fatigue, night sweats, hypoxemia, dyspnea on exertion, rales or ronchi, cyanosis, pneumonia, diarrhea, cryptcoccosis, several viral infections, ulcerating herpes simplex lesions, meningitis, anorexia, inflamed mouth or esophagus, malabsorption, weight loss and poor nutritional status. HIV infection involves multiple organs.

Objectives

1. Prevent additional weight loss from fever, infection, nausea and vomiting. Lean body mass is especially affected.
2. Reduce mealtime fatigue to encourage better intake.
3. Prevent further opportunistic infections, such as oral candidiasis, by strengthening immunity.
4. Where needed, support mechanical ventilation; wean where possible.
5. Lower temperature to normal, when febrile.
6. Correct and treat diarrhea, malabsorption, vomiting, HIV-induced enteropathy.
7. If necessary, hyperaliment to prevent further immunodeficiency.
8. Correct any fluid and electrolyte imbalances.
9. In a child, prevent feeding regression and growth delay.

---

* Human Immunodeficiency Virus (formerly called HTLV-III)

10. Support depleted levels of such nutrients as linolenic acid, selenium, and vitamin B_{12}.
11. Counteract such problems as dysphagia and difficulty in chewing.
12. Alleviate nutritional impact of fatigue, depression, and dyspnea.

Dietary Recommendations

1. Maintain diet as appropriate for condition (e.g., high calorie/high protein diet with adequate nutritional supplementation). Use tube feeding or TPN if warranted by status. Low lactose/low fat TF products may be needed. 1–2 g protein/kg and 35–45 kcal/kg may be useful.
2. Provide adequate fluid and potassium when needed. Increase use of fatty fish for omega-3 fatty acids.
3. Small, frequent feedings are usually better tolerated.
4. In some cases, lactose or gluten are not tolerated. Reduce intake if necessary, but avoid further anorexia where possible by offering some preferred foods and beverages. Sucrose, fat, and d-xylose may also need to be limited.
5. A general multivitamin/mineral supplement may be needed. The diet and supplements should provide adequate vitamins C, B_{12}, copper, selenium, vitamin A, zinc, B-complex, etc.* 2–5 × RDA of all except fat-soluble vitamins may be useful.
6. Nutrient-dense snacks may be beneficial (i.e., ice cream or pudding if tolerated; nonacidic juices for sore mouth; ices made with tolerated juices; sandwiches made with cold meat salads, etc.).
7. In a child, 50–100% above RDA for protein may be necessary (Bentler & Stanish: *JADA* April 1987).

Profile

Ht	Wt	H & H
Pre-illness wt	Wt changes	Platelets
Alb, RBP,	TLC (CD_4 lymphocyte)	Creat
Prealbumin	BP	Transferrin
Gluc	I & O	Diarrhea; stool tests
Temp	ELISA test for Aids	CBC
Liver function tests	IBW	

Side Effects of Common Drugs Used

1. *Antineoplastic agents* (Adriamycin, bleomycin, vincristine) or *interferon*—for Karposi's sarcoma. Numerous side effects occur, including nausea, vomiting, diarrhea, anorexia, stomatitis, and weight loss.
2. *Analgesics*—over time, aspirin may aggravate anemias.

---

* See immune system information, Table 15.1.

3. *Antibiotics*—side effects are specific to the drug used.
4. *Azidothymidine/zidovudine* (AZT)—this anti-infective agent can cause severe bone marrow depletion and anemia. It works better in sequence with acyclovir. Adequate folate and B_{12} may prevent toxicity.
5. *Acyclovir* (zovirax) may cause headache, nausea, anorexia, sore throat, and diarrhea.
6. *Ribavirin* (virazole)—may cause dyspnea and anemia.
7. *Steroids*—sodium retention; potassium, calcium and vitamin C depletion can occur; and protein malnutrition can occur with extended use. Glucose intolerance may also result.
8. *Trimethoprim-sulfamethoxazole* (Bactrim, Septra) may be used for the PCP for about 1 month. The drug may cause hepatitis, azotemia, anorexia, stomatitis, thrombocytopenia. It should be carefully monitored. Folate may be needed.
9. *Antifungals* (amphotericin-B, clotrimazole) may cause nausea, vomiting, diarrhea, and GI distress.

Patient Education

1. Exceptional hand-washing techniques should be used by all caregivers and by the patient.
2. The importance of maintaining a balanced, nutritious diet should be addressed.
3. The diet must be altered whenever necessary; continuing contact with a nutritionist is essential.
4. The role of nutrition in infection and immunity should be discussed.
5. The patient and caregivers should report all weight loss, anorexia and fever to the doctor.
6. Adequate education should address the gradual and likely decline in self-care abilities, as well as alternative therapies and consequences.
7. In home care, TPN may be used. Adequate and continuing education should be offered to caregivers to prevent transmission of the disease and to reduce further likelihood of infection.
8. BF mothers who are HIV positive may want to use formula instead.

Comments

Beware of excesses of iron or zinc, vitamin E and PUFA because of their effects on immunity when taken in large doses. Parenteral iron is not appropriate in cachexic patients, or in sepsis, except in careful consideration by the physician. TPN is contraindicated with sepsis.

For More Information

AIDS Hotline: (800) 342-2437
AIDS Information Hotline, National Gay Task Force: (800) 221-7044

ASCARIASIS

Usual Hospital Stay

4–5 days.

Notation

Intestinal roundworms are the most common intestinal helminth, and are usually found in warm or humid climates, or where personal hygiene is inadequate. Adult worms live in the small intestine, with eggs that pass out in human feces. These eggs become infective within 2–3 weeks. When ingested by humans through fecally contaminated food or water, the eggs hatch and penetrate the intestines. Eventually they reach the heart. Larvae mature within 2–3 months, and adult worms may live for a year or longer. Hemorrhage can occur in lung tissue and cause pneumonitis. Vague abdominal discomfort can occur with SI involvement.

Objectives

1. Prevent or correct protein malnutrition.
2. Prevent blockage, inflammation, volvulus, and bowel perforation.
3. Differentiate symptoms from other disorders.
4. Prevent further complications.

Dietary Recommendations

1. Increase protein if patient is malnourished.
2. Increase or ensure adequate calorie intake.
3. Provide balanced intake of all vitamins and minerals.

Profile

Ht, Wt	IBW/HBW	Stool Exam
ALb	Transferrin	Gluc
H & H	TLC, WBCs	Serum iron
		TIBC

Side Effects of Drugs Commonly Used

Pyrantel pamoate (Povan)—rarely, vomiting or diarrhea may occur.

Patient Education

Discuss the importance of personal hygiene in maintaining a sanitary environment and in preventing reinfestation.

BACTERIAL ENDOCARDITIS

Usual Hospital Stay

Subacute 4–5 days; acute, 18 days.

Notation

Bacterial endocarditis is a bacterial infection of the membrane lining the heart chambers. Symptoms and signs include fever, chills, joint pains, lassitude, and malaise. Acute forms have rapid onset; subacute form begins slowly. Anorexia and weight loss are common side effects.

Most afflicted persons have had a previous heart condition, such as rheumatic fever. Bacterial endocarditis accounts for 2% of all cases of organic heart diseases.

Objectives

1. Restore patient's nutritional status to normal.
2. Replenish electrolytes and fluids.
3. Reduce edema if present.
4. Prevent heart failure, infections, flu, anemia, embolism, and nephritis.

Dietary Recommendations

1. Use a high calorie diet. The patient's need to replenish the stores of protein may require a high protein diet.
2. Ensure intake of an adequate amount of fluids, especially fruit juices.
3. If the patient's appetite is poor, encourage intake of favorite foods.

Profile

Ht	Wt	WBCs, TLC
IBW/HBW	Alb	Temp
H & H	K^+, Na^+	I & O
BP	Edema	

Side Effects of Common Drugs Used

Check specific *antibiotics* for appropriate timing of meals and drugs. Penicillin, erythromycin, and other combinations may be used.

Patient Education

1. Indicate which foods are sources of protein and calories in the diet.
2. Dental care may require special attention. Abscesses should be treated immediately.

BURNS (THERMAL INJURY)

Usual Hospital Stay

3 days, nonsurgical extensive; 17 days nonextensive with skin graft.

Notation

Burns may be caused by electrical, thermal, or radioactive agents. With a first degree burn, simple redness of the epidermis occurs. In a second degree burn, redness and blistering occur. In a third degree burn, skin and tissue destruction occurs. Total burn thickness seems to affect BEE more than body surface area (BSA). Burns are the third leading cause of accidental death in the U.S.

Loss of 1 g of nitrogen is equivalent to a 30 g loss of LBM. Nitrogen balance becomes a matter of life and death in a major body burn. Survival depends on effective nutritional support (10% wt. loss is acceptable; 40–50% can lead to mortality). The GI tract becomes nonfunctional in a 40–50% TBSA burn; use of parenteral support may be needed.

Objectives

1. Relieve pain and conserve heat (to decrease hypermetabolism).
2. Restore fluid and electrolyte balance to prevent shock. Beware of exudate losses, which may be 20–25% total daily nitrogen losses.
3. Prevent renal shutdown from decreased plasma volume, decreased cardiac output and excessive pigment overload (from necrosis, toxins, and hemolysis). Correct SIADH, hypertonic dehydration and overhydration.
4. Minimize catabolism of protein tissues to avoid consequences of protein-calorie malnutrition (impaired immunity, decreased wound healing, decreased vigor and muscle strength, retarded synthesis of blood proteins and hemoglobin, increased likelihood of infection). Patients with burns have an elevated basal metabolism rate 1.5–2 times the normal rate.
5. Promote wound healing and graft retention.
6. Avoid weight losses greater than 10% preburn weight (if that weight corresponds to the patient's IBW).
7. Eventually balance the patient's stores of nitrogen.
8. Correct stress hyperglycemia and overfeeding.
9. Reduce evaporative water losses, especially with occlusive wound dressings.
10. Restore the skin's protection to reduce infection. Sepsis is a major cause of mortality, often 2–3 weeks postinjury.

Dietary Recommendations

1. *Immediately* use IV fluids to prevent gastric distention and paralytic ileus. Gastrostomy TF may also be possible. Prevent overhydration.

2. Gradually use a high calorie, high protein diet with 5–6 small meals and snacks. Protein intake should be 1.5–3 g/kg IBW each 24 hours. Caloric intake should be 40–60 kcal/kg each 24 hours. It is not uncommon to need 4000–5000 kcal. Use 25% protein, 50% CHO, 25% fat (1–2% EFAs). CHO may be given as 5 mg/kg/min. Enteral or parenteral N:calorie ratio would be 1:80–100 in adults; 1:130–150 in children.

3. Tube feed patient if needed. Use Precision HN, Trauma-Cal, or similar products. Increased use of BCAAs has not been proven conclusively to be beneficial in burn patients.

4. Provide adequate fluid intake: encourage intake of fruit juices (cranberry, grapefruit, prune, or orange juice) for adequate supplies of potassium. Water losses may be 10–12× normal in the first few weeks.

5. Supplement the diet with 5–10× RDA of vitamin C; zinc sulfate (2× RDA); ferrous sulfate; and two to three times the RDA for the vitamin B-complex. 2× RDA for vitamins A and D may be useful at first. Vitamins K and B_{12} should be given at least weekly. Be careful about iron and zinc in patients with sepsis.

6. In *children,* vitamins should be given at 5–10× RDAs for a few days, then 2–3× RDAs until recovery. PN levels should be 4 g AAs/kg/day or .52 g N/kg/day; fat at 4–6 g/kg daily.

7. Special snacks may include peanut butter cookies, brownies, cake, shakes, pasteurized eggs in milkshakes or eggnog, protein in broths, and dextrins added to coffee. See "Tips for Adding Protein and Calories to the Diet." 5–6 small meals may be tolerated best.

8. Provide adequate copper (for collagen cross-linkage). Arginine up to 2% of kcal and carnitine may also be beneficial.

9. Add fish often for omega-3 fatty acids (salmon, etc.).

Profile

Ht, wt
Pre-burn IBW/HBW
I & O
BUN
Cl^-
K^+
Urinary N
Urinary creatinine
3-methyl histidine
BEE/REE
Daily wt (beware heavy exudates, edema)

Prealbumin (dec.)
Na^+ ($\downarrow$)
Transferrin
Ca^{++}, Mg^{++}
N balance (amount excreted in g × 6.25 = g protein)
Edema
P_{CO_2}, P_{O_2}
Chol, trig
WBCs, TLC
Temp

Serum catecholamines (inc.)
Urine acetone, sugars
Ceruloplasmin
PO_4
H & H
Alb, RBP
Gluc (inc.)
SGOT (inc.)

Side Effects of Common Drugs Used

1. *Silver nitrate dressings.* Beware of nutrient leaching of sodium, copper, potassium, magnesium, calcium, and B-complex. The patient may need added salt or supplements of potassium and calcium in the diet.
2. *Antacids* are used to prevent Curling's ulcer. *Cimetidine* is also useful. Beware of intestinal obstruction.
3. *Pain medications* may have some effect on GI function and appetite.
4. *Insulin* is used for stress-induced hyperglycemia.

Patient Education

1. Explain the hazards of long-term immobilization: renal calculi, pneumonia, contractures, and decubitus ulcers. Have the patient carefully increase exercise as pain tolerance allows.
2. Stress the importance of fat intake. Fat is high in calories with low volume, and is helpful in normalizing elimination.
3. Explain that adequate intake of fiber is important.
4. The family's attitude toward the patient's dietary intake should be firm but also patient and understanding.
5. A daily kcal intake record is the best way to achieve goals, and to assess intake.
6. Discuss problems to monitor (fever, drainage, etc.).
7. Offer a written care plan for home use.

Comments

Procedures

1. Take a dietary history of the patient's food preferences, allergies, and dislikes.
2. Calculate the percentage of the body that has been burned: head and neck, 9%; each arm, 9%; anterior trunk, 18%; posterior trunk, 18%; each leg, 18%; and perineum, 1%.
3. Assist in feeding the patient and help determine the proper feeding method to use.
4. Avoid painful procedures before the patient's mealtime. Do not interrupt mealtime for laboratory tests.
5. Plan meals to best utilize the protein:calorie ratio (a 1:150 ratio is optimal).
6. Discourage consumption of empty calorie foods or beverages. Medications can be taken with supplements, milk, or juice.
7. Be careful to avoid excesses of linoleic acid, which can depress immunocompetence.
8. Anticipate 2–3 months total for optimal recovery time.
9. In *children,* aggressive nutritional support can improve survival. Weight maintenance is not enough; gain must occur.

Table 15–2.

Common Methods for Calculating Calorie Needs in Burn Patients

1. Curreri's Equation: $[(25 \times \text{wt in kg}) + (40 \times \%\text{TBS burned})]$—may be high
2. BEE $\times$ 1.5—2
3. Indirect Calorimetry: more accurate for individual patients (take RQ twice weekly)
4. 40–60 kcal/kg BW

Table 15–3.

Modular Tube Feeding for Burn Patients*

Polycose (Ross Lab)	533 gms (70 kg adult)	or 114 gms (15 kg child)
Whole egg powder (American Egg Board, Park Ridge, Ill)	144 gms	79 gms
Egg white solids	135 gms	0 gms
Corn oil	0 ml	106 ml
Total kcal	3277 kcal	1753 kcal

* Adapted from Bell, S., et al.: Prediction of total urinary nitrogen from urea nitrogen for burned patients. *JADA* 85:1100, 1985.

NOTES

CANDIDIASIS

Usual Hospital Stay

4–5 days.

Notation

Candida albicans is found in mouth, feces and vagina normally. A greater colonization occurs in debilitated persons, where thrush or vaginitis or cutaneous lesions are common. Persons who are susceptible include patients with hematological malignancy, immunosuppressed patients, postoperative patients, people receiving antibiotic therapy, and people who are obese or have diabetes.

Objectives

1. Prevent or treat systemic infections.
2. Prevent endocarditis, emboli, splenomegaly and other complications.
3. Correct underlying conditions, where possible.

Dietary Recommendations

1. Ensure intake that is balanced for all nutrients, high in quality proteins and adequate in calories.
2. Adequate fluid intake is beneficial.
3. Some research suggests use of yogurt in the diet; no conclusions are evident.

Profile

Ht, wt	Gluc	Transferrin
Wt changes	Underlying conditions	TLC, WBCs
Lesions, symptoms	Alb	H & H
IBW/HBW		

Side Effects of Drugs Commonly Used

1. *Nystatin* or *amphotericin B* may be used to correct the condition. Diarrhea, nausea, stomach pain may occur.
2. Extended use of *antibiotics* may have caused or aggravated the condition.

Patient Education

1. For patients with malignant disease, a discussion about the importance of nutrition in maintaining good health status would be essential.
2. In general, patients who are debilitated will need to understand that meals should be consumed regularly, with smaller and frequent meals and snacks used if large meals are not tolerated. Fasting and skipping of meals should be avoided.

NOTES

ENCEPHALITIS AND REYE'S DISEASE

Usual Hospital Stay

5 days.

Notation

Encephalitis involves an inflammation of brain cells, usually by a virus, such as measles, mumps, mononucleosis or herpes simplex. It may also be caused by the tsetse fly (African sleeping sickness).

Reye's syndrome is a disease of the brain and some abdominal organs (liver, for example), affecting mostly children and teenagers following viral illness. The etiology is unknown, but some linkage to aspirin has been suggested. Symptoms are similar to those of encephalitis.

Symptoms and signs include headache, loss of energy, anorexia, irritability, restlessness, drowsiness, double vision, impaired speech and hearing, possibly even seizures or coma.

Objectives

1. Ease symptoms.
2. Allow natural defense system to work.
3. Assist breathing with respirator if necessary.
4. Control any pernicious vomiting.

Dietary Recommendations

1. NG tube feeding may be needed if patient is comatose.
2. When patient can eat again, a high protein/high calorie diet should be provided, including vitamins and minerals in adequate amounts.
3. Adequate fluid intake will be important.

Profile

Ht, wt	IBW/HBW	EEG
CSF	Na^+, K^+	BP
TLC, WBCs	Fever, Temp	I & O
LDH, CPK (inc.)	Gluc (dec.)	BUN, UA (inc.)
Ammonia (inc.)	SGOT, SGPT (inc.)	Creat

Side Effects of Drugs Commonly Used

Steroids are commonly provided. Long-term use may affect nitrogen balance or cause hyperglycemia. Sodium retention and potassium depletion can also occur. After the diet as necessary.

Patient Education

1. Stress the importance of consuming a balanced diet with adequate fluids.
2. Help patient accept speech therapy or physical therapy if needed.
3. Discuss infection control measures in the environment; use of aspirin, etc.

CHRONIC FATIGUE SYNDROME, (EPSTEIN-BARR VIRUS SYNDROME)

Usual Hospital Stay

4–5 days.

Notation

Chronic fatigue syndrome (CFS), also called the CEBV syndrome, involves severe exhaustion and weakness, headaches, fever, muscle aches, inability to concentrate, and depression. The etiology is unknown, but studies suggest a chronic mononucleosis caused by a herpes virus (perhaps the one known as human B-lymphotrophic virus).

CFS is a vague illness and the symptoms tend to mimic depression, lupus or even cancer. A thorough physical examination is suggested. Research is inconclusive regarding this syndrome; some physicians doubt its existence. A Harvard University study suggests a link to Hodgkin's disease 4 years after diagnosis.

Objectives

1. Improve immunological status; prevent malnutrition.
2. Prevent recurrent attacks, if possible.
3. Lessen severity of attacks.
4. Prevent additional infections and stress.

Dietary Recommendations

1. Adequate protein should be consumed (0.8–1 gm/kg); 35 kcal/kg may be needed.
2. Adequate vitamin and mineral intake should be assured.

Profile

Ht, wt	Antibodies to	TLC, WBCs
EBV levels	measles, herpes	Gluc
Alb	simplex,	Transferrin
H & H	cytomegalovirus	Serum iron
IBW/HBW	Wt changes	TIBC

Patient Education

1. Discuss the importance of maintaining adequate nutritional intake to optimize immunological status.
2. Referral for counseling may be beneficial for some patients.

NOTES

FEVER

Usual Hospital Stay

5–6 days; fever of unknown origin.

Notation

Pyrexia may be acute (with pneumonia, measles, flu or chicken pox) or chronic (with tuberculosis, hepatitis, malaria, etc.). Fever represents disturbed thermoregulation, controlled by the hypothalamus. Fever of unknown origin (FUO) involves illness of 3 weeks duration with a fever over 100.4% F. Testing is needed. FUO is 40% infectious, 20% neoplastic, 15% connective tissue disease, and 25% from undetermined causes.

Objectives

1. Meet increased nutrient needs caused by the patient's hypermetabolic state, calorie needs especially. Each 1°F elevation causes 7% increase in BMR. This equals 12% rise in BEE per 1°C fever above 37°C.
2. Replace nitrogen losses and destroyed tissue.
3. Replenish carbohydrate stores. Normalize electrolyte status.
4. Replace losses from perspiration and facilitate toxin elimination through increased urine output.
5. Prevent water retention from SIADH and hypertonic dehydration.
6. Correct anorexia, nausea, and vomiting where present.

Dietary Recommendations

1. Adults need 30–40 kcal/kg daily, or an estimated 500–600 added kcal per 1°F rise. Infants need an additional 200 kcal/kg and children 100–150 kcal/kg per 1°F rise.

2. Adults need 1.5–2.5 g protein/kg if severe.
3. Adults need adequate carbohydrate to spare protein and restore glycogen in the liver. Ideal N:calorie ratio would be 1:150 with activity.
4. Adults need 10–15 cups fluid per day. Salty broths, fruit juices, and milk can be used.
5. If the fever is acute, the patient may need full liquids. As treatment progresses, a soft to general diet with small, frequent feedings can be used.
6. With longer duration, thiamine and other nutrients should be added.

Profile

Ht	K^+	Temp
IBW/HBW	BP	Na^+
N balance	Wt	Cl^-
I & O	3-methyl histidine	Specific gravity,
TLC, WBCs	Carotenoids ($\downarrow$)	urine ($\uparrow$)
		Alb, RBP

Side Effects of Common Drugs Used

1. *Penicillins* should not be taken with acidic food or fluids such as fruit juice. Penicillin combines with serum albumins; adequate protein repletion is needed.
2. *Erythromycin* should be taken with a full glass of water on an empty stomach. It may cause sore mouth, diarrhea, and nausea.
3. *Tetracycline* should be taken on an empty stomach with a full glass of water. Do *not* give with milk or 2 hours before or after use of calcium-containing foods. Do not use with children as tetracycline can mottle teeth. Be careful with pregnant patients as well.
4. *Anti-pyretics/aspirin* can cause GI distress. Take with food or milk. Avoid alcoholic beverages. Monitor use of aspirin in light of Reye's syndrome.
5. Other medications may require special instructions according to the patient's problem.

Patient Education

1. "*Feed* a cold, *feed* a fever." Discuss how fever affects BMR.
2. Stress the importance of fluid intake.

NOTES

FRACTURE, HIP

Usual Hospital Stay

Surgical, 13 days; medical, 7 days.

Notation

"Broken hip" includes fractures of the femur head (intracapsular), femur neck (extracapsular), and greater Hesser trochanter. Hip fracture is actually more common in populations where intakes of dairy products and calcium are relatively high. *Pathological* fractures involve weakened bones breaking from old age, osteoporosis, and bone cancer. Incidence increases after age 60, especially in women.

Fatigue fractures occur from prolonged stress on normal bones.

Objectives

1. Support formation of the bone matrix. Complete union may take 4–8 months.
2. Supply adequate nutrition for collagen formation and calcium deposition.
3. Prevent side effects of long-term immobilization: renal calculi, decubitus, urinary tract infections, embolus, contractures.
4. In the case of *open reduction with internal fixation,* adequate nutrition is necessary for wound healing and to reduce infectious processes.
5. Maintain optimal systemic functioning.

Dietary Recommendations

1. Use a high protein, high calorie diet. Needs increase by 20–25%.
2. Use adequate levels of calcium, phosphorus, vitamin D, and vitamin C. Encourage these nutrients to be taken in the diet. Be careful of excessive vitamin D, or excessive calcium intake during immobilization. Reduce excessive meat intakes.
3. Ensure adequate fluid intake to excrete calcium excesses.
4. Supply zinc for wound healing after surgical procedures. Watch for fever, pneumonia, and possible embolism.

Profile

Ht	Wt (if possible)	N balance
IBW/HBW	Ca^{++} (serum,	Alb
P, Alk phos (inc.)	urinary)	Gluc
BUN, creat	H & H	WBCs, TLC
I & O	Serum Fe	TIBC

Patient Education

1. Emphasize the importance of nutrition for healing. Indicate which foods are good sources of protein in the diet.
2. Encourage activity and use of physical therapy, once healing has progressed.
3. Refer to appropriate agencies, such as VNA or Meals-on-Wheels, as needed.

Comments

Table 15–4.
Broken Bones—Most Common
1. Forearm (ulna, radius)
2. Hands and feet (carpals, metacarpals, tarsals and metatarsals)
3. Ribs
4. Fingers and thumbs (phalanges)
5. Shin bones (tibia, fibula)
6. Thigh bones (femur)
7. Skull
8. Upper arm (humerus)
9. Collarbone (clavicle)
10. Backbone (spinal bones or vertebrae).

Broken bones result from a physical force greater than stress that can be withstood. Simple fractures involve bones that do not protrude. A compound fracture does allow the bone to protrude. With multiple fractures, BMR may increase by 20% or more for several weeks.

NOTES

FRACTURE, LONG-BONE

Usual Hospital Stay

8–9 days.

Notation

A fracture of this nature is generally an emergency and may be complicated by shock, wound infection, bleeding, or inadequate hydration. Decubiti, calculi, nausea and vomiting from spinal anesthesia may be complicating factors. Traction is generally needed for internal immobilization.

Objectives

1. Meet calorie needs, usually increased by 25%.
2. Provide adequate intake of all vitamins and minerals and nutrients needed to heal the fracture appropriately.
3. Keep nearby joints as active as possible.
4. Prevent complications.

Dietary Recommendations

1. High protein/high calorie intake will be needed.
2. Vitamin D, calcium, phosphorus and vitamin C are especially important for bone formation. Avoid excessive calcium during immobilized period.
3. Zinc will help with wound healing, especially with surgery. Vitamin A is also essential.
4. Progress from liquids to a soft diet as possible.

Profile

Ht, wt	IBW/HBW	TLC
Alb	N balance	Alk phos (elevated)
BUN, Creat	Temp	WBCs
PT	Gluc	H & H
P (elevated)	Ca^{++}	Serum Fe, TIBC

Side Effects of Drugs Commonly Used

Analgesics are used for pain relief. Be careful about GI irritation or depletion of vitamin C and iron levels. *Meperidine* (Demerol) may cause vomiting, nausea, and constipation.

Patient Education

1. The importance of balanced nutrition during healing should be emphasized.
2. Key nutrients and their food sources should be highlighted.
3. Discuss the benefits of activity or physical therapy.

NOTES

HERPES SIMPLEX I AND II

Usual Hospital Stay

Varies with complications.

Notation

Herpes simplex involves a viral infection of skin or mucous membranes (I usually involves oral infections, II usually involves genital/anal infections) with vesicular eruptions of repeated frequency. Oral lesions may be commonly called "cold sores" or "fever blisters" because of their recurrence with periods of stress; they are latent in the nerve cell ganglia of the trigeminal nerve. Herpetic outbreaks are common in HIV-positive patients.

Objectives

1. Reduce inflammation and duration.
2. Lessen recurrences and virulence.
3. Prevent spread or contact to other parts of the body, or to other persons.
4. Reduce stress and febrile states.
5. Prevent further complications, such as encephalitis and aseptic meningitis.

Dietary Recommendations

1. High quality protein/adequate calories will be essential.
2. Some studies suggest that lysine may be important in lessening virulence. Research is not yet conclusive. An adequate diet contains approximately 5–8 g lysine daily.

3. Be aware that lysine supplementation can alter lysine:arginine ratio, which may cause elevated serum cholesterol levels.

Profile

Ht, wt	IBW/HBW	WBC, TLC
Alb	Gluc	I & O
Swollen lymph	Temp	Chol
nodes	H & H	

Side Effects of Drugs Commonly Used

1. *Acyclovir* (Zovirax) has been used with some success (*JAMA 116:672*, 1980).
2. *Aspirin* or *acetaminophen* have been used for fever reduction.
3. *L-lysine monohydrochloride* (1 g daily for 6 months) is used by some physicians. Monitor effects on serum cholesterol.
4. *Interferon* studies are being conducted in some research centers.

Patient Education

1. A well-balanced diet with quality proteins should be discussed. Milk is a food that is naturally high in lysine.
2. Discuss the relationship of nutrition to the immune status.
3. Relaxation and stress reduction techniques should be highlighted.

NOTES

HERPES ZOSTER (SHINGLES)

Usual Hospital Stay

6 days.

Notation

Herpes zoster is an acute viral infection with crops of vesicles, usually confined to a specific nerve tract, with neuralgic pain in the area of the affected nerve. It may be a response to the varicella virus and severity correlates with age. In children, the condition is usually chicken pox or varicella.

Symptoms and signs include pain along the affected nerve tract, fever, malaise, anorexia, enlarged lymph nodes, bacterial infection of the lesions, poor nutritional status, dehydration if prolonged time elapses.

Objectives

1. Prevent further systemic infection; reduce fever.
2. Correct or prevent malnutrition, constipation, and encephalitis.
3. Hydrate adequately.
4. Prevent or correct unplanned weight loss.

Dietary Recommendations

1. A balanced diet with frequent, small feedings may be needed.
2. Increased fiber may be useful to correct constipation.
3. Facial nerves may be affected; alter diet as needed.
4. Adequate vitamin E has been suggested for postzoster neuralgia. Research will be necessary to confirm this finding.

Profile

Ht, wt	IBW/HBW	H & H
Alb	TLC, WBCs	Temp
I & O	Na^+, K^+	Gluc

Side Effects of Drugs Commonly Used

1. *Narcotics* and *analgesics* may be needed to reduce pain.
2. *Prednisone* may be used in some cases; alter sodium intake as necessary. Use is generally not for an extended period of time, but monitor for side effects, such as glucose intolerance.

Patient Education

1. Discuss the need to increase fluid intake.
2. A balanced diet will be essential in recovery.
3. Infectious precautions should be discussed with the patient and family.

NOTES

INFECTION

Usual Hospital Stay

Varies by cause and extent of infection.

Notation

Infection results from the successful invasion, establishment, and growth of microorganisms in a host.

Responses involve general and antigen-specific immunological defense systems.

Objectives

1. Provide adequate nourishment to counteract the patient's hypermetabolic state. Support the body's host defense system.
2. Prevent or correct dehydration, hypoglycemia, complications, anorexia.
3. Replace nutrient losses (potassium, nitrogen, magnesium, phosphorus, zinc, and sulfur).

Dietary Recommendations

1. Use a high protein, high calorie diet. Needs increase 0–20% in mild infections, 20–40% in moderate conditions, 40–60% in sepsis.
2. Increase the patient's fluid intake.
3. Supplement diet with vitamin A, folate, vitamin C and B-complex.
4. Be careful with the use of iron and zinc supplements, as these may serve as nutrients for bacteria. It may be helpful to wait before providing these supplements, especially IV, IM or by TPN.

Profile

Ht	H & H	3-methyl His
IBW/HBW	N balance	Ceruloplasmin (dec.)
Temp	TLC, WBCs	I & O
BUN, Creat	Gluc	Serum zinc
Wt	BP	SGOT ($\uparrow$ in acute
Alb	K^+, Na^+	stages)

Side Effects of Common Drugs Used

1. *Antibiotics.* Administration of antibiotics with or without food is specific to the type of drug used. Avoid caffeine, soda pop and fruit juice when taking *penicillins.* For *tetracycline,* avoid milk and dairy products 2 hours before and after taking the drug. With amoxicillin (*Augmentin*), diarrhea, nausea, and vomiting may occur.

2. *Griseofulvin* for fungal infections should be taken with a high fat meal. Dry mouth, nausea, and diarrhea are common effects.
3. *Cephalosporins* (Ceclor, Duricef) may cause diarrhea, nausea, vomiting, and sore mouth.

Patient Education

1. Emphasize the importance of eating to counteract infection and prevent new infections.
2. Discuss the role of vitamins A, C, and B_6, niacin and riboflavin in maintaining skin and mucous membrane integrity to prevent bacterial invasion and subsequent infections.

NOTES

INFECTIOUS MONONUCLEOSIS

Usual Hospital Stay

4–5 days.

Notation

Infectious mononucleosis is an acute infectious disease, believed to be due to Epstein-Barr (EB) herpes virus, causing gland swellings in the neck and elsewhere (giving it its other name, "glandular fever") with fatigue, malaise, headache, chills, and sometimes one or more other symptoms such as sore throat, fever, abdominal pain, jaundice, stiff neck, chest pain, breathing difficulty, cough, and hepatitis. Incubation is 5–15 days. It is most common between ages 10 and 35.

Objectives

1. Restore fluid balance.
2. Replenish glucose stores. Spare protein.
3. Restore lost weight.
4. Reduce fever. Prevent complications such as myocarditis, hepatitis, encephalitis.

Dietary Recommendations

1. Use a high protein, high calorie diet.
2. Use liquids when swallowing of solid foods is difficult.
3. Use small, frequent feedings to improve overall nutritional quality and quantity.
4. An ideal N:calorie ratio is 1:150 with activity.

Profile

Ht	Alb	Serum agglutination
IBW/HBW	Transferrin	test
H & H	WBCs, TLC	Uric acid (inc.)
N balance	CSF pressure (inc.)	SGOT, SGPT (inc.)
Wt	EB Virus titer	

Side Effects of Drugs Commonly Used

Acyclovir (Zovirax) may be useful in initial infection, preventing the typical persistence. Nausea, anorexia, vomiting may occur.

Patient Education

1. Emphasize the importance of exercise in restoring nitrogen balance.
2. Instruct the patient to modify food textures when swallowing is difficult.
3. Discuss potential for relapse, which may be common. No specific medications are available at this time.
4. Discuss frequent snacking to increase protein and calorie intakes.

NOTES

INFLUENZA

Usual Hospital Stay

4–6 days, varying with complications.

Notation

The flu virus is transmitted by respiratory route, generally in the fall and winter months. Incubation is 1–4 days, with abrupt onset (chills, fever for 3–5 days, malaise, muscular aching, substernal soreness, nasal stuffiness, sore throat, some nausea, nonproductive cough, and headache).

Objectives

1. Reduce fever and relieve symptoms.
2. Prevent complications, such as Reye's syndrome, secondary bacterial infections (especially pneumonia), otitis media, and bronchitis.
3. Promote bed rest, adequate hydration, and calorie intake.
4. Replace fluid and electrolyte losses.

Dietary Recommendations

1. Increase fluids (e.g., salty broths, juices).
2. A high calorie/high protein intake should be encouraged. Small meals and snacks may be better tolerated than 3 large meals.
3. Adequate sodium and potassium should be considered.

Profile

Ht, wt	IBW/HBW	Wt changes
I & O	Temp	TLC
H & H	Alb	Gluc
Proteinuria	WBCs (decreased)	Na^+, K^+

Side Effects of Drugs Commonly Used

1. *Aspirin* should not be used because of the potential for Reye's syndrome in children. Other analgesics and pain relievers can be used.
2. If bacterial infections complicate the disorder, *antibiotics* may be needed.

Patient Education

1. Discuss the need for rest and adequate hydration to promote rapid recovery.
2. Discuss infection control and personal hygiene, if necessary.

NOTES

MENINGITIS

Usual Hospital Stay

7 days, viral meningitis.

Notation

Infection of the meninges causes inflammatory reactions, usually in the pia mater or arachnoid membranes. The condition may be viral or bacterial. Bacterial forms are more likely to be fatal if left untreated. Meningitis can be caused by lung or ear infections, or by a skull fracture.

Symptoms and signs include headache, nuchal rigidity, fever, tachycardia, tachypnea, nausea and/or vomiting, disorientation, diplopia, altered consciousness, photophobia, petechial rash, irritability, malaise, seizure activity, dehydration. It could lead to septic shock, respiratory failure or death.

Objectives

1. Prevent or correct weight loss.
2. Force fluids.
3. Prevent or correct constipation, fever and other symptoms.
4. Correct cerebral edema.
5. In the long term, control obesity, which can occur.

Dietary Recommendations

1. Maintain IVs as appropriate; prevent overhydration.
2. Progress diet, as possible, to high calorie/high protein intake.
3. Unless contraindicated, provide 2–3 liters of fluid.
4. Adequate fiber will be beneficial to correct or prevent constipation.
5. Gradually return to normal caloric intake for age.

Profile

Ht, wt	Prealbumin	H & H
CSF (lumbar puncture)	IBW/HBW	Temp
BP	WBCs (inc.)	Na^+, K^+
Alb, RBP	Gluc	
	I & O	

Side Effects of Drugs Commonly Used

1. *Antibiotics* may be used in bacterial forms, or to prevent complications in viral forms.
2. *Analgesics* may be used for malaise.

Patient Education

1. Discuss methods to promote recovery and emphasize adequate rest.
2. Discuss the role of nutrition in immunological status.

MULTIPLE ORGAN SYSTEMS FAILURE (MOSF)

Usual Hospital Stay

Varies by systems involved.

Notation

MOSF involves two or more systems in failure at the same time (e.g., renal, hepatic, cardiac, or respiratory). The condition always warrants hospitalization, and almost always requires ICU support.

Objectives

1. Stabilize electrolyte and hemodynamic balances. Remove/control sources of failure.
2. Promote prompt and immediate response to all changing parameters.
3. Consider the implications and short-term as well as long-term consequences of all actions (for example, treatments must incorporate a consensus of opinions about which therapy precedes another).
4. Promote recovery and well-being.
5. Prevent further complications and sepsis.
6. Promote wound healing if surgery is required.
7. Provide nutritional support in appropriate mode(s); progress from parenteral to enteral or oral as rapidly as possible to preserve the gut and to promote immune system integrity. Support organs with appropriate substrate.
8. Document all findings and recommendations immediately in order to allow appropriate actions to be initiated.

Dietary Recommendations

1. Often, parenteral therapy may be required to stabilize the patient. If PPN or TPN are prolonged, ensure daily and weekly monitoring of all essential anthropometric and laboratory parameters to assure that all nutrients (especially amino acids, glucose and vitamins) are available as necessary.
2. If and when the patient is weaned to enteral nutrition, assure that the feeding is appropriate for the site of entry (e.g., jejunostomy feedings must be more elemental than gastrostomy feedings). Evaluate affected organ systems and provide a correctly calculated feeding for the patient's diagnosis and condition. For example, a patient with hepatic and renal failure will require a carefully chosen feeding product, site of

administration and monitoring technique. Patients requiring ventilator support may need a higher lipid content in their feeding, even with cardiac failure.

3. Progress, when possible, to oral intake. Wean gradually from both PN and EN to an appropriate oral diet, considering all disorders and parameters. The dietitian should review all available diagnostic information for appropriate interpretation of actions needed.

Profile

Ht, wt, IBW/HBW	Mg^{++}, P, Ca^{++}	Chol, trig
Dry wt, edema, ascites	Gluc, acetone	GFR
	SGOT, SGPT	TLC, WBCs
BUN, creat	I & O	H & H, serum Fe,
Alb, RBP, prealbumin	Serum insulin	TIBC
Na^+, K^+, Cl^-	P_{CO_2}, P_{O_2}	PO_4

Side Effects of Drugs Commonly Used

1. All medications should be reviewed for an assessment of effects on nutritional support. Try to avoid the inclusion of medications with enteral nutrition products because of drug-nutrient interactions, and because the drugs may then be less available to the patient.
2. Review, as well, all vitamin and mineral supplements and enteral products to determine if the potential of hypervitaminosis and mineral toxicities exists. Discuss with the physician where relevant.
3. Insulin may be required, even in nondiabetics, because of the hyperglycemia that occurs with such stress.

Patient Education

1. When possible, discuss implications of the organ system failures in relationship to nutritional support. Include a realistic assessment of the potentials for recovery and use of EN in the home setting, as discussed with the physician.
2. The family should be included in discussions about the nutritional support measures that are taken.
3. As appropriate, prepare the patient for home nutritional needs, TPN/EN/oral intake as planned.
4. Alleviate fears associated with eating or nutritional support therapies.
5. Discuss any signs of problems that should require professional intervention.

Comments

Generally, lactate, pyruvate and alanine levels are higher at death than glucose levels, perhaps signifying retention/accumulation.

PELVIC INFLAMMATORY DISEASE (PID)

Usual Hospital Stay

4 days.

Notation

PID involves inflammation of the pelvic cavity, which may affect the Fallopian tubes (salpingitis) and ovaries (oophoritis).

Symptoms and signs include acute pelvic and abdominal pain, low back pain, fever, prurulent vaginal discharge, nausea and vomiting, UTIs, diarrhea, maceration of the vulva, and leukocytosis.

Objectives

1. Promote good nutritional status to maintain weight and immunity.
2. Increase hydration as tolerated.
3. Lessen diarrhea, nausea and vomiting.

Dietary Recommendations

1. Provide a diet as tolerated with small, frequent feedings until nausea and vomiting subside.
2. Alter fiber and fluid as needed for the patient's status.
3. Increase calories and protein if needed to improve patient's nutritional status.
4. Ensure adequate intake of all vitamins and minerals.

Profile

Ht, wt	IBW/HBW	H & H
Alb	TLC	WBCs
Gluc	Temp	I & O
Nausea, vomiting	Na^+, K^+	

Side Effects of Drugs Commonly Used

1. *Antibiotics* may be used. Monitor specific effects.
2. *Analgesics* are generally used to reduce pain.

Patient Education

1. Discuss the role of nutrition in immunity.
2. If nausea and vomiting are extensive, discuss the need for small meals and omission of fluids at mealtime. Have the patient consume beverages 30 minutes before or at least 1 hour after meals.

POLIOMYELITIS

Usual Hospital Stay

Varies by stage.

Notation

An epidemic virus infection, "infantile paralysis" attacks the motor neurons of the brain stem and spinal cord. It may or may not cause paralysis. It is rare in areas where vaccine is available, but is still a risk. Symptoms and signs include headache, sore throat, fever, neck and back pain.

Objectives

1. Beware of possible choking or aspiration in the bulbar type of paralysis—the patient may be unable to swallow.
2. Provide adequate nourishment.
3. Prevent complications of prolonged immobilization—renal calculi, decubitus ulcers and negative nitrogen balance.
4. Correct electrolyte imbalance.

Dietary Recommendations

1. For the patient with *acute* paralysis, use a high protein, high calorie diet in liquid form. Use IV feeding and tube feeding when needed.
2. Use vitamin supplements in 1–2 × RDAs. Potassium may be needed to replace losses.
3. As treatment progresses, the diet may be changed from a liquid to a soft, bland diet. Reduce tube feeding as oral intake increases.
4. Frequent high-nutrient-density snacks are recommended.

Profile

Ht	Wt	Temp
IBW/HBW	Alb	I & O
H & H	K^+	Na^+
Transferrin	Ca^+	P
N balance	WBC, TLC	

Patient Education

1. Instruct the patient in how to puree or blenderize foods as needed.
2. Discuss appropriate recipes for high calorie/high protein foods.
3. Extra immunization may be needed for persons traveling to tropical areas. Where polio persists, it is transmitted by personal contact, by eating contaminated food, or by drinking contaminated fluids.

RHEUMATIC FEVER (RHEUMATIC HEART DISEASE)

Usual Hospital Stay

5 days.

Notation

Rheumatic fever is a disorder affecting the connective tissues, causing pain, swelling, pyrexia, and carditis. It usually follows 3 weeks after streptococcal infection. Heart murmur may result from damaged valves. Children and adults under 30 are more susceptible.

Objectives

1. Recover lost weight.
2. Reduce fluid retention if present.
3. Prevent complications, such as endocarditis.

Dietary Recommendations

1. Use a full liquid diet for *acute* rheumatic fever.
2. As treatment progresses, gradually change the diet, first to a soft diet and then to a regular diet.
3. Restrict sodium intake if edema is present or if steroids are used.
4. Increase intake of vitamin C, protein, and calories. Include adequate vitamin A as well.

Profile

Ht	Wt	WBC, TLC
IBW/HBW	Na^+	Gluc
K^+	Edema	H & H
Temp	Alb	Serum Fe, TIBC

Side Effects of Drugs Commonly Used

1. *Antibiotics* are used.
2. Restrict sodium if *ACTH* is given.

Patient Education

1. Explain the increased need for calories and protein.
2. Adequate rest, exercise and nutrition are essential.
3. Discuss potential for recurrence.

NOTES

SEPSIS, SEPTICEMIA

Usual Hospital Stay

7–8 days.

Notation

Sepsis is an infection that has spread to other areas; if involving the bloodstream, it is called septicemia. *Septicemia* usually occurs from gram-negative or gram-positive bacteria.

Sepsis can also be a complication of TPN (bacterial or fungal). Decreased glucose tolerance is common. Other symptoms and signs include fever and catabolism of lean body mass.

Objectives

1. Remove infection or drain a local site, as possible.
2. Prevent septic shock, pulmonary edema, liver failure or encephalopathy.
3. Counteract nausea, vomiting, and anorexia.
4. Prevent or counteract TPN complications where affected—hyperglycemia, glycosuria, osmotic diarrhea, hyperosmolar/nonketotic coma, electrolyte abnormalities (dec. potassium, dec. phosphate, elevated chloride).
5. Prevent or correct fluid overload.
6. Decrease hospital stay and prevent death. Of ICU deaths 40% are from sepsis.
7. Keep environment germ-free as far as possible.
8. Meet calorie needs (mild infection elevates RMR by 15–40%; sepsis increases RMR by 40–70% and doubles nitrogen losses).
9. Prevent multiple-organ system failure (MOSF).
10. Promote tissue repair and wound healing.
11. Normalize insulin response; correct insulin resistance.
12. Prevent or correct excess CO_2 production.

Dietary Recommendations

1. Protein should be provided in levels of 1.6–2.5 g/kg daily, with up to 45% BCAAs and a higher % arginine, lower % taurine/methionine/cysteine and lower % aromatic AAs (phenylalanine, tyrosine, threonine).
2. If TPN is used with septic complications, PPN may need to be initiated or tube feeding may be less likely to promote risks.
3. Increase calories to 45 kcal/kg (approx. 350–450 g CHO daily average, and 20% kcal as fat). Check use of xylitol carefully; data is not conclusive.
4. When patient can eat, soft diet or liquids of high-caloric value and nutrient density may be beneficial.
5. MCTs and essential fatty acids may be helpful if LCTs are not tolerated.
6. Vitamins A and C, thiamine, vitamins D and K, and folic acid may become depleted with infection. Supplement or include in dietary intake. Urinary excretion of phosphorus, potassium, magnesium, zinc, and chromium also occurs; monitor signs of malnutrition.

Profile

Ht, wt	BUN, creat, UUN	Temp
I & O	Tachycardia	N balance
BP	Alb, prealbumin,	T_3 (dec.)
Chol (dec.)	RBP	Glucose (altered)
P_{O_2}, P_{CO_2}	K^+, Na^+, Cl^-	Phosphate (dec.)
WBCs, TLC	Glucagon (inc.)	Osm
Transferrin	3-methyl his	5-HIAA (inc.)
Trig (inc.)	Ca^{++}, Mg^{++}	Ketones
IBW/HBW	H & H, serum Fe	Glucagon: Insulin
SGOT ($\uparrow$)		ratio
		Plasma lactate

Side Effects of Common Drugs Used

1. *Antibiotics* are generally used. Nutrient depletion can occur.
2. *Steroids* may be used, causing greater nitrogen depletion and hyperglycemia, sodium retention and potassium losses. Monitor carefully.
3. *Insulin* may be needed.
4. *Dopamine* may be used.
5. Be careful not to give iron and zinc immediately in TPN or PPN solutions because they are both bacterial nutrients.

Patient Education

1. Aseptic techniques will be essential.
2. The need for a well-managed convalescence and gradual refeeding process will be needed to support the patient's resistance and immunity.
3. Reverse the cycle of infection/malnutrition/reinfection/further PCM.

Comment

1. BCAAs are useful for energy without the need to be metabolized to glucose first.
2. Metabolic responses in sepsis include increases in ACTH, aldosterone, catecholamines (with increased gluconeogenesis and glycolysis and proteolysis and lipolysis). Decreased T_3 may reflect the increased tissue levels that occur with tissue degradation. Increased mobilized triglycerides also occur.
3. With sepsis, leukocytic endogenous mediators (LEM) are released by phagocytes when activated; hepatic uptake of amino acids occurs, with protein synthesis; increased prostaglandin synthesis also occurs; fever occurs as well.

NOTES

TOXIC SHOCK SYNDROME

Usual Hospital Stay

4–5 days.

Notation

TSS is an acute bacterial infection caused by *Staphylococcus aureus* and is most often associated with continual use of tampons during menses.

Symptoms and signs include sudden onset of high fever, myalgia, vomiting, watery diarrhea, red rash on palms and soles (with desquamation), decreased circulation to fingers and toes, disorientation, peripheral edema, pulmonary edema, respiratory distress syndrome, and sudden hypotension progressing to shock.

Objectives

1. Treat patient for septic shock or respiratory distress, or for other complications.
2. Control diarrhea and vomiting.
3. Improve well-being.
4. Stabilize hydration and electrolyte balance.

Dietary Recommendations

1. Progress, as tolerated, from clear liquids to diet as usual. Small, frequent feedings are best tolerated.
2. Increase fluids to 3 liters daily unless contraindicated.

Profile

Ht, wt	SGOT, SGPT (inc.)	Na^+, K^+, Cl^-
WBCs (inc.)	Platelets (dec.)	IBW/HBW
BUN, creat. (inc.)	Wt changes	BP
Bilirubin (inc.)	Alb	Gluc
Temp	CPK (inc.)	
Po_2, Pco_2	H & H	

Side Effects of Common Drugs Used

Antibiotics are commonly required.

Patient Education

1. Discuss with patient ways to decrease likelihood of reinfection.
2. Discuss the need for adequate fluid intake and small meals, especially with vomiting or nausea.

NOTES

TRAUMA

Usual Hospital Stay

5–6 days, multiple trauma with complications.

Notation

Trauma is caused by major injury or accidents (50% are related to traffic accidents). Trauma is related to 33% of all hospital admissions, and is a leading cause of death for ages 1–40.

Elevated plasma catecholamines, glucocorticoids, glucagon and glucose are noted. The heart and brain are the organs most affected by shock.

For feeding, use the gut first if possible. TF is a preferred route since it is safer and less expensive than parenteral. Osmolarity should be monitored to be close to 300 mOsm. Predigested formula may be needed for GI injury.

Objectives

1. Assess and monitor extent of injury and resulting problems.
2. Restore hemodynamic and metabolic functions, acid-base balance and fluid balance.
3. Meet elevated BMR requirements (up by 20–45%). Spare proteins and LBM.
4. Determine digestive/absorptive capacity; provide nutrients in the most effective mode.
5. Prevent complications, infection, respiratory failure, shock, sepsis.
6. Promote healing and rapid recovery.
7. Adapt to ileus or fistula if either occurs.
8. Promote rehabilitation; correct anorexia and depression, which are common.
9. Control glucose homeostasis (decrease stress diabetes). High glucose loads can lead to liver dysfunction.
10. Decrease nitrogen losses; promote nitrogen balance.
11. Prevent overfeeding with respiratory distress from increased CO_2 production.
12. Hydrate adequately but do not overhydrate.

Dietary Recommendations

1. *Immediately*—IVs with glucose and potassium, etc. for approximately 24 hours until stabilization; life support measures and careful monitoring are usually provided.
2. Days 2–5 usually entail assessment of needs, with implementation of nutrition in the most effective means (oral, enteral or parenteral). Injury location and extent will dictate the most desirable mode.
3. Days 5–10 are often the *adaptive phase,* with products like Trauma-Cal (50% BCAAs) and lipid emulsions being used where possible. N:kcal ratio is usually given as 1:100 during trauma. 30–35 kcal/kg; 1.5–2 g protein/kg and CHO given as 5 mg/kg/minute should be calculated. The BEE is often 2× normal. A diet providing 50% CHO, 15% protein and 35% fat should be adequate.

4. A slight increase in vitamin/mineral intake should be addressed, with B-complex, zinc and vitamins A and C provided in particular.
5. In the *rehabilitative phase,* the patient has generally returned to normal BMR and can be weaned from PN to EN or oral diet, and from ventilator support. Liquid to regular diets are usually tolerated at this time.

Profile

Ht, wt pretrauma/	WBCs	BEE, Indirect
post-trauma	Trig	calorimetry
Na^+, K^+, Cl^-	PO_4, alk phos	Bilirubin, SGOT
H & H, serum Fe	Serum hormones	(inc.)
Temp	Wt changes	Alb, transferrin
I & O	IBW/HBW	RBP, prealbumin
BP	BUN, creat	N balance
P_{CO_2}, P_{O_2}	Gluc (inc.)	Serum AAs
TLC	Ca^{++}, Mg^{++}	CPK (inc.)

Side Effects of Common Drugs Used

1. *Antibiotics* are generally used to reduce bacterial infection.
2. *Insulin* may be used for hypergycemia.
3. *Barbiturates* are often used for closed head injury. They will decrease BMR.
4. Analgesics, antacids, and other medications may have an impact on nutritional status.

Patient Education

1. The need for specific nutrients should be discussed.
2. Rehabilitation should progress according to individual requirements and injury sites, side effects and complications.

Comments

1. Hyperosmolar diets can cause diarrhea. Begin feedings slowly and advance strength over several days.
2. Avoid infusion of free iron because of the risks of bacterial infection. Packed red cells may be preferred until the patient's condition is more stable.
3. Infusion of 5% human albumin can increase alk. phos. Monitor carefully.
4. Keep in mind that repletion of body fat occurs after repletion of LBM.
5. In children, 4–8% of calories should be from essential fatty acids as from safflower oil.
6. Skeletal muscle is a major source of protein in humans; BCAAs are used here. Nitrogen excretion increases after injury, peaks after 7 days, and

eventually stabilizes. BCAA-enriched formulas may be beneficial in trauma. Exact % of BCAAs is still being tested.
7. According to Chen, "Multiple trauma is a post-trauma complex involving at least 2 injuries, each of which requires hospital admission in its own right." Long bone fractures, pelvis or vertebral fractures and damage to body cavities (head, thorax or abdomen) are generally involved.
8. A needle catheter jejunostomy may be useful in head/neck trauma.
9. Fluid shifts can affect serum levels of albumin and transferrin; keep hydration status in mind when reviewing these parameters.

NOTES

TRICHINOSIS

Usual Hospital Stay

4 days.

Notation

An acute infection caused by roundworm *Trichinella spiralis,* trichinosis is usually acquired by eating encysted larvae in raw or undercooked pork. The disorder has a 4% prevalence in the U.S.

Larvae mature and mate in the small intestine; larvae reaching striated muscle will encyst and live for years. Usual incubation is 5–15 days.

Symptoms and signs include diarrhea, abdominal cramps, malaise; later, low-grade fever, edema, sweating, dyspnea, cough, muscle pain. In non-striated muscle tissues like heart, brain, kidney or lung, death can follow in 4–6 weeks.

Objectives

1. Correctly identify the condition as rapidly as possible; treat as needed.
2. Treat infections and diarrhea if severe.
3. Prevent complications, such as pneumonia and cardiac failure.

Dietary Recommendations

1. Diet as usual can be provided.
2. Ensure an adequate fluid intake, especially with diarrheal losses.
3. Replace electrolytes with broths, juices.
4. With poor appetite, offer small, frequent meals and snacks to correct any weight loss that is undesirable.

Profile

Ht, wt	Alb	Wt changes
Positive skin and	IBW/HBW	Bx skeletal muscle
serological	H & H	Transferrin
tests for	Gluc	Temp
eosinophilia and	TLC, WBCs	Na^+, K^+, Cl^-
leukocytosis	I & O	

Side Effects of Common Drugs Used

Thiabendazole may be used.

Patient Education

Discuss the proper handling and cooking methods for pork and other meats. Discuss use of thermometers.

TYPHOID FEVER

Usual Hospital Stay

4–5 days.

Notation

Typhoid fever is an infectious fever spread by contamination of food, water, or milk with *Salmonella typhi,* which can come from sewage, flies, or faulty personal hygiene. Most infections are found in people who are in contact with carriers who have persistent gallbladder or urinary tract infections. Incubation is 5–14 days. Symptoms include malaise, headache, cough, sore throat, "pea soup" diarrhea, constipation, rose spots, splenomegaly.

The problem has practically been eradicated in areas of proper sanitary practice.

Objectives

1. Reduce fever and prevent irritation.
2. Replace nutrient losses from diarrhea.
3. Replace tissue losses.
4. Prevent complications such as intestinal hemorrhage or shock.

Dietary Recommendations

1. For patients with *acute* fever, use a diet of high protein, high calorie liquids. A low residue diet may be needed temporarily.
2. As treatment progresses, gradually add soft, bland foods. Try small, frequent feedings. Gradually add pectin and other fiber.

Profile

Ht	Wt	$^+$Stool and urine for
IBW/HBW	Temp	Widal test
Alb	H & H	Gluc
I & O	WBCs, TLC	

Side Effects of Drugs Commonly Used

1. *Ampicillin* should be taken 1–2 hours before or after meals. Nausea or vomiting may occur.
2. *Chloramphenicol* may increase the need for riboflavin and vitamins B_6 and B_{12}. Nausea, vomiting or diarrhea may result.

Patient Education

1. Explain which foods are high protein, high calorie sources.
2. Discuss control of future reinfection.

Section 16
Renal Disorders

Chief Assessment Factors

renal insufficiency or failure

uremia

altered BP

bone pain, altered height or LBM

unbalanced $CA^{++}:PO_4$ ratios, lipid and AA levels

presence or history of UTIs

renal dialysis

frequent weight shifts

leg swelling, leg cramps

night urination

abnormal BUN/creatinine

weakness, pallor, anemia

itching

RENAL HORMONAL CONTROL

The kidney produces *renin*, which converts angiotensinogen to angiotensin I. Blood enzymes convert angiotensin I to angiotensin II, which then stimulates

491

the adrenal gland to produce aldosterone. Increased sodium reabsorption results from the aldosterone production.

Antidiuretic hormone from the hypothalamus increases the permeability of the distal and collecting tubules to increase water reabsorption. The kidney accomplishes the final stage of *conversion of vitamin D* to its active form: 1, 25 dihydroxy vitamin D, in the proximal tubule.

Table 16–1.
Human Kidney Functions
1. Waste removal
2. Erythropoietin secretion for RBC production
3. Renin for BP regulation
4. Vitamin D_3 control for Ca:P homeostasis
5. Control of potassium and phosphate
6. Acid-base balance (bicarbonate reabsorption and hydrogen ion secretion).
7. Carnitine synthesis to carry fatty acids from cytoplasm to mitochondria, for heart and skeletal muscle fuel. Lysine and methionine, vitamin C, iron, vitamin B_6 and niacin are needed to produce carnitine (*JADA* 86:644, 1986).

Table 16–2.
Renal Notes
Body water = 2/3 extracellular water + 1/3 intracellular water
Renal Functioning: Decreased—GFR decreases by 50%
Insufficiency—GFR decreases by 75%
Renal Failure—GFR decreases by over 75%
BUN: Creatinine ratio is typically 15:0 (renal function decreases by 50% as creatinine doubles).
End-stage renal disease (ESRD) = less than 10% remaining kidney function

For More Information

National Kidney Foundation
30 East 33rd St.
New York, NY 10016
(800) 622-9010

American Kidney Fund: (800) 638-8299

GLOMERULONEPHRITIS, ACUTE

Usual Hospital Stay

3–4 days.

Notation

After an antigen-antibody complex reaction, some complexes become trapped in the glomeruli. Edema and scarring result, causing *glomerulonephritis,* or inflamed glomeruli. Untreated streptococcal infection can cause GN.

Uremia is the accumulation in the blood of waste substances ordinarily eliminated in the urine. This happens because the kidneys have lost their filtering ability as a result of temporary poisoning or severe kidney disease. Signs and symptoms include a drop in urine volume, urine smell on breath and sweat, itching, vomiting, convulsions, and yellowish-brown skin discoloration.

See also Acute Renal Failure.

Objectives

1. Reduce elevated serum nitrogen levels from breakdown of endogenous proteins.
2. Reduce elevated blood pressure or edema.
3. Spare protein for tissue repair.
4. Improve renal functioning; prevent systemic complications.
5. In children, avoid growth retardation over time.

Dietary Recommendations

1. For patients with *oliguria,* restrict fluid intake to 500–700 ml. Restrict protein intake if needed.
2. For patients with *uremia,* the diet should include protein at 0.2–0.3 g/kg body weight, HBV proteins (eggs and milk); or 2–3 × normal EAAs should be included. Progress as tolerated to 0.5–0.6 g protein/kg. 70% HBV/30% LBV orders are common.
3. If the patient has edema or high blood pressure, restrict sodium intake to 500–1000 mg.
4. Use high calorie diet to spare protein, 35 kcal/kg (60–65% CHO, 25–30% lipid for non-nitrogen kcal).
5. When urinary output is greatly reduced, restrict potassium intake and phosphorus as needed (e.g. 400–500 mg).
6. Some patients could use dialysis to remove waste products.
7. Vitamin D_3, calcium, iron, and multivitamin intake should be increased as appropriate.

Profile

Ht	IBW/HBW	WBCs
H & H	BUN, creat	3-methyl histidine
GFR	BP	Ca^{++}, Phosphorus
K^+, Na^+	Temp	Specific gravity (↑)
Dry Wt	Serum Cu (inc.)	SGOT

| Edema | I & O | Chol ($\uparrow$) |
| Alb, transferrin | CrCl levels | Serum Fe, TIBC |

Side Effects of Common Drugs Used

1. When *diuretics* are used to reduce edema, watch for potassium wasting. Dehydration can elevate BUN; assess carefully.
2. See Hypertension entry for the side effects of antihypertensives.

Patient Education

1. Patients with ascites may become anorexic in the upright position. Have the patient carefully positioned for food intake.
2. Fluid intake should be carefully distributed throughout the patient's waking hours. Check for changes according to diarrhea, etc.
3. Encourage frequent doctor or clinic visits to monitor renal functioning.

NOTES

GLOMERULONEPHRITIS, CHRONIC

Usual Hospital Stay

3–4 days.

Notation

Repeated episodes of nephritis lead to loss of renal tissue and kidney function. Glomeruli disappear and normal filtering is lost. Kidneys can no longer concentrate urine, and more urine is voided in an effort to rid the body of wastes. Protein and blood are lost in the urine. Blood pressure rises, causing vascular changes. CRF may be a result. Decreased proteinuria indicates an improved prognosis, while hypertension can delay improvement. See also Chronic Renal Failure.

Objectives

1. Control hypertension, UTIs and proteinuria.
2. Correct metabolic abnormalities. Improve nutritional status, appetite.

3. Reduce edema.
4. Prevent further catabolism of protein to lower urea production and other protein waste products.
5. Prevent complications, including growth failure in children.

Dietary Recommendations

1. Modify the patient's diet according to progression of the disease.
2. Maintain sufficient levels of protein as long as kidneys can eliminate waste products of protein metabolism. Calculate the usual RDAs, and then add those vitamins and nutrients that have been lost in the urine during the previous 24 hours. As the BUN rises, restrict protein intake to 0.6g/kg, or less. Control meat intake (high protein and phosphorus).
3. Complete the patient's energy requirements with carbohydrates and fat (2000–3000 kcal for adults, or 30–40 kcal/kg dry wt).
4. Restrict sodium intake in patients with edema, or to forestall fluid retention. Carefully monitor sodium levels, since sodium depletion can occur during the diuretic phase of chronic glomerulonephritis. Check potassium and phosphorus levels also.
5. Children with uremia require vitamin D_3 to promote growth and to improve appetite.

Profile

Ht	Dry Wt	Proteinuria
IBW/HBW	Edema	I & O
WBCs	Alb	Creat. clearance*
H & H	BUN, creat*	3-methyl histidine
GFR	BP	Serum Cu (inc.)
K^+, Na^+	Temp	PO_4, alk phos
Chol ($\uparrow$)	Specific gravity ($\downarrow$)	H & H, serum Fe, TIBC

Patient Education

1. The patient should not avoid drinking fluid in order to prevent nocturia.
2. Fluid retention is better controlled by sodium restriction than by fluid restriction. Monitor the patient carefully.
3. Patients with edema are often thirsty despite fluid retention. Edema water is trapped and unavailable for the body's use.
4. Frequent doctor or clinic visits are recommended to evaluate renal functioning.

---

* Once patient is on a controlled diet for protein and phosphorus, especially limiting meat, creatinine fails to be a valid measure of renal function because it is from the diet and muscle.

Comments*

1. *Conservative treatment* promotes protein restriction in order to correct metabolic and hormonal derangements.
2. *Protein restriction* is absolutely contraindicated in protein malnutrition!
3. Dietary protein restriction has its *limitations*—renal dietitian is needed; commitment from patient and family is essential; extra expense is incurred for EAAs, KAAs and low-protein foods; growth and muscle mass may decline; calorie intake is essential to prevent PCM; neoplasm of infections preclude any protein restriction.

* *Giovannetti: Lancet* Nov. 15, 1986).

NOTES

NEPHRITIS (BRIGHT'S DISEASE)

Usual Hospital Stay

3–4 days.

Notation

Kidney inflammation results from a diffuse, progressive lesion affecting the renal parenchyma, interstitial tissue, and renal vascular system. The inflammation can become acute or chronic. It causes include scarlet fever, flu, and tonsillitis. Nephritis may reflect any altered kidney functioning.

Objectives

1. Reduce renal workload to allow healing.
2. Improve or control excretion of waste products such as urea and sodium.
3. Prevent edema resulting from sodium and fluid retention.
4. Prevent uremia from nitrogen retention.
5. Adjust electrolyte levels as needed (e.g., Na^+, K^+, and Cl^-).
6. Prevent systemic complications or net protein catabolism, as from poor intake.

Dietary Recommendations

1. Determine fluid intake (measured output plus 500 ml insensible losses).
2. Restrict sodium intake to 1–2 g if patient has hypertension or edema.
3. In the case of renal failure, protein intake should be low. Use HBV proteins to ensure positive nitrogen balance.
4. Check need for vitamin A, which may be low.

Profile

Ht	Wt or dry wt	P
IBW/HBW	Edema	Na^+
I & O	Alb	SGOT
BUN, creat	BP	Ca^{++}
N balance	K^+	Proteinuria
Cl^-	Urea	Serum Cu (may be
GFR	RBP	dec.)
Chol (may be inc.)	Temp	H & H, serum Fe, TIBC

Patient Education

Ensure that dietary measures are appropriate for the patient's particular needs.

NOTES

NEPHROSCLEROSIS (ARTERIOSCLEROTIC BRIGHT'S DISEASE)

Usual Hospital Stay

3–4 days.

Notation

Nephrosclerosis is caused by hardening of the renal arteries, usually as a result of renal hypertension and generalized atherosclerotic heart disease. Albumin is lost in the urine, nitrogen waste products are retained, and retinal changes occur. Death may occur from circulatory failure or hypertension. Nephrosclerosis usually occurs in persons older than 35 years.

Objectives

1. Reduce the workload of the circulatory system by decreasing excess weight where present.
2. Monitor abnormal protein status and nitrogen retention.
3. Control hypertension.
4. Prevent systemic complications.
5. Control hyperglycemia if patient has diabetes.
6. Decrease elevated serum lipids.

Dietary Recommendations

1. If patient is obese use a low calorie diet.
2. Protein intake should be normal except during periods of nitrogen retention.
3. The diet should be low in cholesterol and saturated fats to lessen atherosclerotic heart disease. Linoleic acid seems to be important.
4. Monitor fluid intake according to the patient's output. Intake should be adequate to eliminate wastes, but controlled when retention occurs.
5. Restrict sodium intake to reduce edema and hypertension.
6. Control CHO intake with diabetes.

Profile

Ht	Wt or dry wt	Creat
IBW/HBW	Alb	SGOT
BP	BUN	Trig
I & O	GFR	K^+
Urea	Edema	Na^+
H & H	Chol (inc.)	Glucose, ketones

Patient Education

Help the patient control specific nutrients as needed (e.g., proteins, sodium, fluid, etc.).

NOTES

NEPHROTIC SYNDROME

Usual Hospital Stay

3 days.

Notation

In nephrotic syndrome (also called nephrosis), massive proteinuria occurs when 3.5 g or more of protein is lost within 24 hours. As much as 30 g could be lost as a result of decreased plasma proteins.

Albumin is especially decreased. Signs and symptoms include weight gain, HLP, edema, chest pains, and weakness. Adults who have nephrotic syndrome usually have some form of glomerulonephritis, with renal failure not far behind. Elevated LDL cholesterol is common as well, from changes in lipoprotein production.

A high protein diet will alter GFR; limit protein to decrease hyperfiltration.

Objectives

1. Replace protein losses, especially albumin.
2. Ensure efficient utilization of fed proteins with use of adequate calories. Prevent muscle catabolism.
3. Reduce edema.
4. Control sodium intake with otherwise uncontrolled HPN.
5. Monitor hypercholesterolemia, elevated triglycerides.
6. Monitor patient for potassium deficits with certain diuretics.
7. Prevent or control renal failure.
8. Correct anorexia.
9. Replace any other nutrients, especially those at risk.

Dietary Recommendations

1. Use a diet of HBV proteins—(1.5 g/kg IBW). Children may need 2–3 g/kg IBW. Use lower levels with renal failure.
2. Carbohydrate intake should be high to spare protein for LBM.
3. The diet should provide 40–60 kcal/kg body weight daily.
4. If the patient has edema, sodium intake should be restricted to 2–4 g.
5. Provide adequate sources of potassium and calcium as tolerated.
6. No fluid restrictions are necessary, unless renal failure occurs.
7. Offer appetizing meals to increase intake. If required, tube feed patient. TPN may also be beneficial.
8. In the case of elevated levels of cholesterol and triglycerides, limit dietary cholesterol and decrease intake of free sugars. Utilize linoleic acid.
9. Replace zinc, vitamin C, folacin, and other nutrients.

Profile

Ht	IBW/HBW	Alb
Chol	Ceruloplasmin (dec.)	BUN
Transferrin (inc.)	SGOT (inc.)	I & O
Wt	Na$^+$	K$^+$
BP	Uremia	GFR
Proteinuria	Alk phos	Edema
Trig (inc.)	Ca^{++}	Creatinine

Side Effects of Common Drugs Used

1. *Diuretics*. Thiazides deplete potassium. Check for replacements.
2. *Corticosteroids*. Sodium restrictions apply. Potassium and nitrogen or calcium losses may result.

Patient Education

1. Help the patient plan appetizing meals.
2. If patient has edema, careful positioning will increase comfort.

NOTES

PYELONEPHRITIS

Usual Hospital Stay

7 days, acute; chronic varies with complications.

Notation

Bacterial invasion of the kidneys (usually from *E. coli*) leads to fibrosis, scarring, and dilatation of the tubules, which impair renal function. Hypertension or some degree of renal failure is usually present in chronic pyelonephritis.

Acute pyelonephritis is usually rapidly corrected with urinary antiinfectives.

Objectives

1. Preserve kidney function.
2. Control blood pressure.
3. Acidify urine to decrease additional bacterial growth.
4. Force fluids unless contraindicated.

Dietary Recommendations

1. Restrict excess sodium to control elevated blood pressure. However, some patients lose excessive amounts of sodium in their urine and must be monitored for depletion.
2. Restrict protein intake if renal function is threatened. Otherwise, use HBV proteins, including foods such as meat, fish, poultry, eggs, and cheese.
3. Restrict potassium when serum K^+ is elevated. Check drugs first.
4. Cranberries, plums, and prunes produce hippuric acid, which helps to acidify urine. Corn, lentils, breads/starches, peanuts, and walnuts also acidify urine.
5. Avoid excesses of caffeine for the diuretic effect.
6. Vitamin A tends to be low; encourage improved intake.

Profile

Ht	Wt
IBW/HBW	BP (inc.)
Alb	BUN
I & O	Edema
K^+, Na^+	Urinary Na^+
Gluc	Creat
RBP	Temp

Side Effects of Common Drugs Used

1. *Urinary anti-infectives.* When allowed, a lot of water and fluids should be ingested. Monitor diabetic responses to glucose changes. *Sulfisoxazole* (Gantrisin) can deplete folacin and vitamin K. Nausea and vomiting may also occur.
2. According to a study in JAMA (12/84), vitamin C is not necessarily effective in lowering urinary pH.
3. *Trimethoprim* (Bactrim/Septra) may cause diarrhea, GI distress, and stomatitis. Use adequate fluid.
4. *Nitrofurantoin* (Furadantin, Macrodantin) should be consumed with food or milk. An adequate protein diet is needed. Nausea, vomiting, anorexia, and diarrhea are common.

Patient Education

1. Indicate which foods are palatable as sources of nutrients for the dietary restrictions, and for the nutrients that tend to be low.
2. Encourage appropriate fluid intake.
3. Discuss acid-ash diets in light of medical treatment first, diet second.

UROLITHIASIS/NEPHROLITHIASIS

Usual Hospital Stay

3 days; less with extracorporeal shock wave lithotripsy (ESWL).

Notation

Kidney stones develop when salt and minerals in urine form crystals that coalesce and grow in size. Annually, 400,000 people are treated for this problem. The major causes of renal stones are hypercalciuria from a high calcium diet, hypervitaminosis D, urinary tract infections, cancer, immobilization, and osteoporosis. Renal stones can also be caused by hypoparathyroidism, renal tubular acidosis, or vitamin A deficiency.

The stones are formed by progressive deposition of crystalline material about an organic nidus. Ten percent of the stones are organic (composed of cystine or uric acid), and 90% are inorganic (composed of calcium, magnesium, ammonium, oxalate, phosphate, or carbonate).

Signs and symptoms include excruciating pain, nausea, vomiting, burning and urinary frequency.

Objectives

1. Determine predominant components and prevent recurrence in calculi-prone patients.
2. Modify diet according to the predominant component—seldom is there a single cause.
3. To increase excretion of salts, dilute urine by increasing fluid volume to at least 2 L per 24 hours.

Dietary Recommendations

1. Fluid intake should be high (8 oz hourly while patient is awake).
2. *Calcium oxalate stones.* Restrict calcium intake to less than 1000 mg. Intake of sodium (with thiazides) should be normal but not high. The diet should include fewer dairy products, nuts, fish, green leafy vegetables, and peanut butter. Use more fiber (a source of phytic acid) and less vitamin D.
3. *Cystine stones.* Use a diet low in cystine, methionine, and cysteine. Protein intake should be lessened, but not severely restricted. Cystine

stones are usually the result of a hereditary defect. Alkalize urine with agents like D-penicillamine.

4. *Uric acid stones.* Resulting from purine metabolism, uric acid stones may require a reduction in foods high in purines (e.g., sardines, etc.). Uric acid stones may also result from gout, leukemia, cancer, etc. Alkalinize urine with citrate or bicarbonate.

5. The use of an acid ash or alkaline ash diet must be specifically determined by the stone's composition. Acid ash is found in foods such as cranberries, plums, prunes, meat, and bread. Alkaline ash is found in foods such as milk and fruit and vegetables. These diets are not well documented in the literature.

Profile

Ht	Urinary Ca^{++}	Urinary stone content
IBW/HBW	(normal, 300–400	K^+, Na^+
P	mg)	BUN, creat
Amylase	Ca^{++}	GFR
Gluc	Uric acid	Serum oxalate levels
Wt	Lactose intolerance	

Side Effects of Common Drugs Used

1. For calcium oxalate or uric acid stones, *allopurinol* and *probenecid* are usually used instead of (or in conjunction with) a purine-restricted diet.
2. *Thiazide diuretics* are sometimes used to flush out the stone. Watch potassium levels; use replacements when needed. Control sodium intake.
3. *D-penicillamine* requires B_6 and zinc supplementation.

Patient Education

1. Use dietary measures that are appropriate for the condition and content of the stone. Discuss the controversy about "ash" diets.
2. Cranberry juice is a favorite beverage used to produce a more acidic urine, but quantity needed to do so is excessive and not practical.
3. Check calcium content of the water supply. Distilled water may be required, since hard water contains more calcium.
4. Vitamin B_6 reduces the production of oxalates by 50% and may help treatment. Include good dietary sources daily.
5. Increase fluid intake adequately.
6. Vitamin C excess does not seem to affect oxalate stone formation even though oxalic acid is a by-product of vitamin C metabolism.

Comment

Table 16–3.
Causes of and Predisposition to Renal Stones
1. Age—more common in middle age
2. Sex—3× more common in males
3. Activity—immobilization or excessive fluid losses from sweating
4. Climate—hot climate and summer months
5. Diminished water intake—during sleep, travel, illness, or from poor habits
6. Genetic disorders—gout, primary hyperoxaluria
7. Metabolic disturbances—bowel, endocrine, renal problems that increase blood and urinary Ca^{++} and oxalate levels
8. Diet—excesses of calcium, oxalate
9. Misuse of medications
10. Urinary tract infection or stagnation from blockage.

NOTES

RENAL FAILURE, ACUTE

Usual Hospital Stay

6–7 days.

Notation

Acute renal failure involves abrupt decline in renal function, with waste retention. ARF occurs when the kidneys fail to function because of circulatory, glomerular, or tubular deficiency resulting from an abrupt cause. ARF in acute care may be reversible, but mortality is still 50–75%.

ARF may be caused by burns, severe crushing injuries, transfusions, antibiotics, nephrotoxicity, anesthesia use, cardiac transplantation, shock, or sepsis. The patient with ARF excretes less than 500 ml of urine daily—at least 600 ml are required to eliminate solute wastes. Toxic accumulation occurs and may be fatal.

Renal failure occurs in the following *three stages:*

1. *Oliguric* (10 days). During the oliguric phase, the patient excretes less than 500 ml daily. Abnormal fluid/electrolyte homeostasis occurs.
2. *Diuretic.* During the diuretic phase, the patient gradually increases output of urine, up to several liters per day.
3. *Recovery* (from 3 months to a year). During the recovery phase, the patient gradually improves, although some loss of function is permanent.

Signs and symptoms include anorexia, nausea, drowsiness, fatigue, itching, poor vision, headache, dyspnea, and weakness.

Dialysis (daily or every other day) may be necessary if other treatments fail.

Objectives

1. Correct underlying abnormality. Postpone dialysis if possible.
2. Maintain homeostasis until kidneys resume adequate functioning.
3. Maintain fluid, electrolyte and mineral balances.
4. Retard progression of renal failure.
5. Prevent or correct uremia, Type IV hyperlipidemia, PCM, sepsis, and pulmonary complications.
6. Lessen workload by reducing wastes (urea, uric acid, creatine, electrolytes). Urea precursors include glutamine, alanine, and other ammonia NAAs. Be aware of osmolarity of formulas.
7. Preserve LBM; control catabolism or weight loss.
8. Preserve phospholipid pathways.
9. Prevent death.

Dietary Recommendations

1. Prevent catabolism. Ensure that the diet provides adequate calories (300:1—kcal:N ratio). Controlyte, polycose, fats, sugars, fruits, low protein starches, and vegetables may be used. Use of fructose in ARF is controversial.
2. Restrict fluid intake to patient output plus 500 ml for insensible losses, etc. Err on the side of giving less rather than more!
3. The diet should provide 0.8 g protein/kg body weight at first, but that amount should increase as kidney function improves (to cope with stress). Use HBV proteins, ration of 2:1 HBV:LBV to provide the proper ratio of essential AAs to nonessential AAs. Include histidine. BCAAs may be beneficial.
4. If unable to eat, as gut function often declines in ARF, TPN or TF may be needed. 50% CHO, 20% protein, 30% fat may be recommended, with appropriate alternatives that are patient-specific.
5. With hypertriglyceridemia, use fewer simple sugars.

6. Supplement for folate, vitamins B_6 and C; add zinc, chromium, vitamin K and vitamin A as needed. Avoid excesses.
7. Restrict intake of potassium during anuric phase. Monitor serum levels closely. During the diuretic phase, too much potassium may be lost. The same is true of sodium. Be careful with salt substitutes.
8. Restrict sodium during anuric phase. During the diuretic phase, too much sodium may be lost; liberalize with vomiting or diarrhea as well.
9. Carnitine supplementation may be needed.

Profile

Ht	H & H	Creatinine clearance
IBW/HBW	BP	Transferrin
BUN over 30	Ca^{++} (dec.)	Wt or dry wt
I & O	Chol, trig (inc.)	pH
Alb	CO_2 (dec.)	Glucose (inc.)
K^+ (inc.)	Uric Acid (inc.)	Azotemia
Urea	SGOT (inc.)	N balance
P (inc.)	Na^+ (dec.)	TLC
GFR	Mg^{++} (inc.)	Oliguria (output 50–
Creat	3-methyl histidine	400 ml/day)
Temp	Alk phos	

Side Effects of Common Drugs Used

1. *Exchange resins* may release excessive amounts of potassium during tissue destruction, so that the patient has no capacity for urinary excretion during renal failure. Excessive sodium retention may occur, with edema. Kayexalate may be used.
2. *Sorbitol* may be given orally or by rectum to increase fluid loss through the GI tract.
3. *Antacids* should be monitored for mineral/electrolyte content (Maalox, Gelusil, Mylanta, etc.).
4. *Insulin* may be needed with hyperglycemia, or with TPN.

Patient Education

1. Show the patient how to monitor dietary intake of restricted nutrients, and explain the side effects of renal failure. Diet prescription should be carefully followed.
2. The patient should monitor fluid status with daily weight measurement.
3. Food labels should be read, and all foods should be measured carefully.

Comments

1. Amin-Aid (American McGaw), a mixture of amino acids and histidine without vitamins, can be used to give 670 nonprotein calories from

carbohydrates, fats, and amino acids. Use with nasogastric tube or for oral intake. Other products may also be available for providing non-protein calories.

2. Acute dialysis may be needed for hyperkalemia, pulmonary edema, uremia with malignant hypertension or seizures, heart failure, or pericarditis.

3. TPN can help to allevaite wasting or prolonged convalescence. Monitor glucose (hyperglycemia) and lipids (decreased triglyceride clearance). Free l-amino acids are better tolerated than protein hydrolysates. Other than folate, most vitamins and minerals should be given in smaller amounts because of renal impairment for clearance.

4. Be careful about protein intake, since protein excess leads to perfusion of remaining glomeruli and, therefore, to their destruction.

RENAL FAILURE, CHRONIC

Usual Hospital Stay

6–7 days.

Notation

Chronic renal failure is characterized by the failure of kidney function to return to normal after acute kidney failure or progressive kidney loss due to renal disease. CRF causes permanent reduction in function.

Causes of chronic renal failure are varied, including hypoparathyroidism, recurrent acute or chronic glomerulonephritis, tubular disease, chronic hypercalcemia, chronic hyperkalemia, vascular diseases (ischemic disease, malignant hypertension, nephrosclerosis), pyelonephritis, renal calculi or neoplasms, collagen diseases, amyloidosis, and diabetes.

Signs and symptoms include severe headache, dyspnea, pitting edema of the hands and legs, failing vision, poor appetite, nausea and vomiting, abdominal pain, mouth ulcers, hiccups, bone and joint pain, fatigue, uremic convulsions, and pericarditis.

Objectives

1. Control uremic symptoms and complications from accumulation of nitrogenous waste.
2. Restore and maintain electrolyte balance; correct acidosis and anemias.
3. Limit further renal impairment. Reduce kidney workload.
4. Minimize tissue catabolism. Negative nitrogen balance is common.
5. Maintain nutritional status, weight, morale, appetite, and LBM.
6. Provide AAs in proportion to minimal RDAs of each.
7. Postpone dialysis if possible.
8. Maintain growth with adequate calories, vitamins, and minerals.

Dietary Recommendations

1. The diet should provide adequate calories to prevent tissue catabolism. Controlyte or Polycose may be used. 25–35 kcal/kg are recommended.
2. If patient has edema, restrict sodium intake to 1.5–2 g sodium. Watch the use of salt substitute if potassium levels are high. Restrict intake of potassium and phosphorus if needed. Liberalize with diarrhea or vomiting.
3. In the severe stages of chronic renal failure, restrict protein intake to 0.6–1.0 g/kg IBW. Three fourths of protein intake should be HBV proteins; 25% LBV proteins.
4. Fluid intake should be equivalent to the patient's output plus 500–1000 ml for insensible losses. Monitor regularly.
5. Amino acid analogs (carbohydrate skeleton of amino acids minus the amino group) may be used. EAAs can be given orally or by keto-acid analogs (alpha-ketoisocaproate, etc.).
6. Carbohydrate intolerance is common. Fructose, galactose, and sorbitol are well tolerated.
7. Provide adequate vitamin B_6, folic acid and vitamin C, with RDA levels for other nutrients. Calcium and carnitine may also be needed.
8. With TPN, be careful not to use excesses of micronutrients because of reduced renal clearance.

Profile

Ht	Edema	Uric acid (inc.)
IBW/HBW	H & H	Mg^{++} (inc.)
Alb	GFR (below 5 ml/min.	Alk phos
Transferrin	consider dialysis)	3-methyl histidine
PO_4 (inc.)	Dry wt	BUN : creat ratio*
Creat	BUN	pH
Azotemia (excess urea	Ca^{++} (dec.)	CO_2
and nitrogenous	I & O	Cl^-
wastes)	BP	Chol, trig
		TSF, MAC, MAMC

Side Effects of Common Drugs Used

1. For drugs to alleviate hypertension, monitor side effects.
2. *Calcium medications* (gluconate, carbonate, or lactate) may help increase calcium intake while not requiring the intake of high phosphorus foods. In renal failure, the patient is unable to convert vitamin D to its active form, and osteodystrophy can result from a lack of calcium utilization. It may also be helpful to supplement the diet with vitamin D.

---

* This ratio is altered by catabolic stress, low urine volume, and altered muscle mass.

3. *Iron supplements* may be needed to treat anemia; or recombinant human erythropoietin can be used.
4. Supplementation with *histidine,* an amino acid essential for renal patients, helps increase hemoglobin levels and promotes maintenance of a positive nitrogen balance.
5. *Phosphate Binders* may be used (at GFR levels 30–50 ml/min, for example).

Patient Education

1. Indicate which food sources must be restricted or used more frequently.
2. Have the patient use more milk and eggs than meat, since meat produces more nitrogenous waste. HBV proteins should be consumed throughout the day.
3. Taste changes may occur in patients with chronic renal failure—foods with sharp, distinct flavors may be needed.
4. Low protein wheat starch, hard candy, and jelly can be used.
5. Discuss that diet adherence is the single most important factor in achieving its therapeutic effectiveness. Dietary restriction is an important element in therapy.
6. Have the patient weigh self daily.
7. Reading food labels and measuring foods will be essential for control.

Comment

Chronic dialysis may be needed for bone disease, neuropathy, malnutrition (especially low albumin or low TLC).

In disturbances of bowel flora in CRF, researchers are currently studying the benefits of *Lactobacillus* as in specialty yogurts.

NOTES

HEMODIALYSIS

Usual Hospital Stay

2 days.

Notation

Hemodialysis is artificial filtering of blood by a machine, a catabolic process. Morbidity is largely related to physical fitness at the start of therapy. Among hemodialysis patients, 50% of deaths are related to CVD, especially type IV HLP. Less protein is lost with hemodialysis than with peritoneal dialysis; nevertheless, amino acid losses still occur.

Objectives

1. Compensate for protein losses. Ensure that protein intake is sufficient for children to grow. 1–2 g protein may be lost per 2 liter exchange.
2. Spare protein adequately to allow for tissue repair and synthesis.
3. Modify electrolytes and fluid balance according to patient's tolerance.
4. Replace lost amino acids, etc., without causing uremic symptoms.
5. Prevent osteopenia, muscle weakness, cardiac arrhythmias, hypertriglyceridemia, as well as viral infections, TB, and neoplasms (more common in CRF with maintenance dialysis).

Dietary Recommendations

1. Intake of protein should be 1–1.2 g/kg dry wt, 70% of which should be HBW proteins.* Urea kinetic modeling may also be used to devise a protein prescription.
2. Limit sodium intake unless there are large losses in dialysate, or through vomiting or diarrhea. 1–2 g sodium is common.
3. Check predialysis levels of potassium and phosphorus. Modify diet accordingly. Dialysis removes very little phosphorus. 2 g potassium is a typical order.
4. Fluid intake should be 500–1000 ml plus the amount equal to previous day's output, or enough to permit a gain of 1–1.5 kg between treatments.
5. Caloric intake should be 30–35 kcal/kg IBW, or a range of 25–50 kcal/kg dependent on patient.
6. Use vitamin supplementation to replace dialysate losses. Water-soluble vitamins are especially necessary, but may not be needed daily. Vitamin B_{12} is not lost, for example. Folic acid, vitamins B_6 and C, calcium, and vitamin D should be monitored. Be careful about zinc and vitamin A excesses. Carnitine may be supplemented, if needed. Use caution with parenteral solutions also, especially for vitamins D, A, and C.

---

* Children need 3–4 g/kg body weight. Watch potassium and phosphorus restrictions because protein foods may be high in these nutrients. Use 100–150 kcal/kg body weight to encourage growth. Fluid intake should be 20 ml/kg body weight plus amount equal to previous day's output.

Profile

Ht	I & O	Urea
IBW/HBW	Edema	Serum Fe, B_{12}, folacin
BP	K^+	Chol, trig
P	Uric acid	N balance
H & H	BUN	TSF; MAC and MAMC
Creatinine, CrCl	Alb	in non-access arm
Gluc	Na^+	SGOT ($\downarrow$)
Ca^{++}	Mg^{++}	
GFR	Alk phos	
Dry wt	Temp	

Side Effects of Drugs Commonly Used

1. *Phosphate binders* (aluminum hydroxide [Alu-cap, Amphojel]) may be used for hyperphosphatemia.
2. *Calcium* and *vitamin D* supplements may be prescribed.
3. *Carnitine* may be needed (2 g/day for example).
4. *Kayexalate* may be needed to deplete excess potassium.
5. Excesses of *vitamin-mineral* supplements should be avoided.

Patient Education

1. Instruct the patient to avoid use of carbonated beverages/phosphates. Meat is high in creatinine and phosphorus and should be controlled.
2. Provide information about dining away from home.
3. Discuss high-calorie, low protein, mineral-controlled foods and supplements.
4. Adequate care must be taken to ingest appropriate levels of protein and calories.
5. Counsel the patient regarding atherogenesis, if relevant.
6. Discuss signs of uremia (N,V, hiccups, fatigue, weakness).
7. Discuss maximum fluid gain (usually 3–4#) between dialysis sessions.
8. *Public Law 92-603* (7/73) provides financial assistance via Medicaid to all persons covered by Social Security who have ESRD with dialysis.

Comment

Table 16–4.

Fluids

Equivalent Measures

30 cc = 1 fluid oz = 2 tablespoons
240 cc = 8 fluid oz = 1 cup
2 cups = 1 lb fluid weight
2.2 lbs = 1 kg fluid wt. or 4 cups liquid

Sample Items
1 whole Popsicle = 90 cc
4 oz soup = 120 cc
6 oz juice = 180 cc
8 oz beverage = 240 cc
12 oz soda pop = 360 cc
16 oz milkshake = 480 cc

NOTES

PERITONEAL RENAL DIALYSIS

Usual Hospital Stay

1 day.

Notation

Peritoneal dialysis involves artificial filtering of the blood by a hyperosmolar solution (with osmosis to remove water and diffusion for glucose exchange/ waste removal). Peritoneal renal dialysis removes metabolic wastes and excess fluid from the body but not so thoroughly that diet therapy is unnecessary. Considerable losses of protein and amino acids occur. Between peritoneal dialysis treatments, the patient must return to a strict renal diet for chronic renal failure. Total calorie intake increases from glucose in dialysate in CAPD. Types include *IPD* (*intermittent*); *CCPD* (continuous cycling—used nearly 100% in children); and *CAPD* (continuous ambulatory). In CAPD, there is fluid in the abdomen nearly 100% of the time; dialysis is done 4× daily; no partner is necessary.

Objectives

1. Compensate for protein losses.
2. Ensure adequate sparing of protein for tissue repair and synthesis.
3. Modify electrolytes and fluid balance according to patient's tolerance.
4. Replace lost amino acids without causing uremic symptoms. 6–12 g protein may be lost in the dialysate.
5. Prevent or correct anorexia, constipation, osteopenia, growth delay.

6. Alter calorie intake according to glucose absorption from the solution (e.g., 20 kcal/liter of 1.5% solution; 60 kcal/liter of 2.5% solution; 126 kcal/liter of 4.5% solution).

Dietary Recommendations

1. Protein intake should be 1.2–1.5 g/kg dry wt daily. Emphasize HBV proteins.
2. Use a high calorie diet—35–45 kcal/kg body weight daily, one-third of which should come from carbohydrates. If wt. loss is needed, use 20–25 kcal/kg BW.
3. Intake of sodium should be liberal, pending assessment of hydration, blood pressure, losses in the dialysate, vomiting, and diarrhea. Usually 2–3 g of sodium daily is used.
4. Adjust potassium and phosphorus intake according to serum levels; 2 g potassium, 1 g phosphorus may be ordered.
5. Fluid intake should be determined by the patient's state of hydration—encourage or restrict according to intake and output. No more than 1 kg should be gained in 1 day.
6. Supplement diet with multivitamins, especially vitamin B_6, folic acid. Monitor needs for calcium vitamin C and vitamin D. Be careful about vitamin A; check serum levels. Monitor parenteral micronutrients carefully.

Profile

Ht	I & O	Na^+
IBW/HBW	Edema	Temp
BP	K^+	Urea
P (inc.)	Uric acid	Serum Fe, folacin, B_{12}
H & H	BUN	Chol, trig
Creatinine	Alb	Mg^{++}
Gluc	TSF, MAC, MAMC	SGOT ($\downarrow$)
Ca^{++}	Alk phos	
Dry Wt	RBP	

Side Effects of Drugs Commonly Used

1. *Calcium carbonate* may act as a phosphate binder.
2. *Phosphate binders* may cause constipation; add fiber as possible. Take phosphate binders with meals. If dialysis does not remove all PO_4, diet may need to be limited in meat, nuts, legumes, and milk.

Patient Education

1. Instruct the patient to use salt substitutes carefully because of their potassium content.

2. Instruct the patient to beware of LBV proteins such as gelatin and corn in excesses.
3. Have the patient use milk sparingly if fluid restriction is necessary.
4. Explain that vegetables may need to be leached before cooking to remove potassium, depending on serum K^+ levels and need.
5. The patient should learn how to recognize significant changes in dry weight or food intake. Discuss actions to be taken. Usually 3–4 lbs between IPD is allowed.

Comments

Continuous ambulatory peritoneal dialysis (CAPD) may be necessary if higher levels of Hgb and Hct are seen. Electrolytes need not be excluded as much. Intake of proteins may be liberalized somewhat. With CAPD, extra glucose can increase weight and triglyceride levels. CHO absorption calculations should be individualized. In cases of peritonitis, 1.5 g protein/kg and 35 kcal/kg IBW should be planned.

CAPD may yield fewer growth problems in children.

Table 16–5.
Conservative Management: Protein Calculations by GFR or CrCl

Glomerular Filtration Rate (ml/min)	Protein Allowances (g/day)
20–50	60–90
15–20	50–70
10–15	40–50
5–10	35–40
less than 5	20 + dialysis!!

Creatinine Clearance	
Dietary Protein	**Creatinine Clearance (ml/min)**
50 g or 1.3 g/kg IBW	20–30
40 g or 1.0 g/kg IBW	15–20
30 g or 0.7 g/kg IBW	10–15
25 g or 0.55 g/kg IBW	5–10

NOTES

RENAL TRANSPLANTATION

Usual Hospital Stay

15–16 days.

Notation

After a renal transplant, the patient has a functioning donor kidney. High doses of glucocorticoid drugs are given to prevent rejection. Persons over 50 with poor health or history of CA cannot receive a transplant. A child must reach 20 kg to receive a parent's kidney. No siblings under 18 are allowed to donate a kidney.

Objectives

1. Normalize the diet to meet the specific needs of the patient.
2. Modify diet according to drug therapy.
3. Watch for abnormalities in calcium or phosphorus metabolism with hyperparathyroidism.
4. Monitor carbohydrate intolerance, but make sure that the diet provides enough carbohydrates to spare proteins.
5. Alleviate rejection episodes. Control infections.
6. Force fluids unless contraindicated.
7. Help patient adjust to lifelong medical regimen.

Dietary Recommendations

1. Daily intake of protein should be appropriate for RDAs (age, sex).
2. Daily intake of sodium should be 2–4 g.
3. Daily intake of calcium should be 1–1.5 × RDA to offset poor absorption.
4. Daily intake of phosphorus should be equal to Ca^{++} intake.
5. Restrict CHO intake with hyperglycemia.
6. Supplement diet with calcium, vitamin D, magnesium, and thiamine as needed. Children especially need adequate calcium for growth.
7. The special diet may be discontinued when drug therapy is reduced to maintenance levels.

Profile

Ht	Dry wt, present wt	Temp
IBW/HBW	H & H	WBCs, TLC
Alb	BUN, creat	Gluc
Ca^{++}	Mg^{++}	N balance
P	I & O	GFR

K+	BP	Alk phos
Na+	TSF, MAC, MAMC	SGOT, SGPT
		Bilirubin

Side Effects of Common Drugs Used

1. *Corticosteroids* are used for immunosuppression. Side effects include increased catabolism of proteins, negative nitrogen balance, decreased glucose tolerance, sodium retention, fluid retention, and impaired calcium absorption.
2. *Cyclosporins* do not retain sodium as much as corticosteroids do. IV doses are more effective than oral doses. Nausea, vomiting, and diarrhea are common side effects.
3. *OKT3* and *FK506* are less nephrotoxic than cyclosporine, but can cause nausea and vomiting.

Patient Education

1. Indicate which foods are sources of protein, calcium, and sodium in the diet.
2. If patient does not prefer milk, show how other sources of calcium may be used in the diet.
3. Alcohol should be avoided unless permitted by the doctor.
4. Discuss control of hyperglycemia where appropriate.
5. Patients should learn self-medication and when to seek medical attention.
6. Discuss problems with long-term obesity and hypercholesterolemia.

For More Information

American Council on Transplantation
700 N. Fairfax Str., Suite 505
Alexandria, VA 22314
(703) 836-4301

INBORN ERRORS OF RENAL METABOLISM: VITAMIN-D-RESISTANT RICKETS, HARTNUP DISEASE, AND POLYCYSTIC KIDNEY DISEASE

Usual Hospital Stay

4–5 days.

Notation

Vitamin-D-resistant rickets is a hypophosphatemia associated with decreased renal tubular reabsorption of P. Vitamin D is abnormally metabolized, and calcium absorption is decreased. Rickets or osteomalacia occurs. Often the occurrence is familial.

Hartnup disease is a rare familial condition characterized by hyperaminoaciduria. It results from the homozygous manifestation of a non-X-linked rare allele. The tryptophan-loading test is used to diagnose the disease. A red, scaly rash is seen on the face, neck, hands, and legs (symptoms resemble those of dietary pellagra). Emotional instability and delirium may exist in affected persons.

Polycystic kidney disease (PKD) is an inherited disorder which causes bilateral cysts in the kidneys and may also affect the liver, pancreas, colon, blood, and heart valves. 1/400 people have PKD, with symptoms of back or side pain, HTN, hematuria, and chronic headaches.

Objectives

1. Correct the malabsorption of vitamin D, calcium, and phosphorus in persons with vitamin-D-resistant rickets.
2. Correct behavioral side effects of persons with Hartnup disease.
3. With PKD, prevent/treat RF, nausea, vomiting, anorexia.

Dietary Recommendations

1. *Vitamin-D-resistant rickets.* The diet should include 4800 IU of 1,25-vitamin D_3 plus oral phosphate in a quantity of 1.5–2 g phosphorus per day. Ensure that the diet provides adequate amounts of calcium. Be careful about toxicity!
2. *Hartnup Disease.* Patient should be given oral nicotinamide therapy (40–200 mg per day) plus a high protein diet or supplements. Oral neomycin should also be given.
3. For PKD, no definite diet is warranted; modify according to symptoms.

Profile

Birthweight, present wt	Serum vitamin D Length	Tryptophan-loading test
Growth %	Alb	IBW/HBW
BUN	Ca^{++}	Creat
H & H	P	Alk phos
Ultrasound	BP	

Patient Education

1. Explain to the patient those measures appropriate to the specific condition.
2. Encourage regular doctor visits and visits to the nutritionist.

Section 17
Enteral and Parenteral Nutrition

ENTERAL NUTRITION

Usual Hospital Stay

Varies by condition.

Notation

Enteral nutrition involves nutritional support via nasogastric tube, orogastric tube, esophagostomy, gastrostomy, duodenostomy, or jejunostomy for patients who are unable to consume adequate nutrients and fluid orally. Enteral nutrition is safer than parenteral nutrition and is also more economical. Enteral nutrition also yields better nutrient utilization by helping to maintain gut mucosal integrity.

Candidates must have a functioning GI tract.

Enteral nutrition has advantages—IgA prevents absorption of enteric antigens. IgA increases with enteral nutrition but not with parenteral.

Objectives

1. Meet 100% RDAs for vitamins. Identify and monitor needs for amino acids, carbohydrate, fat, minerals and water.
2. Assess key factors (such as consciousness, respiratory distress, nausea, vomiting, aspiration tendency, abdominal distention, diarrhea, abdominal cramping, weight changes, esophageal reflexes, hydration status, constipation, abnormal lab values, lactose or gluten intolerances. Alter TF accordingly.

519

3. Monitor feeding tube selection according to placement, patency, type, location (mouth/nose/ostomy). Always use the least invasive method unless the tube will be placed for a long period of time.
4. Feeding content selection includes an evaluation of amount ordered vs. amount tolerated; type of feeding needed by the individual and the disorder; viscosity; calories/ml; feeding temperature; amount of residual from previous feedings; and metabolic utilization potentials.
5. Monitor patient positioning. Head of bed should be elevated 60–90° during feeding. For unconscious patient, turn to left side. Check tube placement. If residuals are greater than 100 ml, hold feeding. Replace aspirate to reduce loss of electrolytes and gastric juices.
6. Utilize feeding at proper temperatures. Remove the feeding from refrigeration 10–15 minutes before feeding. Do not leave extra feeding at room temperature for long.
7. Keep patient on right side or keep head of bed elevated for 30 minutes after feeding to prevent aspiration.
8. Patient should be weighed on the same scale at the same time every other day. Similar clothing should be worn by the patient.
9. Adjust formula, as needed, for constipation, diarrhea, abdominal distention, and other signs of intolerance. Type, volume and concentration may be altered.
10. Fiber-added formulas, like Enrich, may be appropriate with diarrhea or constipation, especially if the formula will be used over time.
11. Adding a few drops of blue food coloring to a formula can help in distinguishing between lung aspirate and TF formula.
12. Calorie goals are often 150:1 in relationship to nitrogen needs. Some conditions will warrant alterations in this pattern (e.g., hepatic or renal failures).
13. Maintenance levels of vitamins, minerals and essential fatty acids must also be provided and monitored, especially if not given with the chosen solution.
14. Correct albumin levels to normal to ↑ GI tolerance to EN.

Dietary Recommendations

1. Calculate BEE and protein and nutrient needs according to age, sex, and medical status. Fluid is often calculated as 1 ml/kcal.
2. Check regularly regarding tolerance and side effects; alter formula content as appropriate.
3. Sample new products to determine costs, taste and convenience for home EN, as well as for institutions.
4. Offer water or flush tubing with water (25–100 ml) every 3–6 hours. Estimate needs at 30–35 ml free H_2O/kg BW, or 1 ml/kg.
5. In catabolic stress, glutamine-rich products may be beneficial, such as "Impact."

Profile

Ht, wt	Na$^+$, K$^+$, Cl$^-$	Pco$_2$, Po$_2$
Alb	Diarrhea	IBW/HBW
Transferrin	BUN, Creat	TLC
Chol, trig	Chest x-ray	PO$_4$
Ca^{++}, Mg^{++}	Temp	Urine acetone
Gluc	PT	Other parameters as
I & O	Nausea, vomiting	needed
H & H	Serum insulin	

Medications

1. Drugs added to the tube feeding can greatly alter absorption of both the drugs themselves and the nutrients of the feeding. Monitor carefully.
2. *Metoclopramide* has been used to prevent GE reflux and aspiration in tube-fed patients. Administration ten minutes prior to insertion seems to increase success rate of intubation. Gastric motility and relaxation of the pyloric sphincter are improved with this drug.
3. Antidiarrheal drugs (kaolin [Kaopectate], Lomotil, etc.) can be used to slow GI motility.

Patient Education

1. Safe preparation of tube feeding, if used at home, is essential. No more than 4-hr supply should be hanging at any time.
2. The patient/caretaker should be taught to review signs and symptoms of intolerance; how to manage simple problems; where to call for guidance; and when to call the physician.
3. At least one follow-up phone call or home visit should be made to the HEN (home enteral nutrition) patient.
4. If banana flakes are added to control diarrhea, monitor signs of hyperkalemia. Discuss this problem with the patient/caretaker.
5. The patient should be allowed/encouraged to maintain social contacts at mealtime.

Table 17–1.
Sample Formulas

1. Blenderized—homemade (watch avidin/biotin problems, Salmonella risks); Compleat, Vitaneed
2. Standard—Ensure, Osmolite, Meritene, Sustacal, Isocal
3. Added Fiber—Enrich, Susta II, Jevity
4. Extra Calories—Ensure Plus, Sustacal HC, Magnacal
5. High Nitrogen—Ensure HN, Ensure Plus HN, Precision HN, Osmolite HN, Isocal HCN
6. Carefully Altered—Precision LR, Travasorb

7. Clear Liquid Additive—Citrotein, Nutrex, Ross SLD, Polycose, Controlyte
8. Predigested—Criticare HN, Travasorb HN, Travasorb STD, Vital HN, Vivonex STD or HN or TEN
9. Disease-Specific—Amin Aid, Hepatic Aid, Pulmocare, Stresstein, Traumacal, Traum-Aid, Travasorb Renal, Travasorb Hepatic.

Table 17–2.
Homemade Blenderized Tube Feeding (Shils/Bloch)
1 cal/ml (2500 ml total volume)

> 10 g strained oatmeal
> 50 g dextri-maltose
> 50 g instant dry milk
> 20 g strained liver
> 568 g strained beef
> 484 g strained green beans
> 402 g strained applesauce
> 85 ml vegetable oil
> 200 ml orange juice
> 300 ml whole milk
> 500 ml water

This product yields 1312 mg calcium, 1518 mg phosphorus, 24 mg iron, 7582 IU vitamin A, 2.67 mg thiamine, 3.7 mg riboflavin, 27 mg niacin, 163 mg vitamin C, 2550 mg sodium, 4150 mg potassium.

Table 17–3.
Phone Numbers for Major Enteral Feeding Companies
American McGaw: Irvine, CA (714) 261-6360
Biosearch Medical: (201) 722-5000
Cambridge Scientific Industries: (800) 638-9566
Lactaid: (609) 645-7500
Mead Johnson: (812) 429-5000
Norwich Eaton: (800) 446-6654
Nutrex: (408) 554-8600
O'Brien Pharmaceuticals: (800) 345-6039
Ross Labs: (614) 227-3333
Sandoz: (612) 925-2100
Travacare: (312) 940-6524

Table 17–4.

Key Enteral Issues*

FEEDING SITE SELECTION

Nasogastric

Nasoduodenal

Nasojejunal

Gastrostomy—surgical incision or endoscopically placed percutaneous gastrostomy (PEG) Jejunostomy

Esophagostomy

FORMULA SELECTION

Substrates—CHO, protein, fat (consider patient's ability to digest and absorb nutrients)

Elemental versus intact formulas—no superiority has been documented for elemental; if not sure of ability to digest fats, use MCTs (e.g. Osmolite or Isocal)

Tolerance factors—osmolality, calorie and nutrient densities, pH, residue content (in general, more free water is needed with a more concentrated formula)

FLUID NEEDS

Generally, 1 ml/kcal (1 cc/kcal) is recommended, unless patient needs fluid restriction

20–40 cc/kg can also be used as an estimation

DELIVERY METHODS†

Patient intolerance is key—ability to meet needs without complications like nausea, vomiting, diarrhea or glucosuria.

Bolus—set amount given every 3–4 hours as a rapid syringe feeding

Intermittent—prescribed amount given every 3–4 hours by drip over 20–30 minutes (beneficial metabolically?)

Continuous—controlled delivery of feeding over 24 hours

Cycled—controlled delivery over 8–16 hours, allowing some rest periods for the patient during the 24 hours.

---

* Adapted from Romberau, J., and Caldwell, M.: *Enteral and Tube Feeding,* Vol. 1. Philadelphia: W. B. Saunders, 1984.

† Cyclic intermittent perhaps best.

For More Information

American Society for Parenteral and Enteral Nutrition
8630 Fenton St., Suite 412
Silver Spring, MD 20910

NOTES

PARENTERAL NUTRITION

Usual Hospital Stay

Varies by condition, but a typical TPN patient requires 10–14 days on the average.

Notation

Parenteral nutrition is used when an oral or enteral mode is inadequate (e.g., short bowel syndrome, malabsorption, fractures, major burns); when it should be avoided (IBD, GI obstruction); or when it is dangerous (with a high risk of aspiration).

Parenteral nutrition refers to the system of feeding which bypasses the GI tract. Central PN, partial PN, and total PN are noted in the literature and available in practice. In general, PN is more expensive than EN and oral modes.

In most cases, gradual weaning from PN to EN or oral nutrition is required. Without weaning, the patient is at greater risk from a sudden depletion of total calories consumed. Note that TPN is never an emergency and is *never without potential risks*.

Objectives

1. Maintain or replete lean body mass, avoiding or correcting malnutrition and its consequences.
2. Determine appropriate patient requirements for calories, protein, vitamins, minerals and fluid. Fat and CHO make the balance of nonprotein calories to be given.
3. Maintain aseptic procedures in all techniques for safe nutritional support.
4. Prevent or correct all side effects of parenteral nutrition (i.e., weight gain over 2 lbs or 1 kg daily indicating SIADH or fluid overload; elevated temperature or sepsis; elevated glucose levels; shortness of breath; tightness of chest; anemia; nausea and vomiting; jaundice; allergy to protein content of the solutions; pneumothorax; cardiac arrhythmias; metabolic bone disease, etc.).
5. Wean back to enteral or oral intake when and if feasible.
6. Manage fluid and extraneous losses as needed.

Dietary Recommendations

1. Calculate needs for parenteral nutrition related to present oral and enteral intake (calories, protein, fluid, vitamins and minerals). Usually 2000–2500 kcal per day can be provided to an adult. 30–35 kcal/kg BW or IBW can be calculated, starting with 20–25 kcal/kg.
2. If tolerated, 4% total kcal should be given as fat to prevent EFAD. A 20% lipid emulsion yields 2 kcal/ml.
3. Be careful not to overfeed because of resulting CO_2 production, etc. Maximum glucose oxidation equals 6 mg/kg/minute.
4. Provide weaning when the patient is ready; use tube feedings for interim nourishment as necessary. Progress to liquids and solids when the patient is ready (e.g., bowel sounds, gag reflex, etc.).
5. Monitor phosphate needs from anabolism, malnutrition, etc.
6. Glutamine infusion may be helpful in IBD or stressed patients but *not* in hepatic encephalopathy.

Profile

Ht, wt, IBW/HBW	BEE/REE	Wt changes
Gluc	Chol, trig	H & H
Alb, prealbumin	Transferrin	Serum Fe, B_{12}
RBP	PT	SGOT, SGPT
K^+, Na^+	Ca^{++}, Mg^{++}	WBCs, TLC
BUN, creat	N balance	I & O
Alk phos	P	Ammonia
Acetone	Amylase, lipase	Urine tests
Chest x-ray	Signs of malnutrition	Other parameters

Patient Education

1. Discuss with patient/caretakers the goals of the parenteral nutrition, especially if home TPN will be used.
2. Teach weaning processes when and if the patient is ready.
3. Home TPN (HPN) requires meticulous catheter care. Infection control measures should be discussed.
4. Solutions, if prepared at home, must be prepared under sterile conditions. For most persons, prepackaged solutions are desirable.
5. Discuss signs and symptoms of systems failure: when to call the doctor, when to call the dietitian, and when to call the pharmacist or nurse.
6. Discuss anxiety, anger or adaptation to PN and oral deprivation.

Comment

1. D_5W = osmolality of 252 mOsm per liter.
   $D_{10}W$ = osmolality of 504 mOsm per liter

$D_{20}W$ = osmolality of 1008 mOsm per liter
$D_{40}W$ = osmolality of 2016 mOsm per liter

2. Dextrose in TPN = 3.4 kcal/g, not 4.
3. Vitamin A is only 1/4–1/3 available because it attaches to the plastic bags. Vitamin E is also a problem. Vitamin D is given as ergocalciferol in PN form. Vitamin K is generally only given weekly.
4. Water-soluble vitamins are often given as: 3 mg thiamine, 100 mg vitamin C, 400 μg folic acid, 5 μg B_{12}, 60 μg biotin, 3.6 mg riboflavin, 4 mg vitamin B_6, 40 mg niacin.
5. Copper may be given as 0.5–1.5 mg; pantothenic acid as 15 mg in adults.

Table 17–5.
Undesirable Practices Affecting the Nutritional Health of Hospital Patients*

1. Failure to record height and weight on admission; lack of weight curves
2. Rotation of staff at frequent intervals
3. Diffusion of responsibility for patient care
4. Prolonged use of glucose and saline intravenous feedings
5. Failure to observe or record patient food intake
6. Withholding meals because of diagnostic tests
7. Use of tube feedings of inadequate amount and uncertain composition especially under unsanitary conditions
8. Ignorance of the composition of nutritional products (vitamins, etc.)
9. Failure to recognize altered needs as a result of injury, illness, trauma, sepsis or surgery
10. Performance of surgery without ascertaining optimal nutritional status and failure to replete stores after surgery
11. Failure to appreciate the role of nutrition in the prevention of, and recovery from, infection; especially with unwarranted reliance on antibiotics
12. Lack of communication between physician and dietitian
13. Delay of nutritional support until the patient is in a state of advanced depletion, which may be irreversible
14. Limited availability of laboratory tests to assess nutritional status.

---

* Adapted from Butterworth, C.: The skeleton in the hospital closet. *Nutrition Today*, March/April 1974, p. 8.

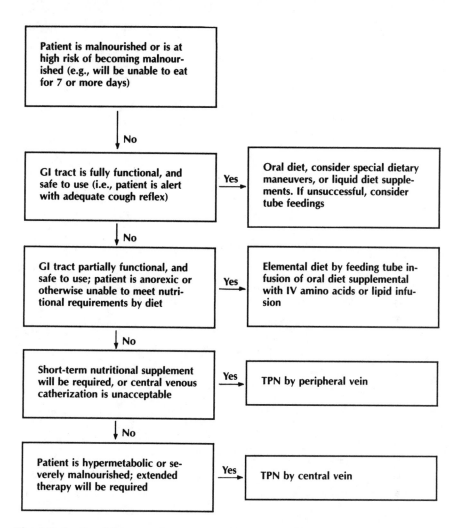

Fig. 17–1. Decision tree for Intervention in Malnutrition.

Reprinted by permission from Willard, M.: *Nutritional Management for the Practicing Physician*. Reading, MA: Addison-Wesley, 1982, p. 42.

Appendix A:
Nutritional Review

CHANGES IN MUSCLE MASS, BONE, AND BODY FAT IN DIFFERENT LIFE STAGES OR DISEASE CONDITIONS

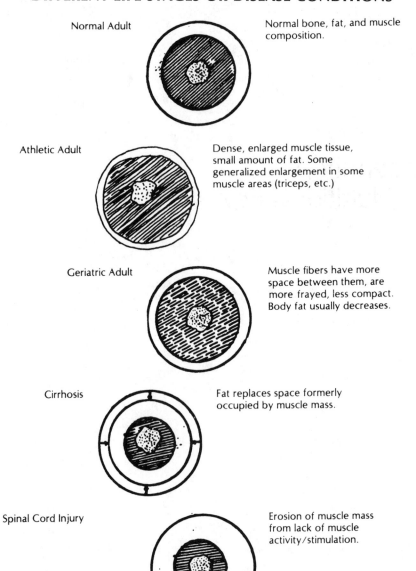

Normal Adult — Normal bone, fat, and muscle composition.

Athletic Adult — Dense, enlarged muscle tissue, small amount of fat. Some generalized enlargement in some muscle areas (triceps, etc.)

Geriatric Adult — Muscle fibers have more space between them, are more frayed, less compact. Body fat usually decreases.

Cirrhosis — Fat replaces space formerly occupied by muscle mass.

Spinal Cord Injury — Erosion of muscle mass from lack of muscle activity/stimulation.

☐ Fat; ▦ Bone; and ▨ Muscle.

Fig. A–1. Changes in muscle mass, bone, and body fat in different life stages or disease conditions. From Brown W.J., et al.: The distribution of body fat in relation to habitual activity. *Ann Hum Biol* **4:**537, 1977

Table A–1.
Carbohydrate and Fiber Classifications
Generally, over 90% CHO is absorbed from a mixed diet.

	FOOD SOURCES
Monosaccharides	
Glucose	Corn syrup, honey, fruits, vegetables
Fructose	Honey, fruits, vegetables
Galactose	Milk sugar
Mannose	Of little nutritional value; found in poorly digested fruit structures
Disaccharides	
Glucose + Fructose = Sucrose	Table sugar, cane or beet sugars, maple sugar, some natural fruits and vegetables
Glucose + Galactose = Lactose	Milk, cream, whey
Glucose + Glucose = Maltose	Malt sugar, sprouting grains, partially digested starch
Polysaccharides	
Insoluble Fibers*—Cellulose	Soybean hulls, fruit membranes, legumes, carrots, other vegetables
—Lignin	Wheat straw, alfalfa stems, tannins, cottonseed hulls
—Cutin	Apple or tomato peels, seeds in berries, peanut or almond skins, onion skins
Soluble Fibers†—Hemicellulose	Corn or barley or oat hulls, wheat and corn brans, soy fiber concentrate
—Pectin	Citrus pulp, apple pulp, sugar beet pulp, cabbage and Brassica foods, legumes, alfalfa leaves, sunflower heads
—Gum	Oats, gum arabic, guar gum from legumes, psyllium from plantains, xanthan from prickly ash trees

---

* Insoluble fibers (bran, cereal, vegetables) have no effect on serum cholesterol but are useful in reducing appendicitis, constipation, diverticulosis, and perhaps colon cancer. Mineral depletion may also occur.
† Soluble fibers (fruit, barley, oat bran, legumes) decrease serum cholesterol by altering related enzymes; stabilize blood glucose levels; help maintain mineral nutriture. They have no effect on fecal bulk or transit time, and may be related to changes in tumor growth in colon (latter is being researched at this time).
Adapted From Crosby, L.: Fiber: Standardized Sources, *Nutr. Cancer* 1:15, 1978; and Howe, P.: *Basic Nutrition in Health and Disease,* 7th ed. Philadelphia: W.B. Saunders, 1981.

FATS, LIPIDS, AND FATTY ACID REVIEW

The usual American diet contains 40% fat by kcals; a better goal is under 35% daily. Fats are carriers for fat-soluble vitamins and essential fatty acids; they are part of cell membranes; insulating agents; organ padding; and rich sources of calories. Generally, 95% of fat from the diet is absorbed.

1–2% of calories should be available as linoleic acid, which prevents EFA deficiency. At risk are people with low body fat stores, very malnourished persons, and premature LBW infants.

Lipase is needed for LCT (triglyceride) breakdown into free fatty acids (FFA). Most fat emulsions contain LCTs and can compromise immune function, elevate serum lipids, impair alveolar diffusion capacity, or decrease reticular endothelial system.

MCTs are transported to the liver via the portal vein, therefore not requiring micelle or chylomicron formation. They are now being investigated for IV fat use.

Table A–2.
Fatty Acids

Family	Fatty Acid	Key Food Sources
omega-3	Linolenic acid (polyunsaturated)	Vegetable oils (soybean, rapeseed) and nuts
	Eicosapentanoic acid* (EPA)	Fish, especially salmon, mackerel, eel, tuna, and herring
	Docosahexanoic acid (DHA)	Fish (same as EPA)
omega-6	Linoleic acid	Vegetable oils
	Arachidonic acid*	Animal tissues
omega-9	Oleic acid (monounsaturated)	Vegetable oils

* EPA and arachidonic acids are transformed into eicosanoids for prostaglandin and leukotriene and thromboxane and prostacyclin synthesis. Thromboxanes are vasoconstrictors (platelets); leukotrienes are for chemotaxis (leukocytes). Drugs like antihypertensives, diuretics, anti-inflammatories and anti-thrombotics interfere with this process. Prostacyclins are vasodilators (blood vessels). The research lately is studying the effects of precursors of these eicosanoids.

From Anderson, P., and Sprecher, H.: Omega-3 fatty acids in nutrition and health. *Ross Dietetic Currents 14(2)*, 1987.

Other important lipids: phospholipids (lecithins, cephalins, sphingomyelins); glycolipids (cerebrosides, gangliosides); sulfolipids; lipoproteins; sterols (cholesterol, steroid hormones, vitamin D, bile salts); and fat-soluble vitamins A, E and K.

Table A–3.
Intravenous Fat Emulsions

Product:	Intralipid	Liposyn
Manufacturer:	Cutter	Abbott
Concentration:	10%	10%
Fat source:	Soybean oil (10%)	Safflower oil (10%)
Component fatty acids:	Linoleic (54%)	Linoleic (77%)
	Oleic (26%)	Oleic (13%)
	Palmitic (9%)	Palmitic (9%)
	Linolenic (8%)	Stearic (2.5%)
Other additives:	Egg yolk phospholipid (1.2%)	Egg yolk phospholipid (1.2%)
	Glycerin (2.25%)	Glycerin (2.5%)
	Water	Water
Kcal/ml:	1.1	1.1
Osmolarity (mOsm/liter):	280	300

Adapted from Schneider, H., et al.: *Nutritional Support of Medical Practice,* 2nd ed. Philadelphia: Harper & Row, 1983, p. 676.

Choline

Choline is a widely distributed phospholipid.

Functions. Lipotrophic agents; some role in short-term memory with neurotransmitter (acetylcholine); component of sphingomyelin; emulsifier in bile; component of pulmonary surfactant (CO_2/O_2 exchange).

Sources. Eggs, soybeans, peanuts, and liver.

Note. Lecithin is one form of choline precursor, as is phosphatidylcholine. Liver can synthesize/resynthesize. Average daily intake is 400–900 mg. High fat intake accelerates a deficiency.

AMINO ACID CLASSIFICATION

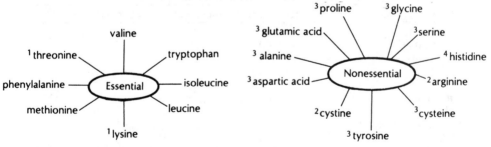

Fig. A–2. Amino acid classification.

[1] *Totally indispensable.* Absolutely no precursors.
[2] *Semi-indispensable.* Can reduce dietary requirement for some other AAs, but in some cases may be indispensable themselves.
[3] *Completely dispensable:* made freely by the body.
[4] Histidine is now considered to be an EAA (for TPN especially. 3-methyl histidine is a good marker of muscle breakdown.
From McMurray, W.C.[2] *Essentials of Human Metabolism,* 2nd ed. Philadelphia: Harper & Row, 1983, p. 209.

To produce the nonessential amino acids from dietary intake of the essentials, it is recommended that the limited amino acids be consumed within 3 hours of each other. Protein synthesis requires 19 AAs. An insufficient amount of any one may impede or slow formation of the polypeptide chain. Foods of high biologic value contain approximately 40% EAAs.

Table A–4.
Individual Essential Amino Acid Requirements and Percentage of Total Protein Needs of Infants and Adults

Amino	Requirements	
	Infant	*Adult*
Isoleucine	6.5%	2.4%
Leucine	9.0%	3.0%
Lysine	5.6%	2.4%
Methionine & cystine	3.0%	3.0%
Phenylalanine & tyrosine	5.3%	3.3%
Threonine	3.9%	1.5%
Tryptophan	1.1%	0.7%
Valine	5.6%	3.0%
Total essential	40%	19%

From *Symposium on Total Parenteral Nutrition*. Chicago, American Medical Association, January 17–19, 1972.

Utilization of EAAs will be curtailed/limited if any single EAA is deficient.

Protein requirement is inversely related to calories when the latter are deficient. Generally, over 90% of protein is absorbed from the diet.

For valine, leucine and isoleucine, the requirement of each is increased by excess of the other BCAAs.

Biologic Value of Food Proteins: 100% would be ideal.

Chemical Score and Net Protein Utilization Values of Common Foods

Protein	New Pattern Chemical Score	NPU Measured in Rats
Whole egg	100	94
Human milk	100	87
Cow's milk	95	82
Soya bean	74	65
Sesame	50	54
Groundnut	65	47
Cottonseed	81	59
Maize	49	52
Millet	63	44
Rice, polished	67	59
Wheat, whole	53	48

Adapted from Joint FAO/WHO Ad Hoc Expert Committee, Energy and Protein Requirements: WHO Tech. Rep. No. 522, Geneva, 1973, p. 67.

Table A–5.
Total Parenteral Nutrition: Essential Amino Acids and Protein Needs (mg/kg) by Body Weight in Humans

Requirements	Infants	Children (10–12 years)	Adults
Histidine	25	—	—
Isoleucine (BCAA)	111	28	12
Leucine (BCAA)	153	49	16
Lysine	96	59	12
Methionine and cystine	50	27	10
Phenylalanine and tyrosine	90	27	16
Threonine	66	34	8
Tryptophan	19	4	3
Valine (BCAA)	95	33	14
	Total: 680	261	91

From McMurray, W.: *Essentials of Human Metabolism*, 2nd ed. Philadelphia: Harper & Row, 1983.

Average Total Protein Needs

Infants. 1700 mg/kg body weight (40% essential).
Children. 700 mg/kg body weight (36% essential).
Adults. 425 mg/kg body weight (19% essential).
Oral and parenteral sources of essential amino acids are currently considered to be the same for required intake.

Table A–6.
Mineral and Vitamin Needs in Total Parenteral Nutrition

Mineral	Child	Adult
Sodium	3–5 mEq/kg	60 + mEq
Potassium	2–5 mEq/kg	60 + mEq
Calcium	1–4 mEq/kg	10–15 mEq
Phosphate	0.7–3 mmol/kg	20–50 mmol
Magnesium	0.3–2 mEq/kg	8–20 mEq

From Butterworth, C. E. Jr., Weinsier, R.: Handbook of Clinical Nutrition, p. 98. St. Louis, C. V. Mosby Co., 1981.

Mineral	Child	Adult (Stable)
Zinc	100–300 μ/kg	2.5–4 mg
Copper	20 μ/kg	0.1–1.5 mg
Chromium	0.14–0.12 μ/kg	10–15 μg
Manganese	2–10 μ/kg	0.15–0.8 mg
Iodine	5 μ/kg	500–100 μg

From American Medical Association: Guidelines for Trace Element Preparations for Parenteral Use. *JAMA* 241:2051, 1979.

Recommended Intravenous Vitamin Allowances and Contents of Commercial Preparations

	Recommended Daily Allowance		MVI (Multivitamin Infusion) Concentrate (2.5 ml)	Berocca-C (2 ml)	Folbesyn (2 ml)	Betalin Complex F.C. (2 mil)	Solu-B-Forte (1 mil)
	Newborns and Infants	Adults					
Thiamin (mg)	0.04	1.5	25	10	10	12.5	25
Riboflavin (mg)	0.4	1.7	5	10	10	3	5
Niacin (mg)	5	.9	50	80	75	50	125
Pyridoxine (mg)	0.3	2.0	7.5	20	5	5	5
Vitamin B_{12} (µg)	0.3	2.0	—	—	15	—	—
Folate (µg)	25	200	—	—	3,000	—	—
Pantothenate (mg)	2	4	12.5	20	10	2.5	50
Biotin (µg)	10	30	—·	200	—	—	—
Ascorbate (mg)	30	60	250	100	300	75	100
Vitamin A (µg)	375	1000	1,500	—	—	—	—
D_3 Cholecalciferol (µg)	7.5	5	12.5	—	—	—	—
Vitamin E (mg)	3	10	2.5	—	—	—	—
Vitamin K (µg)	5	80	—	—	—	—	—

From Butterworth, C.E., Jr., and Weinsier R.: Handbook of Clinical Nutrition, St. Louis: C.V. Mosby, 1981, p. 96; based on data from Wretlind, A.: Nutr Betab *14 (Suppl.)*:1, 1972; updated for 1989 RDAs.

MINERALS

Boron

Roles. Mineral metabolism in animals and man.
Sources. Drinking water; fruits, tubers, legumes.
Note. Protein foods and grains are low.

Calcium

Roles. Bones, teeth; nerve irritability; muscle contraction; heart rhythm; blood coagulation; enzymes; osmotic pressure; intercellular cement. 60% is bound to protein, mostly albumin. 30–60% absorption occurs with intakes of 400–1,000 mg.
Sources. Milk, cheese, other dairy/milk products; dried fruit; green leafy vegetables; molasses; tofu. Phytates and excessive protein decrease absorption.

Calcium Substitutes for Milk

1 cup oysters = 226 mg
3 oz salmon = 167 mg
3 oz sardines = 372 mg
1 cup almonds = 332 mg
1 cup Brazil nuts = 260 mg
1 cup dates = 130 mg

1 cup peanuts = 107 mg
1 cup pork and beans = 138 mg
1 cup dried apricots = 100 mg
1 cup cranberry sauce = 104 mg
1 tablespoon blackstrap molasses = 137 mg

Chloride

Roles. Digestion (HCl in stomach); acid-base balance; O_2/CO_2 exchange in RBCs; fluid balance.
Sources. Table salt. Salt substitutes containing KCl.

Chromium

Roles. Insulin molecule; some inhibition of vascular disorders from aortic plaque; fatty acid and cholesterol metabolism; normal glucose metabolism; nucleic acid stability. Absorption ranges from 1–22%.

Sources. Brewer's yeast, whole grains; eggs; vegetable oil; shortening; nuts; meats; dairy products.

Note. Phytates and oxalates can decrease absorption.

Cobalt

Roles. Treatment of some anemias; part of structure of vitamin B_{12}; some role in immunity.

Sources. Green, leafy vegetables; seafood, meats, grains, cereals.

Note. Cow's milk is very low. Over 50% of dietary cobalt is absorbed.

Copper

Roles. Skeletal development; immunity; formation of red blood cells; phospholipid synthesis; electron transport; pigmentation; aortic elasticity; connective tissue formation; CNS structure; deficiency may yield anemia, aortic aneurysms, elevated cholesterol levels. Copper is tightly bound to ceruloplasmin.

Sources. Liver, kidney; nuts; legumes; oysters; yeast; cocoa; and eggs.

Note. Milk is low in copper. Daily intake of copper in the United States is 2–5 mg; however, many persons have a lower intake than this because fresh foods are low in copper. About 30–40% of oral intake is absorbed. Deficiency is rare in adults, except with estrogen use. Absorption is enhanced by acid, decreased by calcium. Excesses may oppose vitamin A absorption. Requirement is increased by excessive zinc intake.

Fluoride

Roles. Prevention of calcified aortas, dental caries, collapsed vertebrae, osteoporosis (some controversy exists in regard to fluoride's etiologic role in osteoporosis); formation of hydroxyapatite; and enamel growth.

Sources. Gelatin; organ meats; seafood; infant foods to which bone meal has been added; dairy products; cereals, grains. 80–90% of oral intake is absorbed.

Note. Excess can result in mottling of teeth or neurological problems.

Iodine

Roles. Energy metabolism; proper thyroid functioning; normal growth and reproduction; prevention of goiter.

Sources. Seaweed and seafoods; cream (in milk); eggs, plant leaves (broccoli, spinach, turnip greens); cranberries; legumes.

Note. Excess may depress thyroid activity, or can lead to hyperthyroidism.

Iron

Roles. Responsible for carrying oxygen to cells through hemoglobin and myoglobin; skeletal muscle functioning; cognitive functioning; leukocyte functions and immunity.

Sources. Lean meat; eggs; dried beans; dried fruits; molasses; liver; dried peas; cocoa; baking chocolate; green vegetables (leaf lettuce, spinach); outer layer of grains; potatoes (especially if eaten frequently).

Note. Oxalic, tannic, and phytic acids can reduce absorption; sulfur amino acids and vitamin C increase absorption. Serum iron is largely bound to transferrin. 15–25% of oral intake of heme iron is absorbed (meat, fish, poultry); 2–20% of oral intake of nonheme iron is absorbed (legumes, grains, and fruit).

Magnesium

Roles. Nerve transmission; muscle contraction; protein synthesis; enzyme activation (ADP, ATP); glucose utilization; prevention of atherosclerosis; bone matrix; normal Na^+/K^+ pump.

Sources. Cocoa, chocolate; nuts; soybeans, dried beans, peas; beet greens; whole grains, especially wheat germ or bran.

Note. Intake from a meal may be 45–55% absorbed. Beware of excess phytates.

Manganese

Roles. Polysaccharide and fatty acid metabolism; enzyme activation; skeletal development; some role in hypertension is possible; fertility and reproduction.

Sources. Tea, coffee; blueberries; beans; dry legumes; nuts; wheat germ; spinach.

Note. Souces of manganese are plant foods, not animal foods. Beware of excess calcium or magnesium supplementation. Manganese and iron complete for pathways. Less than 5% is absorbed from diet.

Molybdenum

Roles. Flavoproteins; copper antagonist; component of sulfite oxidase and xanthine oxidase.

Sources. Legumes; cereal grains; dark green/leafy vegetables; animal organs; meats.

Note. 30–70% of intake is absorbed.

Nickel

Roles. Growth, reproduction; iron and zinc metabolism; hematopoiesis; DNA and RNA; enzyme activation.

Sources. Grains, vegetables.

Note. Less than 10% is absorbed. It is transported by serum albumin.

Phosphorus

Roles. Energy metabolism (ADP, ATP); fat, amino acid and CHO metabolism; Ca^{++} regulation; vitamin utilization; bones and teeth; osmotic pressure; DNA coding; buffer salts; fatty acid transport; oxygen transport and release; leukocyte phagocytosis; microbial resistance.

Sources. Meat; fish; eggs; dried beans and nuts; whole grains; enriched breads; milk, cheese; peas, corn.

Note. Excessive intake of soft drinks increases phosphorus intake, often causing an unbalanced intake of calcium. 70% of oral intake is absorbed.

Potassium

Roles. Nerves and muscles; glycolysis; glycogen formation; protein synthesis and utilization; acid-base balance; cellular enzyme functioning.

Sources. Fruits and vegetables. Each of the foods listed below contains over 500 mg per serving.

1 teaspoon cream of tartar (on cereal, etc.)
1 cup prune or tomato juice
1 1/4 cup orange or citrus juice
one medium banana (1 small banana, 400 mg)
seven to eight dates or four figs
seven large prunes or 1/2 cup dark raisins
six fresh apricots
1 1/2 cups milk (any kind)

1/2 cantaloupe
1 cup broccoli
3/4 cup winter squash
1 large white or sweet potato
1/2 avocado (600 mg)
2 tablespoons molasses
1/2 cup nuts
3/4 cup dry beans, cooked
1/2 teaspoon salt substitute (most brands)

Note. Excess can lead to muscular weakness, arrhythmias or death.

Selenium

Roles. Protein biosynthesis; sparing of vitamin E; growth; nonspecific antioxidant; protein matrix of teeth; protection against mercury toxicity; glutathione peroxidase; fertility; liver function; heart muscle function.

Sources. Most foods if grown in selenium-rich soil, seafood, meats, dairy products, kidney, liver, and wheat germ. Over 50% dietary intake is absorbed.

Silicon

Roles. Normal bone growth and calcification; normal collagen and connective tissue formation (especially in the presence of Ca^{++}); development of atherosclerosis with decreased silicon in aorta is experimental.

Sources. Most foods—only minute amounts are needed. Grains and beer are good sources.

Sodium

Roles. Nerves; muscles; acid-base balance; glucose transport into cells. Sodium is the major extracellular fluid cation.

Sources. Milk, cheese, eggs; meat, fish, poultry; beets, carrots, celery, spinach, chard; seasoned salts; baking powder and soda; table salt (NaCl); many drugs and preservatives; some drinking water.

Note. Over 95% from a mixed diet is absorbed. Excess may lead to HPN, heart failure, or edema.

Sulfur

Roles. Amino acids (methionine, cystine, cysteine); thiamine molecule; coenzyme A; biotin; connective tissue metabolism; penicillin; sulfa drugs.

Sources. Meat, poultry, fish; eggs; legumes; Brassica family vegetables (broccoli, cabbage, etc.).

Vanadium

Roles. Possible role in growth, lipid metabolism, and reproduction.
Sources. Leafy green vegetables, cereal grains.

Zinc

Roles. ACTH-stimulated steroidogenesis in adrenals; fat, CHO, protein and nucleic acid metabolism; CO_2 transport; amino acid breakdown from peptides; oxidation of vitamin A; reproduction; growth; enzymes,* wound healing; catalyst for hydrogenation; taste acuity; immunity; night vision; sexual maturation.

Sources. Seafoods (especially oysters); milk, liver; oatmeal; whole corn; wheat germ; yeast; whole wheat or rye bread; meat, fish; fruits; eggs; green, leafy vegetables.

Note. In children with zinc deficiency, severe growth depression is seen. The average American diet contains 10–15 mg daily. Animal sources are better utilized—vegetarians need to be monitored for zinc deficiency. Phytates and excess fiber can decrease absorption by forming complexes. Phosphate salts also decrease absorption. 10–40% from meals is absorbed.

---

* Such as alkaline phosphatase, carboxypeptidase and alcohol dehydrogenase.

Table A–7.
Adverse and Toxic Effects of Excessive Intakes of Mineral Nutrients

Nutrient	Excessive Acute Oral or Enteral Intake	Excessively Elevated Circulating Concentration	Excessive Tissue/Total-Body Accumulation
Calcium	Bitter taste	Lethargy Somnolence Coma Anorexia Constipation Subcutaneous fat necrosis	Renal (interstitial) calcification Nephrolithiasis (kidney stones)
Magnesium	Laxative effect Diarrhea	Transient hypocalcemia Respiratory paralysis Cardiac arrest	None known
Iron	Nausea Vomiting Metallic taste Discolored (black) stools	Increased susceptibility to disseminated Gram-negative septicemias Dizziness Peripheral vascular collapse Anaphylaxis (to iron *dextrans*)	Hemosiderosis Splenomegaly Negative chromium balance Increased susceptibility to intracellular infections Hemochromatosis (only with *genetic* predisposition)
Zinc	Nausea Vomiting Metallic taste Epigastric distress Gastric erosion	Sweating Dizziness Tachycardia Hyperamylasemia	T cell dysfunction Phagocytic dysfunction Elevated LDL/HDL ratio in serum lipid pattern
Copper	Nausea Vomiting Gastrointestinal hemorrhage	Hemolytic anemia Jaundice	Chronic hepatic cirrhosis Acute hepatic necrosis Jaundice
Manganese	None known	None known	Schizophrenia-like psychotic disorder Parkinson's disease-like neurologic disorder
Selenium	None known	Peripheral vascular collapse	Weakened fingernails and toenails Dental enamel defects Hair loss Dermatitis Generalized tremor Garlicky odor of breath
Chromium	**For chromates** Nausea and vomiting **For chromic salts** None known	Increased insulin sensitivity and hypoglycemia (*theoretical*)	None known
Molybdenum	None known	None known	Hypercupruria Genu valgum (in India)
Nickel	Allergic reactions (dermatitis or rash)	Allergic reactions (dermatitis or rash)	None known
Silicon	Gritty taste	None known	None known
Phosphorus	Hypocalcemia (with possible resultant tetany)	None known	None known

Adapted with permission from: *Nutritional Support Services 5(6),* June, 1985. Prepared by Noel Solomons, M.D.

FAT-SOLUBLE VITAMINS

Vitamin A (retinol, retinal, retinoic acid)

Two beta-carotene molecules are equivalent to one molecule of vitamin A. Carotene is found in deep yellow, orange, or dark green fruits and vegetables such as carrots, broccoli, sweet potatoes, collards, peaches, apricots, and papaya. 9–17% of dietary carotene is absorbed. It may have a role in cancer prevention.

Functions. Vision; growth; prevention of early miscarriage; antiinfection; corticosterones; weight gain; proper bone, tooth, and nerve development; membrane functions; epithelial tissue integrity.

Sources. Fish liver oils; egg yolk; animal livers.

Note. 7–65% of vitamin A from the diet is absorbed. RBP is used to evaluate transport. Stress can increase excretion. Zinc or protein deficiency can decrease transport.

Vitamin D (Ergocalciferol, Cholecalciferol)

Functions. Utilization of calcium and phosphorus; volume and acidity of gastric secretions; growth of soft tissues; bone calcification; prevention of rickets; tooth formation; effects on PTH and renal/intestinal phosphate absorption.

Sources. Cod liver oil; sunshine; eggs (one yolk = 27 IU); liver; salmon; sardines; fish roe; tuna (3 1/2 oz = 200–300 IU); herring (3 1/2 oz = 330 IU); vitamin-D-fortified milk (8 oz = 100 IU).

Note. 90% of dietary intake is absorbed. Bile salts are required for absorption. There is decreased production with aging. Active metabolite = 1,25 dihydroxyvitamin D_3.

Vitamin E (Alpha-Tocopherol)

Functions. Antioxidant; vitamin K antagonist; role with selenium; intracellular respiration; hemopoietic agent; roles in muscular, vascular, reproductive, and CNS systems; some role in reproduction; neutralizes free radicals.

Sources. Salad oils; shortening; margarine; fruits and vegetables; grain products; most meats.

Note. Normal requirements increase with the use of PUFAs. Normal needs are 15 mg daily, but with PUFAs normal requirements double daily. Overall 20–40% is absorbed with meals. Bile and pancreatic secretions are needed.

Excessive intake does not appear to cause hypervitaminosis, but has caused isolated cases of dermatitis, fatigue, pruitus ani, acne, vasodilation, hypoglycemia; GI symptoms; impaired coagulation; muscle damage.

Vitamin K (Phytylmenaquinone, Menaquinone)

First isolated from alfalfa, vitamin K is also known as "menadione."

Functions. Antihemorrhagic factor; normal blood coagulation; possibly bone mineralization.

Sources. Plant foods are better sources of vitamin K, including kale, Brussel sprouts, spinach, cauliflower, and cabbage; lettuce (if eaten in large amounts); fish, and hog liver.

Note. Because men hemorrhage more often than women, it may be necessary to review male patient intake of vitamin K. 50% of the bodily requirement is made by intestinal bacteria. A sterile gut or malabsorption can create deficiency. Vitamin K absorption is optimal with bile and pancreatic juice. 10–70% of dietary intake is usually absorbed. Beware, vitamin E excesses can reduce absorption. Warfarin (coumadin) blocks regeneration of active, reduced vitamin K, thus prolonging clotting time (PT).

WATER-SOLUBLE VITAMINS

Thiamine (Vitamin B₁)

A "morale" vitamin, thiamine is spared by fat, protein, sorbitol, and vitamin C. As calorie intake from protein and fat increases, the thiamine requirement decreases. Some nutrients are thiamine-sparing; others destroy the nutrient. Thiamine is generally beneficial to cardiac patients; thiamine deficiency is also common in alcoholics. High CHO diets, pregnancy, lactation, increased BMR, and antibiotic use will increase needs.

Functions. Prevents beriberi; role in cell respiration; RNA and DNA formation; protein catabolism; growth; appetite; normal muscle tone in cardiac and digestive tissues; neurological functioning; CHO metabolism as coenzyme in energy-producing Krebs cycle, TPP at pyruvic acid step. Magnesium, manganese, riboflavin, and vitamin B₆ are synergists. Acetylcholine synthesis requires thiamine.

Sources. Pork; yeast; dried legumes; organ meats; rolled oats; whole wheats; nuts; cornmeal; brown rice; enriched flours and breads/cereals; dried milk; wheat germ; dried egg yolk or whole egg; green peas.

Note. Two slices of bread or one slice of bread and one serving of cereal will provide 15% of the daily RDA. Extent of absorption varies widely. Thiamine hydrochloride is the common supplemental form.

Riboflavin (Vitamin B₂)

As protein intake increases, the need for riboflavin decreases. Riboflavin is spared by dextrins and starch, and is found in greater amounts in protein foods. Cheilosis gives a magenta-colored tongue.

Functions. Cell respiration; oxidation-reduction; conversion of tryptophan to niacin; component of retinal pigment; involvement in all metabolisms (especially fat); purine degradation; adrenocortical function; coenzyme in electron transport as FAD/FMN.

Sources. Milk; cheese; eggs; legumes, peanuts; fish; glandular meats and animal muscles.

Note. Daily requirements are affected by body size, BMR, growth, activity excesses, and fat metabolism. Beware of excesses of niacin and methylxanthines.

Niacin (Vitamin B₃)

Sixty mg of tryptophan is equivalent to 1 mg of niacin. The diet supplies 31% of niacin intake as tryptophan. Milk and eggs are good sources of tryptophan but not niacin. Nicotinic acid is one form of niacin; it is often used as a vasodilator. Nicotinamide is less vasodilating.

Functions. Prevention of pellagra (along with other B-complex vitamins); used to treat TB with INH; part of nicotinamide adenine dinucleotide (NAD) in metabolism; use of CHO, protein, and fat; growth; conversion of vitamin A to retinol; lowering of serum cholesterol and triglycerides.

Sources. Yeast; organ meats; meat, poultry; salt water fish; nuts and legumes.

Note. Niacin requirements are related to protein and calorie intake. One sign of pellagra is Casal's collar, a rough, red dermatitis.

Pyridoxine (Vitamin B₆)

Widely distributed throughout the diet; deficiency is rare. Infants need three times as much as adults do. Needs increase with increased protein intake, decrease with fatty acids, or decrease with other B-complex vitamins. High protein intakes may even deplete vitamin B₆ levels.

Functions. Protein metabolism; coenzymes (-ases); conversion of tryptophan to niacin; fat metabolism and some relationship to atherosclerosis; CHO metabolism; synthesis of folic acid; glandular and endocrine functions; nerve and brain energy; antibodies; may work against dental caries in the PG patient; role in dopamine and serotonin metabolism; glycogen phosphorylase.

Sources. Muscle and organ meats; fish; whole grain cereals; legumes and peanuts; molasses; yeast; bananas; corn; cabbage; yams.

Note. Vitamin B₆ can be made by enteric bacteria in healthy persons. 96% of dietary vitamin B₆ is absorbed.

Cobalamin (Vitamin B₁₂)

Vitamin B₁₂ is not found in plant foods. Watch persons on a vegetarian diet. Known as a "growth stimulator," "extrinsic factor." For best metabolism, riboflavin, niacin, magnesium, and vitamin B_6 are needed. Cyanocobalamin is the typical, active form.

Functions. Coenzymes; blood cell formation; nucleoproteins; nutrient metabolism; growth; nerve tissue; thyroid functions; metabolism; transmethylation; myelin formation.

Sources. Liver, kidney; muscle meats; eggs; cheese; milk; and fish.

Folic Acid (Folacin)

Folic acid can be made in the intestines with help from biotin, protein, and vitamin C. Deficiency is common, especially during pregnancy, with oral contraceptive use, in alcoholics, teens or the elderly.

Functions. Prevents megaloblastic and macrocytic anemias; growth; hemoglobin; amino acid metabolism.

Sources. Liver; deep green vegetables (broccoli, etc.); legumes, nuts; whole grains; kidney. Think "foliage" for folic acid.

Note. Pteroylglutamic acid is the pharmacological form. 25–50% of dietary folacin is bioavailable. Some drugs interfere with utilization, such as sulfasalazine (Azulfidine), phenytoin (Dilantin), methotrexate.

Pantothenic Acid (Vitamin B_5)

Pantothenic acids is digested "from everywhere." Deficiency is rare, but patient's complaint may include the burning feet syndrome.

Functions. Coenzyme A; metabolism; synthesis of cholesterol and fatty acids; adrenal gland activity; acetyl transfer; antibodies; normal serum glucose; electrolyte control and hydration; prevents premature graying in some animals; heme synthesis; choline to acetylcholine.

Sources. Liver, organ meats; egg yolks; legumes; peanuts; yeast; salmon; mushrooms; broccoli, kale; avocado; whole grains; lean muscle meats; poultry.

Note. Needs increased by 1/3 in pregnancy and lactation. 50% is bioavailable from the diet.

Biotin (Vitamin H)

Synthesized by intestinal bacteria. "Anti-raw egg white" factor.

Functions. Coenzyme in CO_2 fixation; deamination; decarboxylation; synthesis of fatty acids; CHO metabolism; oxidative phosphorylation; leucine catabolism; carboxylation of pyruvic acid to oxaloacetate.

Sources. Liver, kidney; milk; egg yolk; yeast; nuts; legumes; chocolate; fish; some fruits and vegetables.

Note. Raw egg white decreases biotin availability with its content of avidin. Be wary of extended antibiotic use. Probably 50% of dietary biotin is absorbed from the small intestine.

Ascorbic Acid (Vitamin C)

No more than 1 g/day is stored in liver tissue. An excretion of 50% is normal. Men are found to have lower serum levels than women. Excesses do not produce a hypervitaminosis but are linked to oxalate stones and grout in susceptible persons. Smoking decreases serum levels.*

Functions. Hydroxylation (hydroxyproline to proline) in collagen formation; wound healing; norepinephrine metabolism; lowering of serum cholesterol; changes ferric iron to ferrous iron; prevention of infection; intracellular respiration; intercellular structures of bone, teeth, and cartilage; prevention of scurvy; thought to defer aging with collagen turnover process; reducing agent; elevation of HDL cholesterol in the elderly.

Sources. Citrus fruits; strawberries; green peppers; tomatoes; cantaloupes; currants, gooseberries; liver; plant leaves (e.g., broccoli); baked potato.

---

* Increasing the intake of vitamin C is not recommended for smokers: increased intake removes greater amounts of nicotine, and the patient may decide to smoke *more* cigarettes.

Note. New RDAs do suggest an increased intake of vitamin C; research is ongoing.

Table A–8.

Vitamins: Risk Factors, Deficiency, and Signs and Symptoms of Hypervitaminosis

Risk Factors	Signs and Symptoms of Deficiency	Signs and Symptoms of Hypervitaminosis
Vitamin A		
Anorexia nervosa	Thickened bone	Transient hydrocephalus
Appendicitis	Loss of lung elasticity	Precocious skeletal growth
Burns	Epithelial keratinization	Irritability, fatigue,
Biliary obstruction	Impaired hearing	increased intracranial
Cirrhosis	Dryness of cornea,	pressure
Celiac disease	conjunctiva, night	Anorexia, vomiting
Colitis	blindness, Bitot's spots	Dry and pruritic skin
Cystic fibrosis	Urinary calculi	Loss of body hair
Drugs	Keratinization of salivary	Nystagmus
Cholestyramine	glands	Gingivitis, fissures on
Mineral oil		tongue
Neomycin		Hepatosplenomegaly
Hookworm		Lymph node enlargement
Hepatitis, infectious		Slow clotting time
Giardiasis		Increased serum alkaline
Kwashiorkor		phosphatase
Malignant disease		
Malaria		
Pancreatic disease		
Pneumonia		
Premature infants		
Prostatic disease		
Rheumatic fever		
Tropical sprue		
Zinc deficiency		
Vitamin D		
Biliary obstruction	Skeletal deformities:	Muscle weakness, joint
Celiac disease	fractures, osteoporosis,	pain, premature closure
Cystic fibrosis	osteomalacia,	of sutures
Drugs	osteodystrophy	Anorexia, vomiting, thirst,
Bile salt binders	Muscle weakness and loss	polyuria
Glucocorticoids	of tone	Fatigue, lassitude,
Phenobarbital	Hypocalcemic tetany	headaches
Diphenylhydantoin	Delayed dentition	Abnormal ECG, shortened
Primidone	Aminoaciduria	QT interval
Glutethimide	Decreased calcium and	Increased calcium and
Diphosphorates	phosphorus	phosphorus
Mineral oil	Increased alkaline	Decreased magnesium,
End-organ failure	phosphatase	and increased
Fanconi's syndrome		cholesterol
Hepatic disease		
Primary hypophosphatemia		
Hypoparathyroidism		
Intestinal malabsorption		

(continued)

Table A–8.
Vitamins: Risk Factors, Deficiency, and Signs and Symptoms of Hypervitaminosis (Continued)

Risk Factors	Signs and Symptoms of Deficiency	Signs and Symptoms of Hypervitaminosis
Vitamin D (Continued)		
Lack of exposure to sunlight		
Liver disease		
Lymphatic obstruction		
Pancreatitis		
Parathyroid surgery		
Postmenopause		
Premature infants		
Renal disease		
Regional ileitis		
Small bowel resection		
Tropical sprue		
Vitamin E		
Biliary cirrhosis	Increased creatinuria	Possible high blood pressure
Bronchopulmonary dysplasia	Increased hemolysis of red blood cells	Increased phosphorus
Cystic fibrosis	Muscle weakness	
Drugs	Decreased serum lipid levels	
Cholestyramine	Steatorrhea	
Clofibrate	Infants: anemia, decreased levels of tocopherol, edema of legs, labia, scrotum	
Contraceptives		
Triiodothyronine		
Excess dietary polyunsaturated fatty acids		
Malabsorption syndromes		
Malnutrition		
Pancreatitis		
Premature infants		
Retrolental fibroplasia		
Steatorrhea		
Vitamin K		
Drugs	Cutaneous purpura	Transient hyperprothrombinemia
Anticoagulant therapy	Ecchymosis	Synthetic vitamin K excess
Antibiotics (neomycin)	Retinal hemorrhage	Hemorrhage
Cholestyramine	Gastrointestinal bleeding	Kernicterus
Mineral oil	Epistaxis	Vomiting
Hepatocellular disease	Hematuria	Porphyrinuria
Infants	Postoperative hemorrhage	Albuminuria
Premature: hepatic immaturity		Prolonged clotting time
Term: insufficient intestinal synthesis, inadequate intake		

Table A-8.
**Vitamins: Risk Factors, Deficiency, and Signs and Symptoms of
Hypervitaminosis** (*Continued*)

Risk Factors	Signs and Symptoms of Deficiency	Signs and Symptoms of Hypervitaminosis
Vitamin K (*Continued*)		
Hepatic biliary obstruction		
Malabsorption syndromes		
Small bowel disease		
Thiamine		
Alcoholism	Children	Allergies
Carbohydrate, high oral intake	Aphonia	Edema
Chronic colitis	Cardiopathy	Fatty liver
Fever	Polyneuritis	Herpes
Malignant disease	Adults	Nervousness
Pregnancy, lactation (low oral intake)	Central nervous system changes	Sweating
Sprue	Peripheral neuritis	Tachycardia
Thyrotoxicosis	Vomiting, diarrhea	Tremors
Parenteral glucose alimentation		Vascular hypotension
Riboflavin		
Alcoholism	Eyes: burning, dim vision, photophobia	Essentially nontoxic
Chronic infections	Mouth: magenta tongue	
Drugs	Skin: angular stomatitis, cheilosis, seborrheic dermatitis	
Broad spectrum antibiotics		
Chloramphenicol		
Gastrectomy (subtotal, total)		
Low oral intake during childhood, pregnancy, and lactation		
Malignant disease		
Vitamin B$_6$		
Alcoholism	Anemia	Limited toxicity
Drugs:	Cultaneous Peripheral neuritis	
Cycloserine	Infants: convulsive seizures, diarrhea, hyperactivity	
Hydantoin		
Hydralazine		
Isoniazid		
Oral contraceptives		
Penicillamine		
Elderly		
Infants of preeclamptic mothers or mothers deficient in B$_6$		
Pregnancy		

(continued)

Table A–8.
Vitamins: Risk Factors, Deficiency, and Signs and Symptoms of Hypervitaminosis (*Continued*)

Risk Factors	Signs and Symptoms of Deficiency	Signs and Symptoms of Hypervitaminosis
Niacin		
Alcoholism	Achlorhydria	Low blood pressure
Chronic diarrhea	Dermatitis	Burning, itching skin
Cirrhosis	Diarrhea	Fatty liver
Diabetes mellitus	Loss of memory	Peripheral vasodilatation
Malignant disease	Pigmentation	Decreased serum
Tuberculosis	Retarded growth	cholesterol
		Stimulated central nervous system
		Increased cerebral blood flow
		Increased pulse rate
		increased respiratory rate
Pantothenic Acid		
Alcoholism	Cardiovascular changes	Essentially nontoxic
Elderly women	Depression	
Liver disease	Digestive disorders	
Pregnancy	Greater susceptibility to infection	
	Neuromotor disturbances	
	Physical weakness	
Vitamin B$_{12}$		
Disorders of gastric mucosa	Anemia, megaloblastic	Polycythemia
Genetic defects	Gastrointestinal tract changes	
Apoenzymes	Leukopenia	
Absence of transcobalamin II	Nerve damage, peripheral neuropathy	
Absence of ileal receptors	Diminished sense of position and vibration	
Intestinal infections	Poor growth	
Malabsorption secondary to	Sore, smooth tongue	
Gastrectomy, total	Splenomegaly	
Ileal disease or resection	Thrombocytopenia	
Prolonged daily intake of megadose B$_{12}$ (greater than 1 g per day)		
Strict vegetarians		
Biotin		
Excessive dietary intake of raw egg whites	Anorexia	Essentially nontoxic
Genetic dependency:	Anemia	
Beta-methyl-crotonyglycinuria	Dermatitis: fine, non-pruritic; scalp, cheeks, neck, groin, and gluteal region	
Propionic lacidemia		

Table A–8.
Vitamins: Risk Factors, Deficiency, and Signs and Symptoms of Hypervitaminosis (*Continued*)

Risk Factors	Signs and Symptoms of Deficiency	Signs and Symptoms of Hypervitaminosis
Biotin (*Continued*)		
Inadequate parenteral provision	Hypesthesias Hypercholesterolemia Lassitude Muscular pain	
Folic Acid		
Alcoholism Drugs Aspirin Cycloserine Diphenylhydantoin Methotrexate Oral contraceptives Primidone Pyrimethamine Hematologic diseases: Pernicious anemia Sickle cell anemia Thalassemia Hypovitaminosis B_{12} Malabsorption syndromes Malignant disease Pregnancy	Anemia: megaloblastic, pernicious Central nervous system changes Glossitis Hepatomegaly Hyperpigmentation Intestinal disturbances Leukopenia Sprue Thrombocytopenia	No toxicity reported
Vitamin C		
Alcoholism Achlorhydria Burns Chronic diarrhea Diabetes Infants: maternal intake greater than 400 mg per day during pregnancy Malignant disease Nephrosis Severe trauma Surgical wounds Tuberculosis	Edema Hyperkeratotic papules especially on buttocks, calves Perifollicular hemorrhage Scorbutic bone formation Teeth and gum defects Weakness	Essentially nontoxic except possible kidney stones in gout patients

From Nutrition: *Nurs. Clin. N. Am. 18*:30, 1983.

1989 RECOMMENDED DIETARY ALLOWANCES

The following tables have been approved by the National Academy of Sciences for distribution. They include tables on (a) recommended energy intakes, together with mean heights and weights; (b) the recommended dietary allowances for protein, fat-soluble vitamins, water-soluble vitamins, and minerals; and (c) estimates of adequate and safe intakes of selected vitamins, trace elements, and electrolytes.

Table A–9.
Weights for Height of Adults in the United States*

Height cm (in)	Weight, kg (lb)					
	Males, by Percentile			Females, by Percentile		
	15th	50th	85th	15th	50th	85th
147 (58)				45 (99)	55 (122)	72 (159)
152 (60)				49 (107)	60 (132)	75 (164)
157 (62)	57 (125)	64 (142)	76 (168)	51 (112)	60 (132)	77 (170)
163 (64)	58 (129)	67 (148)	79 (174)	54 (118)	63 (139)	79 (175)
168 (66)	61 (134)	71 (158)	83 (183)	55 (122)	64 (141)	81 (179)
173 (68)	65 (143)	76 (167)	88 (195)	59 (130)	67 (148)	83 (184)
178 (70)	67 (149)	79 (173)	93 (206)	61 (133)	69 (152)	78 (171)
183 (72)	73 (161)	83 (183)	99 (218)			
188 (74)	77 (171)	88 (194)	99 (217)			
193 (76)	85 (187)	103 (227)	106 (234)			

* Unpublished data from NHANES II (1976–1980) provided by the National Center for Health Statistics. Values rounded to nearest whole number. Subjects were ages 18 to 74 years. Height determined without shoes. Weight includes clothing weight, ranging from an estimated 0.09 to 0.28 kg (0.20 to 0.62 lb).
From *Recommended Dietary Allowances,* 10th ed. Washington, DC: National Academy of Sciences, 1989.

Table A–10.
Weight and Height of Males and Females Up to 18 Years in the United States*

	Males, by Percentile						Females, by Percentile					
	Weight, kg (lb)			Height, cm (in)			Weight, kg (lb)			Height, cm (in)		
Age	5th	50th	95th	5th	50th	95th	5th	50th	95th	5th	50th	95th
Months												
1	3.16	4.29 (9.4)	5.38	50.4	54.6 (21.5)	58.6	2.97	3.98 (8.8)	4.92	49.2	53.5 (21.1)	56.9
3	4.43	5.98 (13.2)	7.37	56.7	61.1 (24.1)	65.4	4.18	5.40 (11.9)	6.74	55.4	59.5 (23.4)	63.4
6	6.20	7.85 (17.3)	9.46	63.4	67.8 (26.7)	72.3	5.79	7.21 (15.9)	8.73	61.8	65.9 (25.9)	70.2
9	7.52	9.18 (20.2)	10.93	68.0	72.3 (28.5)	77.1	7.00	8.56 (18.8)	10.17	66.1	70.4 (27.7)	75.0
12	8.43	10.15 (22.3)	11.99	71.7	76.1 (30.0)	81.2	7.84	9.53 (21.0)	11.24	69.8	74.3 (29.3)	79.1
18	9.59	11.47 (25.2)	13.44	77.5	82.4 (32.4)	88.1	8.92	10.82 (23.8)	12.76	76.0	80.9 (31.9)	86.1
Years												
2	10.49	12.34 (27.1)	15.50	82.5	86.8 (34.2)	94.4	9.95	11.80 (26.0)	14.15	81.6	86.8 (34.2)	93.6
3	12.05	14.62 (32.2)	17.77	89.0	94.9 (37.4)	102.0	11.61	14.10 (31.0)	17.22	88.3	94.1 (37.0)	100.6
4	13.64	16.69 (36.7)	20.27	95.8	102.9 (40.5)	109.9	13.11	15.96 (35.1)	19.91	95.0	101.6 (40.0)	108.3
5	15.27	18.67 (41.1)	23.09	102.0	109.9 (43.3)	117.0	14.55	17.66 (38.9)	22.62	101.1	108.4 (42.7)	115.6
6	16.93	20.69 (45.5)	26.34	107.7	116.1 (45.7)	123.5	16.05	19.52 (42.9)	25.75	106.6	114.6 (45.1)	122.7
7	18.64	22.85 (50.3)	30.12	113.0	121.7 (47.9)	129.7	17.71	21.84 (48.0)	29.68	111.8	120.6 (47.5)	129.5
8	20.40	25.30 (55.7)	34.51	118.1	127.0 (50.0)	135.7	19.62	24.84 (54.6)	34.71	116.9	126.4 (49.8)	136.2
9	22.25	28.13 (61.9)	39.58	122.9	132.2 (52.0)	141.8	21.82	28.46 (62.6)	40.64	122.1	132.2 (52.0)	142.9
10	24.33	31.44 (69.2)	45.27	127.7	137.5 (54.1)	148.1	24.36	32.55 (71.6)	47.17	127.5	138.3 (54.4)	149.5
11	26.80	35.30 (77.7)	51.47	132.6	143.3 (56.4)	154.9	27.24	36.95 (81.3)	54.00	133.5	144.8 (57.0)	156.2
12	29.85	39.78 (87.5)	58.09	137.6	149.7 (58.9)	162.3	30.52	41.53 (91.4)	60.81	139.8	151.5 (59.6)	162.7
13	33.64	44.95 (98.9)	65.02	142.9	156.5 (61.6)	169.8	34.14	46.10 (101.4)	67.30	145.2	157.1 (61.9)	168.1
14	38.22	50.77 (111.7)	72.13	148.8	163.1 (64.2)	176.7	37.76	50.28 (110.6)	73.08	148.7	160.4 (63.1)	171.3
15	43.11	56.71 (124.8)	79.12	155.2	169.0 (66.5)	181.9	40.99	53.68 (118.1)	77.78	150.5	161.8 (63.7)	172.8
16	47.74	62.10 (136.6)	85.62	161.1	173.5 (68.3)	185.4	43.41	55.89 (123.0)	80.99	151.6	162.4 (63.9)	173.3
17	51.50	66.31 (145.9)	91.43	164.9	176.2 (69.4)	187.3	44.74	56.69 (124.7)	82.46	152.7	163.1 (64.2)	173.5
18	53.97	68.88 (151.5)	95.76	165.7	176.8 (69.6)	187.6	45.26	56.62 (124.7)	82.47	153.6	163.7 (64.4)	173.6

* Data in this table have been used to derive weight and height reference points in the present report. It is not intended that they necessarily be considered standards of normal growth and development. Data pertaining to infants 2 to 18 months of age are taken from longitudinal growth studies at Fels Research Institute. Ages are exact, and infants were measured in the recumbent position. The measurements were based on some 867 children followed longitudinally at the Institute between 1929 and 1975. Data pertaining to children between 2 and 18 years of age were collected between 1962 and 1974 by the National Center for Health Statistics and involve some 20,000 individuals comprising nationally representative samples in three studies conducted between 1960 and 1974. In these studies, children were measured in the standing position with no upward pressure exerted on the mastoid processes. In the ninth edition of this report, data for children up to 6 years of age were taken from longitudinal growth studies in Iowa and Boston, where children were measured in the recumbent position. This explains the systematically smaller heights for 2- to 5-year-old children in this current table compared with those represented in previous editions. In this table, actual age is represented.

Adapted from Hamill et al., in *Recommended Dietary Allowances*, 10th ed. Washington, DC: National Academy of Sciences, 1989.

Table A–11.
Food and Nutrition Board, National Academy of Sciences—National Research Council Recommended Dietary Allowances,[a] Revised 1989

Designed for the maintenance of good nutrition of practically all healthy people in the United States

Category	Age (years) or Condition	Weight[b] (kg)	Weight[b] (lb)	Height[b] (cm)	Height[b] (in)	Protein (g)	Vitamin A (µg RE)[c]	Vitamin D (µg)[a]	Vitamin E (mg alpha-TE)[e]	Vitamin K (µg)
Infants	0.0–0.5	6	13	60	24	13	375	7.5	3	5
	0.5–1.0	9	20	71	28	14	375	10	4	10
Children	1–3	13	29	90	35	16	400	10	6	15
	4–6	20	44	112	44	24	500	10	7	20
	7–10	28	62	132	52	28	700	10	7	30
Males	11–14	45	99	157	62	45	1,000	10	10	45
	15–18	66	145	176	69	59	1,000	10	10	65
	19–24	72	160	177	70	58	1,000	10	10	70
	25–50	79	174	176	70	63	1,000	5	10	80
	51+	77	170	173	68	63	1,000	5	10	80
Females	11–14	46	101	157	62	46	800	10	8	45
	15–18	55	120	163	64	44	800	10	8	55
	19–24	58	128	164	65	46	800	10	8	60
	25–50	63	138	163	64	50	800	5	8	65
	51+	65	143	160	63	50	800	5	8	65
Pregnant						60	800	10	10	65
Lactating	1st 6 months					65	1,300	10	12	65
	2nd 6 months					62	1,200	10	11	65

[a] The allowances, expressed as average daily intakes over time, are intended to provide for individual variations among most normal persons as they live in the United States under usual environmental stresses. Diets should be based on a variety of common foods in order to provide other nutrients for which human requirements have been less well defined.
[b] Weights and heights of reference adults are actual medians for the U.S. population of the designated age, as reported by NHANES II. The median weights and heights of those under 19 years of age were taken from Hamill et al. (1979). The use of these figures does not imply that the height-to-weight ratios are ideal.
[c] Retinol equivalents. 1 retinol equivalent = 1 µg retinol or 6 µg beta-carotene.
[d] As cholecalciferol. 10µg cholecalciferol = 400 IU of vitamin D.
[e] alpha-Tocopherol equivalents. 1 mg d-alpha tocopherol = 1 alpha-TE.
[f] 1 NE (niacin equivalent) is equal to 1 mg of niacin or 60 mg of dietary tryptophan.
From *Recommended Dietary Allowances*, 10th ed. Washington, DC: National Academy of Sciences, 1989.

Water-Soluble Vitamins — Vitamin C (mg)	Thiamin (mg)	Riboflavin (mg)	Niacin (mg NE)	Vitamin B6 (mg)	Folate (µg)	Vitamin B12 (µg)	Minerals — Calcium (mg)	Phosphorus (mg)	Magnesium (mg)	Iron (mg)	Zinc (mg)	Iodine (µg)	Selenium (µg)
30	0.3	0.4	5	0.3	25	0.3	400	300	40	6	5	40	10
35	0.4	0.5	6	0.6	35	0.5	600	500	60	10	5	50	15
40	0.7	0.8	9	1.0	50	0.7	800	800	80	10	10	70	20
45	0.9	1.1	12	1.1	75	1.0	800	800	120	10	10	90	20
45	1.0	1.2	13	1.4	100	1.4	800	800	170	10	10	120	30
50	1.3	1.5	17	1.7	150	2.0	1,200	1,200	270	12	15	150	40
60	1.5	1.8	20	2.0	200	2.0	1,200	1,200	400	12	15	150	50
60	1.5	1.7	19	2.0	200	2.0	1,200	1,200	350	10	15	150	70
60	1.5	1.7	19	2.0	200	2.0	800	800	350	10	15	150	70
60	1.2	1.4	15	2.0	200	2.0	800	800	350	10	15	150	70
50	1.1	1.3	15	1.4	150	2.0	1,200	1,200	280	15	12	150	45
60	1.1	1.3	15	1.5	180	2.0	1,200	1,200	300	15	12	150	50
60	1.1	1.3	15	1.6	180	2.0	1,200	1,200	280	15	12	150	55
60	1.1	1.3	15	1.6	180	2.0	800	800	280	15	12	150	55
60	1.0	1.2	13	1.6	180	2.0	800	800	280	10	12	150	55
70	1.5	1.6	17	2.2	400	2.2	1,200	1,200	320	30	15	175	65
95	1.6	1.8	20	2.1	280	2.6	1,200	1,200	355	15	19	200	75
90	1.6	1.7	20	2.1	260	2.6	1,200	1,200	340	15	16	200	75

Table A–12.
Estimated Safe and Adequate Daily Dietary Intakes of Selected Vitamins and Minerals*

Category	Age (years)	Vitamins	
		Biotin (µg)	Pantothenic Acid (mg)
Infants	0–0.5	10	2
	0.5–1	15	3
Children and adolescents	1–3	20	3
	4–6	25	3–4
	7–10	30	4–5
	11+	30–100	4–7
Adults		30–100	4–7

Category	Age (years)	Trace Elements†				
		Copper (mg)	Manganese (mg)	Fluoride (mg)	Chromium (µg)	Molybdenum (µg)
Infants	0–0.5	0.4–0.6	0.3–0.6	0.1–0.5	10–40	15–30
	0.5–1	0.6–0.7	0.6–1.0	0.2–1.0	20–60	20–40
Children and adolescents	1–3	0.7–1.0	1.0–1.5	0.5–1.5	20–80	25–50
	4–6	1.0–1.5	1.5–2.0	1.0–2.5	30–120	30–75
	7–10	1.0–2.0	2.0–3.0	1.5–2.5	50–200	50–150
	11+	1.5–2.5	2.0–5.0	1.5–2.5	50–200	75–250
Adults		1.5–3.0	2.0–5.0	1.5–4.0	50–200	75–250

* Because there is less information on which to base allowances, these figures are not given in the main table of RDA and are provided here in the form of ranges of recommended intakes.

† Since the toxic levels for many trace elements may be only several times usual intakes, the upper levels for the trace elements given in this table should not be habitually exceeded.

From *Recommended Dietary Allowances*, 10th ed. Washington, DC: National Academy of Sciences, 1989.

Appendix B:
Dietetic Process, Forms, and Counseling Tips

For More In-Depth Information: Grant and DeHoog, *Nutritional Assessment and Support*, 4th ed., 1990, Seattle, WA.

PATIENT EDUCATION AND COUNSELING TIPS

Chief Assessment Factors

1. Socioeconomic factors.
2. Cultural, religious beliefs and background.
3. Age and sex of patient and significant others (SO).
4. Birth order and family involvement of the patient.
5. Occupation.
6. Medical status and prior medical history.
7. Marital status; number and ages of children.
8. Cognitive status; educational level; readiness to learn.
9. Emotional status (stress, acceptance of illness or chronic disease or condition).
10. Instructor's ability to teach; awareness and use of teaching/learning principles and adult learner theories.

Principles of Learning

1. Information must be valued.
2. The pace should be adequate for the learner (i.e., small steps).
3. The environment should be conducive to learning (e.g., free of distractions and stress) and the patient should be ready to learn (e.g., free of pain).
4. Information must be meaningful, relevant and organized. The material should be logical in sequence.
5. The counselor must be truly interested in sharing the information.
6. Adequate follow-up should be available for reinforcement of facts and principles.

Principles of Teaching

1. The counselor must *listen* first to the patient.
2. Small segments of information should be presented in understandable language.
3. An organized plan should be used to teach.
4. Feedback should be used with each step.
5. Good eye contact should be maintained with the patient.
6. Appropriate teaching tools or audio-visual aids should be used as appropriate.
7. Questions must be allowed for clarification.
8. Praise and positive reinforcement should be offered to the learner. Carl Rogers emphasizes "unconditional positive regard" for all persons.

Counseling Tips

1. Knowledge does not automatically ensure compliance. Behavioral change takes time and encouragement.
2. Trial and error will be common for the patient in learning new behaviors.
3. Increase in self-esteem comes with improvement in behavior.
4. Independence should be fostered appropriately by the counselor.

NOTES

THE DIETETIC PROCESS

Assessment

Establish data base and problem list. Read medical history, review lab data and medications, and conduct physical assessment for nutritional problems or review physical exam as conducted by physician. Prioritize levels of care.

Take a home-based diet history or record a typical daily intake (3–7 day records are more accurate when available). Determine calorie and protein requirements. Select appropriate diet and feeding mode.

Plan

Establish a nutritional care plan to give directional stimulus to treatment efforts. Consider nutritional problems and determine the course of action for the following:

1. *Treatment.* Procedures and dietary adjustment to meet goals, including oral, EN or PN modes.
2. *Diagnoses.* Request more data—food diary, tests, possibly a home visit, nutrient or calorie intake analyses.
3. *Education.* Explain the relation of diet to disorder and disease, plus the patient's/client's role in management. Use a client-centered approach.

Explain the diet—dietary principles, ways to change and improve habits, written materials, sample menus, meal patterns.

Formulate objectives with the patient and the physician. Contact family when appropriate. Determine goals (i.e., maintenance, anabolism, etc.)

Implementation

Carry out plans. Consult with physician about other needed referrals. Complete anthropometric measurements. Participate in medical rounds. Evaluate food-drug interactions; counsel accordingly. Coordinate transitional feedings. Monitor food intake, nitrogen balance, etc.

Evaluation

Document evaluation with progress notes. Test knowledge of patient/client and family members. Determine changes that have occurred—weight, dietary behavior, laboratory data. Interpret/identify nutritional deficiency. Make a nutritional diagnosis, as appropriate. Evaluate plan/outcome.

Reassessment

Monitor and evaluate nutritional status of patient to determine any new steps that should be completed to allow the patient to succeed in his or her nutritional goals (as either inpatient or outpatient). Identify necessary changes in care (nutrient or fluid needs, mode of intake).

Discharge Planning

Determine needs for home services—EN, TPN or oral. Educate patient or family or caretakers accordingly. Refer to other agencies where appropriate. Document services; submit copy to agency, physician or program.

ROLE OF THE REGISTERED DIETITIAN ON THE HEALTH TEAM

1. Assess needs and status. Listen to patient, family, and physician. Establish nutritional diagnosis.*
2. Establish a *nutritional care plan*, pending completion of a home-based or recent nutritional history. Evaluate previous nutritional practices, knowledge of diet and of normal nutrition, and need for further instructions. Establish a realistic goal with the physician; consult with the physician as needed regarding special nutritional supplements or feeding methods.
3. Chart pertinent information from the nutritional care plan.
4. Give formal diet instructions when needed. Include the definition of the diet, an explanation of the relation between diet and disease, an ex-

---

* See also: Kight, M.: Working with diagnosis-related groups (DRGs): diagnosis in the practice of selected health-medical team members. *NSS* 5(2); 39, Feb., 1985.

planation of the dietary treatment specific to the patient, instructions in how to follow the diet in other settings, and instruction of family members and significant other persons.

5. Consult with the physician about other necessary referrals.
6. Maintain medical team communication by making rounds or attending conferences.
7. Conduct group classes and outpatient conferences when needed. Use appropriate A-V aids, and teaching tools.
8. Monitor the patient's nutritional progress: portion control, ingredient control, meal quality, delivery system (oral, EN, PN).
9. Audit nutritional care—when feasible, give a follow-up call to the patient after discharge, or conduct a home visit. Evaluate which goals, if any, have been met. Monitor efficacy of therapy and nutritional interventions.
10. Manage and evaluate resources, plans, and outcomes. A multidisciplinary case-management approach is best.

RD Actions

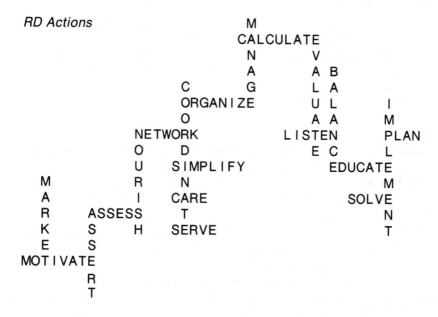

NOTES

NUTRITIONAL ASSESSMENT

Factors required for a thorough nutritional assessment include the following:*
1. *Clinical Assessment.* Physical exam, dietary intake
2. *Anthropometric Assessment.* Weight for height, mid-arm muscle circumference, skinfold thickness
3. *Hematological Assessment.* Hemoglobin, red cell morphology, ferritin, other stores
4. *Biochemical Assessment.* Albumin, transferrin, creatinine--height index, zinc, other parameters
5. *Immune Status.* Delayed cutaneous hypersensitivity, total lymphocyte count, T-cells
6. *Miscellany.* Hand grip strength, darkness adaptation, taste acuity.

---

* From Chandra, R.K.: *Contemporary Nutrition* 11:12, 1986.

Global Assessment*

1. *History.* Wt. loss 6 mos.; changes in dietary intake; significant GI symptoms; functional GI capacity; metabolic demands of disease.
2. *Physical Exam.* Loss of subcutaneous fat, muscle wasting, edema, ascites.

---

* From Detsky, A., et al.: *JPEN* 11:8, Jan./Feb., 1987.

Table B–1.
Common Calculations and Factors Related to Basal Metabolic Rate, Calorie and Protein Requirements

Basal metabolic rate = energy expenditure at rest; kilocalories required to maintain minimal physiological functioning (i.e., heart beating, breathing, etc.)

Factors Affecting Basal Metabolic Rate and Calorie Needs
1. *Age.* Infants need more kilocalories per square meter of body surface than do any other age groups. BMR declines after maturity.
2. *Body Size.* Total BMR relates to body size, with large persons requiring more kilocalories for basal and activity levels.
3. *Body Composition.* Lean tissue is more active than fatty tissue. An obese person generally has a lower metabolic rate than a lean person.
4. *Climate.* A damp or hot climate decreases BMR, a cold climate increases BMR. Changes are slight.
5. *Hormones.* Thyroxine increases BMR; sex hormones and adrenalin alter BMR mildly; low zinc intake may lower BMR.
6. *Fever.* BMR increases by 7% for each degree Fahrenheit above normal.
7. *Growth.* BMR increases during anabolic stages (pregnancy, childhood, teen years, as well as anabolic stages of wound healing).

Healthy Persons—Calculations of Calories*

	SEDENTARY	MODERATE	ACTIVE
Overweight	20–25 kcal/kg	30 kcal/kg	35 kcal/kg
Normal Weight	30 kcal/kg	35 kcal/kg	40 kcal/kg
Underweight	30 kcal/kg	40 kcal/kg	45–50 kcal/kg

Healthy Body Weight (HBW): less strict than "ideal" body weight.

Feeding programs should support a patient being within 10–15 lbs. of healthy/ideal body weight tables.

---

* Adapted from Goodhart, R.S., and, Shils, M.E.: *Modern Nutrition in Health and Disease*, 6th ed. Philadelphia: Lea & Febiger, 1980.

Determination of Weight Changes: Nonplanned weight loss can affect morbidity and mortality

$$\% \ Weight \ change = \frac{usual \ weight - actual \ weight}{usual \ weight} \times 100\%$$

Severe weight changes = over 2% in 1 week
over 5% in 1 month
over 7.5% in 3 months
over 20% in unlimited period of time
over 40% usually incompatible with life

Various methods are used to determine basal metabolic rate (BMR) and calorie or protein needs in sick individuals. Several of the most common methods include the following calculations:

METHOD A

1. *Harris-Benedict Equation: BEE (1919)*

    Men BEE (kcal) = [66 + 13.7 × wt. (kg) + 5 × ht (cm) − 6.8 × age (yrs)]

    Women BEE (kcal) = [655 + 9.6 × wt. (kg) + 1.7 × ht (cm) − 4.7 × age (yrs)]

    Note: For some conditions, the BEE has been overestimated when actual resting energy expenditure (REE) is measured by indirect calorimetry. In other cases, the BEE has underestimated patient needs. A "best guess" by other parameters may be needed.

2. *Add Activity and Injury Factors: (rank Cerra, 1983)*

Sedentary Patients Weight Maintenance	1.2 × BEE	
Patients Out of Bed	1.3 × BEE	
Anabolism or Moderate Stress	1.5 × BEE	(Minor Surgery; Infection)

563

Cancer or Sepsis	1.6 × BEE	
Severe Stress, Major Surgery,	1.75 × BEE	
Severe Sepsis		
Extreme Stress, Burns, Trauma	2–2.5 × BEE	(20% TBS burns, etc.)

3. *Total Energy Expenditure (TEE)* = BEE × Activity and Injury Factors

---

METHOD B†

Calorie needs = 28 kcal/kg in *starvation;* 150:1 NPC:N and 1 g AAs/kg daily with diet @ 15% AAs, 55–60% CHO, 25% fat.

32 kcal/kg in *elective surgery;* 150:1 NPC:N and 1.5 g AAs/kg daily with diet @ 20% AAs, 50% CHO, 30% fat.

40 kcal/kg in *polytrauma;* 100:1 NPC:N and 2 g AAs/kg daily with diet @ 40% CHO, 35% fat, 25% protein.

50 kcal/kg in *sepsis;* 80:1 NPC:N and 2.5 g AAs/kg daily with diet @ 30% AAs, 70% CHO and 0% fat.

METHOD C

Indirect Calorimetry: Calculation of energy expenditure by measuring gas exchange ($\dot{V}_{O_2}$ and $\dot{V}_{CO_2}$ represent intracellular metabolism). It is helpful for ICU patients.

For REE: MMC Horizon Metabolic Cart, Sensor Medics, Anaheim, CA

REE also includes SDA for digestion and absorption (5–10% greater than BEE), and is considered relativity equivalent in clinical context. BEE and REE are estimations.

Harris & Bendict (1919) practiced calorimetry to evaluate BEE (energy to fuel basic life functions at rest in a thermally neutral environment, 10 or more hours after eating). The study was done in *healthy* persons.

REE can be normal to 30% below normal in partial starvation.

Note: If energy is not provided in adequate amounts, protein tissues become a substrate.

Protein Needs/Degree of Illness:

Method A

No illness	100% basal needs
Mild illness	130% basal needs
Moderate illness	160% basal needs
Severe illness	200% basal needs

Method B

mild stress	35 kcal/kg + 1 g protein/kg
moderate stress	45 kcal/kg + 1.5 g protein/kg

---

† From Shronts, E.: *Calorie Sources. Nutrition Support Services* 5:1, 26, 1985.

Amino acids (AA) = 1 g/kg × 4 kcal = AA calories
NPC = total kcals less AA kcals
NPC kcals for a patient are often based on 40% fat, 60% CHO

Normal Nitrogen needs = 1 g N/300 kcal.

Illness Nitrogen needs = 1 g N/120–180 kcal.

Note: 6.25 g protein = 1 g nitrogen

Therefore, estimated nitrogen requirements × 6.25 = estimated protein needs in grams.

Defer weight repletion until a patient's critical episode subsides. Prevent overfeeding, which can cause fluid overload, increased CO_2 production, and hepatic aberrations. Keep in mind that postinsult needs generally normalize again in 20–50 days.

RQ = CO_2 production/O_2 consumption (fat = 0.7; protein = 0.8; CHO = 1)

Nutrient Calorie Yields: CHO yields approximately 3.94 kcal/g orally

Protein yields approximately 4 kcal/g orally

Fat yields approximately 9 kcal/g orally.

Some authors indicate even higher yield of fat, such as 11 kcal/g.

Alcohol yields approximately 7 kcal/g orally.

CHARTING NOTES

Using the "SOAP" method of charting will permit the dietitian to communicate his or her role on the health care team. The following guidelines may be used to develop effective notes:

S—*Subjective* information regarding current status as reported by the patient or others (e.g., nausea, difficulty with chewing and swallowing, notable food habits that affect dietary treatment, comments about usual food intake elsewhere). Actual comments from the patient may be included by enclosing them in quotation marks.

O—*Objective* and measurable data from the recording of the patient's weight, height, ideal weight, lab data, dietary orders, drug orders, etc.; or from documented medical notes and records. Known and observed eating habits and facts are part of these data.

A—*Assessment* of patient's S & O by dietitian. For example, the dietitian may respond to the patient's statements about eating excessive amounts of sweets and elevated blood glucose levels by writing that "Dietary intake exceeds the order for 1200-kcal ADA diet." The assessment should make the **P** (Plans) section a natural consequence for activity.

P—*Plans* and recommended follow-up.

Treatment. Alterations in diet; changes in consistency of diet; supplemental feedings; prosthetic feeding aid; mode of feeding.

Diagnosis. Request for more diagnostic tests; completion of an actual food diary for several days.

Education. Diet classes; personalized instructions to patients and significant others.

Progress Notes

Patient Progress. Dietary intake (calorie counts, gross nutrient inadequacies); problems with eating or feeding; food acceptance or rejection due to dislikes, allergies, intolerances, poor appetite, environmental factors, cultural factors, food quality; understanding of modified diet instructions being presented.

Specific Dietary Information. Unusual diet patterns; composition of calculated diets; significant nutrient deficiencies in diets as ordered, comments about multiple nutrient restrictions that are difficult or unacceptable to the patient; precautions in the use of the diet; composition of tube feeding when not specifically ordered; suggestions for change in a diet order with given rationale; nourishments and supplements as part of the diet regimen; explanation or interpretation of an unusual diet prescription.

Information Related to Diet Instructions. Record of initial instructions and patient responses; patient progress in accepting and understanding the diet; ability to follow a diet order; suggested referrals to outside agencies or programs; appointments made to outpatient nutrition counseling services.

Nutrition History. Comments about the recorded history of the patient, including an interpretation of such observations.

Follow-up. Outcomes of nutritional services. Suggested changes.

SAMPLE LAB FACTS

Each facility has its own values according to lab procedures. The following ranges are estimated and sample values.

Normal Serum Values

Coagulation Tests: Bleeding time = 1–3 min/Ivy; 2–4 min Duke
 Coagulation time = 6–10 min
 Erythrocyte Sedimentation Rates = 0–10 mm/hr
  (males); 0–15 mm/hr (females)
 Prothrombin time = 11–16 sec control; 70–110%
  of control value

Amylase = 60–180 Somogyi units/dl
Bilirubin, total = 0.15–1.0 mg/dl
Calcium = 8.5–10.5 mg/dl
Carotene = 48–200 μg/dl

Ceruloplasmin = 27–37 mg/dl
Chloride = 96–108 mEq/liter
CO_2 = 24–32 mEq/liter
Copper = 70–155 µg/dl
Creatinine = 0.7–1.4 mg/dl
Glycohemoglobin = 5.5–8.5%
Glucose, fasting = 65–110 mg/dl
Lipase = under 1.5 units
Lipids: total serum = 450–850 mg/dl
       cholesterol = 120–210 mg/dl (20–30% HDL, 60–70% L
       triglycerides = 10–190 mg/dl
       total fatty acids = 190–240 mg/dl
       phospholipids = 60–350 mg/dl
Magnesium = 1.5–2.5 mEq/liter or 1.8–3 mg/dl
Nitrogen balance = goal of 1–4 g/24 hrs. (UUN)
Nitrogen, nonprotein, serum = 15–35 mg/dl
Osmolality, serum = 285–295 mOsm/liter
Oxygen, blood capacity =16–24 volume % (varies with Hgb)
pH, arterial, plasma = 7.35–7.45
Phenylalanine, serum = less than 3 mg/dl
Phosphatase, serum: acid = 0.5–2 Bodansky units
             alkalne = 2–4.5 Bodansky units (30–135 u/liter)
Phosphate, inorganic, serum 3–4.5 mg/dl
Phosphorus = 2.5–4 mg/dl
Potassium, serum = 3.5–5.5 mEq/liter
Proteins, serum: total = 6–8 g/dl
       albumin = 3.5–5.5 g/dl (45–55% total)
       globulin = 1.5–3 g/dl
       prealbumin = 10–40 mg/dl
       retinol-binding protein = 37.2 µg/dl
       transferrin = 200–400 mg/dl
Sodium, serum = 136–145 mEq/liter
Sulfates, serum, inorganic = 0.5–1.5 mg/dl
Transaminases (liver, muscle, brain): SGOT (AST) = 5–40 units/ml
                          SGPT (ALT) = 5–35 units/ml
Urea nitrogen (BUN) = 10–20 mg/dl
Uric acid = 4.0–9.0 mg/dl
Vitamin A = 125–150 IU/dl or 20–80 µg/dl
Vitamin B_6 = 3.6–18.0 µg/liter
Vitamin B_{12} = 200–900 ng/liter
Vitamin C = 0.6–2 mg/dl
Zinc = 0.75–1.4 µg/ml or up to 79 mg/dl
CPK = 0–145 u/liter
LDH = 200–680 u/ml

****

Blood Cell Values

Erythrocyte count = 4.5–6.2 million/mm^3 (males)
= 4.2–5.4 million/mm^3 (females)
Ferritin = 20–300 ng/ml (males); 20–120 ng/ml = (females)
Folate = 2–20 ng/ml
Iron = 75–175 µg/dl Males; 65–165 µg/dl Females
Iron-binding capacity, total = 240–450 µg/dl (18–59% saturation)
Hematocrit = 40–54% (males); 37–47% (females)
Hemoglobin = 14–17 g/dl (males); 12–15 g/dl (females)
Mean cell volume (MCV) = 80–94 cu/microns
Mean cell hemoglobin (MCH) = 26–32 picograms
Mean cell hemoglobin concentration = 32–36%
White blood cells = 4.8–11.8 thousand/mm^3
Lymphocytes = 24–44% total WBC's
TLC = % lymphocytes × WBC/100; normal = >2000/mm^3 deficient = <900/mm^3

****

Normal Urine Values

Acetone = 0
Aldosterone = 6–16 µg/24 hrs
Ammonia = 20–70 mEq/liter
Amylase = 260–950 Somogyi units/24 hrs
Calcium, normal diet = less than 250 mg/24 hrs
Creatine = less than 100 mg/24 hrs (higher in pregnancy, in children)
Creatinine = 15–25 mg/kg BW in 24 hrs
Estrogens = 4–25 µg/24 hrs. (males); 4–60 µg/24 hrs (females) (higher in PG)
Hemoglobin, myoglobin = 0
5-hydroxyindoleacetic acid (5-HIAA) = 0
Osmolality = 300–800 mOsm/kg
Oxalate = 20–60 mg/24 hrs
pH = 4.6–8 with average of 6 (diet dependent)
Protein = less than 30 mg/24 hrs (0 qualitative)
Specific gravity = 1.003–1.030
Sugar = 0
Vanillylmandelic acid (VMA) = 1.8–8.4 mg/24 hrs

****

Stool Values

Fat = less than 7 g/24 hrs in a 3-day period
Nitrogen = less than 2.5 g/day

****

Other Specific Tests

Renal Values: GFR = 110–150 ml/min (males); 105–132 ml/min (females)
Urea clearance = 40–65 ml/min standard; 60–100 ml/min maximum

Thyroid Values: T_3 (concentration) = 50–210 ng/dl serum
T_4 (concentration) = 4.8–13.2 μg/dl serum
TSH = less than or equal to 0.2 micro-U/liter
Radioactive Iodine Uptake = 9–19% in one hr; 10–50%/24 hrs
Protein-bound iodine = 3.6–8.8 μg/dl

Sources: Pemberton, C., Gastineau, G. (Editors), *Mayo Clinic Diet Manual.* Philadelphia: W.B. Saunders, 1981; Medical Associates Laboratories, Pittsburgh, PA.

SAMPLE TECHNICIAN CARE PLAN CARD—HOSPITAL

DATES	DIET ORDERS; TESTS & SURGERY		
		PREFERENCES	
		BEVERAGES:* C T S M Sk J 7-Up Cocoa	
		DISLIKES:	
		ALLERGIES:	
		COMMENTS:	NOURISHMENTS:

MENUS: Self_____ Tech _____Family_____

DIET ACCEPTED: Yes_____No_____   HANDICAPS

NAME: AGE: ROOM#:

_____

*C = coffee; T = tea; S = Sanka; M = milk; SK = skim milk; J = juice.

HOSPITAL NUTRITION HISTORY AND CARE PLAN FORM

MEDICAL DIAGNOSES/CLINICAL PROBLEMS

ADDRESSOGRAPH

NO.

OTHER STAFF MEMBERS

INIT.

UNIT TECHNICIAN

INIT.

RESPONSIBLE DIETITIAN

INIT.

CL. PROB. NO.	EXPECTED PATIENT OUTCOMES	NUTRITION INTERVENTIONS	INIT./DATE	EVALUATION	INIT./DATE

DIET INSTRUCTIONS:

LABS	DATE	DATE	DATE	DATE	DATE
BS					
Sodium					
Potassium					
Chloride					
HGB					
HCT					

	DATE	DATE	DATE	DATE	DATE
Albumin					
BUN					
Creat.					
T. Pro.					
Chol.					
Trig.					
Amylase					

Phos.		
Ht.		
Wt.		
%		
IBW/HBW		
Other		

DRUGS	INTERACTION

571

HOSPITAL NUTRITION HISTORY AND CARE PLAN

SUBJECTIVE:

Date Interviewed _____

Home Diet _____ Compliance G F P

Present Appetite G F P Home Appetite G F P

Recent Surgery, illness or stress _____

Meals/day _____ Snacks _____

Meals eaten home _____ Away _____ Where _____

Recent weight _____ #_____ 's Y N

Bowel Habits: Normal Constipated Diarrhetic

Dental: Chewing Swallowing

Dentures: Y N Partials

Physical Limitations; _____

Life Style: _____

	B	L	D	10	PM	HS
Meat						
Bread						
Veg.						
Fruit						
Fat						
Milk						
W 2% S						

NOURISHMENTS:

AM

PM

HS

MEAL PATTERN/FOOD HABITS

FOOD GROUPS	DAY	WK.	USUAL EATING PATTERN
Milk			
Cheese			
Meat/Poultry			
Eggs			
Veg.			
Starch Veg.			
Fruits			
Starch			
Fats			
Dessert			
Sugar/Candy			
Alcohol			
Beverage			
Meals Out			

DIET HISTORY

1. Who Shops
2. Who Cooks
3. No. In Household
4. No. Eating Together
5. Meal Eaten Where
6. Occupation
7. Activity Level
8. Exercise
   How Often
9. Religious Influence
10. Cultural Influence
11. Sodium Intake—Table
    Cooking
    Salty Foods
12. Dietetic Products
13. Supplements/Vitamins

ALLERGIES:

INTOLERANCES:

Previous Hx:

Adapted with permission from Food and Nutrition Services Department, Aliquippa Hospital, Aliquippa, PA, 1986.

SAMPLE TECHNICIAN CARE PLAN CARD—NURSING HOME

Beverage Preference:* Breakfast—C T S M J   Lunch—C T S M J   Dinner—C T S M J

	Ex.	Good	Fair	Poor	FAVORITE FOODS	FOODS DISLIKED
Ability to Communicate						
Ability to Chew						
Ability to Swallow						
Appetite						ALLERGIES
Present Food Intake						

Other Factors: Dentures   yes____no____
                Alert—   yes____no____   Dx:_____
                Feed Self—   yes____no____   Handicaps:_____
                Ambulate—   yes____no____   Chart entries:_____
                Dining Room—   yes____no____   Religious
                                                     background: P____C____J____other____

Birthdate_____

	Last	First	Age	Sex	Room#	Diet
NAME						

*C = coffee; T = milk, S = Sanka; M = Milk; J = juice

For Dietary cardexes, kept by Technicians.

SAMPLE NUTRITIONAL ASSESSMENT FORM—NURSING HOME

NURSING HOME   NUTRITIONAL ASSESSMENT FORM

                                                    Initial____Annual____

Patient's Name_____Adm. Date____Age____Sex____Room____

Diagnoses_____Diet_____

Meds/Insulin_____Weight____Ht____Ideal Wt____BEE/REE_____Protein Needs_____

Religious/Ethnic Background: Protestant____Catholic____Jewish____Other_____

Activity Level: Bedridden____Bed to Chair____Ambulatory____To Physical Therapy____

GI Function: Normal Elimination__Diarrhea__Uses Antidiarrheal meds __Colostomy/Ileostomy__

   Constipation____Uses laxatives____Good appetite____Anorexia____Ulcers____Incontinent____

   Use antacids____Feeds self____Cannot feed self____Food allergies_____

Abilities/Limitations: Chewing problems – yes____no____Swallowing problems – yes____no____

   Good communication____Aphasic____Hearing problems – normal____deaf____hearing aid____

   Attentive____Confused____Taste alterations – yes____no____Fever present – yes____no____

BP Elevated____Other Problems:

Part 1

Physical Assessment

	Normal	Abnormal	Severe	Comments
WEIGHT FOR AGE	At ideal, or normal for age.	Thin____Obese____	Morbidly obese____ Emaciated____	
HAIR	Firmly attached Normal distribution Lustrous, shiny.	Thin, sparse. Dull, dry.	Depigmented. Easily pluckable.	Chemotherapy?
EYES	Bright, clear. Pink conjunctiva.	Sunken. Dull. Poor sight. Pale, dry.	Blind. Night blindness.	
LIPS	Good color, moist.	Swollen, red. Dry, cracked.	Fissured, bleeding.	
GUMS	Pink, firm.	Sore, spongy. Red, swollen.	Bleed easily.	
TONGUE	Pink. Papillae present.	Purple, magenta. White, grey coating. Smooth, slick.	Beefy red. Burning. Fissured.	
TEETH	Straight, clean.	Dentures in good repair. Missing teeth, loose teeth or chipped teeth.	Edentulous. Poorly fitted or loose dentures. Caries.	
SKIN	Smooth, slightly moist. Good color.	Pale, dry, scaly. Bruises easily. Hyperpigmented.	Pellagrous dermatitis. Decubiti.	
LEGS	Well-developed; firm muscles	Calf tenderness. Flaccid muscles.	Edema. Bowlegs.	
HANDS & NAILS	Normal, smooth.	Brittle, thin nails. Atrophied fine muscles.	Spoon-shaped nails.	
MUSCULOSKELETAL	Normal muscular and bone development.	Calf muscle tenderness. Wasted appearance.	Paralysis. Osteoporosis. Bone Fractures.	
NEUROLOGICAL	Normal reflexes, abilities.	CVA. Limited reflexes. Listlessness. Irritability.	Comatose. Seizures.	

Evaluations: Nutritional Status: Normal_____Abnormal because of_____

_____

Recommendations/Goals:_____

_____

Signed:_____

Date:_____

Part 2

DIETARY MASTER PLAN OF CARE—EXTENDED CARE FACILITY

Problem	Plan of Action	Goal
1. Needs assistance at meal-time	1. Nursing will cut meat, open milk, arrange food. Dietary should mark meal cards with appropriate color to indicate feeding assistance needed.	1. Adequate intake of basic foods. Adequate fluid and calorie intake. Meet energy and nutrient needs of patient.
2. Cannot self-feed	2. Spoon feeding by Nursing will be needed.	2. Adequate intake of basic foods so that fluid, calorie, protein and nutrient needs are met.
3. Cannot swallow (dysphagia)	3. Tube feeding will be administered by nursing. Progress as tolerated to thick pureed diet.	3. Tube feeding should be calculated to provide adequate calories, protein, and nutrients to meet needs of patient. Adequate fluid intake.
4. Blind	4. Tray arranged by nursing. May require bowls from Dietary if patient wishes to feed self.	4. Adequate intake of basic foods so that fluid, calorie, protein, and nutrient needs are met.
5. No teeth or poorly fitting dentures or difficulty in chewing	5. Modify food consistency (moisture) or texture (chopping, mincing) to meet patient needs. Either mechanical soft diet or pureed foods. Be aware of weight losses.	5. Adequate intake of basic foods in altered form to insure that calories, fluid, protein, and nutrient needs are met.
6. Poor appetite or refuses to eat or poor calorie intake	6. Offer encouragement at mealtimes. Assist if needed. Spoon fed if necessary. If severe, may tube feed. Offer preferred foods and/or provide nutritional supplement between meals (by Nursing). Suggest occupational therapy group feeding ("lunch bunch"). Identify causation, treatments.	6. Increase intake of calories, protein, fluids, and other nutrients to meet needs. Correct anorexia, weight loss.
7. Fluid retention (edema)	7. Control sodium content of diet. Offer diet as ordered by physician. (May be "no added salt," 2–3 g sodium diet, or other restriction.) Check/monitor albumin, I & O.	7. Lessen edema. Prevent further complications. Control sodium intake through diet. Correct protein malnutrition, if evident.

Problem	Intervention	Goal
8. Will not complete meals	8. Encourage self-help. If patient falls asleep, remind patient to finish meals.	8. Monitor feeding process to insure adequate intake of fluid, protein, calories and other nutrients.
9. Dietary inadequacy	9. Encourage foods from all four basic food groups. (If patient refuses citrus fruits, vitamin C may be lacking. If milk, calcium is at risk. If meats, protein may be lacking. If vegetables, vitamins and fiber may be low.) Encourage dessert last.	9. Monitor dietary intake to improve intake of food groups so that nutrients are no longer lacking. Evaluate and maintain calorie levels.
10. Buying foods from snack machines while on modified diet	10. Ask Nursing to watch patient so that snacks are not brought in by family or purchased by patient. Discuss problem with the patient to explain role of the diet in treatment plan.	10. Reduce cheating on diet. Increase adherence to diet.
11. Elevated blood sugar or uncontrolled diabetes	11. Control intake of calories and concentrated sweets. Follow calorie-controlled diet as ordered by doctor. Offer substitutes when diet is not consumed.	11. Adhere to diabetic diet. Adequate intake of protein, calories, fluid, and nutrients. Limit side effects of diabetes.
12. Constipation	12. Add fiber and fluid unless contraindicated. Crushed bran can be added to hot cereal for pureed diets. Milk or prune juice may also be helpful if tolerated. Add activity if feasible. If TF, use Enrich, Jevity, or similar product.	12. Alleviate constipation. Prevent obstruction.
13. Decubitus ulcer	13. Add extra protein and calories to meals and snacks. Add a supplement or tube feed if necessary.	13. Heal ulcer. Prevent further skin breakdown.
14. Significant weight loss, especially rapid	14. Add snacks or supplements between meals. Use nutrient-dense foods at mealtime. Weigh regularly (once weekly) with same clothing.	14. Promote return to healthy/ideal body weight. Prevent morbidity/mortality.

SAMPLE NUTRITIONAL CARE AUDIT

Patient's Unit Code Number_____

Type of chart: general/disease-specific/RD-specific_____

Dates of Hospitalization:_____Length of Stay_____

Patient's Name:_____Age_____Sex_____

Physician's Name(s)_____Nursing Unit_____

Provisional Diagnosis_____

Final Diagnosis_____

1. PHYSICIAN'S CARE:

   Documented on History and Physical: Yes   No

       Patient's diet at home   _____   _____

       Patient's recent appetite or intake?   _____   _____

       Changes in weight status?   _____   _____

       Previous nutritional problems?   _____   _____

       Diseases requiring nutritional intervention?   _____   _____

       Other nutrition-related statement?   _____   _____

       Explain_____

   _____

   Other chart notes regarding intake, appetite, weight changes,
   fluid restrictions, lab tests that suggest the need for nutritional
   intervention?   _____   _____

   Explain_____

   Surgical procedures affecting nutritional status:_____

   _____

   Tests done which required dietary preparation?_____

   _____

   Drugs ordered_____

   _____

   Abnormal lab values affecting nutritional outcomes:_____

   _____

   Use of parenteral nutrition for more than 2 days: Yes_____No_____if yes,

       describe:_____

   _____

2. NURSING CARE: Recorded ht_____Admitting wt_____Discharge wt_____

       # times wt. was recorded_____Notes about appetite, wt. changes, visits by

       dietary, etc._____

3. OTHER ANCILLARY SERVICES AFFECTING NUTRITION:

   Physical Therapy_____

   Occupational Therapy_____

   Social Services_____

   Home Health Services_____

   Pharmacy_____

   Respiratory Therapy_____

   Speech Pathology_____

Criteria: Check if included in note. Write "N.A." if not applicable.	DATE:____ RD:____ DIET:____	DATE:____ RD:____ DIET:____	DATE:____ RD:____ DIET:____	DATE:____ RD:____ DIET:____	DATE:____ RD:____ DIET:____
Format: Used proper place for notes. Used date, time, signature.					
S Included diet history information.					
As appropriate, included patient statements.					
Included diet followed at home (if any).					
Statement about recent appetite/nausea.					
Eating problems; chewing difficulties.					
O Ht., wt. and IBW, TSF, MAC, MAMC.					
Lab data and reference to drugs ordered.					
Diet order stated.					
Weight changes.					
BMR factors: fever, tachycardia, exudates; BEE and prot/kcal needs for age, sex, etc.					
Calorie counts; or estimated intake.					
A % IBW or % Usual weight.					
Nutrient deficiencies in diet as ordered.					
Evaluation of diet or diet hx.					
Patient acceptance of diet ordered.					
Patient understanding of diet instructions.					
Verification of diet as appropriate for pt.					
Recommendations for anticipated problems.					
P Instructions					
Consult/refer to other professional/agency					
Obtain weight; obtain calorie counts.					
Recommend alternate feedings/supplements/route.					
Request change in diet.					
Short-term and long-term goals indicated.					

Criteria: Check if included in note. Write "N.A." if not applicable.	RD:____ DATE:____ DIET:	RD:____ DATE:____ DIET:	RD:____ DATE:____ DIET:	RD:____ DATE:____ DIET:	RD:____ DATE:____ DIET:
I-E-R*Nutritional breakdown of calculated diet (or other modification/feeding) recorded.					
Stated that diet copy/written handouts were given to pt. or significant other.					
Stated course of nutritional care while hospitalized.					
Stated whether or not pt. selects own menu (esp. for modified diets).					
Plans for discharge noted: referred to Nutrition Counseling Service, etc.					
Pt. and/or significant other attended Class.					
Measurable patient outcomes noted (wt. loss or gain; able to state foods to avoid, etc.)					

OTHER COMMENTS:_____

OVERALL OPINION OF NUTRITIONAL CARE WHILE HOSPITALIZED:_____
_____

SUGGESTIONS FOR IMPROVEMENT OF CARE:_____
_____

SIGNATURE OF REVIEWER: _____DATE OF REVIEW_____

_____

*I = Implementation; E = Education; R = Replan.

SAMPLE OUTCOME AUDITS—PATIENT EDUCATION

All Patients

1. Pt. is able to identify the basic four food groups and can select his/her menu accurately.
2. Pt. is able to explain importance of his/her diet to his/her health.
3. Pt. is able to plan one day's menus and snacks from his/her dietary pattern.
4. Pt. is able to incorporate economic/ethnic food choices into his/her prescribed diet.
5. Pt. has been following _____ diet at home for _____ period of time. Pt. is able to describe elements of this diet with accuracy.
6. Pt. expresses recognition of the need to lose/gain weight.
7. Pt. is allergic to _____ foods, as documented by _____ (tests, observation, family etc.)
8. Pt. likes/refuses to eat _____ (foods, beverages).

Liquid Diets

1. Pt. requests progression to solid foods at this time.
2. Pt. is able to tolerate only clear/full liquids at this time.

Protein Diets

1. Pt. can identify _____ foods that contain protein of high biologic value.
2. Pt. can name _____ foods to include/omit in diet to increase/decrease protein content of meals and snacks.

Mineral Diets (Iron, Potassium, Calcium, etc.)

1. Pt. is able to name _____ foods that are high/low in _____ (mineral).
2. Pt. is able to accurately select menus choices for days that include/exclude foods that are high in _____ (mineral).
3. Pt. is able to plan menus for _____ days at home that are high/low in _____ (in mineral).

Vegetarian Diet

1. Pt. is able to identify correctly _____ (2–3) complementary protein foods.
2. Pt. is able to plan menus for _____ days that provide adequate protein for age and sex.

Tube Feeding

1. Pt. does/does not tolerate specific tube feeding as ordered.
2. Pt. will receive _____ calories in _____ (product used), dilution _____ (where no specified order is given).
3. S.O. is able to prepare tube feeding as ordered for use at home (when home feedings are ordered).

Bland

1. Pt. is able to identify _____ foods to avoid on the bland diet.
2. Pt. is able to explain the rationale for excluding caffeine-containing beverages and food items.
3. Pt. is able to verbalize the reasoning for modifying eating habits when he/she is under stress.

Post-Gastrectomy or Dumping Syndrome (for any reason)

1. Pt. is able to verbalize the effects of diet on the dumping syndrome.
2. Pt. is able to explain _____ guidelines to be followed to prevent the dumping syndrome.
3. Pt. is able to tolerate meals when beverages are served 30 minutes prior to or following meals.

High Fiber

1. Pt. is able to verbalize _____ foods that can be used to increase fiber in his/her diet.
2. Pt. is able to explain the role of fiber in his/her particular disorder.
3. Pt. is able to describe the purpose of adequate fluids in the dietary regimen.

Low Fat

1. Pt. is able to name _____ foods that he/she must omit for the low fat diet.
2. Pt. is able to explain the role of fat in his/her condition.

Low Cholesterol

1. Pt. is able to describe simple definitions for cholesterol, saturated fat, polyunsaturated fat, monounsaturated fat.
2. Pt. is able to identify _____ foods that have a high cholesterol content.
3. Pt. is able to name _____ vegetable oils that may be used on the diet.
4. Pt. is able to describe 3 cooking methods that are acceptable for the dietary regimen.

Hyperlipidemia Diets

1. Pt. is able to explain the principal restrictions for his/her diet regarding calories, carbohydrate, fat, alcohol and cholesterol.
2. Pt. is able to plan _____ day menus within dietary restrictions.
3. Pt. is able to discuss the role of soluble fiber.

Hypoglycemia Diet

1. Pt. is able to verbalize the reasons for eating frequently.
2. Pt. is able to describe the reactions that can occur when concentrated carbohydrates are eaten, or with omission of meals.
3. Pt. is able to describe the role of protein and fats in the diet.

Diabetic Diets

1. Pt. is able to explain the relationship of diet to side effects of diabetes.
2. Pt. is able to name _____ foods that are high in simple sugars.
3. Pt. is able to categorize correctly _____ into the proper food group lists.
4. Pt. is able to verbalize a simple definition of diabetes.
5. Pt. is able to describe the role of medications to food intake.
6. Pt. is able to explain the rationale for following a prudent diet to prevent complications of atherosclerosis.
7. Pt. is able to explain how proper spacing of meals affects his/her disorder.
8. Pt. is able to describe the symptoms of ketoacidosis and insulin shock, and can name foods to take or avoid for each condition.
9. After looking at several food labels, Pt. is able to point out ingredients that mean "sugar" or carbohydrate.

Reducing Diets

1. Pt. is able to verbalize his/her primary motivation for losing weight.
2. Pt. is able to describe his/her realistic goal for weight loss—either short-term or long-term, including a timetable.
3. Pt. is able to list _____ foods that are low-calorie and may be eaten as snacks.
4. Pt. is able to categorize _____ foods into the proper food group category.
5. Pt. is able to demonstrate the proper technique for recording food intake at home.
6. Pt. has shown _____ weight loss over _____ (time).

Cardiac Care

1. Pt. is able to name three beverages that are high in caffeine.
2. Pt. is able to describe the modifications in his/her diet that will be needed to prevent further coronary complications.

Sodium Restrictions

1. Pt. is able to name _____ foods that are naturally high in sodium.
2. Pt. is able to name _____ foods that have been processed or prepared with excesses of sodium.
3. Pt. is able to explain the difference between "salt" and "sodium" in foods.
4. Pt. is able to list _____ seasonings that can be used at home, in place of salt and salt-containing seasonings.
5. Pt. is able to plan menus for _____ days that will be low in sodium for home use.
6. Pt. is able to identify the salt substitutes that he/she can use for his/her condition.

Gliadin-Free/Gluten-Restricted Diet

1. Pt. is able to examine food labels and to name the ingredients that he/she must avoid for his/her condition.
2. Pt. is able to list 5 gluten-containing products that must be avoided on the diet.
3. Pt. is able to plan menus for _____ days that can be used at home.

Lactose Intolerance

1. Pt. is able to name _____ foods or beverages that he/she should avoid for his/her condition.
2. Pt. is able to plan menus for _____ days that are nutritionally complete for calcium, but are lactose-restricted.

Renal Diets

1. Pt. is able to describe the dietary restrictions that are needed for his/her diet in regard to protein, sodium, potassium, fluid, calories, and phosphorus.
2. Pt. is able to plan menus for _____ days that are balanced for the restricted nutrients.
3. Pt. is able to name _____ free foods that he/she can eat as desired.

COMMON ABBREVIATIONS

AA	amino acid
abd.	abdomen, abdominal
ABW	average body weight
ACE	angiotensin-converting enzyme
ADA	American Dietetic Association
alb	albumin
alk phos	alkaline phosphatase
amts.	amounts
ARF	acute renal failure
ASHD	atherosclerotic heart disease
ATP	adenosine triphosphate
BCAAs	branched-chain amino acids
BEE	basal energy expenditure
BF	breast-feeding, breast-feeder
BMR	basal metabolic rate
BP	blood pressure
BS	blood sugar
BSA	body surface area
BUN	blood urea nitrogen
BW	body weight
bx	biopsy
c	cup
C	coffee
CA	cancer
Ca, Ca^{++}	calcium
CABG	coronary artery bypass grafting
CBC	complete blood count
CF	cystic fibrosis
CHD	congenital heart disease
CHF	congestive heart failure
CHO	carbohydrate
chol	cholesterol
circum.	circumference
Cl, Cl^-	chloride
CNS	central nervous system
CO_2	carbon dioxide
CPK	creatine phosophokinase
CPR	cardiopulmonary resuscitation
CrCl	creatine clearance
CRP	C-reactive protein
CT	computed tomography
Cu	copper
CVA	cerebrovascular accident

DAT	diet as tolerated
dec.	decreased
decaf.	decaffeinated
def.	deficiency
DJD	degenerative joint disease
dl	deciliter
DM	diabetes mellitus
DNA	deoxyribonucleic acid
DOB	date of birth
dx	diagnosis
D_5W	5% dextrose solution in water
ECG	electrocardiogram
EEG	electroencephalogram
EFAs	essential fatty acids
e.g.	for example
elec.	electrolytes
elim.	eliminate, elimination
EN	enteral nutrition
esp.	especially
ESRD	end-stage renal disease
ETOH	ethanol/ethyl alcohol
Fe, Fe^{++}	iron
F & V	fruits and vegetables
FSH	follicle-stimulating hormone
FTT	failure to thrive
FUO	fever of unknown origin
g	grams(s)
GA	gestational age
GBD	gallbladder disease
GE	gastroenteritis
gest.	gestational
GFR	glomerular filtration rate
GI	gastrointestinal
gluc	glucose
GN	glomerular nephritis
GTT	glucose tolerance test
H & H	hemoglobin & hematocrit
HBV	high biologic value
HBW	healthy body wt.
HCl	hydrochloric acid
Hct	hematocrit
HDL	high-density lipoprotein
Hgb A_1C	hemoglobin A_1C test (glucose)
HLP	hyperlipoproteinemia or hyperlipidemia
HPN, HTN	hypertension

ht	height
hx	history
I	infant
I & O	intake and output
IBW	ideal body weight
IDDM	insulin-dependent diabetes mellitus
i.e.	that is
IEM	inborn error of metabolism
inc.	increased
I.U.	international units
IUD	intrauterine device
IV	intravenous
J, jc	juice
K, K$^+$	potassium
kcal	food kilocalories
kg	kilogram(s)
L	liter(s)
LBM	lean body mass
LBV	low biological value
LBW	low birthweight
LCT	long-chain triglycerides
LDH	lactic acid dehydrogenase
LDL	low-density lipoproteins
L.E.	lupus erythematosus
LGA	large for gestational age
LH	luteinizing hormone
LI	large intestine
lytes	electrolytes
M	milk
MAC	mid-arm circumference
MAMC	mid-arm muscle circumference
MAO	monoamine oxidase
MBF	meat-base formula
MCH	mean cell hemoglobin
MCT	medium-chain triglycerides
MCV	mean cell volume
meds	medications
MI	myocardial infarction
Mg, Mg^{++}	magnesium
mg	milligram(s)
μg	micrograms
mm	millimeter(s)
mos.	months
MOSF	multiple organ systems failure
MSG	monosodium glutamate

N	nitrogen
N & V	nausea & vomiting
Na, Na$^+$	sodium
NEC	necrotizing enterocolitis
NG	nasogastric
NIDDM	non-insulin-dependent diabetes mellitus
NP	non-protein (as in NP calories)
NPO	nil per os (nothing by mouth)
O_2	oxygen
OCs	oral contraceptives
OJ	orange juice
OK	okay, suitable
OT	occupational therapist
oz	ounce(s)
P	phosphorus
PCM	protein-calorie malnutrition
P_{CO_2}	partial pressure of carbon dioxide
PG	pregnant, pregnancy
PKU	phenylketonuria
PN	parenteral nutrition
P_{O_2}	partial pressure of oxygen
prn	pro re nata (as needed)
prot.	protein
PT	pro-time or Physical Therapy
PTH	parathormone
PTT	prothrombin time
PUFA(s)	polyunsaturated fatty acid(s)
PVD	peripheral vascular disease
RAST	radioallergosorbent test
RBC	red blood cell count
RDAs	recommended dietary allowances
RDS	respiratory distress syndrome
REE	resting energy expenditure
RQ	respiratory quotient
Rx	treatment
S	Sanka
sed. rate	sedimentation rate
SGA	small for gestational age
SGOT	serum glutamic-oxaloacetic transaminase
SGPT	serum glutamic-pyruvic transaminase
SI	small intestine
SIADH	syndrome of inappropriate antidiuretic hormone
SIDS	sudden infant death syndrome
SOB	shortness of breath
sub.	substitute

Sx	symptoms
T	tablespoon(s); tea
t	teaspoon(s)
TB	tuberculosis
temp.	temperature
TF	tube feeding; tube-fed
TIBC	total iron-binding capacity
TLC	total lymphocyte count
TPN	total parenteral nutrition
trig	triglyceride(s)
TSF	triceps skinfold
UA	uric acid
UTIs	urinary tract infections
UUN	urine urea nitrogen
vit.	vitamin(s)
VMA	vanillylmandelic acid
$\dot{V}O_{2max}$	maximum oxygen uptake
vs.	versus
WBC	white blood cell count
wt	weight
yrs.	years
Zn	zinc
#	pounds (lbs)
24°	24 hours
↑	high, elevated or increased
↓	low or decreased
√	check

SELECTED CLEARINGHOUSE AND INFORMATION CENTERS

Alcohol
National Clearinghouse for Alcohol
Information
P.O. Box 2345
Rockville, MD 20852
(301) 468-2600
Arthritis
Arthritis Information Clearinghouse
P.O. Box 9782
Arlington, VA 22209
(703) 558-4999
Cancer
Cancer Information Clearinghouse
National Cancer Institute
Office of Cancer Communications
9000 Rockville Pike, Bldg. 31,
Room 10A18
Bethesda, MD 20205
(301) 496-5583
Consumer Information
Consumer Information Center
Room G-142, 18th and F Streets,
NW
Washington, DC 20405
Diabetes
National Diabetes Information
Clearinghouse
Box: NDIC
Bethesda, MD 20892
(301) 468-6344
Digestive Diseases
National Digestive Diseases
Education and Information
Clearinghouse
1255 23rd St. NW, Suite 275
Washington, DC 20037
Family Planning
National Clearinghouse for Family
Planning Information
P.O. Box 2225
Rockville, MD 20852
(301) 881-9400
Handicapped
Clearinghouse on the Handicapped
400 Maryland Avenue, SW
3119 Switzer Bldg.
Washington, DC 20202
(202) 245-0080

Health Indexes
Clearinghouse on Health Indexes
National Center for Health Statistics
Division of Epidemiology and Health
Promotion
3700 East-West Highway, Room
2-27
Hyattsville, MD 20782
Health Information
National Health Information
Clearinghouse
P.O. Box 1133
Washington, DC 20013-1133
(207) 429-9091/(800) 336-4797
Health Promotion and Education
Center for Health Promotion and
Education
Centers for Disease Control
1600 Clifton Road, Bldg. 1, SSB-249
Atlanta, GA 30333
(404) 329-3492
High Blood Pressure
High Blood Pressure Information
Center
120–80 National Institutes of Health
Bethesda, MD 20205
(703) 558-4880
Maternal and Child Health
National Center for Education in
Maternal and Child Health
3520 Prospect Street, Ground Floor
Washington, DC 20057
(202) 625-8400
Medications
Food and Drug Administration (FDA)
Office of Consumer Affairs, Public
Inquiries
5600 Fishers Lane (HFE-88)
Rockville, MD 20857
(301) 443-3170
Mental Health
National Clearinghouse for Mental
Health Information
Public Inquiries Section
5600 Fishers Lane, Room 15C-05
Rockville, MD 20857
(301) 443-4513

Nutrition and Food
Food and Nutrition Information
Center
National Agricultural Library Bldg.,
Room 304
10301 Baltimore Blvd.
Beltsville, MD 20705
(301) 344-3719
Rehabilitation
National Rehabilitation Information
Center
4407 Eighth Street, NE
Washington, DC 20017-2299
(202) 635-5822

Smoking
Office on Smoking and Health
Technical Information Center
5600 Fishers Lane, Park Bldg.,
Room 116
Rockville, MD 20857
(301) 443-1690

AMERICAN DIETETIC ASSOCIATION PRACTICE GROUPS

* Public Health Nutrition
* Gerontological Nutrition
* Dietetics in Developmental and Psychiatric Disorders
* Vegetarian Nutrition
* Renal Dietitians
* Pediatric Nutrition
* Diabetes Care and Education
* Dietitians in Nutrition Support
* Dietetics in Physical Medicine and Rehabilitation
* Sports and Cardiovascular Nutritionists
* Dietitians in General Clinical Practice
* Consulting Dietitians—Private Practice
* Consultant Dietitians in Health-Care Facilities
* Dietitians in Business and Communications
* ADA Members with Management Responsibilities in Health-Care Delivery Systems
* School Nutrition Services
* Dietitians in College and University Foodservice
* Clinical Nutrition Management
* Technical Practice in Dietetics
* Dietetic Educators of Practitioners
* Nutrition Education of Health Professionals
* Nutrition Education of the Public
* Nutrition Research

FOR MORE INFORMATION, OR TO CONTACT A PRACTICE GROUP, WRITE:

The American Dietetic Association
216 W. Jackson Blvd., Suite 800
Chicago, Illinois 60606-6995
(800) 877-1600

RATIONALE FOR DIAGNOSTIC-RELATED GROUP TABLES

In the United States, medical costs have soared higher than other expenses in cost-of-living evaluations. To curb the excessive growth in medical charges, Diagnostic-Related Groupings (DRGs) were established by the federal government as reasonable costs per diagnosis, recognizing regional differences as well as differences in size of the facilities.

With awareness that nutritional status affects immunity, wound healing, and other factors related to medical care, a sample population was selected to create the tables. The typical *length of stay* for an uncomplicated procedure also varies, with a certain payment allowed up to the typical length of stay. It is good practice for the hospitals to admit and discharge patients expediently, and to provide excellent care, especially to be paid for the services rendered.

Many authors have described the impact of DRGs on hospital malnutrition, and vice versa. For example, in some institutions it has been possible to obtain more money per case when malnutrition is listed as a co-morbidity factor or a complication. However, some of the reimbursements have *not* increased because of the patient's age.

Although the DRGs affect medicare patients, it is believed by some economists that other third-party payors will follow the same trend. It is possible that, if DRGs continue to lead in hospital payment systems, one day all hospital charges will be predictable in advance. Payments in this method are '''prospective'' rather than retrospective. Thus, the "Prospective Payment System" (PPS) has had a significant impact on health-care services in the United States.

It is likely that the trend to "cost-justify" all services (including nutritional services) will continue. The reader must remember that malnourished patients have longer lengths of stay at higher costs, as well as more deaths. The goal of each health provider (physician, dietitian, nurse, pharmacist, etc.) must include assurance that the patient will have a satisfactory or improved nutritional status during hospitalization and that rapid discharge to home, other rehabilitative or skilled nursing center, or other site will be appropriate within a reasonable time frame.

The tables of DRGs listed on the next few pages are not complete, but are samples of the codes and lengths of stay that would be permitted for persons of a particular age. The actual DRG codes are assigned by the institution and are scrutinized intermittently by the government. For more information, contact the medical records, admitting or fiscal departments of the local hospitals for localized information.

SAMPLE DIAGNOSTIC-RELATED GROUPINGS (DRGs)*

CONDITION AND ICD-9-CM INTERNATIONAL CODE	DRG CODE EXAMPLE
Pregnancy (650)	#373
Infertility (628.9)	#369
Dental difficulties/oral disorders:	#185
Edentulism (525.1)	
Broken or wired jaw (802.2)	
Mouth ulcers (528.9)	
Tongue disorders (529.9)	
Periodontal disease (523.9)	#185
Skin disorders:	#284
Acne (706.1)	#284
Psoriasis (696.1)	#273
Chronic urticaria (708.9)	#284
Infantile eczema (692.9)	#284
Acrodermatitis enteropathica (686.8)	#278
Dermatitis herpetiformis (692.9)	#284
Decubitus ulcer (707.0)	#271
Vitamin deficiencies:	#297
Xerophthalmia (264.7)	#47
Cheilosis (266.0)	#297
Scurvy (267)	#297
Food Allergy/allergic reactions	#447
Asthma (493)	#97
Food poisoning (005.9)	#183
Meniere's syndrome	#73
Biliary atresia (751.61)	#208
Cerebral palsy (343.9)	#35
Cleft palate (749)	#52 Surgical #74 Medical
Congenital heart disease	#137
Cystic fibrosis (277)	#298
Cystinosis (270)	#299
Down's syndrome (758)	#429
Failure to thrive (783.4)	#298
Inborn errors of CHO metabolism	#299
Hirschsprung's disease (751.3)	#190
Homocystinuria (270.4)	#299
Low birthweight infant (765.1)	#385
Maple syrup urine disease (270.3)	#299
Necrotizing entercolitis	#184
Phenylketonuria (270.1)	#299
Prader-Willi syndrome (759.8)	#385
Tyrosinemia (270.4)	#299
Wilson's disease (275.1)	#299
Alzheimer's disease (331.0)	#429
Amyotrophic lateral sclerosis (335.20)	#12
Anorexia nervosa (307.1)	#428
Coma (780.0)	#27

* Length-of-stay information is noted by each diagnosis.

Depression (311)	#426
Epilepsy (345.9)	#25
Huntington's chorea (333.4)	#12
Multiple sclerosis (340)	#13
Myasthenia gravis (358)	#12
Neurological trauma/spinal cord injury (952.9)	#9
Parkinson's disease (332)	#12
Psychosis	#430
Bronchial asthma	#96
Acute respiratory failure (799.1)	#87
Pneumonia/bronchitis	#90
Chronic obstructive pulmonary disease (496)	#88
Cor pulmonale (416.9)	#145
Pulmonary embolus (415.1)	#78
Tuberculosis (011.9)	#80
Atherosclerosis or Ischemic heart disease (414)	#132
Cerebrovascular disease (436)	#131
Congestive failure and shock (428)	#127
Heart valve disorder	#136
Hyperlipoproteinemias (272.4)	#299
Hypertension (401.9)	#134
Myocardial infarction (410.9)	#121
Peripheral vascular disease (443.9)	#130
Achalasia (530.3)	#183
Heartburn/esophagitis (553.3)	#183
Dyspepsia (536.8)	#183
Gastric retention (536.8)	#183
Gastritis/gastroenteritis (535.5)	#183
Pernicious vomiting (536.2)	#183
Peptic ulcer/complications (533.9)	#176
Gastrectomy or vagotomy (43.89)	#155
Diarrhea (558.9)	#183
Dysentery (009.0)	#183
Malabsorption syndrome (579.9)	#183
Gluten-induced enteropathy (579.0)	#183
Tropical sprue (579.1)	#183
Lactose malabsorption (271.3)	#183
Constipation (564)	#183
Irritable colon (564.1)	#183
Diverticular diseases (562.11)	#183
Enteritis or Crohn's disease (555.9)	#179
Intestinal fistula (569.81)	#189
Ileitis (558.9)	#183
Ulcerative colitis/ileostomy (556)	#149
Ileostomy, permanent (46.23)	#149
Colostomy (46.10)	#149
Anal procedures such as hemorrhoidectomy (49.46)	#157
Intestinal lipodystrophy (Whipple's disease)	#188
Pancreatitis (577.0)	#204
Pancreatic insufficiency (577.8)	#204
Zollinger-Ellison syndrome (251.5)	#176
Cholecystitis (574.0)	#208
Cholecystectomy (574.0)	#195

Jaundice (782.4)	#464
Hepatitis (573.3)	#206
Biliary cirrhosis (571.6)	#207
Alcoholic liver disease (571.3)	#202
Alcohol dependence (305)	#436
Ascites (789.5)	#464
Hepatic cirrhosis (571.5)	#202
Liver transplant	#191
Hepatic encephalopathy and/or coma (572.2)	#206
Type I diabetes mellitus (250.01)	#295
Type II diabetes mellitus (250.00)	#294
Ketaoacidosis and/or coma (250.11)	#294
Hypoglycemia (251.2)	#297
Hyperinsulinism (251.1)	#301
Addison's disease (255.4)	#301
Hyperthyroidism (242.9)	#301
Hypothyroidism (244.9)	#301
Goiter (240.9)	#301
Diabetes insipidus (253.5)	#301
Gout (274.9)	#245
Cushing's syndrome (255.0)	#301
Parathyroid disorders (252)	#301
Altered calcium metabolism (275.4)	#297
Gestational diabetes (648.8)	#372
Pregnancy-induced hypertension (642.4)	#372
Obesity (278.0)	#297
Underweight or general debility (269.9)	#297
Kwashiorkor (260)	#297
Marasmus (261)	#297
Muscular dystrophy (359.1)	#256
Osteoarthritis (715.9)	#245
Osteomalacia (268.2)	#245
Osteoporosis (733)	#245
Rheumatoid arthritis (714)	#242
Scleroderma	#241
Systemic lupus erythematosus (710)	#241
Nutritional anemias (281)	#395
Iron-deficiency anemia (280.9)	#395
Sickle-cell anemia (282.6)	#395
Brain tumor	#10
Cancer (such as leukemia 209.9 or lymphoma 202.8)	#403
Radiotherapy	#409
Chemotherapy	#410
Electrolyte imbalances (K^+, Ca^{++}, Mg^{++}, Na^+) 275-6	#297
Amputation (84.17)	#114
Appendectomy/complications (47)	#164
Bowel surgery	#148
Jejuno-ileal bypass (45.91)	#288
Gastric bypass or stapling (44.31)	#288
Craniotomy	#1
Retinal cataract surgery	#36

Hysterectomy, abdominal (68.4)	#353
Coronary bypass with cardiac catheterization (36.10)	#106
Total hip arthroplasty (81.59)	#209
Tonsillectomy/adenoidectomy (28.3)	#57–58
Acquired immune deficiency syndrome	#423
Bacterial endocarditis (421)	#126
Burns (949)	#457
Fever, unknown origin (780.6)	#419
Fracture, hip (821)	#210 Surgical #236 Medical
Infectious mononucleosis (075)	#421
Poliomyelitis (045.9)	#20
Rheumatic fever (390)	#241
Typhoid fever (002)	#423
Glomerulonephritis, acute (580.9)	#332
Glomerulonephritis, chronic (582.9)	#332
Nephritis (583.9)	#332
Nephrosclerosis (403.9)	#332
Nephrotic syndrome (581.9)	#326
Pyelonephritis, chronic (590.0)	#320
Urolithiasis (592.9)	#323
Renal failure, acute (584.9)	#316
Renal failure, chronic (585)	#316
Renal dialysis: hemodialysis (39.95)	#317
Renal dialysis: peritoneal (54.98)	#317
Post-renal transplantation (55.69)	#302
Vitamin-D resistant rickets (275.3)	#299
Hartnup disease (270)	#299

Note: This chart was created to serve as a guide for planning nutritional care during a limited hospitalization. From *Federal Register 53*:(190), 9/30/88.

BIBLIOGRAPHY

Key to Journal Abbreviations:

Adv Nut Res	Advanced Nutrition Research
AJCN	American Journal of Clinical Nutrition
AJPH	American Journal of Public Health
Am Coll Surg	American College of Surgeons
Am Fam Phys	American Family Physician
Am J Card	American Journal of Cardiology
Am J Dis Child	American Journal of Diseases of Children
Am J Epid	American Journal of Epidemiology
Am J Gastro	American Journal of Gastroenterology
Am J Hematol	American Journal of Hematology
Am J Hosp Pharm	American Journal of Hospital Pharmacy
Am J Kid Dis	American Journal of Kidney Diseases
Am J Med	American Journal of Medicine
Am J Nurs	American Journal of Nursing
Am J OB and Gyne	American Journal of Obstetrics and Gynecology
Am J Psych	American Journal of Psychiatry
Am J Surg	American Journal of Surgery
Anes	Anesthesiology
Ann Hum Biol	Annals of Human Biology
Ann Int Med	Annals of Internal Medicine
Ann Neuro	Annals of Neurology
Ann NY Acad Sci	Annals of the New York Academy of Sciences
Ann Thor Surg	Annals of Thoracic Surgery
Arch Dis Child	Archives of Diseases of Childhood
Arch Gen Psych	Archives of General Psychiatry
Arch Int Med	Archives of Internal Medicine
Arch Neuro	Archives of Neurology
Arch Orthop Tr Surg	Archives of Orthopedics and Trauma Surgery
Arch Surg	Archives of Surgery
Brit J Psychiatry	British Journal of Psychiatry
Brit J Surg	British Journal of Surgery
Brit Med J	British Journal of Medicine
Cancer Bull	Cancer Bulletin
Cancer Detect Prev	Cancer Detection and Prevention
Cancer Res	Cancer Research
Clin Chest Med	Clinics in Chest Medicine
Clin Endo	Clinical Endocrinology
Clin Gastro	Clinical Gastroenterology
Clin Nutr	Clinical Nutrition

Clin Nutr Man	Clinical Nutrition Manual
Clin Perinat	Clinics in Perinatology
Clin Plast Surg	Clinics in Plastic Surgery
Comp Ther	Comprehensive Therapy
Contemp Surg	Contemporary Surgery
Crit Care Curr	Critical Care Currents
Crit Care Med	Critical Care Medicine
Crit Care Nurs	Critical Care Nursing
Crit Care Quarterly	Critical Care Quarterly
Dairy Sci	Dairy Science
Dig Dis and Sci	Digestive Diseases and Science
Dis Colon Rectum	Diseases of the Colon and Rectum
DNA Newsletter	Dietitians in Nutrition Support Newsletter
FDA Consumer	Food and Drug Administration Consumer
Fed Proc	Federal Proceedings
Gastro	Gastroenterology
Hosp Form	Hospital Formulary
Hosp Pract	Hospital Practice
JADA	Journal of the American Dietetic Association
JAMA	Journal of the American Medical Association
J Am Coll Nut	Journal of the American College of Nutrition
J Am Geriatric Soc	Journal of the American Geriatric Society
J Antimicro Chemo	Journal of Antimicrobial and Chemotherapy
J Appl Phys	Journal of Applied Physiology
J Clin Endo and Metab	Journal of Clinical Endocrinology and Metabolism
J Clin Invest	Journal of Clinical Investigation
J Clin Path	Journal of Clinical Pathology
J Dent Assoc	Journal of the American Dental Association
J Gen Int Med	Journal of General Internal Medicine
J Hosp Infec	Journal of Hospital Infections
J Neurosurg	Journal of Neurosurgery
J Nut	Journal of Nutrition
J Nut Ed	Journal of Nutrition Education
JOGN Nursing	Journal of Obsterical and Gynecological Nursing
J Ped Nursing	Journal of Pediatric Nursing
J Ped Surg	Journal of Pediatric Surgery
J Peds	Journal of Pediatrics
JPEN	Journal of Parenteral and Enteral Nutrition
J Psychosocial Nurs	Journal of Psychosocial Nursing

J R Soc Health	Journal of the Royal Society of Health
J Repro Med	Journal of Reproductive Medicine
J Respir Dis	Journal of Respiratory Diseases
J Rheum	Journal of Rheumatology
J Surg Res	Journal of Surgical Research
J Trauma	Journal of Trauma
Kid Int	Kidney International
Mayo Clin Proc	Mayo Clinic Proceedings
MCN	Maternal and Child Nursing
Med Clin N Am	Medical Clinics of North America
Med Times	Medical Times
NEJM	New England Journal of Medicine
NSS	Nutrition Support Services
Nurs Clin N Am	Nursing Clinics of North America
Nutr Rev	Nutrition Reviews
Onc Nurs Forum	Oncology Nursing Forum
Ped Clin N Am	Pediatric Clinics of North America
Peds	Pediatrics
Postgrad Med	Postgraduate Medicine
Pract Cardio	Practical Cardiology
Proc for Soc for Exp Biol and Med	Proceedings for the Society for Experimental Biology and Medicine
Psychol Med	Psychological Medicine
Psychopharmacol Bull	Psychopharmacological Bulletin
Sci Am	Scientific American
Sem Onc	Seminars in Oncology
Surg	Surgery
Surg Clin N Am	Surgical Clinics of North America
Surg Forum	Surgical Forum
Surg Gyne and OB	Surgery in Gynecology and Obstetrics
Top Clin Nutr	Topics in Clinical Nutrition
W J Med	Western Journal of Medicine

GENERAL MEDICINE, NUTRITIONAL TEXTS AND JOURNALS

Alpers, D., Clouse, R., and Stenson, W.: *Manual of Medical Therapeutics*. Boston: Little, Brown and Co., 1983.

American Dietetic Association: *Handbook of Clinical Dietetics*. New Haven: Yale University Press, 1981.

American Medical Association: Symposium on Total Parenteral Nutrition, January 17–19, 1972.

Ballinger, W., et al.: *Manual of Surgical Nutrition*. Philadelphia: W.B. Saunders Co., 2nd ed., 1982.

Blackburn, G., Bistrian, B., Maini, B., et al.: Nutritional and Metabolic Assessment of the Hospitalized Patient. *JPEN 1*:17, 1977.

Bodinski, L.: *Nurses' Guide to Diet Therapy*. New York: John Wiley & Sons, 2nd ed., 1987.

Braunwald, E., Isselbach, K., Petersdorf, R., et al.: *Harrison's Principles of Internal Medicine*, 11th ed. New York: McGraw-Hill Book Co., 1987.

Brown, W.: The Distribution of Body Fat in Relation to Habitual Activity. *Ann Hum Biol 4*:537, 1977.

Brunnstrom, S.: *Clinical Kinesiology*. Philadelphia: F.A. Davis Co., 1972.

Butterworth, G., and Blackburn, G.: Hospital Malnutrition. *Nutrition Today* 10(2), March-April 1975, pp. 4–8.

Campbell, J., and Frisse, M.: *Manual of Medical Therapeutics*, 24th ed. Boston: Little, Brown and Co., 1983.

Cerra, F.: *Pocket Manual of Surgical Nutrition*. St Louis: C.V. Mosby Co., 1984.

Chernoff, R., and Vanderveen, T.: Interrelationships of Dietary and Pharmacy Services in Nutrition Support. Columbus: Ross Laboratories, *Ross Roundtables on Medical Issues*, 4th Report, March, 1983.

Cooper, J.: Food-Drug Interactions. *U.S. Pharmacist* Nov.-Dec. 1976, 17–28.

Feldman, J., Lee, E., and Castleberry, C.: Catecholamine and Serotonin Content of Foods: Effect on Urinary Excretion of Homovanillic and 5-Hydroxyindolacetic Acid. *JADA 87*:1031, 1987.

Gastineau, C. (ed.): *Dialogues in Nutrition*. Evansville, IN: Mead Johnson Company, 1977.

Golden, M., et al.: The Relationship Between Dietary Intake, Weight Change, Nitrogen Balance and Protein Turnover in Man. *AJCN 30*:1345, 1977.

Goodman, L.: *Goodman and Gilman's The Pharmacological Basis of Therapeutics*. New York: Macmillan Publishing Co., Inc., 1985.

Grant, A., and DeHoog, S.: *Nutritional Assesment and Support*, 3rd ed. Northgate Station, Seattle, 1985.

Guthrie, H.: *Introductory Nutrition*, 7th ed. St. Louis: C.V. Mosby Co., 1986.

Guyton, A.: *Textbook of Medical Physiology*, 3rd ed. Philadelphia: W.B. Saunders Co., 1986.

Hamilton Smith, C., and Bidlack, W.: Dietary Concerns Associated With Use of Medications. *JADA 84*:901, 1984.

Harris, J., and Benedict, F.: *A Biometric Study of Basal Metabolism in Man*. Washington, D.C.: Carnegie Institute of Washington. Publication #279. 1919.

Hayes, J., and Borzelleca, J.: Nutrient Interaction with Drugs and Other Xenobiotics. *JADA 85*:335, 1985.

Herbold, N., and Ward, R.: *Nutrition in Clinical Care*, 2nd. ed. New York: McGraw-Hill Book Co., 1982.

Holman, S.: *Essentials of Nutrition for the Health Professional*. Philadelphia: J.B. Lippincott Co., 1987.

Howard, P., and Hannaman, K.: Warfarin Resistance Linked to Enteral Nutrition Products. *JADA 85*:713, 1985.

Koplan, J., et al.: Nutrient Intake and Supplementation in the United States (NHANES II), *Am J Public Health 76*:287, 1986.

Lang, C. (ed.): *Nutritional Support in Critical Care*. Rockville, MD: Aspen Publishers, 1987.

Leonard, T., Watson, R., and Mohs, M.: The Effect of Caffeine on Various Body Systems: A Review. *JADA 87*:1048, 1987.

MacInnis, P., and Swanbon, G.: The Malnutrition Dilemma in the DRG System. *NSS 7*:22, Feb., 1987.

McCabe, B.: Dietary Tyramine and Other Pressor Amines and MAOI Regimens: A Review. *JADA 86*:1059, 1986.

McBean, L.: Food Versus Pills Versus Fortified Foods. *Dairy Council Digest*. Rosemont, IL: National Dairy Council. 58(2), March–April 1987.

Mead Johnson Nutritional Division: *A Guide to Nutritional Care*. Evansville, IN: Mead Johnson, 1980.

Nursing Clinics of North America: Nutrition. *Nurs Clin N Am 18*:1, 1983.

Papper, S. (ed.): *Manual of Medical Care of the Surgical Patient*. Boston: Little, Brown and Co., 1976.

Paige, D. (ed.): *Manual of Clinical Nutrition*. Pleasantville, NJ: Nutrition Publications, Inc., 1983.

Pemberton, C., and Gastineau, C. (eds.): *Mayo Clinic Diet Manual* 5th ed. Philadelphia: W.B. Saunders Co., 1981.

Physicians' Desk Reference for Drug Therapy. Oradell, NJ: Medical Economics Company, 42nd ed. 1988.

Pike, R., and Brown, M.: *Nutrition: An Integrated Approach*, 3rd ed. New York: John Wiley & Sons, Inc., 1985.

Raicyzk, G., and Pinto, J.: Drug-Nutrient Interactions—Troublesome Combinations and Susceptible Patients. *Consultant* 85–102, July 1986.

Robinson, G., Goldstein, M., and Levine, G.: Impact of Nutritional Status on DRG Length of Stay. *JPEN 11*:49, Jan.–Feb. 1987.

Roe, D.: Therapeutic Effects of Drug-Nutrient Interactions in the Elderly. *JADA 85*:174, 1985.

Roe, D.: *Drug-Induced Nutritional Deficiencies*, 2nd ed. Westport, CT: AVI Publishing Co., Inc., 1985.

Roubenoff, R., et al.: Malnutrition Among Hospitalized Patients. *Arch Int Med 147*:1462, 1987.

Schneider, H., Anderson, C., and Coursin, D.: *Nutritional Support Of Medical Practice*, 2nd ed. Philadelphia: Harper & Row Publishers, Inc., 1983.

Shils, M. (ed.): *Defined Formula Diets for Medical Purposes*. Chicago: American Medical Association, 1977.

Shils, M. and Young, Y. (eds.): *Modern Nutrition in Health and Disease*. 7th ed. Philadelphia: Lea & Febiger, 1988.

Simko, M., Cowell, C., and Gilbride, J.: *Nutrition Assessment*. Rockville, MD: Aspen Publishers, Inc., 1984.

Suitor, C., and Hunter, M.: *Nutrition: Principles and Application in Health Promotion*. Philadelphia: J.B. Lippincott Co., 1980.

The Nutrition Foundation, Inc.: *Nutrition Reviews' Present Knowledge in Nutrition*, 5th ed. Washington, D.C.: Nutrition Foundation, Inc., 1984.

Thomas, C. (ed.): *Taber's Cyclopedic Medical Dictionary*, 15th ed. Philadelphia: F.A. Davis Co., 1985.

Tilkian, S., et al. (eds.): *Clinical Implications of Laboratory Tests*, 3rd ed. St. Louis: C.V. Mosby Co., 1983.

Tucker, S., et al.: *Patient Care Standards*, 3rd ed. St. Louis: C.V. Mosby Co., 1984.

Tuckerman, M. and Turco, S.: *Human Nutrition*. Philadelphia: Lea & Febiger, 1983.

Wallach, J.: *Interpretation of Laboratory Tests*, 4th ed. Boston: Little, Brown and Co., 1986.

Weigley, E.: Average? Ideal? Desirable? A Brief Overview of Height-Weight Tables in the United States. *JADA 84*:417, 1984.

Weiner, B.: Cardiovascular Drugs, Part 1 and Part 2. *R.D.* New York: Biomedical Information Corporation/Norwich-Eaton Pharmaceuticals. Volume 1(5) and Volume 2(1), 1981–82.

Weintraub, M., and Standish, R.: Lovastatin and Related Compounds: New Approaches to the Treatment of Hypercholesterolemia. *Hosp Form 22*:27, January 1987.

Weissman, C., et al.: Resting Metabolic Rate of the Critically Ill Patient: Measured Versus Predicted. *Anes 64*:673, 1986.

West, J.: *Best and Taylor's Physiological Basis of Medical Practice*. 11th ed. Baltimore: Williams & Wilkins, 1985.

Willard, M.: *Nutrition for the Practicing Physician*. Menlo Park, CA: Addison-Wesley Publishing Company, Inc., 1982.

LIFE-CYCLE NUTRITION

General References

Beal, V.: *Nutrition in the Life Cycle*. New York: John Wiley & Sons, 1980.

Califano, J.: America's Health-Care Revolution: Health Promotion and Disease Prevention. *JADA 87*:437, 1987.

Grant, A., and DeHoog, S.: *Nutritional Assessment and Support*, 4th ed. Seattle, 1990.

Levy, A., and Schucker, R.: Patterns of Nutritional Intake Among Dietary Supplement Users: Attitudinal and Behavioral Correlates. *JADA 87*:754, 1987.

Mayo Clinic Diet Manual, 6th ed. Philadelphia: B.C. Decker, 1988.

National Academy of Sciences: *Recommended Dietary Allowances*, 9th ed. National Research Council, 1980.

Owen, A., and Frankle, R.: *Nutrition in the Community: The Art of Delivering Services*, 2nd ed. St. Louis: C.V. Mosby Co., 1986.

U.S. Departments of Agriculture and Health and Human Services: *Nutrition and Your Health: Dietary Guidelines for Americans*, 2nd ed. Washington, D.C.: U.S. Government Printing Office, 1985.

U.S. Preventative Services Task Force: Nutritional Counseling. *Am Fam Phys 40*:125, 1989.

Prenatal Nutrition

Abrams, B., and Laros, R.: Prepregnancy Weight, Weight Gain and Body Weight. *Am J Ob and Gyne 154*:503, 1986.

Adams, S., Barr, G., and Huenemann, R.: Effect of Nutritional Supplementation in Pregnancy. *JADA 72*:144, 1978.

Alan Guttmacher Institute: *Teenage Pregnancy: The Problem that Hasn't Gone Away.* New York: Alan Guttmacher Institute, 1981.

Alfin-Slater, R., et al.: *Nutrition and Motherhood*. Van Nuys, CA: PM Inc, 1982.

Alfin-Slater, R., et al.: Special Issue: Pregnancy. *Nutrition and the M.D. VI*(11):1–, Nov., 1980.

American Dietetic Association: Position of the American Dietetic Association: Nutrition Management of Adolescent Pregnancy. *JADA 89*:104, 1989.

American College of Obstetrics and Gynecology: *Assessment of Maternal Nutrition*. Chicago: American College of Obstetrics and Gynecology, 1978.

Bachman, J.: Prenatal Care of the Normal Pregnant Woman. *Primary Care 10*(2):145, June, 1983.

Belizan, J., and Villar, J.: The Relationships Between Calcium Intake and Edema-, Proteinuria- and Hypertension-Gestosis: An Hypothesis. *AJCN 33*:2202, 1980.

Brown, J.: Improving Pregnancy Outcomes in the U.S.: The importance of Preventative Nutrition Services. *JADA 89*:631, 1989.

Brown, J.: *Nutrition for Your Pregnancy: The University of Minnesota Guide*. New York: New American Library, 1983.

Bothwell, T., and Finch, C.: *Iron Metabolism*. Boston: Little, Brown and Co., 1962, p. 309.

Butterfield, K.: Perinatal Care. *Leaders Alert Bulletin*. White Plains, NY: National Foundation March of Dimes, 1980.

California State Department of Health: *Nutrition During Pregnancy and Lactation*. California Health Department, 1975.

Carroll, P.: Safe Ingestion of Aspartame during Pregnancy. *Top Clin Nutr 5*:1, 1990.

Carruth, B.: Adolescent Pregnancy and Nutrition. *Contemporary Nutrition. 5*(10), Oct. 1980.

Committee on Nutrition of the Mother and PreSchool Child: Unusual Dietary Practices and Their Consequences in Pregnancy. *Nutrition Today* Jan.–Feb. 1983, 18–19.

Corruccini, C.: *Food Guides: Their Development, Use and Specific Changes Suggested for Nutrition During Pregnancy and Lactation*. Maternal and Child Health Branch, California Department of Health, June, 1977.

Drife, J.: Weight Gain in Pregnancy: Eating for Two or Just Getting Fat? *Brit Med J 293*:903, 1986.

Durnin, J., et al.: Is Nutritional Status Endangered by Virtually No Extra Intake During Pregnancy? *Lancet 2*:823, 1985.

Endres, J., et al.: Older Pregnant Women and Adolescents: Nutrition Data After Enrollment in WIC. *JADA 87*:1011, 1987.

Frisancho, A., et al.: Maternal Nutritional Status and Adolescent Pregnancy Outcome. *AJCN 38*:739, 1983.

Harrison, G., Undal, J., and Morrow, G.: Maternal Obesity, Weight Gain in Pregnancy and Infants' Birth Weight. *Am J Ob and Gyne 136*:411, 1980.

Heslin, J.: Third Trimester Nutrition. *Childbirth Educator*. Winter 1983–84, 38–46.

Hess, M., and Hunt, A.: *Pickles and Ice Cream*. New York: McGraw-Hill Book Company, 1982.

Horner, R., et al.: Pica Practices of Pregnant Women. *JADA 91*:34, 1991.

Huber, A., et al.: Folate Nutriture in Pregnancy. *JADA 88*:791, 1988.

Jacobson, H.: Advances in Knowledge of Fetal and Maternal Nutrition. *Food and Nutrition News 58*(4), Sept.–Oct. 1986. Chicago: National Livestock and Meat Board.

Jacobson, H.: Maternal Nutrition in the 1980s. *JADA 80*:216, 1982.

Lackey, C.: Pica During Pregnancy. *Contemporary Nutrition 8*(11), Nov. 1983, Minneapolis: General Mills Nutrition Department.

Loris, P., et al.: Weight Gain and Dietary Intake of Pregnant Teenagers. *JADA 85*:1296, 1985.

Lu, J., et al.: Intakes of Vitamins and Minerals by Pregnant Women with Selected Clinical Symptoms. *JADA 78*:477, 1981.

Luke, B., et al.: A Consideration of Height as a Function of Prepregnancy Nutritional Background and Its Potential Influence on Birthweight. *JADA 84*:176, 1984.

Mitchell, M., and Lerner, E.: Weight Gain and Pregnancy Outcome in Underweight and Normal Weight Women. *JADA 89*:634, 1989.

Mitchell, M., and Lerner, E.: Factors That Influence the Outcome of Pregnancy in Middle-Class Women. *JADA 87*:731, 1987.

Mukherjee, M., et al.: Maternal Zinc, Iron, Folic Acid and Protein Nutriture and Outcome of Human Pregnancy. *AJCN 40*:496, 1984.

604

National Dairy Council: Nutrition and Pregnancy Outcome. *Dairy Council Digest 54.(3), May–June 1983.* Rosemont, IL: National Dairy Council.

Orstead, C., et al.: Efficacy of Prenatal Nutrition Counseling: Weight Gain, Infant Birthweight and Cost-effectiveness. *JADA 85:40,* 1985.

Parham, E., et al.: The Association of Pregnancy Weight Gain with the Mother's Post-partum Weight. *JADA 90:* 550, 1990.

Pederson, A.: Weight Gain Patterns during Twin Gestation. *JADA 89:* 642, 1989.

Perkin, J.: Maternal Influences on the Development of Food Allergy in the Infant. *Top Clin Nutr 5:*6, 1990.

Phillips, M.: *Food for the Teenager during Pregnancy.* Rockville, MD: Department of Health, Education and Welfare. Publication #HSA-77-5706, 1977.

Pitkin, R.: Nutrition in Pregnancy. *Dietetic Currents 4(1),* Jan.–Feb. 1977. Columbus: Ross Laboratories.

Pugliese, M.: Fear of Obesity: A Cause of Short Stature and Delayed Puberty. *NEJM 309:*513, 1983.

Rosso, P.: Nutrition and Maternal-Fetal Exchange. *AJCN 34:*744, 1981.

Saha, N.: Energy Equation in Pregnancy. *Lancet 1:*102, 1986.

Schneck, M., et al.: Low-Income Pregnant Adolescents and Their Infants: Dietary Findings and Health Outcomes. *JADA 90:*555, 1990.

Schulman, P.: Hyperemesis Gravidarum: An Approach to the Nutritional Aspects of Care. *JADA 80:*577, June, 1982.

Smithells, R., et al.: Further Experience of Vitamin Supplementation for Prevention of Neural Tube Defect Recurrences. *Lancet 1:*1027, 1983.

Splett, P., et al.: Prenatal Nutrition Services: A Cost Analysis. *JADA 87:*204, 1987.

Story, M., and Alton, I.: Nutritional Issues and Adolescent Pregnancy. *Contemporary Nutrition 12(1),* 1987, Minneapolis: General Mills Nutrition Department.

Streissguth, A., et al.: Comparison of Drinking and Smoking Patterns During Pregnancy over a Six-Year Interval. *Am J Ob and Gyne 145:*716, 1983.

Suitor, C.: Perspectives on nutrition during pregnancy: Part I. Weight Gain. Part II. Nutrient Supplements. *JADA 91:*96, 1991.

Sutter, C., and Ott, D.: Maternal and Infant Nutrition Recommendations: A Review. *JADA 84:*572, 1984.

United States Department of Health and Human Services: *Prenatal Care.* Rockville, MD: Department of Health and Human Services. Publication #HRSA-83-5070, 1983.

Weigley, E.: Nutrition and the Older Primigravida. *JADA 82:*529, 1983.

Worthington-Roberts, B., and Weigle, A.: Caffeine and Pregnancy Outcome. *JOGN Nursing* Jan.–Feb. 1983, 21–24.

Worthington-Roberts, B.: Nutrition and Maternal Health. *Nutrition Today* Nov.–Dec. 1984, 6–19.

Worthington-Roberts, B.: Nutritional Support of Successful Reproduction: An Update. *J Nut Ed 19:*1, 1987.

Worthington-Roberts, B., Vermeersch, J., and Williams, S.: *Nutrition in Pregnancy and Lactation.* St. Louis: C.V. Mosby Co., 1985.

Wright, J., et al.: Alcohol Consumption, Pregnancy and Low Birthweight. *Lancet 1:*663, 1983.

Postpartum Nutrition and Lactation

American Academy of Pediatrics, Committee on Drugs: The Transfer of Drugs and Other Chemicals into Human Breast Milk. *Peds 72:*375, 1983.

American Academy of Pediatrics, Committee on Nutrition: Fluoride Supplementation: Revised Dosage Schedule. *Peds 63:*150, 1979.

American Academy of Pediatrics: *Handbook on Nutrition*. Elk Grove, IL: American Academy of Pediatrics, 1985.

American Academy of Pediatrics: Task Force on Promotion of Breast Feeding: The Promotion of Breast Feeding. *Peds 69*:654, 1982.

American Dietetic Association: Position Paper: Promotion of Breast-feeding. *JADA 86*:1850, 1986.

Arena, J.: Contamination of the Ideal Food. *Nutrition Today* Winter 1970, pp. 2–8.

Auerbach, K., and Guss, E.: Maternal Employment and Breast-feeding. *Am J Dis Child 138*:958, 1984.

Axelson, M., et al.: Primiparas' Beliefs about Breast-feeding. *JADA 85*:77, 1985.

Barron, S., et al.: Factors Influencing Duration of Breastfeeding among Low-income Women. *JADA 88*:1557, 1988.

Byrne, J., Thomas, M., and Chan, G.: Calcium Intake and Bone Density of Lactating Women in their Late Childbearing Years. *JADA 87*:883, 1987.

Cunningham, A.: Breast-feeding and Health. *J Peds 110*:658, 1987.

Department of Health and Human Services: On Human Milk and Breast-feeding, Video Teleconference on Maternal and Infant Health. April 7, 1983. Bethesda, MD: National Infant-Child Health Department.

Filer, L.: Maternal Nutrition in Lactation. *Clin Perinat 2*(2):353, 1975.

Finberg, L.: Human Milk Feeding and Vitamin D Supplementation. *J Peds 99*:228, 1981.

Fomon, S.: Breast-feeding and Evolution. *JADA 86*:317, 1986.

Fomon, S., et al.: Cow Milk Feeding in Infancy: Gastrointestinal Blood Loss and Iron Nutritional Stores. *J Peds 98*:540, 1981.

Goldman, A., et al.: Immunologic Factors in Human Milk During the First Year of Lactation. *J Peds 100*:563, 1982.

Greer, F., et al.: Bone Mineral Content and Serum 25-Hydroxy Vitamin D Concentration in Breast-fed Infants With and Without Supplemental Vitamin D: One-Year Follow-Up. *J Peds 100*:919, 1982.

Hambraeus, L., et al.: Nutritional Availability of Breast Milk Protein. *Lancet 2*:167, 1984.

Hecht, A.: Advice on Breast-feeding and Drugs. *FDA Consumer* Nov., 1979, 21–22.

Hitchcock, N., et al.: Growth of Healthy Breast-fed Infants in the First Six Months. *Lancet 1*:64, 1981.

Koetting, C.A., and Wardlaw, G.M.: Wrist, Spine and Hip Bone Density in Women with Variable Histories of Lactation. *AJCN 48*:1479, 1988.

Koop, C.: *Follow-Up Report: The Surgeon General's Workshop on Breast-feeding and Human Lactation*. Rockville, MD: Department of Health and Human Services. Publication #HRS-D-MC-85-2, 1985.

Koop, C.: *Report of the Surgeon General's Workshop on Breast-feeding and Human Lactation*. Washington, D.C.: Department of Health and Human Services. Publication #HRS-D-MC-84-2. June 11–12, 1984.

Lawrence, R.: *Breast-feeding: A Guide for the Medical Profession*. St. Louis: C.V. Mosby Co., 1980.

Leung, A., and Sauve, R.S.: Breastfeeding and Breast Milk Jaundice. *J. of the Royal Society of Health 109*:213, 1989.

Lockhart, J.: Breast Milk. *Contemporary Nutrition 4*(1), Jan. 1979. Minneapolis: General Mills Nutrition Department.

Lonnerdal, B., and Forsum, E.: Casein Content of Human Milk. *AJCN 41*:113, 1985.

McCarthy, M.: Dietitians as Lactation Educators/Consultants. *JADA 86*:88, 1986.

Natow, A.: Nutrition for the Nursing Mother. *In No Nonsense Nutrition for Your Baby's First Year*. Boston: CBI Publishing, 1978.

Potter, J., and Nestel, P.: The Effects of Dietary Fatty Acids and Cholesterol on the Milk

Lipids of Lactating Women and the Plasma Cholesterol of Breast-fed Infants. *AJCN* 29:54, 1976.

Potter, S., et al.: Does Infant Feeding Method Influence Maternal Postpartum Weight Loss? *JADA 91*:441, 1991.

Psiaski, D., and Olson, C.: Current Knowledge on Breast-feeding. Ithaca, NY: Cornell University. Dec. 1977.

Robyn, C., et al.: Advances of Physiology of Human Lactation. *Ann NY Acad Sci 484*:66, 1986.

Rogers, C., et al.: Weaning from the Breast: Influences on Maternal Decisions. *Pediatric Nursing 13*(5):341, 1987.

Ross Laboratories: Observations Regarding the Diet of Lactating Women; Suggested Foods for the Lactating Mother; and How Lactation Affects the RDAs. Columbus: Ross Laboratories, 1976.

Sahu, S.: Drugs and the Nursing Mother. *Am Fam Phys 24*:137, 1981.

Schoensiegel, B.: The Expanded Role of the Dietitian as Lactation Educator or Consultant. *Topics in Clinical Nutrition 2*:21, Jan., 1987.

Infant Nutrition

Alfin-Slater, R., et al.: Infant and Children's Diseases, Special Issue. *Nutrition and the M.D. IX*(11), Nov., 1983.

Allegheny County Health Department: Infant Feeding Practices: Considerations in the Use of Skim or Two Per Cent Milk. Pittsburgh, PA: Allegheny County Health Department, April, 1979.

American Academy of Pediatrics, Committee on Nutrition: The Use of Whole Cow's Milk in Infancy. *Contemporary Nutrition 10*(6), June, 1985, Minneapolis: General Mills Nutrition Department.

Avery, G.: *Neonatology: Pathophysiology and Management of the Newborn*, 3rd ed. Philadelphia: J.B. Lippincott Co., 1987.

Blumenthal, S.: Hypertension: Prevention, Diet and Treatment in Infancy and Childhood Symposium. Bethesda, MD: Biomedical Information Corporation, May 25, 1983.

Broussard, A.: Anticipatory Guidance: Adding Solids to the Infant's Diet. *JOGN Nursing* July–Aug. 1984, 239–241.

Consumers Union: Is Baby Food Good Enough for Baby? *Consumer Reports* Sept. 1986, 593–599.

Fomon, S.: Bioavailability of Iron in Commercially Prepared Dry Infant Cereals. *J Peds 110*:660, 1987.

Fomon, S.: *Infant Nutrition*, 2nd ed. Philadelphia: W.B. Saunders Co., 1974.

Fomon, S., Filer, L., et al.: Recommendations for Feeding Normal Infants. *Peds 63*(1), Jan. 1979.

Fomon, S., and Ziegler, E.: Skim Milk in Infant Feeding. Rockville, MD: U.S. Department of Health, Education and Welfare, August, 1977.

Ford, K., and Labbok, M.: Who is Breastfeeding? Implications of Associated Social and Biochemical Variables for Research on the Consequences of Method of Infant Feeding. *AJCN 52*:451, 1990.

Gaull, G.E.: Taurine in Pediatric Nutrition: Review and Update. *Ped 83*:433, 1989.

Hopkins, H.: Next to Mother's Milk. *FDA Consumer* July–August, 1980.

Hungerford, N.: Making Your Own Baby Food. Tucson, AZ: Tucson Medical Center, Nutrition Services Department, October 1979.

Infant Formula Council: *Infant Feeding and Nutrition*. Atlanta, GA: Infant Formula Council, 1982.

Ivens, B., and Weil, W.: *Teddy Bears and Bean Sprouts: The Infant and Vegetarian Nutrition*. Fremont, MI: Gerber Products Company, 1984.

Krakauer, L., et al. Nutrition. *Yearbook of Sports Medicine*. Chicago: Year Book Medical Publishers, Inc., 1984, p. 177.

Leventhal, E., et al.: Does Breast-feeding Protect Against Infections in Infants Less Than Three Months of Age? *Peds 78*:896, 1986.

Lifschitz, C., and Carrazza, F.: Effect of Formula Carbohydrate Concentration on Tolerance and Macronutrient Absorption in Infants with Severe, Chronic Diarrhea. *J Peds 117*;378, 1990.

Maisels, M., and Gifford, K.: Normal Serum Bilirubin Levels in the Newborn and the Effect of Breast-feeding. *Peds 78*:837, 1986.

Mead Johnson Company: Good Infant Nutrition. Evansville, IN: Mead Johnson Company, 1978.

Natow, A.: Your Baby's First Year and You. Pamphlet derived from *No Nonsense Nutrition for Your Baby's First Year*. Boston: CBI Publishing, 1978.

National Dairy Council: Controversies Related to Infants and Children. *Dairy Council Digest 57*(4), July–Aug. 1986.

Owen, G.: Nutrition of Low Birth Weight Infants: Enteral Feeding. *Clin Nutr 2*(5):9, Sept.–Oct. 1983. Pleasantville, NJ: Nutrition Publications, Inc.

Paige, D.: Infant Growth and Nutrition. *Clin Nutr 2*(5):14, Sept.–Oct. 1983. Pleasantville, NJ: Nutrition Publications, Inc.

Picciano, M.: Nutrient Needs of Infants. *Nutrition Today 22*:8, 1987.

Powell, G.F.: Nonorganic Failure to Thrive in Infancy: An Update on Nutrition, Behavior and Growth. *J Am Coll Nutr* vol. 7, Oct. 1988, p. 345.

Rosso, P.: Nutrient Needs of the Human Fetus. *Clin Nutr 2*(5):4, Sept.–Oct. 1983. Pleasantville, NJ: Nutrition Publications, Inc.

Sampson, H.A.: Infantile Colic and Food Allergy: Fact or Fiction? *J Peds 115*:583, 1989.

Satter, E.: *Child of Mine*. Palo Alto, CA: Bull Publishing Company, 1983.

Satter, E.: The Feeding Relationship. *JADA 86*:352, 1986.

Schwartz, N., and Barr, S.: Mothers—Their Attitudes and Practices in Perinatal Nutrition. *J Nut Ed 9*:169, 1977.

Specker, B.: Cyclical Serum 25-Hydroxyvitamin D Concentrations Paralleling Sunshine Exposure in Exclusively Breast-fed Infants. *J Peds 110*:744, 1987.

Weber, C.: *A Mother's Handbook: Combining Breast-feeding with Work or School*. Madison, WI: Wisconsin Nutrition Project.

Willis, J.: Good Nutrition for the High-Chair Set. *FDA Consumer 19*(7):5, 1985. Department of Health and Human Services Publication #FDA-86-2208.

Winick, M.: Infant Formula: Formula or Breast-feeding? *The Professional Nutritionist 12*(2), Spring 1980, San Francisco: Foremost-McKesson, Inc.

Childhood Nutrition

Agras, W., et al.: Does a Vigorous Feeding Style Influence Early Development of Adiposity? *J Peds 110*:799, 1987.

American Dietetic Association: Position of the American Dietetic Association: Child Nutrition Services. *JADA 87*:217, 1987.

American Dietetic Association: Position of the American Dietetic Association: Nutritional Standards in Day-Care Programs for Children. *JADA 87*:503, 1987.

Beal, V.: Nutrition and Growth Patterns of Young Children. *Contemporary Nutrition 7*(10): October 1982, Minneapolis: General Mills Nutrition Department.

Birch, L.: Dimensions of Preschool Children's Food Preferences. *J Nut Ed 11*(2):77, 1979.

Cook, C., and Payne, I.: Effect of Supplements on the Nutrient Intake of Children, *JADA 74*:130, 1979.

Goldberg, A.C.: Cholesterol Control in Children: Is It Necessary? *Hosp Med Jun* 1989, 73.

Hertzler, A.: Children's Food Patterns—A Review. I. Food Preferences and Feeding Problems. *JADA 83:*551, 1983.

Hertzler, A.: Children's Food Patterns—A Review. II. Family and Group Behavior. *JADA 83:*555, 1983.

Hussey, G., and Klein, M.: A Randomized, Controlled Trial of Vitamin A in Children with Severe Measles. *NEJM 323:*160, 1990.

Levy, R., et al.: *Primary Prevention of Atherosclerosis in Childhood: The Role of Lipids.* New York: Biomedical Information Corporation, 1985.

Natow, A., and Heslin, J.: *No-Nonsense Nutrition for Kids.* New York: McGraw-Hill Book Company, 1985.

Pollitt, E., Haas, J., and Levitsky, D.A.: International Conference on Iron Deficiency and Behavioral Development. *AJCN 50(Supp.)* 565, 1989.

Satter, E.: *Child of Mine.* Palo Alto, CA: Bull Publishing Co., 1986.

Satter, E.: Relating Research to Practice. *Nutrition News 50*(1), Feb., 1987. Rosemont, IL: National Dairy Council.

Story, M., and Brown, J.: Do Young Children Instinctively Know What To Eat? The Studies of Clara Davis Revisited. *NEJM 316:*103, 1987.

Yperman, A., and Vermeersch, J.: Factors Associated with Children's Food Habits. *J Nut Ed 11*(2):77, 1979.

Adolescent Nutrition

Beaudette, T.: *Nutrition in Practice: Adolescent Nutrition.* Minneapolis: Doyle Pharmaceuticals, 1981.

Heald, F.: Nutrition in Adolescence. *Clinical Nutrition 2*(5): 19, Sept.–Oct., 1983. Pleasantville, NJ: Nutrition Publications, Inc.

McBean, L.: Adolescent Nutrition: Issues and Challenges. *Dairy Council Digest 58*(4):July–Aug. 1987.

Moses, N., et al.: Fear of Obesity among Adolescent Girls. *Peds 83:*393, 1989.

National Dairy Council: Nutrition Concerns During Adolescence. *Dairy Council Digest 52*(2):7, March–April 1981.

Thomsen, P., Terry, R., and Amos, R.: Adolescents' Beliefs About and Reasons for Using Vitamin-Mineral Supplements. *JADA 87:*1063, 1987.

Truswell, A., and Darnton-Hill, I.: Food Habits of Adolescents. *Nutrition Reviews 39:*73, 1981.

Wharton, R., and Crocker, R.: Adolescent Obesity. *Children Today 13:*12, Nov.–Dec. 1984.

Nutrition in Athletes

Askew, W.: Nutrition for Top Sports Performance. *Dietetic Currents 8:*3, May–June, 1981. Columbus: Ross Laboratories.

American Dietetic Association: *Sports Nutrition.* Chicago: American Dietetic Association, 1986.

American Heart Association: *Nutrition for Sports and Dance.* Alameda County, CA: American Heart Association, 1984.

Clark, N.: Physically Fit/Nutritionally Sound? Lecture at the Pennsylvania Dietetic Association, Hershey, PA, April, 1987.

Eichner, E.: The Anemias of Athletes. *The Physician and Sportsmedicine 14:*122, 1986.

Elliott, D., and Goldberg, L.: Nutrition and Exercise. *Med Clin N Am 69*(1): 71, 1985.

Graves, K., et al.: Nutrition Training, Attitudes, Knowledge, Recommendations, and Resource Utilization of High School Coaches and Trainers. *JADA 91:*321, 1991.

Hoffman, C., and Coleman, E.: An Eating Plan and Update on Recommended Dietary Practices for the Endurance Athlete. *JADA 91:*325, 1991.

Kershan, A.: Carbohydrate, Fat and Protein Metabolism as Demanded by the Athlete. *Nutrition and the M.D.* January, 1976.

Kris-Etherton, P.: Nutrition and the Exercising Female. *Nutrition Today* March–April 1986, pp. 6–16.

Kris-Etherton, P.: Nutrition, Exercise and Athletic Performance. *Food nd Nutrition News 57:*3, May–June 1985. Chicago: National Livestock and Meat Board.

National Dairy Council: Diet, Exercise and Health. *Dairy Council Digest.* Rosemont, IL: National Dairy Council. *56:*3, May–June 1985.

Nelson, M., et al.: Diet and Bone Status in Amenorrheic Runners. *AJCN 43:*910, 1986.

O'Neil, F., et al.: Research and Application of Current Topics in Sports Nutrition. *JADA 86:*1007, 1986.

Perron, M., and Endres, J.: Knowledge, Attitudes and Dietary Practices of Female Athletes. *JADA 85:*573, 1985.

Puhl, J.: Iron and Exercise Interactions. *Contemporary Nutrition 12*(2), 1987, Minneapolis: General Mills Nutrition Department.

Serfass, R.: Nutrition for the Athlete. *Contemporary Nutrition 2:*5, May, 1977. Minneapolis: General Mills Nutrition Department.

Serfass, R.: Nutrition for the Athlete, 1982. *Contemporary Nutrition 7:*4, April 1982. Minneapolis: General Mills Nutrition Department.

Town, G., and Wheeler, K.: Nutritional Concerns for the Endurance Athlete. *Dietetic Currents 13*(2), 1986, Columbus: Ross Laboratories.

Van Handel, P.: Nutrition for Sports: an Olympic Overview. *Dairy Council Digest 55*(2):12. Rosemont, IL: National Dairy Council, 1984.

Vitale, J.: Nutrition in Sports Medicine. *Clinical Orthopedics and Related Research 198:*158, Sept., 1985.

Nutrition for Adulthood

Abraham, G.: Nutritional factors in the Etiology of Premenstrual Tension Syndromes. *J Repro Med 28:*446, 1983.

American Dietetic Association: The American Dietetic Association's Nutritional Recommendations for Women. *JADA 86:*1663, 1986.

American Dietetic Association: Position of the American Dietetic Association: Physical Fitness and Athletic Performance for Adults. *JADA 87:*933, 1987.

Beaudette, T.: Premenstrual Syndrome: Is It Nutrition-Related? *Nutrition Forum 4*(8):49, Aug., 1987.

Flegal, K.M., et al.: Secular Trends in Body Mass Index and Skinfold Thickness with Socioeconomic Factors in Young Adult Women. *AJCN 48:*535, 1988.

Frisch, R.: Fatness and Fertility. *Sci Am, 258:*88, 1988.

Gillespie, A., and Achterberg, C.: Comparison of Family Interaction Patterns Related to Food and Nutrition. *JADA 89:*509, 1989.

Grunewald, K.: Weight Control for Young College Women: Who Are the Dieters? *JADA 85:*1445, 1985.

Goe, G., and Abraham, G.: Effect of a Nutritional Supplement, Optivite, on Symptoms of Premenstrual Tension. *J Repro Med 28:*527, 1983.

Hubert, H., et al.: Life-Style Correlates of Risk Factor Change in Young Adults: An Eight-Year Study of Coronary Heart Disease Risk Factors in the Framingham Offspring. *Am J Epidem 125:*812, 1987.

Kimman, E., et al.: Amenorrhea Associated with Carotenemia. *JAMA 249:*926, 1983.

Long, P. *The Nutritional Ages of Women.* New York: Macmillan Publishing Co., Inc., 1986.

National Dairy Council: Nutrition and Women's Health Concerns. *Dairy Council Digest* *57*(1):1–6, Jan.–Feb. 1986.

Ohlson, M., and Harper, L.: Longitudinal Studies of Food Intake and Weight of Women from Ages 18–56 Years. *JADA 69:*626, 1976.

Wallace, R., et al.: Contrasting Diet and Body Mass Among Users and Nonusers of Oral Contraceptives and Exogenous Estrogens: The Lipid Research Clinics Program Prevalence Study. *Am J Epid 125:*854, 1987.

Willis, J.: The Gender Gap at the Dinner Table. *FDA Consumer.* Rockville, MD: Department of Health and Human Services. Publication #FDA-84-2197, June, 1984.

Nutrition in the Elderly

Alfin-Slater, R., et al.: The Immune Function and Aging, and Special Edition for the Elderly. *Nutrition and the M.D.13*(8), August 1987.

Alfin-Slater, R., et al.: Nutrition for the Elderly, Special Edition. *Nutrition and the M.D.* 6(2), February 1985.

American Dietetic Association: Position of the American Dietetic Association: Nutrition, Aging and the Continuum of Health Care. *JADA 87:*344, 1987.

Andres, R., and Hallfrisch, J.: Nutrient Intake Recommendations Needed for the Older American. *JADA 89:*1739, 1989.

Blumberg, J.: Drug-Induced Malnutrition in the Geriatric Patient. *Nutrition and the M.D.* 13(8), August 1987.

Cashman, M., and Wightkin, W.: Geriatric Malnutrition: Recognition and Prevention. *Comp Ther 13*(3):45, 1987.

Cerrato, P.: Hidden Malnutrition in Geriatric Patients. *RN 48:*60, 1985.

Chauhan, J., et al.: Age-Related Olfactory and Taste Changes and Interrelationships Between Taste and Nutrition. *JADA 87:*1543, 1987.

Chernoff, R.: Aging and Nutrition. *Nutrition Today* March–April 1987, pp. 4–11.

Colucci, R., et al.: Nutritional Problems of Institutionalized and Free-Living Elderly. *Comp Ther 13:*20, 1987.

Delahanty, L.: Geriatric Team Dynamics: The Dietitian's Role. *JADA 84:*1353, 1984.

Fisher, J., and Johnson, M.A.: Low Body Weight and Weight Loss in the Aged. *JADA 90:*1697, 1990.

Gambert, S.: *Handbook of Geriatrics.* New York: Plenum Medical, 1987.

Institute of Food Technologists: Nutrition and the Elderly. A Scientific Status Summary of IFT's Expert Panel on Food Safety and Nutrition. *Food Technology 40:*81, 1986.

Karkeck, J.: Assessment of Nutritional Status in the Elderly. *NSS 4*(10):23, October, 1987.

Kasim, S.: Cholesterol Changes with Aging: Their Nature and Significance. *Geriatrics 42;*73, 1987.

Kohrs, M.: New Perspectives on Nutritional Counseling for the Elderly. *Contemporary Nutrition 8:*3, March 1983. Minneapolis: General Mills Nutrition Department.

Leaf, A.: The Aging Process: Lessons from Observations in Man. *Nutr Rev 46:*40, 1988.

Lipschitz, D., Mitchell, C., and Thompson, C.: The Anemia of Senescence. *Am J Hematol 11:*47, 1981.

Matthews, L.: Setting Goals in Nutrition Care Planning. *J Nutr for the Elderly 6:*47, 1986.

McCarter, R., and Masoro, E.: Dietary Deprivation and Longevity. *Nutrition International 3:*75, 1987.

McCauley, K., and Nelson, R.: Nutrition and the Elderly: Helping the Elderly Help Themselves. *Comp Ther 11:*8, 1985.

McIntosh, W., et al.: The Relationship between Beliefs about Nutrition and Dietary Practices in the Elderly. *JADA 90:*671, 1990.

Minaker, K.: Aging and Diabetes Mellitus as Risk Factors for Vascular Disease. *Am J Med 82* (Suppl. 1B):47, 1987.

Mitchell, C., and Lipschitz, D.: Arm Length Measurement as an Alternative to Height in Nutritional Assessment of the Elderly. *JPEN 6:*226, 1982.

Mitchell C., and Lipschitz, D.: Detection of Protein-Calorie Malnutrition in the Elderly. *AJCN 35:*398, 1982.

Mitchell, C., and Lipschitz, D.: The Effect of Age and Sex on the Routinely Used Measurements Used to Assess the Nutritional Status of Hospitalized Patients. *AJCN 36:*340, 1982.

National Dairy Council: Nutrition and the Elderly. *Dairy Council Digest 54(4):*19, July–Aug. 1983. Rosemont, IL: National Dairy Council.

National Dairy Council: Nutrition, Longevity and Aging. *Dairy Council Digest 50(4):*19, July–Aug. 1979. Rosemont, IL: National Dairy Council.

Raab, D., and Raab, N.: Nutrition and Aging: An Overview. *The Canadian Nurse 58:*24, March, 1985.

Ranno, B., Wardlaw, G., and Geiger, C.: What Characterizes Elderly Women Who Overuse Vitamin and Mineral Supplements? *JADA 88:*347, 1988.

Roe, D.: *Geriatric Nutrition*, 2nd ed. Englewood Cliffs, NJ: Prentice-Hall Inc., 1987.

Ross Laboratories: Aging and Nutrition. *Dietary Modifications in Disease*. Columbus, OH: Ross Laboratories.

Rowe, D.: Aging—A Jewel in the Mosaic of Life. *JADA 72:*478, 1978.

Runyan, T.: Age-Related Biological Changes Important in Nutrition. *In Nutrition Today*. St. Louis: C.V. Mosby Co., 1976.

Russell, R.: Evaluating the Nutritional Status of the Elderly. *Clin Nutrition Manual (Clin Nutr Supplement) 2:*4, 1983.

Russell, R., and Whinston-Perry, R.: Geriatric Nutrition: Considerations Essential to Accurate Measurement. *Consultant* August 1984, 67–77.

Schneider, E., et al.: RDAs and the Health of the Elderly. *NEJM 314:*157, 1987.

Shannon, B., and Smicklas-Wright, H.: Nutrition Education in Relation to the Needs of the Elderly. *J Nut Ed 11:*85, 1979.

Shuran, M., and Nelson, R.: Updated Nutritional Assessment and Support of the Elderly. *Geriatrics 41:*48, 1986.

Sleen, B.: Body Composition and Aging. *Nutr Rev 46:*45, 1988.

Solomons, N.: Trace Elements in Nutrition of the Elderly—Established RDAs for Iron, Zinc and Iodine. *Postgrad Med 79:*231, 1986.

Steffee, W.: Nutritional Support of Elderly Patients: The Problems and Clark, N.: Proposed Answers. *In Clinical Consultations in Nutritional Support 2(4):*1, October 1982.

Steffee, W., and Clark, N.: Nutritional Support of Elderly Patients. I and II. *Clinical Nutrition Manual, Clin Nut 2* (Suppl.): 1, 1982.

Stiedman, M., Jansen, C., and Harrill, I.: Nutritional Status of Elderly Men and Women. *JADA 73:*132, 1978.

Wade, J.: Practical Aspects of Tube Feeding. *Clinical Consultations in Nutritional Support 2(4):*11, October, 1982.

Walsh, R.: Cardiovascular Effects of the Aging Process. *Am J Med 82* (Suppl 1B): 34, 1987.

Yen, P.: Fat, Cholesterol and a Healthy Older Heart. *Geriatric Nursing* July–Aug. 1984, pp. 254–257.

Zoller, D.: The Physiology of Aging. *Am Fam Phys 36:*112, July, 1987.

DIETARY PRACTICES AND MISCELLANEOUS CONDITIONS

Allman, R., et al.: Pressure Sores Among Hospitalized Patients. *Ann Int Med 105:*337, 1986.

American Dietetic Association: Position of the American Dietetic Association. *JADA 88:*351, 1988.

American Dietetic Association: Position Paper on the Vegetarian Approach to Eating. *JADA 77:*61, 1980.

Bibby, B., et al.: Oral Food Clearance and the pH of the Plaque and Saliva. *J Dent Assoc 112:*333, 1986.

Bock, S., and Atkins, F.: Patterns of Hypersensitivity during Sixteen Years of Double-blind, Placebo-controlled Food Challenges. *J Peds 117:*561, 1990.

Bunce, G., and Hess, J.: Cataract—What Is the Role of Nutrition in Lens Health? *Nutrition Today Nov./Dec.:*6, 1988.

Butkus, S., and Mahan, L.: Food Allergies: Immunological Reactions to Food. *JADA 86:*601, May, 1986.

Center for Disease Control: Progress toward Achieving the 1990 Objectives for the Nation for Fluoridation and Dental Health. *JAMA 264;*1804, 1990.

Cohen, B.: Common Dermatoses of Childhood. *Am Fam Phys 32:*186, 1985.

Durr, E.: Nutritional Intervention for Patients with Pressure Sores. *NSS 6*(10):28, Oct. 1986.

Dwyer, J.T.: Health Aspects of Vegetarian Diets. *AJCN (supp.):*712, 1988.

Dwyer, J.: Vegetarianism. *Contemp Nut.* Minneapolis: General Mills Nutrition Dept. 4(6), June, 1979.

Fanelli, M., and Kuczmarski, R.: Food Selections for Vegetarians. *Dietetic Currents 10*(1) *Jan.–Feb. 1983. Columbus: Ross Laboratories.*

Feldman, J.: Histaminuria from Histamine-Rich Foods. *Arch Int Med 143:*2099, Nov., 1983.

Fothersby, K., and Hunter, J.: Symptoms of Food Allergy. *Clin Gastro 14:*615, 1985.

Freeland-Graves, J., et al.: Health Practices, Attitudes and Beliefs of Vegetarians and Nonvegetarians. *JADA 86:*913, 1986.

Grandjean, A.: The Vegetarian Athlete. *The Physician and Sportsmedicine 15:*191, May, 1987.

Geissler, C.: The Nutritional Effects of Tooth Loss. *AJCN 39:*478, 1984.

Greene, J., Louie, R., and Wycott, S.: Preventative Densistry: Periodontal Diseases, Malocclusion, Trauma, and Oral Cancer. *JAMA 263:*421, 1990.

Hartbarger, J.: *Eating for the Eighties: A Complete Guide to Vegetarian Nutrition.* Philadelphia: W.B. Saunders Co., 1985.

King, J.: Nutrition During Oral Contraceptive Treatment. *Contemporary Nutrition 2*(1), Jan. 1976. Minneapolis: General Mills Nutrition Department.

Hunan, K., and Schesle, L.: Albumin vs. Weight as a Predictor of Nutritional Status and Pressure Ulcer Development. *Ostomy/Wound Manag 33:*447, 1991.

Leinhas, J., McCaskil, C., and Sampson, H.: Food Allergy Challenges. *JADA 87:*614, 1987.

Melnick, S.L., et al.: Epidemiology of Acute Necrotizing Ulcerative Gingivitis. *Epidemiologic Reviews 10:*191, 1988.

Metcalfe, D.: Diseases of Food Hypersensitivity. *NEJM 321:*235, 1989.

Michaelsson, G.: Diet and Acne. *Nutrition Review 39:*104, 1981.

National Dairy Council: Food Poisoning. *Dairy Council Digest 58:*1, 1987. Rosemont, IL: National Dairy Council.

National Dairy Council: The Role of Diet and Nutrition in Oral Health. *Dairy Council Digest 57*(3), May–June, 1986.

Nizel, A.: *Nutrition in Preventive Dentistry*, 2nd ed. Philadelphia: W.B. Saunders Co., 1981.

Novotny, J.: Adolescents, Acne and the Side-Effects of Accutane. *Ped Nursing 15:*247, 1989.

Ofstehage, J., and Magilvy, K.: Oral Health and Aging. *Geriatric Nursing* Sept.–Oct., 1986.

Passero, P., et al: Temporomandibular Joint Dysfunction Syndrome. *Physical Therapy 65:*1207, 1985.

Perkin, J., and Hartje, J.: Diet and Migraine: A Review of the Literature. *JADA 83:*459, 1983.

Puangco, M., Davis, H., and Karp, W.: Evaluation of Dietary Screening Tools Appropriate for Dental Practices. *JADA 86:*1717, 1986.

Resnicow, K., et al.: Diet and Serum Lipids in Vegan Vegetarians: A Model for Risk Reduction. *JADA 91:*447, 1991.

Sampson, H.A., et al.: Spontaneous Release of Histamine from Basophils and Histamine-releasing Factor in Patients with Atopic Dermatitis and Food Hypersensitivity. *NEJM 321:*228, 1989.

Sampson, H.A.: Food Allergies and the Infant at Risk. *JAMA 260:*3507, 1988.

Sampson, H., Buckley, R., and Metcalfe, D.: Food Allergy. *JAMA 258(20):*2886, 1987.

Settipane, G.: The Restaurant Syndromes. *Arch Int Med 146:*2129, 1986.

Shoub Nelson, M., and Jovanovic, L.: Pregnancy, Diabetes and Jewish Dietary Law: The Challenge for the Pregnant Diabetic Woman who Keeps Kosher. *JADA 87:*1054, 1987.

Siegel, S.: The Jewish Dietary Laws, rev. ed. New York: United Synagogue Commission on Jewish Education, 1982.

Thompson, T., Dwyer, J., and Palmer, C.: Nutritional Remedies for Temporomandibular Joint Dysfunction: Fact or Fiction? *Nutrition Today 26:*37, 1991.

Tucker, S., et al.: Acquired Zinc Deficiency: Cutaneous Manifestations Typical of Acrodermatitis Enteropathica. *JAMA 235:*2399, 1976.

Taylor, S.: Food Allergies and Sensitivities. *JADA 86:*599, 1986.

Watts, V., et al.: When Your Patient Has Jaw Surgery. *RN* Oct. 1985, pp. 44–47.

White-Graves, M., and Schiller, M.R.: History of Foods in the Caries Process. *JADA 86:*241, 1986.

Williams, R.: Periodontal Disease. *NEJM 322:*373, 1990.

SPECIAL PEDIATRIC DISORDERS

Acosta, P.: Phenylketonuria—Impact of Nutrition Support on Reproductive Outcomes. *Nutrition Today 26:*43, 1991.

Adamkin, D.: Nutrition in Very, Very Low Birth Weight Infants. *Clin Perinat 13:*419, 1986.

American Dietetic Association: Infant and Child Nutrition: Concerns Regarding the Developmentally Disabled. *JADA 78:*443, 1981.

American Dietetic Association: Position Paper: Nutrition in Comprehensive Program Planning for Persons with Developmental Disabilities. *JADA 87:*1068, 1987.

Anderson, D.: Nutritional Care for the Premature Infant. *Topics in Clinical Nutrition 2:*1, Jan., 1987.

Bavin, R., and Peck, M.: Nutritional Assessment of the Hospitalized Child. *NSS 5*(11):41, Nov., 1985.

Beall, R., and Keramides, S.: Cystic Fibrosis: A Summary of Symptoms, Diagnosis and Treatment. CF Foundation: Rockville, MD, 1984.

Bell, L., Chao, E., and Milne, J.: Dietary Management of Maple Syrup Urine Disease: Extension of Equivalency Systems. *JADA 74:*357, 1979.

Bell, L., and Sherwood, W.: Current Practices and Improved Recommendations for Treating Hereditary Fructose Intolerance. *JADA 87:*722, 1987.

614

Bennish, M., et al.: Hypoglycemia during Diarrhea in Childhood. *NEJM 322*:1357, 1990.

Bier, D., et al.: The Prader-Willi Syndrome—Regulation of Fat Transport. *Diabetes 26*:874, 1977.

Brady, M., et al.: Specialized Formulas and Feedings for Infants with Malabsorption or Formula Intolerance. *JADA 86*:191, 1986.

Calvert, S., and Davis, F.: Nutrition of Children with Handicapping Conditions. *Dietetic Currents 4*(3): May–June 1977, Columbus: Ross Laboratories.

Charney, E., et al.: Management of the Newborn with Myelomeningocele: Time for a Decision-Making Process. *Pediatrics 75*(1):58, 1985.

Cooke, R., and Nicholads, G.: Nutrient Retention in Preterm Infants Fed Standard Infant Formulas. *J Peds 108*:448, 1986.

Cooper, A., and Heird, W.: Nutritional Assessment of the Pediatric Patient including the Low Birth Weight Infant. *AJCN 35*:1132, 1982.

Crump, I.: *Nutrition and Feeding of the Handicapped Child.* Boston: Little, Brown and Co., 1987.

Duggan, M., and Milner, R.: The Maintenance Energy Requirement for Children: An Estimate Based on a Study of Children with Infection-Associated Underfeeding. *AJCN 43*:870, 1986.

Eibl, M., et al.: Prevention of Necrotizing Entercolitis in Low-birth-weight Infants by IgA-IgG Feeding. *NEJM 319*:1, 1988.

Endert, C., and Wooldridge, N.: Nonorganic Failure to Thrive. *Dietetic Currents 14*(1):1987. Columbus: Ross Laboratories.

Ernst, J., et al.: Growth Outcome of the Very-Low-Birthweight Infant at One Year. *JADA 82*:44, 1983.

Farrell, P.: Nutrition in Cystic Fibrosis. *Contemporary Nutrition 8*(6): Aug. 1983. Minneapolis: General Mills Nutrition Department.

Folk, C., and Greene, H.: Dietary Management of Type I Glycogen Storage Disease. *JADA 84*:794, 1984.

Fonkalsrad, E., and Bray, G.: Vagotomy for Treatment of Obesity in Childhood Due to Prader-Willi Syndrome. *J Ped Surg 16*:888, 1981.

Fomon, S.: *Infant Nutrition*, 2nd ed. Philadelphia: W.B. Saunders Co., 1974.

Friedman, A., et al.: Rapid Onset of Essential Fatty Acid Deficiency in the Newborn. *Peds 58*:640, 1976.

Gasch, A.: Use of the Traditional Ketogenic Diet for Treatment of Intractable Epilepsy. *JADA 90*:1433, 1990.

Goldbloom, R.: Failure to Thrive. *Ped Clin N Am 29*:151, 1982.

Griffiths, M., et al.: Metabolic Rate and Physical Development in Children at Risk of Obesity. *Lancet* July 14, 1990.

Grossman, D.: Wilson's Disease: A Genetic Disorder of Copper Metabolism. *J Neuroscience Nurisng 19*(4): 216, 1987.

Hanson, J.: Fetal Alcohol Syndrome. *JAMA 235*:1458, 1976.

Hendricks, K.: Liver Disease and Nutrition in the Child. *Topics in Clinical Nutrition 2*:79, Jan., 1987.

Holsclaw, D., et al.: *Energy, Growth and Cystic Fibrosis Nutrition: Target 100% Plus.* Springhouse, PA: McNeil Laboratories, 1986.

Homer, M.: Selective Treatment. *A J Nurs* March 1984, pp. 309–312.

Hopwood, N., Holzman, I., and Drash, A.: Fructose-1, 6-Diphosphatase Deficiency. *Am J Dis Child 131*:418, 1977.

Hunt, M., et al.: Phenylketonuria, Adolescence and Diet. *JADA 85*:1328, 1985.

Iber, F.: Fetal Alcohol syndrome. *Nutrition Today* Sept.–Oct., 1980, p. 4.

Jaeger, P.: Anticytinuric Effects of Glutamine and of Dietary Sodium Restriction. *NEJM 315*:1120, 1986.

James, J.: Longitudinal Study of the Morbidity of Diarrheal and Respiratory Infections in Malnourished Children. *AJCN 25*:690, 1972.

Janssen, F., et al.: Evaluation of Clinical and Biological Parameters in Marasmic Kwashiorkor Children Treated by Parenteral Nutrition. *JPEN 7*:26, 1981.

Jeffcoate, W., et al.: Endocrine Fucntion in the Prader-Willi Syndrome. *Clin Endo 12*:81, 1980.

Jostworth, B., and Ross Laboratories: *Developmental Disabilities: Mental and Physical.* Columbus: Ross Laboratories, 1982.

Kane, R.E., Hobbs, P.J., and Black, P.G. Comparison of Low, Medium and High Carbohydrate Formulas for Nighttime Enteral Feedings in Cystic Fibrosis Patients. *JPEN 14*:47, 1990.

Kaufman, S., et al.: Nutritional Support for the Infant with Extrahepatic Biliary Atresia. *J Peds 110*:679, 1987.

Kelts, D., and Jones, E.: *Manual of Pediatric Nutrition.* Boston: Little, Brown and Co., 1984.

Kerner, J.: *Manual of Pediatric Nutrition.* New York: John Wiley & sons, 1983.

Killam, P., et al.: Behavioral Pediatric Weight Rehabilitation for Children with Myelomeningocele. *MCN 8*:280, July–Aug., 1983.

Kliegman, R., and Fanaroff, A.: Neonatal Necrotizing Entercolitis: A Nine-Year Experience. I. Epidemiology and Uncommon Observations. *Am J Dis of Children 135*:60, 1981.

Koch, R.: *Phenylketonuria: A Guide to Dietary Management.* Evansville, IN: Mead Johnson Company, 1981.

Laurance, B., et al.: Prader-Willi Syndrome After Age 15 Years. *Arch Dis in Childhood 56*:181, 1981.

Lemire, R.: Neural Tube Defects. *JAMA 259*:558, 1988.

Lipton, M., and Mayo, J.: Diet and Hyperkinesis—An Update. *JADA 83*:132, 1983.

Lloyd, M., and Olsen, W.: A Study of the MOlecular Pathology of Sucrase-Isomaltase Deficiency. *NEJM 316*:438, 1987.

Luder, E.: Nutritional Care of Patients with Cystic Fibrosis. *Top Clin Nutr 6*:39, 1991.

Martin, S., and Acosta, P.: Osmolalities of Selected Enteral Products and Carbohydrate Modules Used to Treat Inherited Metabolic Disorders. *JADA 87*:48, 1987.

McLaurin, R., and Warkany, J.: Management of Spina Bifida and Associated Anomalies. *Comp Therapy 12*:60, 1986.

McLone, D., et al.: CNS Infections as a Limiting Factor in the Intelligence of Children with Myelomeningocele. *Peds 70*(3):338, 1982.

Michaels, K., et al.: Dietary Treatment of Tyrosinemia Type I. *JADA 73*:507, 1978.

Michel, S., and Mueller, D.: Practical Approaches to Nutritional Care of Patients with Cystic Fibrosis. *Top Clin Nutr 2*:10, Jan., 1987.

Milunsky, A., et al.: Multivitamin/Folic Acid Supplementation in Early Pregnancy Reduces the Prevalence of Neural Tube Defects. *JAMA 262*:2847, 1989.

Mulinare, J., et al.: Periconceptional Use of Multivitamins and the Occurrence of Neural Tube Defects. *JAMA 260*:3141, 1988.

Noel, M., et al.: Dietary treatment of Maple Syrup Urine Disease (Branched Chain Ketoaciduria). *JADA 69*:63, 1976.

Ohio Neonatal Nutritionists: *Nutritional Care for High-Risk Newborns.* Philadelphia: George F. Stickley Co., 1985.

Otte, K., et al.: Nutritional Repletion in Malnourished Patients with Emphysema. *JPEM 13*:152, 1989.

Peterson, K., et al.: Team Management of Failure to Thrive. *JADA 84*:810, 1984.

Pomerance, H., and Krall, J.: The Relationship of Birth Size to the Rate of Growth in Infancy and Childhood. *AJCN 39*:95, 1984.

Reynolds, J.: Enteral and Parenteral Nutrition of Low Birthweight Infants. *Contemporary Nutrition 10*(3), March 1985. Minneapolis: Genera Mills Nutrition Department.

616

Riesenberg, D.: Progress in Research, Therapy of Prader-Willi Syndrome. *JAMA* *255*:3211, 1986.

Rizzo, W., et al.: Adrenoleukodystrophy: Dietary Oleic Acid Lowers Hexacosanoate Levels. *Ann Neuro 21*:232, 1987.

Roche, A.: Growth Assessment of Handicapped Children. *Public Health Currents 19*:25, 1979. Columbus: Ross Laboratories.

Sadeghi-Nejad, A., and Senior, B.: Adrenomyeloneuropathy Presenting as Addison's Disease in Childhood. *NEJM 322*:13, 1990.

Sanders, K.D., et al.: Growth Response to Enteral Feeding by Children with Cerebral Palsy. *JPEN 14*:23, 1990.

Scarff, T.: Non-Invasive Neurodiagnostic Tests for Patients with Spina Bifida. *Spina Bifida Therapy 1*(1):5, July 1978.

Schleichkarn, J.: *Coping with Cerebral Palsy: Answers to Questions Parents Often Ask.* Baltimore: University Park Press, 1984.

Schriver, C.: Cystinuria. *NEJM 315*:1155, 1986.

Schwartz, S., et al.: Enteral Nutrition in Infants with Congenital Heart Disease and Growth Failure. *Peds 86*:368, 1990.

Shepherd, R., et al.: Malnutrition in Cystic Fibrosis: The Nature of the Nutritional Deficit and Optimal Management. *Nutrition Abstracts and Reviews 54*:1009, 1984.

Shepherd, R., et al.: Nutritional Rehabilitation in Cystic Fibrosis: Controlled Studies of Effects of Nutrition on Growth Retardation, Body Protein, Turnover and Course of Pulmonary Disease. *J Peds 109*(95):788, 1986.

Siddiqi, S.: Acute Necrotizing Enterocolitis. Lecture at the Fifth Annual Regional Perinatal Symposium—Fetal and Neonatal Nutrition. Sponsored by Ross Laboratories. Monroeville, PA, May 16, 1979.

Signore, J.: Ketogenic Diet Containing Medium-Chain Triglyceride. *JADA 62*:285, 1973.

Solomons, N.: Rehabilitating the Severely Malnourished Infant and Child. *JADA 85*:28, 1985.

Solomons, N., et al.: Some Biochemical Indices of Nutrition in Treated Cystic Fibrosis Patients. *AJCN 34*:462, 1981.

Sondel, S., et al.: Oral Nutritional Supplementation in Cystic Fibrosis. *NSS 7*(4):20, April, 1987.

Sonies, B., et al.: Swallowing Dysfunction in Nephropathic Cystinosis. *NEJM 323*:565, 1990.

Sternfeld, L.: How to Help a Baby with Developmental Delay. *Baby Talk 44*(4), April, 1979.

Suskind, R.: *Textbook of Pediatric Nutrition.* New York: Raven Press, 1981.

Trerin, W.R., and Stanley, C.A.: Massive Hepatomegaly, Steatosis, and Secondary Plasma Carnitine Deficiency in an Infant with Cystic Fibrosis. *Peds 83*;993, 1989.

Vohr, B., et al.: Somatic Growth of Children of Diabetic Mothers with Reference to Birth Size. *J Peds 97*:196, 1980.

Warman, N., and Zitarelli, M.: Nonorganic Failure to Thrive: Etiology, Evaluation and Treatment. *Topics in Clinical Nutrition 2*:31, Jan., 1987.

Williams, J.: Nutritional Goals in Gycogen Storage Disease. *NEJM 314*:709, 1986.

Wilson, P., et al.: Metabolic Rate and Weight Loss in Chronic Obstructive Lung Disease. *JPEN 14*:7, 1990.

Wodarski, L.: Nutritional Intervention in Developmental Disabilities: An Interdisciplinary approach, *JADA 85*:218, 1985.

Zachman, R.D.: Retinol (Vitamin A) and the Neonate: Special Problems of the human Premature Infant. *AJCN 50*:413, 1989.

Zipf, W., et al: Pancreatic Polypeptidase Responses to Protein Meal Challenges in Obese But Otherwise Normal Children and Obese Children with Prader-Willi Syndrome. *J Clin Endo and Metab 57*(5):1074, 1983.

NEUROLOGICAL AND PSYCHIATRIC CONDITIONS

Adams, P., et al.: Effect of Pyridoxine Hydrochloride (Vitamin B_6) upon Depression Associated with Oral Contraception. *The Lancet 1*:897, 1973.

American College of Physicians, Health and Public Policy Committee: Eating Disorders: Anorexia Nervosa and Bulimia. *Nutrition Today* March-April, 1987.

American Dietetic Association: Position of the A.D.A.: Nutrition Intervention in the Treatment of Anorexia Nervosa and Bulemia Nervosa. *JADA 88*:68, 1988.

American Dietetic Association: Position of the A.D.A.: Nutrition Intervention in Treatment and Recovery from Chemical Dependency. *JADA 90*:1274, 1990.

Biery, J., Willford, J., and McMullen, E.: Alcohol Craving in Rehabilitation: Assessment of Nutrition Therapy. *JADA 91*:463, 1991.

Bruch, H.: Anorexia Nervosa. *Nutrition Today.* Sept.-Oct. 1978, pp. 14–18.

Carlson: *Dietetics in Physical and Rehabilitative Medicine* ADA *Newsletter* 6(2), 1987.

Chouinard, G., et al.: Supersensitivity Psychosis and Tardive Dyskinesia: A Survey of Schizophrenic Outpatients. *Psychopharmacology Bulletin 22*:891, 1986.

Chouinard, G., Young, S., et al.: Tryptophan-Nicotinamide Combination with Depression (letter). *The Lancet 1*:249, 1977.

Claggett, M.: Nutritional Factors relevant to Alzheimer's Disease. *JADA 89*:392, 1989.

Clifton, G., et al.: Assessment of Nutritional Requirements of Head-Injured Patients. *J Neurosurg 64*:895, 1986.

Clifton, G., et al.: Enteral Hyperalimentation in Head Injury. *J Neurosurg 62*:186, 1985.

Cohen, E., and Wurtmen, R., Brain Acetylcholine: Control by Dietary Choline. *Science 191*:561, 1976.

Collins, C.S., et al.: Red Blood Cell Uptake of Supplemental Folate in Patients on Anticonvulsant Drug Therapy. *AJCN 48*:1445, 1988.

Cuellar, R., and Van Thiel, D.: Gastrointestinal Consequences of the Eating Disorders: Anorexia Nervosa and Bulimia. *Am J Gastroenterology 81*(12):113, 1986.

Davis, K., et al.: Choline Chloride in the Treatment of Huntington's Disease and Tardive Dyskinesia: A Preliminary Report. *Psychopharmacol Bull 13*:37, 1977.

Drake, M.A.: Symptoms of Anorexia Nervosa in Female University Dietetic Majors. *JADA 89*:97, 1989.

Farley, D.: Eating Disorders—When Thinness Becomes an Obsession. *FDA Consumer*, May, 1986, HHS (FDA) 86-2211.

Frezza, M., et al.: High Blood Alcohol Levels in Women: The Role of Decreased Gastric Alcohol Dehydrogenase Activity and First-pass Metabolism. *NEJM 322*:95, 1990.

Gannon, M., and Mitchell, J.: Subjective Evaluation of Treatment Methods by Patients Treated for Bulimia. *JADA 86*(4):520, 1986.

Gold, P., et al.: Abnormalities in Plasma and Cerebrospinal Fluid Arginine Vasopressin in Patients with Anorexia Nervosa. *NEJM 308*:1117, 1983.

Gray, G.: Nutrition and Dementia. *JADA 89*:1795, 1989.

Gray, G., and Gray, L.: Nutritional Aspects of Psychiatric Disorders. *JADA 89*:1492, 1989.

Harris, F., and Phelps, C.: Anorexia Nervosa, in M. Hershen and A. Bellack (eds.) *Handbook of Clinical Behavior Therapy with Adults.* New York: Plenum Publishing Corp., 1985, pp. 269–291.

Hsu, G., and Holder, D.: Bulimia Nervosa: Treatment and Short-Term Outcomes, *Psychol Medicine 16*:65, 1986.

Hsu, G.: Outcome of Anorexia Nervosa. *Arch Gen Psychiatry 37*:1041, 1980.

Hsu, G.: The Treatment of Anorexia Nervosa. *Am J Psych 143*:573, 1986.

Kann, R., and Butcher, S.: Head Injury and Neurological Patients. Lecture for the Pittsburgh Dietetic Association, Pittsburgh, PA, February 1986.

Kapoor, S.: Treatment for Significant Others of Bulemic Patients May Be Beneficial. *JADA 88*:349, 1988.

Kaye, W., Gwitsman, H., George, D., et al.: Elevated Cerebrospinal Fluid Levels of Immunoreactive Corticotropin-Releasing Hormone in Anorexia Nervosa: Relation to State of Nutrition, Adrenal Function and Intensity of Depression. *J Clin Endo and Metab* 64(2):203, 1987.

Kaye, W., et al.: Caloric Intake Necessary for Weight Maintenance in Anorexia Nervosa: Nonbulimics Require Greater Caloric Intake than Bulimics. *AJCN* 44:453, 1986.

Kaye, W., et al.: Relationship of Mood Alterations to Bingeing Behavior in Bulimia. *Brit J Psychiatry* 149:479, 1986.

Kirkley, B.: Bulimia: Clinical Characteristics, Development and Etiology. *JADA* 86:468, 1986.

Kiecolt-Glaser, J., and Dixon, K.: Postadolescent Onset: Male Anorexia. *J Psychosocial Nurs* 22(1):11, 1984.

Krey, S., Palmer, K., and Porcelli, K.: Eating Disorders: The Clinical Dietitian's Changing Role. *JADA* 89:41, 1989.

Langan, S., and Farrell, P.: Vitamin E, Vitamin A and Essential Fatty Acid Status of Patients Hospitalized for Anorexia Nervosa. *AJCN* 41:1054, 1985.

Le Marchand, L., et al.: Relationship of Alcohol Consumption to Diet: A Population-based Study in Hawaii. *AJCN* 49:567, 1989.

Lieberman, D.A.: Nutritional Management of the Patient with Parkinson's Disease. *Top Clin Nutr* 4:1, 1989.

Miller, C.A.: Nutritional Needs and Care in Amyotrophic Lateral Sclerosis. *Top Clin Nutr* 4:15, 1989.

National Dairy Council: Eating Disorders. *Dairy Council Digest* 56:1, Jan.–Feb., 1985.

National Institute of Nutrition: An Overview of the Eating Disorders Anorexia Nervosa and Bulemia Nervosa. *Nutrition Today* May/Jun:27, 1989.

Ott, L., et al.: Brain Injury and Nutrition. *Nutr Clin Pract* 5:68, 1990.

Perl, M., et al.: TPN and the Anorexia Nervosa Patient. *NSS* 1(10):6, 1981.

Pincus, J., and Barry, K.: Influence of Dietary Protein on Motor Fluctuations in Parkinson's Disease. *Arch Neuro* 44:270, 1987.

Podell, S.: Intermittent Tube Feedings and Gastroesophageal Reflex Control in Head-injured Patients. *JADA* 89:102, 1989.

Podell, R.: Nutritional Supplementation with Megadoses of Vitamin B_6: Effective Therapy, Placebo or Potentiator of Neuropathy? *Postgrad Med* 77:113, 1985.

Position Paper: Eating Disorders: Anorexia Nervosa and Bulimia. *Ann Int Med* 105:790, 1986.

Raymond, C.: Long-Term Sequelae Pondered in Anorexia Nervosa. *JAMA* 257:3324, 1987.

Rud, E., and Longenecker, J.: Nutrition, the Brain, and Alzheimer's Disease. *Nutrition Today* Jul/Aug:11, 1988.

Scheinberg, L.: *M.S.: Guide for Patients and Families.* New York: Raven Press, 1987.

Sheard, N., and Zersil, S.: Are We Considering the Brain When Delivering Enteral/Parenteral Nutrition? *NSS* 3(9):25, 1983.

Simpson, D.: Nutritional Support of the Coma Patient. *NSS* 3(4):21, 1983.

Sitrin, M., et al.: Vitamin E Deficiency and Neurologic Disease in Adults with Cystic Fibrosis. *Ann Int Med* 107(1):51, 1987.

Smith, B.: Diet Adjunct to the Clinical Treatment of Parkinson's Disease. *Nutrition Today* Jan/Feb:25, 1991.

Stool, E., and Miner, M.: Nutritional Management After Severe Head Injury in Children. *NSS* 3(3):71m 1983.

Story, M.: Nutritional Management and Dietary Treatment of Bulimia. *JADA* 86:517, 1986.

Swark, R.L., and Grimsgaard, A.: Multiple Sclerosis: The Lipid Relationship. *AJCN* 48:1387, 1988.

Thomas, D., et al.: Tryptophan and Nutritional Status of Patients with Senile Dementia. *Psychol Med 16:297*, 1986.

Turner, W.: Nutritional Considerations in the Patient with Disabling Brain Disease. *Neurosurgery 16:707*, 1985.

Vazquez, K.: Urinary Creatinine Excretion in Spinal Cord Injured Patients. *Nutrition 3:214*, 1986.

Viscocan, B.: Nutritional Management of Alcoholism. *JADA 83:693*, 1983.

Waters, D., et al.: Metabolic Studies in Had Injury Patients: A Preliminary Report. *Surgery 100:531*, 1986.

Winston, D.: Treatment of Severe Malnutrition in AN with Enteral Tube Feeding. *NSS 7(6):24*, 1987.

Wolfe, M., and Jensen, R.: Zollinger-Ellison Syndrome: Current Concepts in Diagnosis and Management. *NEJM 317:1200*, 1987.

Wurtman, R., et al.: Facilitation of Levadopa-induced Dyskinesias by Dietary Carbohydrates. *NEJM 319:1288*, 1988.

PULMONARY DISORDERS

Anderson, L., and Price, C.: Nursing Care of Patients with Pulmonary Insufficiency. Columbus: Ross Laboratories. *Crit Care Currents 4(4)*, 1986.

Armstrong, J.: Nutrition and the Respiratory Patient. *NSS6(3):8*, March, 1986.

Askanazi, J., et al.: Respiratory Changes Induced by the Large Glucose Loads of Total Parenteral Nutrition. *JAMA 234:1444*, 1980.

Askanazi, J., et al.: Nutrition and the Respiratory Patient. *Crit Care Med 10:163*, 1982.

Aubier, M., et al.: Effect of Hypophosphatemia on Diaphragmatic Contractility in Patients with Acute Respiratory Failure. *NEJM 313:420*, 1985.

Basili, H., and Deitel, M.: Effect of Nutritional Support on Weaning Patients off Mechanical Ventilators. *JPEN 5:161*, 1981.

Belford Budd, C.: Nutritional Care of Patients with *Pneumocystis carinii* Pneumonia. *NSS 2(12):12*, Dec., 1982.

Benatar, S.: Fatal Asthma. *NEJM 314:423*, 1986.

Brandstetter, R., et al.: Lactose Intolerance Associated with Intal Capsules. *NEJM 315:1613*, 1986.

Brown, S., and Light, R.: When C.O.P.D. Patient are Malnourished. *J Respir Dis 36* 1983.

Covelli, H., et al.: Respiratory Failure Precipitated by High Carbohydrate Loads. *Ann Int Med 95:579*, 1981.

Dark, D., Pingleton, S., and Kerby, G.: Hypercapnea During Weaning: A Complication of Nutritional Support. *Chest 88:141*, 1985.

Deitel, M., et al.: Nutritional Management of Ventilator-Dependent Patients. *NSS 3(2):9*, Feb., 1983.

Donohue, J.: Status Asthmaticus: Immediate Therapy and Measures that Prevent Recurrence. *Consultant*, p. 43. July, 1986.

Driver, A., McAlevy, M., and Smith, J.: Nutritional Assessment of Patients with Chronic Obstructive Pulmonary Disease and Acute Respiratory Failure. *Chest 82:568*, 1982.

Ferguson, M., Little, A., and Skinner, D.: Current Concepts in the Management of Postoperative Chylothorax. *Ann Thor Surg 40:542*, 1985.

Fiaccadori, E., et al.: Hypercapnic-hypoxemic Chronic Obstructive Pulmonary Disease (C.O.P.D.): Influence of Severity of C.O.P.D. on Nutritional Status. p. 680.

Goldstein, S., et al.: Metabolic Demand, Ventilation and Muscle Function During Repletion of Malnourished COPD and Surgical Patients. *Anes 63:A276*, 1985.

Goldstein, S., et al.: Fucntional Changes During Nutritional Depletion in Patients with Lung Disease. *Clin Chest Med 7:141*, 1986.

Goldstein, S., and Geare, J.: Nutritional Complications in Respiratory Disease. *Dietitians in Critical Care Newsletter*, pp. 8–11, 1986.

Guenter, C., and Welch, M.: *Pulmonary Medicine*, 2nd ed. Philadelphia: J.B. Lippincott Co., 1982.

Gross, N.: Asthma or Chronic Bronchitis? A Diagnostic Problem in Adults. *Pract Cardio* 12(10):129, Sept., 1986.

Hunter, A.: Clinical Signs of Nutritional Status in COPD Patient.s *Pract Cardio* 9(11):173, 1983.

Irwin, M., and Openbrier, D.: A Delicate Balance: Strategies for Feeding Ventilated COPD Patients. *AJN* 85:274, 1985.

Ireton-Jones, C., and Turner, W.: The Use of Respiratory Quotient to Determine the Efficiency of Nutritional Support Regimens. *JADA* 87:180, 1987.

Keim, N., et al.: Dietary Evaluation of Outpatients with COPD. *JADA* 86:902, 1986.

Leong, E., Beno, M., and Libby, G.: Nutritional Care of the Ventilator-Dependent Patient: Role of the Dietitian. *NSS* 3(7):24, July, 1983.

Olbrantz, K., et al.: Pneumothorax Complicating Enteral Feeding Tube Placement. *JPEN* 9:210, 1985.

Park, R., et al.: Gastrointestinal Manifestations of Cystic Fibrosis: A Review. *Gastro* 81:1143, 1981.

Petty, R.: Future Trends in the Management of Asthma and COPD. *Am J Med* 79:38, 1985.

Pingleton, S., and Harmon, G.: Nutritional Management in Acute Respiratory Failure *JAMA* 257:3094, 1987.

Robinson, C.: The Management of Chylothorax. *Ann Thor Surg* 39:90, 1985.

Rogers, R., et al.: Nutrition and COPD: State of the Art Minireview. *Chest* 85:63, 1984.

Ross Laboratories: *Specialized Nutrition for Pulmonary Patients*. Columbus: Ross Laboratories, G416, Dec., 1984.

Rothkopf, M.M., et al.: Nutritional Support in Respiratory Failure. *Nutr Clin Pract* 4:166, 1989.

Shepherd, R., et al.: Changes in Body Composition and Muscle Protein Degradation During Nutritional Supplementation in Nutritionally Growth-Retarded Children with Cystic Fibrosis. *J Ped Gastroenterology and Nutrition* 2:439, 1983.

Skeie, B., et al.: The Beneficial Effects of Fat on Ventilation and Pulmonary Fucntion. *Nutrition* 3:149, 1987.

Teba, L., Dedhia, H., Bowen, R., and Alexander, J.: Chylothorax Review. *Crit Care Med* 13:49, 1985.

Unge, G., et al: Effects of Dietary Tryptophan Restriction on Clinical Symptoms in Patients With Endogenous Asthma. *Allergy* 38:211, 1983.

Wilson, D., et al.: Metabolic Rate and Weight Loss in C.O.P.D. *JPEN* 14:7, 1990.

Wilson, D., et al.: Nutritional Aspects of C.O.P.D. *Clin Chest Med* 7:643, 1986.

Wotton, S.: The Brighter Side of Cystic Fibrosis. *Nursing Times* 80:58, 1984.

CARDIOVASCULAR DISORDERS

Abel, R., et al.: Malnutrition in Cardiac Surgical Patients: Results of a Prospective Randomized Evaluation of Early Postoperative Parenteral Nutrition. *Arch Surg* 111:45, 1976.

Abel, R.: Nutrition and the Heart. *In* Fischer, J. (ed.): *Surgical Nutrition*. Boston: Little, Brown and Co., 1983, pp. 619–641.

Aberg, H., et al.: Serum Triglycerides Are a Risk Factor for Myocardial Infarction But Not for Angina Pectoris. *Atherosclerosis* 54:89, 1985.

Allred, C., et al.: An Educational and Behavioral Approach for the Primary Prevention of Premature Cardiovascular Disease. *JADA* 84:1042, 1984.

American Heart Association: *Heart Facts*. Dallas: American Heart Association, 1986.

American Heart Association: Risk Factors and Coronary Disease: A Statement for Physicians. *Circulation 62:*445A, 1980.

Anda, R., et al.: Dietary and Weight Control Practices among Persons with Hypertension: Findings from the 1986 Behavioral Risk Factor Surveys. *JADA 89:*1265, 1989.

Anderson, J., and Clark, J.: Dietary Fiber: Hyperlipidemia, Hypertension, and Coronary Heart Disease. *Am J Gastro 81*(10):907, 1986.

Anderson, J., and Clark, J.: Nutrition Management of Hyperlipidemia and Diabetes. *Food and Nutrition News 59*(4):1, Sept.-Oct., 1987.

Anderson, J., et al.: Hypocholesterolemic Effects of Oat Bran or Bean Intake for Hypercholesterolemic Men. *AJCN 4*(6):1146, Dec., 1984.

Anderson, J., and Gustafson, N.: Intensive Management of Hypercholesterolemia. *Practical Cardiology 12:*59, 1986.

Anderson, J.N., and Fustafson, N.J.: Hypcholesteremic Effects of Oat and Bran Products. *AJCN 48(Suppl.):*749, 1988.

Antila, H., et al.: Serum Iron, Zinc, Copper, Selenium, and Bromide Concentrations after Coronary Bypass Operation. *JPEN 14:*85, 1990.

Austin, MA., et al.: Vascular Prostacyclin Is Increased in Patients Ingesting Omega-3 PUFA before Coronary Artery Bypass Graft Surgery. *Circulation 82:*428, 1990.

Axelsson, K., et al.: Eating Problems and Nutritional Status during Hospital Stay of Patients with Severe Stroke. *JADA 89:*1092, 1989.

Baicich, R.: Potassium Supplementation. *NSS 7:*29, August, 1987.

Bak, A., and Grobbee, B.: The Effect on Serum Cholesterol Levels of Coffee Brewed by Filtering or Boiling. *NEJM 321:*1432, 1989.

Ballard-Barbash, R., and Calloway, C.: Marine Fish Oils: Role in Prevention of Coronary Artery Disease. *Mayo Clin Proc 62:*113, 1987.

Barker, D.J.P., et al.: Fetal and Placental Size and Risk of Hypertension in Adult Life. *Br Med J 301:*259, 1990.

Bell, L., et al.: Cholesterol-Lowering Effects of Psyllium Hydrophilic Mucilloid. *JAMA 261:*3419, 1989.

Benafante, R., and Reed, D.: Is Elevated Serum Cholesterol Level a Risk Factor for Coronary Heart Disease in the Elderly? *JAMA 262:*393, 1990.

Blankenham, D.H., et al.: The Influence of Diet on the Appearance of New Lesions in Human Coronary Arteries. *JAMA 263:*1646, 1990.

Bloom, E., et al.: Does Obesity Protect Hypertensives Against Cardiovascular Disease? *JAMA 256:*2972, 1986.

Blum, C.B., and Levy, R.I.: Current Therapy for Hypercholesterolemia. *JAMA 261:*3582, 1989.

Boeckner, K., et al.: A Risk-reduction Nutrition Course for Adults. *JADA 90:*260, 1990.

Brown, H.: Nutritional Treatment of the Patient with Acute Myocardial Infarction. *Cardiac Rehabilitation 7*(3):45, Fall, 1976.

Brunzell, J., and Austin, M.: Plasma Triglyceride Levels and Coronary Disease. *NEJM 184:*147, 1991.

Byrne, J., et al.: Assessment of a Cardiovascular Education Program. *JADA 83:*569, 1983.

Castelli, W., et al.: Incidence of Coronary Heart Disease and Lipoprotein Cholesterol Levels: The Framingham Study. *JAMA 256:*2835, 1986.

Connor, S., et al.: The Cholesterol-saturated Fat Index for Coronary Prevention: Background, Use, and a Comprehensive Table of Foods. *JADA 89:*807, 1989.

Criqui, M.: Epidemiology of Atherosclerosis: An Update Overview. *Am J Cardiol 57:*18C, 1986.

DeBakey, M., et al.: Diet, Nutrition, and Heart Disease. *JADA 86:*729, 1986.

Egan, B.: Nutritional and Lifestyle Approaches to the Prevention and Management of Hypertension. *Comp Ther 11:*15, 1985.

622

Ernst, N.: NIH Consensus Development Conference on Lowering Blood Cholesterol to Prevent Heart Disease: Implications for Dietitians. *JADA 85:*586, 1985.

Fischer, J.: Symposium: Nutritional Support in Cardiac, Hepatic and Renal Failure. *Contemp Surg 19:*77, 1981.

Ernst, N., et al.: The National Cholesterol Education Program: Implications for Dietetic Practitioners From the Adult Treatment Panel Recommendations. *JADA 88:*1401, 1988.

Flynn, M., et al.: Dietary "Meats" and Serum Lipids. *AJCN 35:*935, 1982.

Food and Drug Administration: The Case for Moderating Sodium Consumption. *FDA Consumer.* Department of Health and Human Services Publication #82-2158, October, 1981.

Fowler, N.: Congestive Heart Failure and Its Management. Part II. *Hosp Med Mar.:* 23, 1988.

Freedman, D.S., et al.: Body Fat Distribution and Male/Female Differences in Lipids and Lipoproteins. *Circulation 81:*1498, 1990.

Freis, E.D.: Critique of the Clinical Importance of Diuretic-induced Hypokalemia and Elevated Cholesterol Level. *Arch Int Med 149:*2640, 1989.

Grady, K., and Herold, L.: Comparison of Nutritional Status in Patients before and after Heart Transplantation. *J Heart Transplant 7:*123, 1988.

Grimm, R., et al.: The Influence of Oral Potassium Chloride on Blood Pressure in Hypertensive Men on a Low-sodium Diet. *NEJM 322:*569, 1990.

Gruchaw, H.W., et al.: Calcium Intake and the Relationship of Dietary Sodium and Potassium to Blood Pressure. *AJCN 48:*1463, 1988.

Grundy, S.: Comparison of Monounsaturated Fatty Acids and Carbohydrates for Lowering Plasma Cholesterol. *NEJM 314:*745, 1986.

Grundy, S., et al.: Rationale of the Diet-Heart Statement of the American Heart Association. *Circulation 65:*839A, 1982.

Harris, W.: Health Effects of Omega-3 Fatty Acids. *Contemporary Nutrition 10(8),* August, 1985. Minneapolis: General Mills Nutrition Department.

Healy, M., et al.: The Role of Metals In Cardiovascular Disease. *Nursing Times* January 12, 1983, pp. 41–43.

Hemry, M.A.: Cardiac Rehab: Still Running or Standing Still? *Am J Nurs 88:*1196, 1988.

Heymsfield, S.B., and Casper, K.: Congestive Heart Failure: Clinical Management by Use of Continuous Nasoenteric Feeding. *AJCN 50:*539, 1989.

Heymsfield, S., et al.: Nutritional Support in Cardiac Failure. *Surg Clin N Am 6:*635, 1981.

Hoeg, J., et al.: An Approach to the Management of Hyperlipidemia. *JAMA 255:*512, 1986.

Humble, C.: Oats and Cholesterol: The Prospects for Prevention of Heart Disease. *Am J Pub Health 81:*159, 1991.

Hynak-Hankinson, M., et al.: Dysphagia Evaluation and Treatment: The Team Approach, Part I. *NSS 4(5):*33, May, 1984.

Hynak-Hankinson, M., et al.: Dysphagia Evaluation and Treatment: The Team Approach, Part II. *NSS 4(6):*30, June, 1984.

Hypertension Prevention Trial Research Group: The Hypertension Prevention Trial: Three-year Effects of Dietary Changes on Blood Pressure. *Arch Int Med 150:*137, 1990.

Kannel, W.: Nutrition and the Occurrence and Prevention of Cardiovascular Disease in the Elderly. *Nutr Rev 46:*62, 1988.

Keys, A.: Olive Oil and Coronary Heart Disease. *The Lancet 1:*983, April 25, 1987.

Khaw, K-T., and Barrett-Connor, E.: Dietary Potassium and Stroke-Associated Mortality. *NEJM 316:*235, 1987.

Khaw, K.T., and Garrett-Connor, E.: The "Association" between Blood Pressure, Age, and Dietary Sodium and Potassium: A Population Study. *Circulation 77:*53, 1988.

Kottke, B.: Hyperlipoproteinemia: The Case for Individualized Care. *Consultant*, November, 1986, 160–169.

Kris-Etherton, P.: Support for the Diet-Heart Issue. *J Nut Ed 18*:29, 1985.

Kris-Etherton, P., et al.: The Effect of Diet on Plasma Lipids, Lipoproteins, and Coronary Heart Disease. *JADA 88*:1373, 1988.

Kromhout, D., et al.: The Inverse Relationship Between Fish Consumption and 20-Year Mortality From Coronary Heart Disease. *NAJM 312*:1205, 1985.

Kumar, M., and Coulston, A.: Nutritional Management of the Cardiac Transplant Patient. *JADA 83*:463, 1983.

Kuske, T., and Feldman, E.: Hyperlipoproteinemia, Atherosclerosis Risk and Dietary Management. *Arch Int Med 147*:357, 1987.

LaCroix, A., et al.: Coffee Consumption and The Incidence of Coronary Heat Disease. *NAJM 315*:978, 1986.

La Rosa, J.: A.H.A. Medical/Scientific Statement: Special Report: The Clinical Lipid Specialist. *Circulation 82*:1548, 1990.

Leonard, T., et al.: The Effects of Caffeine on Various Body Systems, *JADA 87*:1048, 1987.

Levin, M.: Restoring the Flow, *Diabetes Forecast 61*:47, Nov.-Dec. 1984.

Levy, R.: Cholesterol and Cardiovascular Disease: No Longer Whether, but Rather When, In Whom and How? *Circulation 72*:686, 1985.

Levy, R.: Current Status of the Cholesterol Controversy. *Am J Med 74*:1, 1983.

Lipid Research Clinics Coronary Primary Prevention Trial Results. I. Reduction in Incidence of Coronary Heart Disease. *JAMA 251*:351, 1984.

Lipid Research Clinics Coronary Primary Prevention Trial Results. II. The Relationship of Reduction in Incidence of Coronary Heart Disease to Cholesterol-Lowering. *JAMA 251*:365, 1984.

Luft, F.: Dietary Sodium, Potassium and Chloride Intake and Arterial Hypertension. *Nutrition Today May/Jun*:9, 1989.

Lyle, R., et al.: Blood Pressure and Metabolic Effects of Caclium Supplementation in Normotensive White and Black Men. *JAMA 257*:1772, April 3, 1987.

MacMahon, S., Wilcken, D., and MacDonald, G.: The Effect of Weight Reduction on Left Ventricular Mass. *NEJM 314*:334, 1986.

Marsh, A.: Processes and Formulations that Affect the Sodium Content of Foods. *Food Technology* July 1983, pp. 45–49.

Matthews, L.: Enteral Nurition in the Geriatric Stroke Patient. *NSS 6*:22, Nov. 1986.

McCann, B., et al.: Promoting Adherance to Low-fat, Low-cholesterol Diets: Review and Recommendations. *JADA 90*: 1383, 1990.

McCarron, D., et al.: Blood Pressure and Nutrient Intake in the United States. *Science 224*:1392, 1984.

McCarron, D., Morris, C., and Bukoski, R.: The Calcium Paradox of Essential Hypertension. *Am J Med 82*(Suppl. 1B): 27, 1987.

McMurry, M., et al.: Family-oriented Nutrition Intervention for a Lipid Clinic Population. *JADA 91*:57, 1991.

McNamara, D.: Dietary and Serum Cholesterol and Coronary Heart Disease. *Nutrition and the M.D.* XI(1):1–6, Jan., 1985.

Melsink, R., and Katan, M.: Effect of a Diet Enriched with Monosaturated or Polyunsaturated Fatty acids on Levels of Low-density and High-density Lipoprotein Cholesterol in Healthy Women and Men. *NEJM 321*:436, 1989.

Mensink, R., and Katan, M.: Effect of Monounsaturated Fatty Acids Versus Complex Carbohydrates on High Density Lipoproteins in Healthy Men and Women. *The Lancet 1*;122, Jan. 17, 1987.

Miller, R.: How to Ignore Salt and Still Please the Palate. *FDA Consumer* Department of Health and Human Services Publication #FDA 82-2165, April, 1982.

Mondeika, T.: Cholesterol Content of Shellfish. *JAMA 254*:2970, 1985.

Myers, M.: Caffeine and Cardiac Arrhythmias. *Ann Int Med 184*:147, 1991.

National Center for Health Statistics, National Heart, Lung, and Blood Institute Collaborative Lipid Group: Trends in Serum Cholesterol Levels Among U.S. Adults Aged 20–74 Years. *JAMA 257*:937, 1987.

National Institutes of Health Consensus Development Conference Summary. Treatment of Hypertriglyceridemia. *Arteriosclerosis 4*:296, 1984.

National Institutes of Health: A Consensus Report: NIH Consensus Development Conference Statement—Lowering Blood Cholesterol. *Nutrition Today* Jan.-Feb. 1985, pp. 13–16.

National Institutes of Health: *Report of the Working Group on Critical Patient Behaviors in the Dietary Management of High Blood Pressure.* NIH Publication #83-2269. December, 1982.

Nestel, P.: Fish Oil Alternates: The Cholesterol-Induced Risk in Lipoprotein Cholesterol. *AJCN 43*(5):752, 1986.

Nestel, P., et al.: Suppression by Diets Rich in Fish Oil of Very Low Density Lipoprotein Production in Man. *J Clin Invest 74*:82, 1984.

Newman, W., et al.: Relation of Serum Lipoprotein Levels and Systolic Blood Pressure to Early Atherosclerosis: The Bogalusa Heart Study. *NEJM 314*:138, 1986.

O'Keefe, C., Hahn, D., and Betts, N.: Physicians' Perspectives on Cholesterol and Heart Disease. *JADA 91*:189, 1991.

Olendzki, M., et al.: Evaluating Nutrition Intervention in Atherosclerosis: Some Theoretical and Practical Considerations. *JADA 79*:9, 1981.

Phillipson, B., et al.: Reduction of Plasma Lipids, Lipoproteins and Apoproteins by Dietary Fish Oils in Patients with Hypertriglyceridemia. *NEJM 19*:1210, 1985.

Pittman, J., and Cohen, P.: The Pathogenesis of Cardiac Cachexia. *NEJM 271*:403, 1964.

Poindexter, S., et al.: Nutrition in Congstive Heart Failure. *Nutrition in Clinical Practice 1*:83, April 1986.

Posner, B., et al.: Preventive Nutrition Intervention in CHD: Risk Assessment and Formulating Dietary Goals. *JADA 86*:1395, 1986.

Raab, C., and Tillotson, J.: *A Manual on Nutrition Counseling for the Reduction of Cardiovascular Disease Risk Factors.* Public Health Service, National Institutes of Health. NIH Publication #83-1528, 198.

Rausch, E.: Diet as Adjunct Therapy in Congestive Heart Failure. *J Ped Nursing 33*:20, 1983.

Resnick, L.: Uniformity and Diversity of Calcium Metabolism in Hypertension. *Am J Med 82*(Suppl. 1B):16 Jan. 26, 1987.

Riccardella, D., and Dwyer, J.: Salt Substitutes and Medicinal Potassium Sources: Risks and Benefits. *JADA 85*:471, 1985.

Rosenberg, L., et al.: Coffee Drinking and Nonfatal Myocardial Infarction in Men under 55 Years of Age. *Am J Epid 128*:570, 1988.

Ross, R.: The Pathogenesis of Atherosclerosis—An Update. *NEJM 314*:488, 1986.

Sachs, F.M.: Dietary Fats and Blood Pressure: A Critical Review of the Evidence. *Nutr Rev 47*:291, 1989.

Saperia, G., and Alpert, J.: Diet in the Coronary Care Unit. *Practical Cardiology 9*:57, 1983.

Schectman, J., Elinsky, E., and Bartman, B.: Primary Care Clinician Compliance with Cholesterol Treatment Guidelines. *J Gen Int Med 6*:121, 1991.

Schmieder, R., and Messerli, F.: Is There a Direct Relationship Betwee Obesity and Hypertension? *Pract Cardio 12*:68, May 1, 1986.

Schnuman, B.: Soluble versus Insoluble Fiber—Different Physiological Responses. *Food Technology 41*:81, 1987.

Schroeder, J., and Hunt, S.: Cardiac Transplantation—Update 1987. *JAMA 258*(21):3142, 1987.

Sebranek, J., et al.: Physiological Role of Dietary Sodium in Human Health and Implications of Sodium Reduction in Muscle Foods. *Food Technology* July 1983, pp. 51–59.

Shah, M., et al.: Hypertension Prevention Trial: Food Pattern Changes Resulting from Intervention on Sodium, Potassium, and Energy Intake. *JADA* 90:69, 1990.

Singh, R., and Cameron, E.: A Hypothesis: Does Magnesium Theapy Have a Role in Ischemic Heart Disease and Sudden Death? *Pract Cardio* 9:180, 1982.

Sowers, M., Wallace, R., and Lemke, J.: The Association of Intakes of Vitamin D and Calcium with Blood Pressure Among Women. *AJCN* 42:135, 1985.

Stamler, R., et al.: Nutritional Therapy for High Blood Pressure, JAMA 257:1484, 1987.

Stampfer, M., et al.: A Prospective Study of Moderate Alcohol Consumption and the Risk of Coronary Disease and Stroke in Women. *JADA* 319:267, 1988.

Stroy, J.: Dietary Fiber and Lipid Metabolism. *Proc for Soc for Exp Biol and Med* 180:447, 1985.

Swain, J.F., et al.: Comparison of the Effects of Oat Bran and Low-fiber Wheat on Serum Lipoprotein Levels and Blood Pressure. *NEJM* 322:147, 1990.

Taylor, W., et al.: Cholesterol Reduction and Life Expectancy: A Model Incorporating Multiple Risk Factors. *Ann Int Med* 106:605, 1987.

Trevisan, M., et al.: Consumption of Olive Oil, Butter and Vegetable Oils and Coronary Heart Disease Risk Factors. *JAMA* 263:1432, 1989.

United States Department of Halth and Human Services, Working Group on Hypertension: Statement on Hypertension in Diabetes Mellitus. *Arch Int Med* 147:830, 1987.

University of Iowa College of Medicine: *Model Workshop on Nutrition Counseling in Hyperlipidemia.* NIH Publication #80-1666, August 1980.

Uusitupa, M.I.J., et al.: 5-Year Incidence of Atherosclerotic Vascular Disease in Relation to General Risk Factors, Insulin Level, and Abnormalities in Lipoprotein Composition in Non-insulin-dependent Diabetics and Nondiabetic Subjects. *Circulation* 82:27, 1990.

Van Gaal, L., and DeLeeuw, I.: Effects of Smoking on Lipid Parameters During Therapeutic Weight Loss. *Atherosclerosis* 60:287, 1986.

Van Horn, L., et al.: Serum Lipid Response to Oat Product Intake with a Fat-Modified Diet. *JADA* 86:759, 1986.

VonBorstel, R.: Biological Effects of Caffeine Metabolism. *Food Technology* 37:40, Sept., 1983.

Wassertheil-Smoller, S., et al.: Effective Dietary Intervention in Hypertensives: Sodium Restriction and Weight Reduction. *JADA* 85:423, 1985.

Watt, P., et al.: Hypercholesterolemia in Patients Undergoing Coronary Bypass Surgery: Are They Aware, Under Treatment, and under Control? *Heart and Lung* 17:205, 1988.

Weinberger, M.: Dietary Sodium and Blood Pressure. *Hospital Practice* August 15, 1986, pp. 55–64.

Weinsier, R., and Norris, D.: Recent Developments in the Etiology and Treatment of Hypertension: Dietary Calcium, Fat and Magnesium. *AJCN* 42:1331, 1985.

Wenger, N.: Guidelines for Dietary Management After Myocardial Infarction. *Geriatrics* August, 1979, pp. 75–83.

Wood, D., et al.: Linoleic and Eicosapentanoic Acids in Adipose Tissue and Platelets and Risk of Coronary Heart Disease. *The Lancet* 1:177, Jan., 1987.

Yetiz, J., and Del Tredici, A.: Bringing the Cholesterol Message to the Public: Dietitians Must be Proactive in Nutrition Counseling. *JADA* 90:1383, 1990.

GASTROINTESTINAL DISORDERS

Alm, L.: Effect of Fermenation on Lactose, Glucose and Galactose-Intolerant Individuals, *Dairy Sci 65*:346, 1982.

Alun, J., et al.: Crohn's Disease: Maintenance of Remission By Diet. *The Lancet 1*:177, July, 1985.

Ambrose, N., et al.: Clinical Impact of Colectomy and Illeorectal Anastomosis in the Management of Crohn's Disease. *Gut 25*:223, 1984.

Anderson, C., and Cerda, J.: Diets for Patients with Esophageal and Gastric Disorders. *Consultant May*, 1986, pp. 25–33.

Anderson, M.: Preventive Maintenance of the GI Tract, Part I. *Postgrad Med 80*:106, 1986.

Avery, M., and Snyder, J.: Oral Therapy for Acute Diarrhea: The Underused Simple Solution. *NEJM 323*:891, 1990.

Baillie, J., and soltis, R.: Systemic Complications of Inflammatory Bowel Disease. *Geriatrics 40*:53, 1985.

Bank, S.: Chronic Pancreatitis: Clinical Features and Medical Management. *Am J Gastro 81*:153, 1986.

Barot, L., et al.: Caloric Requirements in Patients with Inflammatory Bowel Disease. *Ann Surg 195*:214, 1982.

Brauer, P.M., et al.: Economic Impact of Nutrition Counseling in Patients with Crohn's Disease in Canada. *J Can Diet Assoc 49*:236, 1988.

Brauer, P., et al.: Diet of Women with Crohn's Disease and Other GI Diseases. *JADA 82*:659, 1983.

Bhutta, T.: Oral Rehydration for Diarrhea. *NAJM 307*:952, 1982.

Boeckman, C., and Taylor, R.: Bowel Lengthening for Short-Gut Syndrome. *J Ped Surg 16*:996, 1981.

Brandt, L.: Managing GI Disorders of Aging: Noncardiac Chest Pain and Rectal Bleeding. *Geriatrics 41*:20, 1986.

Burkit, D.: Dietary Fiber: Is It Really Helpful? Geriatrics 37:119, 1982.

Burt, M., and Brennan, M.: Nutritional Support of the Patients with Esophageal Cancer. *Sem Onc 11*:127, 1984.

Butcher, S.: Practical Aspects of the Control of Diarrhea in Tube-Fed Patients With Use of a Bulk Laxative. *DNS Newsletter VIII*(6):12, May, 1987.

Castell, D., and Frank, B.: How to Treat Heartburn with Diet Therapy. *Nutrition Today* May-June, 1969, pp. 12–21.

Cello, J., et al.: Management of the Patient with Hemorrhaging Esophageal Varices. *JAMA 256*:1480, 1986.

Clark, C.: Medical Complications for Gastric Surgery for Peptic Ulcer. *Comp Ther 7*:26, 1981.

Chernoff, R., and Dean, J.: Medical and Nutritional Aspects of Intractable Diarrhea. *JADA 76*:161, 1980.

Cowan, G., et al.: Short Bowel Syndrome: Causes and Clinical Consequences. *NSS 4*(9):25, 1984.

Cravo, M., et al.: Nutritional Support in Crohn's Disease: Which Route? *Am J Gastro 86*:317, 1991.

Cummings, J., et al.: Role of the Colon in Ileal-Resection Diarrhea *The Lancet 1*:344, 1973.

Davidson, J., and Sawyers, J.: Crohn's Disease of the Esophagus. *Am Surg 49*:168, 1983.

Deitel, M., et al.: Nutritional Support in Inflammatory Bowel Disease. *Contemp Surg 19*:33, 1981.

Dobbins, J., and Binder, H.: Importance of the Colon in Enteric Hyperoxaluria. *NEJM 296*:288, 1977.

Donaldson, R.: Management of Medical Problems in Pregnancy—Inflammatory Bowel Disease. *NEJM 312*:1616, 1985.

Elliott, J.: Swallowing Disorders in the Elderly: A Guide to Diagnosis and Treatment. *Geriatrics 43*:95, 1988.

Fabricius, P., et al.: Crohn's Disease in the Elderly. *Gut 26*:461, 1985.

Faller, M., et al.: Nutritional Implications and Dietary Management of Postprotocolectomy and Ileal Reservoir Construction. *JADA 86*:1235, 1986.

Fazio, V.: Regional Enteritis (Crohn's Disease): Indications for Surgery and Operative Strategy. *Surg Clin North Am 63*:27, 1983.

Feldman, M.: Bicarbonate, Acid and Duodenal Ulcer. *NEJM 316*:408, 1987.

Fleming, A.: Zinc Nutrition in Crohn's Disease. *Dig Dis and Sci 26*(10):865, 1981.

Flier, J., and Underhill, L.: Pathogenesis of Peptic Ulcer and Implications for Therapy. *NEJM 322*:909, 1990.

Freedman, P., et al.: Crohn's Disease of the Esophagus: Case Report and Review of the Literature. *Am J Gastroenterology 79*:835, 1984.

Fuchs, G.: Malnutrition and Nutritional Support in Inflammatory Bowel Disease. *NSS 5*(6):28, 1985.

Gee, M., et al.: Nutritional Status of Gastroenterology Outpatients: Comparison of Inflammatory Bowel Disease with Functional Disorders. *JADA 85*:1591, 1985.

Gee, M., et al.: Protein-Energy Malnutrition in Gastroenterology Outpatients: Increased Risk in Crohn's Disease. *JADA 85*:1466, 1985.

Goldsmith, G., and Patterson, M.: Irritable Bowel Syndrome: Treatment Update. *Am Fam Phys 31*:191, 1985.

Gorbach, S.: Travelers Diarrhea. *NEJM 307*:881, 1982.

Graham, D.Y., et al.: Spicy Food and the Stomach: Evaluation by Videoendoscopy. *JAMA 260*:3473, 1988.

Graham, T.: Gastrointestinal Disorders. Internal Medicine Board Review, University of Pittsburgh School of Medicine, March 14, 1983.

Granaderos, C.: Nutritional Assessment and Management of Patients with Short Bowel Syndrome. *DNS Newsletter VIII*(6), May 1987.

Grant, D., et al: Loop Ileostomy for Anorectal Crohn's Disease. *Can J Surg 29*:32, 1986.

Haas, P., et al.: The Prevalence of Hemorrhoids. *Dis Colon Rectum 26*:435, 1983.

Hamilton, I., et al.: Intestinal Permeability in Celiac Disease: The Response to Gluten Withdrawal and Single Dose Gluten Challenge. *Gut 23*:202, 1982.

Hamilton, S.: Colorectal Carcinoma in Patients with Crohn's Disease. *Gastroenterology 89*:398, 1985.

Hardy, T., et al.: Management of Inflammatory Bowel Disease: An Effective and Concise Approach. *Dis Colon Rectum 23*:244, 1980.

Harper, P., et al.: Crohn's disease in the Elderly: A Statistical Comparison with Younger Patients Matched for Sex and Duration of Disease. *Arch Int Med 146*:753, 1986.

Harries, A., et al.: Controlled Trial of Supplements on Nutrition in Crohn's Disease. *Lancet 1*:887, April 23, 1983.

Harries, A., et al.: Influence of Nutritional Status on Immune Functions in Patients with Crohn's Disease. *Gut 25*:465, 1984.

Hawker, P., et al.: Management of Enterocutaneous Fistulae in Crohn's Disease. *Gut 24*:284, 1983.

Hermann-Zaidins, M.: Diarrhea. *DNS Newsletter, VIII*(6):11, May, 1987.

Hermann-Zaidins, M.: Malabsorption in Adults: Etiology, Evaluation and Management. *JADA 86*:1171, 1986.

Hodges, P., et al.: Protein-Energy Intake and Malnutrition in Crohn's Disease. *JADA 84*:1460, 1984.

Hodges, P., et al.: Vitamin and Iron Intake in Patients with Crohn's Disease. *JADA 84*:52, 1984.

Hofman, A., and Poley, J.: Role of Bile and Malabsorption on Pathogenesis of Diarrhea and Steatorrhea in Patients with Ileal Resection. *Gastro 62:*918, 1972.

Imes, S., Pinchbeck, B., and Thomson, A.: Diet Counseling Modifies Nutrient Intake of Patients with Crohn's Disease. *JADA 87:*457, 1987.

Jackson, M., and Eastwood, G.: Diagnosis: Crohn's Disease. *Hosp Med Mar:* 121, 1991.

Jeejeebhoy, K.: Therapy of the Short Gut Syndrome. *Lancet 1:*1427, June 25, 1983.

Jones, V., et al.: Crohn's Disease: Maintenance of Remission by Diet. *The Lancet 2;*177, July 27, 1985.

Kaldor, P.: Stress Ulcers. *Critical Care Nursing Currents 3*(3), 1985. Columbus: Ross Laboratories.

Kennedy, H., et al.: Water and Electrolyte Balance in Subjects with a Permanent Ileostomy. *Gut 24:*702, 1983.

Kind, C., and Toskes, P.: Small Intestine Bacterial Overgrowth. *Gastro 76:*1035, 1979.

Kirschner, B., et al.: Lactose Malabsorption in Children and Adolescents with Inflammatory Bowel Disease. *Gastro 81:*829, 1981.

Kirschner, B., et al.: Reversal of Growth Retardation in Crohn's Disease with Therapy Emphasizing Oral Nutritional Restitution. *Gastro 80:*10, 1981.

Klurfeld, D.: The Role of Dietary Fiber in Gastrointestinal Disease. *JADA 87:*1172, 1987.

Kolata, G.: Brain Receptors for Appetite Discovered. *Science 218:*460, 1982.

Korman, S.H.: Pica as a Presenting Symptom in Childhood Celiac Disease. *AJCN 51:*139, 1990.

Krasinski, S., et al.: The Prevalence of Vitamin K Deficiency in Chronic Gastrointestinal Disorders. *AJCN 41:*639, 1985.

Latimer, P., et al.: Gastric Stasis and Vomiting: Behavioral Treatment. *Gastro 83:*684, 1982.

Lee, E.: Aim of Surgical Treatment of Crohn's Disease. *Gut 25:*217, 1984.

Levine, G.: Nutritional Support in Gastrointestinal Disease. *Surg Clin North Am 61:*701, 1981.

Littman, A.: Lactase Deficiency: Diagnosis and Management. *Hospital Practice* January 30, 1987, pp. 111–124.

Logan, R., et al.: Reduction of Gastrointestinal Protein Loss by Elemental Diet in Crohn's Disease of the Small Bowel. *Gut 22:*383, 1981.

Louridice, T., and Lang, J.: Treatment of Radiation Enteritis: A Comparison Study. *Am J Gastroenterology 78:*481, 1983.

Maton, P.: The Carcinoid Syndrome. *JAMA 260:*1602, 1988.

Matuchansky, C.: Nutritional Support and Gastrointestinal Function. *Gastro 8:*7, 1984.

McCauley, K.: Medium-Chain Triglycerides: Enteral Use. *NSS* 4(4):50, April, 1984.

Meyer, B., and Cerda, J.: Malabsorption: Pathophysiological Considerations and Diagnosis. *Comp Ther 11:*49, 1985.

Miholic, J., et al.: Nutritional Consequences of Total Gastrectomy: The Relationship between Mode of Reconstruction, Postprandial Symptoms, and Body Composition. *Surg 108:*488, 1990.

Moghissi, K., et al.: Esophageal Problems: Use of Nutritional Support. *In* Dietel, M. (ed.): *Nutrition in Clinical Surgery.* Baltimore: Williams & Wilkins, 1985, p. 303.

Moore, F.: Current Thoughts on Malabsorption: Parenteral, Enteral and Oral Feeding. *JADA 86:*1169, 1986.

Motil, K., et al.: Mineral Balance During Nutritional Support in Adolescents with Crohn's Disease and Growth Failure. *J Ped 107:*473, 1985.

Muller, J., et al.: Preoperative Parenteral Feeding in Patients with Gastrointestinal Cancer. *Lancet 1:*68, 1982.

National Dairy Council: Nutritional Importance of Lactose and Lactase Activity. *Dairy Council Digest 56*(5): Sept–Oct., 1985. Rosemont, IL: National Dairy Council.

Nunan, T., et al.: Intestinal Calcium Absorption in Patients After Jejunal-Ileal Bypass or Small Intestinal Resection and the Effect of Vitamin D. *Digestion 34:*9, 1986.

O'Grady, J., et al.: Hyposplenism and Gluten-Sensitivity Enteropathy. *Gastro 87:*1326, 1984.

Olson, G., and Gallo, G.: Gluten in Pharmaceutical and Nutritional Products. *Am J Hosp Pharm 40:*121, 1983.

Miglioli, M., et al.: Optimal Nutritional Indexes in Gastroenterology. *JPEN 11*(6):126S, 1987.

O'Sullivan, P.: Review of the GI Tract for the R.D. *DNS Newsletter VIII*(6):2–3, May, 1987.

Palmer, E.: Chronic Idiopathic Gastritis: Clinical Implications. *Hosp Med Feb:*56, 1989.

Penny, W., et al.: Relationship Between Trace Elements, Sugar Consumption and Taste in Crohn's Disease. *Gut 24:*288, 1983.

Pereira, J., and Horrigan, F.: Understanding Adult-Acquired Megacolon. *Geriatric Nursing* Jan.-Feb. 1987, 16–19.

Purdum, P., and Kirby, D.: Short-bowel Syndrome: A Review of the Role of Nutrition Support. *JPEN 15:*93, 1991.

Rathgeber, M.: Nutrition and Ostomies. *DNS Newsletter VIII*(6):5, May, 1987.

Raymond, J., and Becker, J.: Ileoanal Pull-Through: A New Surgical Alternative to Ileostomy and a New Challenge in Diet Therapy. *JADA 86:*663, 1986.

Reber, H., et al.: Management of External Gastrointestinal Fistulas. *Ann Surg 188:*460, 1978.

Recker, R.: Calcium Absorption and Achlorhydria. *NEJM 313:*70, 1985.

Rhodes, J., and Rose, J.: Does Food Affect Acute Inflammatory Bowel Disease? The Role of Parenteral, Elemental and Exclusion Diets. *Gut 27:*471, 1986.

Rombeau, J., et al.: Preoperative Total Parenteral Nutrition and Surgical Outcome in Patients with Inflammatory Bowel Disease. *Am J Surg 143:*139, 1982.

Rombeau, J., et al.: Experience with a New Gastrostomy-Jejunal Feeding Tube. *Surgery 93:*574, 1983.

Rosenthal, S., et al.: Growth Failure and Inflammatory Bowel Disease: Approach to Treatment of a Complicated Adolescent Problem. *Peds 72:*481, 1983.

Schwabe, A.: Dietary Management of the Irritable Bowel Syndrome. *Nutrition and the M.D. 13:*7, July, 1987.

Schwartz, R., et al.: Apparent Absorption and Retention of Ca, Cu, Mg, Mn, and Zn from a Diet Containing Bran. *AJCN 43:*444, 1986.

Sciarrette, G., et al.: Hydrogen Breath Test Quantification and Clinical Correlation of Lactose Malabsorption in Adult Irritable Bowel Syndrome and Ulcerative Colitis. *Dig Dis Sci 29:*1098, 1984.

Seashore, J., et al.: Total Parenteral Nutrition in Crohn's Disease. Is It a Primary or Supportive Mode of Therapy? *Dis Colon Rectum 26:*275, 1982.

Simpson, D., and Loftus, J.: A Program to Establish Natural Normal Bowel Elimination in the Comatose Enteral Tube-Fed Patient. *NSS 5*(9):37, Sept., 1985.

Shiau, F., et al.: Stool Electrolytes and Osmolality Measurements in the Evaluation of Diarrheal Disorders. *Ann Int Med 102:*773, 1985.

Skikne, B.: Role of Gastric Acid in Food Iron Absorption. *Gastro 81:*1068, 1981.

Sleisinger, M.: How Should We Treat Crohn's Disease? *NEJM 302:*1024, 1980.

Smidy, P., et al.: Fecal Loss of Fluid, Electrolytes, and Nitrogen in Colitis Before and After Ileostomy. *Lancet 1:*14, 1960.

Solomons, N., et al.: Zinc Deficiency in Crohn's Disease. *Digestion 16:*87, 1977.

Spencer, H., et al.: Effect of Small Doses of Aluminum-Containing Antacids on Calcium and Phosphorus Metabolism. *AJCN 36;*32, 1982.

Steiger, E.: Morbidity and Mortality Related to Home Parenteral Nutrition in Patients with Gut Failure. *Am J Surg 145:*102, 1983.

Steinberg, S.: Zince Deficiency in Crohn's Disease. *Comp Ther 11:*34, 1985.

Timmcke, A.: Granulomatous Appendicitis: Is It Crohn's Disease? Report of a Case and Review of the Literature. *Am J Gastroenterology 81*:283, 1986.

Valero, V., et al.: Liver Abscess Complicating Crohn's Disease Presenting as Thoracic Empyema. Case Report and Review of the Literature. *Am J Med 79*:659, 1985.

Van Kalmthout, P., et al.: Severe Copper Deficiency Due to Excessive Use of an Antacid Combined with Pyloric Stenosis. *Dig Dis and Sci 27*:859, 1982.

Vuoristo, M., and Miettinen, T.: Increased Biliary Lipid Secretion in Celiac Disease. *Gastro 88*:134, 1985.

Wallace, C.: Gastroesophageal Reflux. *Comp Ther 9*:57, 1983.

Wilson, J.: Gastrointestinal Dysfunction in the Critically Ill: Nutritional Implications. *Comp Ther 11*:45, 1985.

Wolever, T., et al.: Ileal Loss of Available Carbohydrate in Man: Comparison of a Breath Hydrogen Method with Direct Measurement Using a Human Ileostomy Model. *Am J Gastroenterology 81*:115, 1986.

Wytock, D., and DiPalma, J.: All Yogurts Are Not Created Equal. *AJCN 47*:454, 1988.

Young, E.: Short Bowel Syndrome: High Fat Versus High Carbohydrate Diet. *Gastro 84*:872, 1985.

PANCREATIC, HEPATIC, AND BILIARY DISORDERS

Achord, J.: Cirrhosis: Making Sure of the Diagnosis. *Consultant 22*:40, 1982.

Berk, P.: Fulminant Hepatic Failure Can Be Life-Threatening. *Consultant 21*:182, 1981.

Boudeman, K., et al.: Pancreatic Disease: Special Feeding Problems. *NSS 5*(11):22, Nov., 1985.

Cerra, F., et al.: Disease-Specific Amino Acid Infusion (F080) in Hepatic Encephalopathy: A Prospective, Randomized, Double-Blind, Controlled Study. *JPEN 9*:288, 1985.

Cobert, B.: Answers to Questions on Liver Function Testing. *Hospital Medicine 19*(12):13, 1983.

DiCecco, S., et al.: Assessment of Nutritional Status of Patients with End-stage Liver Disease Undergoing Liver Transplantation. *Mayo Clin Proc 64*:95, 1989.

DiMagno, E.: Medical Treatment of Pancreatic Insufficiency. *Mayo Clinic Proceedings 54*:435, 1979.

Dinga, M.: Nutrition in Liver Transplantation. *DNS Newsletter VIII*(6):5, May, 1987.

Dirks, I.: Intravenous Fat Emulsions as a Complication of TPN. *NSS 4*:41, 1984.

D'Souga, A., and Floch, M.: Calcium Metabolism in Pancreatic Disease. *AJCN 26*:52, 1973.

Enloe, C.: The Pancreas. *Nutrition Today*, pp. 20–23, March-April 1982.

Francis, D., et al.: Occurrence of Hepatitis A, B and Non-A/Non-B in the United States. *Am J Med 76*:69, 1984.

Freund, H., et al.: Infusion of Branched-Chain Enriched Amino Acid Solution in Patients with Hepatic Encephalopathy. *Ann Surg 196*:209, 1982.

Gitlin, N.: Nutritional Support in Liver Disease. *NSS 4*(6):14, June, 1984.

Goff, D., and Lorenzo, A.: Nutritional Therapy of Hepatic Encephalopathy. *NSS 4*:53, 1984.

Gore, R.: Ultrasound and CT Scanning in the Evaluation of Ascites. *Med Times 112;*65, 1984.

Grant, J., et al.: Total Parenteral Nutrition in Pancreatic Disease. *Ann Surg 200*:627, 1984.

Hasse, J.: Role of the Dietitian in the Nutrition Management of Adults after Liver Transplantation. *JADA 91*:473, 1991.

Horst, D., et al.: Comparison of Dietary Protein with an Oral Branched-Chain-Enriched Amino Acid Supplement in Chronic Port-Systemic Encephalopathy: A Randomized Controlled Trial. *Hepatology 4*:279, 1984.

631

John, W., et al.: Resting Energy Expenditure in Patients with Alcoholic Hepatitis. *JPEN* 13:124, 1989.

Kappas, A., and Alvares, A.: How the Liver Metabolizes Foreign Substances. *Sci Am* June, 1975, pp. 27–32.

Keith, J.: Hepatic Failure: Etiology, Manifestations and Management. *Crit Care Nurs* 5(1):60, 1985.

Keohane, P., et al.: Enteral Nutrition in Malnourished Patients with Hepatic Cirrhosis and Acute Encephalopathy. *JPEN* 7(4):346, 1983.

Kirby, D., and Craig, R.: The Value of Intensive Nutritional Support in Pancreatitis. *JPEN* 9:353, 1985.

Krevsky, B., and Godley, J.: Nutritional Support in Advanced Liver Disease. *NSS* 5(8):8, August, 1985.

Levy, M., and Wexler, M.: Salt and Water Balance in Liver Disease. *Hosp Pract* 19:57, 1984.

Mendenhall, C., et al.: Veterans Administration Cooperative Study on Alcoholic Hepatitis. II. Prognostic Significance of Protein-Calorie Malnutrition. *AJCN* 43:213, 1986.

Merli, M., et al.: Optimal Nutritional Indexes in Chronic Liver Disease. *JPEN* 11:1305, 1987.

Mueller, K.: Total Parenteral Nutrition in Acute Pancreatitis. *DNS Newsletter, VIII*(6):1, May, 1987.

Palumbo, J.D., et al.: Blood Carnitine Status after Orthotropic Liver Transplantation in Patients with End-stage Liver Disease. *AJCN* 50:504, 1989.

Pastides, H., et al.: A Case-control Study of the Relationship between Smoking, Diet and Gallbladder Disease. *Arch Int Med* 150:1409, 1990.

Pitchumoni, C., et al.: Nutrition in the Pathogenesis of Alcoholic Pancreatitis. *AJCN* 33:631, 1980.

Press, O., Press, N., and Kaufman, S.: Evaluation and Management of Chylous Ascites. *Ann Int Med* 96:358, 1982.

Roslyn, J., et al.: Parenteral Nutrition-Indueced Gallbladder Disease: A Reason for Early Cholecystectomy. *Am J Surg* 148:58, 1984.

Schiff, L., and Schiff, E.: *Diseases of the Liver*, 6th ed. Philadelphia: J.B. Lippincott Co., 1987.

Sherwin, R., et al.: Hyperglucagonemia in Laennec's Cirrhosis: The Role of Portalsystemic Shunting. *NEJM* 290:239, 1974.

Shronts, E., Teasley, K., Thoele, S., and Cerra, F.: Nutritional Support of the Adult with Liver Transplantation. *JADA* 87:441, 1987.

Silberman, H., et al.: The Safety and Efficacy of a Lipid-Based System of Parenteral Nutrition in Acute Pancreatitis. *Am J Gastroenterology* 77:494, 1982.

Simko, V.: Nutritional Therapy for Liver Diseases. *Comp Ther* 11:62, 1985.

Small, D.: The Formation and Treatment of Gallstones. *In* Schiff, L., and Schiff, E. (eds.): *Diseases of the Liver*, 5th ed. Philadelphia: J.B. Lippincott Co., 1982, pp. 151–166.

Smith, R.H., and Mekhijan, H.: Dietary Habits of Patients with Cholelithiasis: Do We Need to Instruct? *JADA* 87:209, 1987.

Sokol, R., et al.: Vitamin E Deficiency in Adults with Chronic Liver Disease. *AJCN* 41:66, 1985.

Strauss, E., et al.: Treatment of Hepatic Encephalopathy: A Randomized Clinical Trial Comparing a Branched Chain-Enriched Amino Acid Solution to Oral Neomycin. *Nutr Supp Serve* 6:18, 1986.

Wolfe, M., and Jensen, J.: Zollinger-Ellison Syndrome—Current Concepts in Diagnosis and Treatment. *NEJM* 317(19):1200, 1987.

Wright, R.: *Liver and Biliary Disease*. Philadelphia: W.B. Saunders Co., 1985.

Zieve, L.: The Mechanism of Hepatic Coma. *Hepatology* 1:360, 1981.

ENDOCRINE DISORDERS

Adrogue, H., et al.: Diabetic Ketoacidosis: A Practical Approach. *Hosp Pract Feb.* 15:83, 1989.

American Diabetes Association: Principles of Nutrition and Dietary Recommendations for Individuals with Diabetes Mellitus. *Diabetes Care* Jan.-Feb., 1987.

American Diabetes Association: *The Physician's Guide to Type II Diabetes (NIDDM): Diagnosis and Treatment.* New York: American Diabetes Association, 1984.

American Dietetic Association: Diabetes Care and Education Practice Group. *Diabetes Mellitus and Glycemic Responses to Different Foods: A Summary and Annotated Bibliography.* Chicago: American Dietetic Association, 1985.

Anderson, E., et al.: Effects of a High-Protein and Low-Fat versus Low-Protein and High-Fat Diet on Blood Glucose, Serum Lipoproteins and Cholesterol Metabolism in NIDDM. *AJCN* 45:406, 1987.

Anderson, J., and Gustafson, N.: Diabetes Mellitus Type II—Nutrition Can Be Your Primary Treatment. *Consultant* 27:40, 1987.

Anderson, J.: Hyperlipidemia and Diabetes: Nutrition Considerations. *In* Jovanovic, L., and Peterson, C. (eds.): *Nutrition and Diabetes.* New York: Alan Liss, Inc., 1985, pp. 133–159.

Beebe, C., et al.: Nutritional Management for Individuals with Noninsulin-dependent Diabetes Mellitus in the 1990's: A Review by the Diabetes Care and Education Dietetic Practice Group. *JADA* 91:196, 1991.

Borneman, M., et al.: Insulin-Induced Hypoglycemia in Type I Diabetics. *The Diabetes Educator* 10:25, Fall, 1984.

Butler, P.C., et al.: Effects of Meal Ingestion on Plasma Amylin Concentration in NIDDM and Nondiabetic Humans. *Diabetes* 39:752, 1990.

Christensen, N., et al.: Quantitative Assessment of Dietary Compliance in Patients with Insulin-Dependent Diabetes Mellitus. *Diabetes* 6:245, 1983.

Colagiuri, S., et al.: Metabolic Effects of Adding Sucrose and Aspartame to the Diet of Subjects with NIDDM. *AJCN* 50:474, 1989.

Comi, R., and Gordon, P.: Approach to Hypoglycemia in Adults. *Comp Ther* 13:38, 1987.

Coordinator, National High Blood Pressure Program, National Heart, Lung and Blood Institute: Statement of Hypertension in Diabetes Mellitus. *Arch Int Med* 147:830, 1987.

Coulston, A., Hollenbeck, C., et al.: Deleterious Metabolic Effects of High-Carbohydrates, Sucrose-Containing Diets in Patients with NIDDM. *Am J Med* 82:213, 1987.

Crapo, P., et al.: Carbohydrate in the Diabetic Diet. *J Am Coll Nutrition* 5:31, 1986.

Durr, J., et al.: Diabetes Insipidus in Pregnancy Associated with Abnormally High Circulating Vasopressinase Action. *NEJM* 316:1070, 1987.

Eckerling, L., and Kohrs, M.: Research on Compliance with Diabetic Regimens: Application to Practice. *JADA* 84:805, 1984.

Eisenbarth, G.: Type I Diabetes: A Chronic Autoimmune Disease. *NEJM* 314:1360, 1986.

Evanoff, G., et al.: The Effect of Dietary Protein Restriction on the Progression of Diabetic Nephropathy—A 12-Month Follow-Up. *Arch Int Med* 147:492, 1987.

Etzwiler, D.: Diabetes Management—The Importance of Patient Education and Participation. *Postgrad Med* 80:67, 1986.

Ferris, A., et al.: Lactation Outcome in IDDM Women. *JADA* 88:317, 1988.

Franz, M.: Exercise and the Management of Diabetes Mellitus. *JADA* 87:874, 1987.

Freinkel, N., et al.: Gestational Diabetes Mellitus: Heterogenicity of Maternal Age, Weight, Insulin Secretion, HLA Antigens, and Islet Cell Antibodies and the Impact of Maternal Metabolism on Pancreatic B-cell and Somatic Development in the Offspring. *Diabetes 34*(Suppl. 2):1, 1985.

Gentry, P., and Miller, P.F.: Nutritional Considerations in a Patient with Gastroparesis. *Diabetes Educator 25*:374, 1989.

Gerich, J.: Pathogenesis and Differentiation of the Dawn and Somogyi Phenomena in Patients with Diabetes Mellitus. *Pract Cardio 13*:83, 1987.

Gisinger, C., et al.: Effect of Vitamin E Supplementation on Platelet Thromboxane A_2 Production in Type I Diabetic Patients: Double blind Crossover Trial. *Diabetes 37*:1260, 1988.

Gobbe, S.: Gestational Diabetes. *NEJM 315*:1025, 1986.

Goldstein, D.: Should Glycosylated Hemoglobin Be Used for Monitoring of Diabetes Control? *Pract Cardio 9*:187, 1983.

Haire-Joshu, D.: Diabetes: Controlling the Insulin Balance. *Am J Nursing* 1239, Nov., 1986.

Harold, M., et al.: Effect of Dietary Fiber in Insulin-Dependent Diabetics: Insulin Requirements and Serum Lipids. *JADA 85*:1455, 1985.

Hollenbeck, C., and Coulston, A.: The Role of Dietary Fiber in the Nutritional Management of Diabetes Mellitus. *Pract Card 13*:49, 1987.

Hollingsworth, D.: Diabetes Mellitus—Newest Approaches for a Successful Pregnancy. *Consultant*, August, 1984, p. 29.

Horwath, C., and Worsley, A.: Dietary Habits of Elderly Persons with Diabetes. *JADA 91*:553, 1991.

Huzar, J., and Cerrato, P.: The Role of Diet and Drugs. *R N Apr*: 46, 1989.

Jenkins, D.: Diet and Diabetes: A Common Approach. *J Am Coll Nut 4*:407, 1985.

Jenkins, D., et al.: Decrease in Postprandial Insulin and Glucose Concentration by Guar and Pectin. *Ann Int Med 86*:20, 1977.

Jenkins, D., et al.: Glycemic Responses to Foods: Possible Difference Between Insulin-Dependent and Non-Insulin Dependent Diabetes. *AJCN 40*:971, 1984.

Kabad, U.: Nutritional Therapy in Diabetes: Rationale and Recommendations. *Postgrad Med 79*:145, 1986.

Kennedy, W., et al.: Effects of Pancreatic Transplantation on Diabetic Neuropathy. *NEJM 322*:1031, 1990.

Khachadurian, A.: Hyperuricemia and Gout: An Update. *Am Fam Phys 24*:143, 1981.

Kozlovsky, A., et al.: Effects of Diets High in Simple Sugars on Urinary Chromium Losses. *Metabolism 35*:515, 1986.

Kreisberg, R.: Aging, Glucose Metabolism and Diabetes: Current Concepts. *Geriatrics 42*:67, 1987.

Kritz-Silverstein, D., et al.: The Effect of Parity on the Later Development of NIDDM or Impaired Glucose Tolerance. *NEJM 321*:1214, 1989.

Levine, M., and Kleeman, C.: Hypercalcemia: Pathophysiology and Treatment. *Hosp Pract* July 15, 1987, pp. 93–110.

Marcus, M., and Wing, R.: Eating Disorders in Patients with Diabetes Mellitus. *Pract Card 13*:115, 1987.

Martin, D.: Type II Diabetes: Insulin versus Oral Agents. *NEJM 314*:1314, 1986.

Mintz, D., et al.: Diabetes Mellitus and Pregnancy. *Diabetes Care 1*:49, 1978.

Mobarhan, D., et al.: Enteral Feeding in a Diabetic Patient with Gastroenteropathy. *NSS 3*(12), Dec., 1983.

Morgensen, C.E.: Microalbuminuria as a Predictor of Clinical Diabetic Nephropathy. *Kidney Int 31*:673, 1987.

Nelson, R.: Hypoglycemia: Fact or Fiction. *Mayo Clin Proc 60*:844, 1985.

National Institutes of Health Consensus Development Conference on Diet and Exercise in NIDDM. Bethesda, MD, Dec. 8–10, 1986.

Nuttall, F., et al.: Individualized Diets for Diabetic Patients. *Ann Int Med 99*:204, 1983.

Olefsky, J., and Crapo, P.: Fructose, Xylitol, Sorbitol. *Diabetes Care 3*:390, 1980.

Orchard, T., et al.: Prevalence of Complications in IDDM by Sex and Duration: Pittsburgh Epidemiology of Diabetes Complications Study II. *Diabetes 39:*1116, 1990.

Paige, M.S., and Heins, J.M.: Nutritional Management of Diabetic Patients during Intensive Insulin Therapy. *Diabetes Educator 14:*505, 1988.

Piziak, V.: Hypoglycemia. *Resident and Staff Physician: Problems in Primary Care 32*(8):11PC–18PC, 1986.

Powers, M.: *Handbook of Diabetes Management,* 1st ed. Baltimore: Aspen Publishers, 1987.

Rapp, S., et al.: Food Portion Size Estimation by Men with Type II Diabetes. *JADA 86:*249, 1986.

Reaven, G.: Dietary Therapy for NIDDM. *NEJM 319:*862, 1988.

Reiser, S., Metabolic Effects of Dietary Pectins Related to Human Health. *Food Technology 41:*91, 1987.

Rosenstock, J., et al.: Reduction in Cardiovascular Risk Factors with Intensive Diabetes Treatment in IDDM. *Diabetes Care 10:*729, 1987.

Rossetti, L., et al.: Glucose Toxicity. *Diabetes Care 13:*610, 1990.

Schafer, R.G.: Implementation of Low-protein Diets for Treatment of Persons with Early Diabetic Nephropathy. *Diabetes Educator 15:*231, 1989.

Schiller, M., et al.: Motivational Techniques of Dietitians Counseling Individuals with Type II Diabetes Mellitus. *JADA 87:*37, 1987.

Selby, J., et al.: The Natural History and Epidemiology of Diabetic Nephropathy. *JAMA 263:*1954, 1990.

Simpson, H., et al.: The Dietary Management of Diabetes. *Adv Nut Res 7:*39, 1985.

Waldause, W., et al.: Effect of Stress Hormones on Splanchnic Substrate and Insulin Disposal After Glucose Ingestion in Healthy Humans. *Diabetes 36:*127, 1987.

Walker, J.D., et al.: Restriction of Dietary Protein and Progression of Renal Failure in Diabetic Nephropathy. *Lancet 2;*1421, 1989.

Wolever, T., and Jenkins, D.: The Use of the Glycemic Index in Predicting the Blood Glucose Response to Mixed Meals, *AJCN 43:*167, 1986.

Wood, F., and Bierman, E.: Is Diet the Cornerstone in Management of Diabetes? *NEJM 315:*1224, 1986.

Wylie-Rosett, J.: Evaluation of Protein in Dietary Management of Diabetes Mellitus. *Diabetes Care 11:*143, 1988.

Zucker, A., and Chernow, B.: Diabetes Insipidus and the Syndrome of Inappropriate Antidiuretic Hormone. *Critical Care Quarterly 6:*74, 1983.

WEIGHT CONTROL AND MALNUTRITION

American Dietetic Association: Position of the A.D.A.: Very-low-calorie Weight Loss Diets. *JADA 90:*722, 1990.

American Dietetic Association: Position of the A.D.A.: Optimal Weight as a Health Promotion Strategy. *JADA 89:*1814, 1989.

Bistrian, B.: Nutritional Assessment and Therapy of Protein-Calorie Malnutrition in the Hospital. *JADA 71:*393, 1977.

Bistrian, B., Blackburn, G., et al.: Therapeutic Index of Nutritional Depletion in Hospitalized Patients. *Surg Gyne Ob 141:*512, 1973.

Bistrian, B., Blackburn, G., Vitale, J., et al.: Prevalence of Malnutrition in General Medical Patients. *JAMA 235:*1567, 1976.

Bistrian, B., Sherman, M., Blackburn, G., et al.: Cellular Immunity in Adult Marasmus. *Arch Intern Med 137:*249, 1977.

Brownell, K.: A Program for Managing Obesity. *Dietetic Currents.* Columbus: Ross Laboratories. *13*(3), 1986.

Burgert, S., and Anderson, C.: An Evaluation of Upper Arm Measurements Used in Nutritional Assessment. *AJCN 32:*2136, 1979.

Burton, B., and Foster, W.: Health Implications of Obesity: An NIH Consensus Development Conference. *JADA 85*:1117, 1985.

Cahill, G.: Starvation in Man. *NEJM 282*:668, 1970.

Dieguez, C., and Scanlon, M.: The Search for a Hormonal Switch for Obesity. *Brit Med J 294*:1371, May 30, 1987.

DiLorenzo, C., et al.: Pectin Delays Gastric Emptying and Increased Satiety in Obese Subjects. *Gastro 95*:1211, 1989.

Elliott, D., et al.: Obesity: Pathophysiology and Practical Management. *J Gen Int Med 2*:188, May-June 1987.

Faintuch, J., et al.: Anthropometric Assessment of Nutritional Depletion After Surgical Injury. *JPEN 3*:369, 1979.

Fitzwater, S., et al.: Evaluation of a Long-term Weight Changes after a Multidisciplinary Weight Control Program. *JADA 89*:421, 1989.

Foster, G.D., et al.: Controlled Trial of the Metabolic Effects of a Very-low-calorie Diet: Short and Long-term Effects. *AJCN 51*:167, 1990.

Frankle, R.: Obesity—Family Matter: Creating New Behaviors. *JADA 85*:598, 1985.

Frisancho, A.: Triceps Skinfold and Upper Arm Muscle Size Norms for Assessment of Nutritional Status. *AJCN 27*:1052, 1974.

Gray, G., and Gray, L.: Validity of Anthropometric Norms Used in the Assessment of Hospitalized Patients. *JPEN 3*:366, 1979.

Horton, E.: Metabolic Aspects of Exercise and Weight Reduction. *Medicine and Science in Sports and Exercise 18*:10, 1985.

Ingenbleek, Y., et al.: Measurement of Prealbumin as Index of Protein-Calorie Malnutrition. *The Lancet 2*:106, 1972.

Ingenbleek, Y., et al.: The Role of Retinol-Binding Protein in Protein-Calorie Malnutrition. *Metabolism 24*:633, 1975.

Kaminski, M., et al.: Correction of Mortality with Serum Transferrin and Energy. *JPEN 1*:27A, 1977.

Kern, P., et al.: The Effects of Weight Loss on the Activity and Expression of Adipose-tissue Lipoportein Lipase in Very Obese Humans. *NEJM 322*:1053, 1990.

Keys, A., Brozek, J., et al.: *Biology of Human Starvation.* Minneapolis: University of Minnesota Press, 1950.

King, A.C., et al.: Diet vs. Exercise in Weight Maintenance: The Effects of Minimal Intervention Strategies on Long-term Outcomes in Men. *Arch Int Med 149*:2741, 1989.

Law, D., et al.: Immunocompetence of Patients with Protein-Calorie Malnutrition. *Ann Intern Med 79*:545, 1973.

Leaf, D.: Overweight: Assessment and Management Issues. *Am Fam Phys 42*:653, 1990.

Leevy, C., et al.: Incidence and Significance of Hypovitaminemia in a Randomly Selected Municipal Hospital Population. *AJCN 17*:259, 1965.

Levine, A., and Morley, J.: The Shortening Pathways to Appetite Control. *Nutrition Today* Jan.–Feb. 1983.

Manson, J., et al.: A Prospective Study of Obesity and Risk of Coronary Heart Disease in Women. *NEJM 322*:882, 1990.

Manson, J., et al.: Body Weight and Longevity. *JAMA 257*:253, 1987.

Miller, A., and Blyth, C.: Estimation of Lean Body Mass and Fat from Basal Oxygen Consumption and Creatinine Excretion. *J Appl Phys 5*:73, 1952.

Morrow, S., and Mona, L.: Effect of Gastric Balloons on Nutrient Intake and Weight Loss in Obese Subjects. *JADA 90*:718, 1990.

Murray, M., et al.: Nutritional Assessment of Intensive-care Unit Patients. *Mayo Clin Proc 63*:1106, 1988.

Omizo, S., and Oda, E.: Anorexia Nervosa: Psychological Considerations for Nutritional Counseling. *JADA 88*:49, 1988.

636

Piziak, V., Management of Obesity. *Comp Ther 13*(1):7, 1987.

Rothchild, M., et al.: Albumin Synthesis. *NEJM 286*:748, 1972.

Ryan, R., et al.: Relationship of Body Composition to Oxygen Consumption and Creatinine Excretion in Healthy and Wasted Men. *Metabolism 6*:365, 1957.

Sankey, J., et al.: Nutritional Support in Morbid Obesity with Respiratory Complications. *NSS 6*(3):12, 1986.

Satter, E.: The Feeding Relationship: Implications for Obesity. *Food and Nutrition News 59*(3), 1987. Chicago: National Livestock and Meat Board.

Schulz, L.: Brown Adipose Tissue. Regulation of Thermogenesis and Implications for Obesity. *JADA 87*:761, 1987.

Segal, K.R., et al.: Comparison of Thermic Effects of Constant and Relative Caloric Loads in Lean and Obese Men. *AJCN 51*:14, 1990.

Stark, R.: Body Mass Index. *The Bariatrician* Winter, 1987.

Stensland, S., and Margolis, S.: Simplifying the Calculation of Body Mass Index for Quick Reference. *JADA 90*:856, 1990.

Stunkard, A., et al.: An Adoption Study of Human Obesity. *NEJM 314*:193, 1986.

Wadden, et al.: Responsible and Irresponsible use of Very-low-Calorie Diets in the Treatment of Obesity. *JAMA 263*:83, 1990.

Webb, J., and Birmingham, C.: Cardiac Effects of Dieting. *Practical Cardiology 13*(10):105, 1987.

Weddle, D., et al.: Inpatient and Post-discharge Course of the Malnourished Patient. *JADA 91*:307, 1991.

Weinsier, R., et al.: Hospital Malnutrition: A Prospective Evaluation of General Medical Patients During the Course of Hospitalization. *AJCN 32*:418, 1979.

Whitehead, R., et al.: Serum Albumin and the Onset of Kwashiorkor. *The Lancet 1*:63, 1973.

Wood, E.: Weight Loss Maintenance 1 Year after Individual Counseling. *JADA 90*:1256, 1990.

Wurtman, J.: The Involvement of Brain Serotonin in Excessive Carbohydrate Snacking by Obese Carbohydrate Cravers. *JADA 84*:1004, 1984.

MUSCULOSKELETAL, ARTHRITIC, AND COLLAGEN DISORDERS

Alfin-Slater, R., et al. (eds.): Osteoporosis Issue. *Nutrition and the M.D. XI*(3), March, 1985.

Allen, L.: Calcium and Osteoporosis. *Nutrition Today.* May-June 1986, pp. 6–10.

Blotzer, J.: Accurate Laboratory Tests in Rheumatic Diseases. *Geriatrics 39*:63, 1984.

Cauley, J.A., et al.: Endogenous Estrogen Levels and Calcium Intakes in Postmenopausal Women: Relationships with Cortical Bone Measures. *JAMA 260*:3150, 1988.

Cohen, S.: The Gastrointestinal Manifestations of Scleroderma: Pathogenesis and Management. *Gastro 79*:155, 1980.

Ehrlich, G.: Diffuse Collagen Disease. *JAMA 251*:1595, 1984.

Fanelli, M.: Promoting Women's Health. *Dietetic Currents 12*(4), 1985. Columbus: Ross Laboratories.

Flores, R., et al.: Familial Occurrence of Progressive Systemic Sclerosis and SLE. *J Rheum 11*:321, 1984.

Hall, F., et al.: Bone Mineral Screening for Osteoporosis. *NEJM 316*:212, 1987.

Jaffe, G.: Historical Perspective on Diet and Arthritis. *Dietitians in Critical Care Newsletter VI*(4):3, June, 1984.

Kowsari, B., et al.: Assessment of the Diet of Patients with Rheumatoid Arthritis and Osteoarthritis. *JADA 82*:657, 1983.

Kremer, J., et al.: Fish-Oil Fatty Acid Supplementation in Active Rheumatoid Arthritis:

A Double-Blind, Placebo-Controlled, Cross-over Study. *Arch Int Med 106:497*, 1987.

Lezak, M.: *Neuropsychological Assessment*. New York: Oxford University Press, 1983.

Maddern, G., et al.: Abnormalities of Esophageal and Gastric Emptying in Progressive Systemic Sclerosis. *Gastro 87:922*, 1984.

Mascioli, E., and Blackburn, G.: Nutrition and Rheumatic Disease. *In* Kelley, W., et al.: *Textbook of Rheumatology. Philadelphia:* W.B. Saunders Co., 1985.

Massey, L., and Strang, M.: Soft Drink Consumption, Phosphorus Intake and Osteoporosis. *JADA 80:581*, 1982.

McCullough, M., and Hsu, N.: Metabolic Bone Disease in Home Total Parenteral Nutrition. *JADA 87:915*, 1987.

McKenna, M., and Frame, B.: Privational Vitamin D Deficiency. *Comp Ther 13(1):54*, 1987.

Meenan, R., et al.: Measuring Health Status in Arthritis. *Arthritis and Rheumatism 23:146*, 1980.

National Dairy Council: Diet and Bone Health. *Dairy Council Digest 53(5)*, Sept.-Oct., 1986, Rosemont, IL: National Dairy Council.

National Institute of Arthritis, Musculoskeletal and Skin Diseases: *Osteoporosis: Cause, Treatment, Prevention*. NIH Publication #86-2226, May, 1986.

National Institutes of Health: *Diet and Arthritis: An Annotated Bibliography*. Arlington, VA: National Arthritis, Musculoskeletal and Skin Diseases Clearinghouse, May 1986, NIH Pub. #86-2226.

National Institutes of Health: *Osteoporosis: Consensus Development Conference Statement*. Bethesda, MD: DHHS. 5(3), 1984.

Nordin, B., et al.: A Prospective Trial of the Effect of Vitamin D Supplementation on Metacarpal Bone Loss in Elderly Women. *AJCN 42:470*, 1985.

Panush, R., et al.: Food-Induced (Allergic) Arthritis: Inflammatory Arthritis Exacerbated by Milk. *Arthritis and Rheumatism 29:220*, 1986.

Podell, R.: Systemic Lupus Erythematosus: Does Diet Play A Causative Role? *Postgraduate Medicine 75:251*, 1984.

Riggs, B., and Melton, L.: Involutional Osteoporosis. *NEJM 314:1676*, 1986.

Riggs, B.: Osteoporosis: 'First Step' Diet Treatment. *Geriatrics 41(7):77*, 1986.

Riggs, B., et al.: Treatment of Primary Osteoporosis with Fluoride Therapy, *JAMA 243:446*, 1980.

Riis, B., et al.: Does Calcium Supplementation Prevent Postmenopausal Bone Loss? *NEJM 316:173*, 1987.

Ruden, R.: Scleroderma. *Dietitians in Critical Care Newsletter VI (4):3*, June, 1984.

Santora, A.: Role of Nutrition and Exercise in Osteoporosis. *Am J Med 82* (Suppl. 1B):73, 1987.

Sledge, E.: *Nutrition and Lupus*. Birmingham, AL: Lupus Foudnation of America, 1987.

Spencer, H., and Kramer, L.: Factors Contributing to Osteoporosis. *J Nut 116:316*, 1986.

Spencer, H.: Osteoporosis: Goals of Therapy. *Hosp Pract* March 1982, pp. 131–148.

Stern, J.: Dealing With Your Diet. *Muscular Dystrophy Association Magazine*. March, 1986, pp. 13–16.

Touger-Decker, R.: Nutritional Consideration in Rheumatoid Arthritis. *JADA 88:327*, 1988.

Touger-Decker, R.: Case Study: Scleroderma. *Dietitians in Critical Care Newsletter VI(4):1*, June, 1984.

Trace Element Losses During Bed Rest. *Nutr Rev 46:379*, 1988.

Walden, O.: The Relationship of Dietary and Supplemental Caclium Intake to Bone Loss and Osteoporosis. *JADA 89:397*, 1989.

Ziff, M.: Diet in the Treatment of Rheumatoid Arthritis. *Arthritis and Rheumatism 26;457*, 1983.

ANEMIAS AND BLOOD DISORDERS

Austin, C.: Nutritional Management of the Anemias in the Life Cycle. *DNS Newsletter* *VIII*(5):8, 1987.

Beck, W.: *Hematology*, Boston: MIT Press, 1985.

Beissner, R.: Clinical Assessment of Anemia. *Postgrad Med 80*:83, 1986.

Beuthler, E.: The Common Anemias. *JAMA 259*:2433, 1988.

Bloem, M.W., et al.: Vitamin A Intervention: Short-term Effects of a Single, Oral, Massive Dose on Iron Metabolism. *AJCN 51*:76, 1990.

Clementz, G.L., and Schade, S.G.: The Spectrum of Vitamin B_{12} Deficiency. *Am Fam Phys 41*:150, 1990.

Cook, J.: Determinants of Nonheme Iron Absorption in Man. *Food Technology 37*(10):124, 1983.

Cook, J., and Monsen, E.: Vitamin C, the Common Cold and Iron Absorption. *AJCN 30*:235, 1977.

Cook, J. and Monsen, E.: Food Iron Absorption in Human Subjects. III. Comparison of the Effect of Animal Protein on Nonheme Iron Absorption. *AJCN 29*:859, 1976.

Crosby, W.: Hemochromatosis: The Missed Diagnosis. *Arch Int Med 146*:1209, 1986.

Finch, C., and Cook, J.: Iron Deficiency. *AJCN 39*:471, 1984.

Hallberg, L.: Bioavailable Nutrient Density: A New Concept Applied in the Interpretation of Food Iron Absorption Data. *AJCN 34*:2242, 1981.

Herbert, V.: Therapeutic Treatment of Nutritional Anemias. *DNS Newsletter VIII*(5):4, 1987.

Herbert, V.: The Nutritional Anemias. *Hosp Pract* March, 1980, pp. 65–88.

Isaacs, B.: Understanding the Pathway for the Diagnosis of Nutritional Anemias. *DNS Newsletter VIII*(5):4, 1987.

Morck, T., Lynch, S., and Cook, J.: Inhibition of Food Iron absorption by Coffee. *AJCN 37*:416, 1983.

Raper, N., Rosenthal, J., and Wotecki, C.: Estimates of Available Iron in Diets of Individuals 1 Year Old and Older in the Nationwide Food Consumption Survey. *JADA 84*:783, 1984.

Reed, J., et al.: Nutrition and Sickle Cell Disease. *Am J Hematol 24*:441, 1987.

Rubens, S.: Anemias: An Overview. *DNS Newsletter VIII*(5):4, 1987.

LEUKEMIAS, LYMPHOMAS, AND CANCER

Aker, S., Lenssen, P., et al.: Nutritional Assessment in the Marrow Transplant Patient. *NSS 3*(10):22, 1983.

American College of Physicians: Position Paper: Parenteral Nutrition Patients Receiving Cancer Chemotherapy. *Ann Int Med 110*:734,

American Dietetic Association: Issues in Feeding the Terminally Ill Adult. *JADA 87*:78, 1987.

Balducci, L., and Hardy, C.: Cancer and Nurition: A Review. *Comp Ther 13*:60, 1987.

Beaudette, T.: *Nutrition in Practice: Diet, Nutrition and Cancer*. Minneapolis: Doyle Pharmaceutical Company. *1*(2), Aug.-Sept. 1981.

Beer, W., et al.: Clinical and Nutritional Implications of Radiation Enteritis. *AJCN 41*:85, 1985.

Blackburn, G., et al.: The Effect of Cancer on Nitrogen, Electrolyte and Mineral Metabolism. *Cancer Research 37*:2348, 1977.

Bounous, G., et al.: Dietary Protection During Radiation Therapy. *Strahlentherapie 149*:476, 1979.

Bowers, D.: Nutritional Support of the Bone Marrow Transplant Patient. *DNS Newsletter VIII*(5):5, 1987.

Bright-See, E.: Dietary Fiber and Cancer. *Nutrition Today Jul/Aug*:4, 1988.

Butrum, R.R., Clifford, C.K., and Lanza, E.: NCI Dietary Guidelines: Rationale. *AJCN 48 (Suppl.)*:888, 1988.

Byham, L.: Dietary Fat and Natural Killer Cell Function. *Nutrition Today Jan/Feb*:31, 1991.

Cannon-Albright, L., et al.: Common Inheritance of Susceptibility to Colonic Adenomatous Polyps and Associated Colorectal Cancers. *NEJM 319*:533, 1988.

Chlebowski, R.: Critical Evaluation of the Role of Nutritional Support with Chemotherapy. *Cancer 55*:268, 1985.

Cimino, J.: Feeding Patients with Advanced Cancer. *Dietetic Currents 10*(5), Sept.-Oct. 1983. Columbus: Ross Laboratories.

Colitz, G., et al.: Diet and Lung Cancer: A Review of the Epidemiologic Evidence in Humans. *Arch Int Med 147*:157, 1987.

Creasy, W.: *Diet and Cancer*. Philadelphia: Lea & Febiger, 1985.

Crosley, M.: Watch Out for Nutritional Complications of Cancer. *RN* March 1985, pp. 22–27.

Del Regato, J., Spjut, H., and Cox, J.: *Cancer: Diagnosis, Treatment and Prognosis*, 6th ed. St. Louis: C.V. Mosby Co., 1985.

Dempsey, D., and Mullen, J.: Macronutrient Requirements in the Malnourished Cancer Patient. *Cancer 55*:290, 1985.

Desmond, S.: Diet and Cancer: Should We Change What We Eat? Medical Staff Conference, University of California San Francisco. *Western Journal of Medicine 146*:73, 1987.

deVries, E., Mulder, N., et al.: Enteral Nutrition by Nasogastric Tube in Adult Patients Treated with Intensive Chemotherapy for Acute Leukemia. *AJCN 35*:1490, 1982.

Driedger, L., and Burstall, C.: Bone Marrow Transplantation: Dietitians' Experience and Perspective. *JADA 87*:1387, October, 1987.

Dvorak, H.: Tumors: Wounds That Do Not Heal. *NEJM 315*:1650, 1986.

Frame, R., et al.: The Dentist, the Nutritionist and the Cancer Patient. *NSS 4*(9):10, 1984.

Freudenheim, J.L., et al.: A Case-control Study of Diet and Rectal Cancer in Western New York. *Am J Epid 131*:612, 1990.

Gallagher, P., and Tweedle, D.: Taste Threshold and Acceptability of Commercial Diets in Cancer Patients. *JPEN 7*:361, 1984.

Galloway, D.: Experimental Colorectal Cancer: The Relationship of Diet and Fecal Bile Acid Concentration of Tumor Induction. *Brit J Surg 73*:233, 1986.

Gildea, J., et al.: A Systematic Approach to Providing Nutritional Care to Cancer Patients. *NSS 2*:24, 1982.

Graham, S., et al.: Dietary Epidemiology of Cancer of the Colon in Western New York. *Am J Epid 128*:490, 1988.

Greenwald, P., et al. Dietary Fiber in the Reduction of Colon Cancer Risk. *JADA 87*:1178, 1987.

Grindel, C., et al.: Food Intake of Women with Breast Cancer During Their First Six Months of Chemotherapy. *Onc Nurs Forum 16*:401, 1989.

Harvey, K., et al.: Nutritional Assessment and Patient Outcome During Oncological Therapy. *Cancer 43*:2065, 1979.

Hearne, B., et al.: Enteral Nutritional Support in Head and Neck Cancer: Tube versus Oral Feeding During Radiation Therapy. *JADA 85*:670, 1985.

Heber, D., et al.: Malnutrition and Cancer: Mechanisms and Therapy, Part I. *Nutritional International 2*:184, 1986.

Heber, D., et al.: Metabolic Abnormalities in the Cancer Patient. *Cancer 55*:225, 1985.

Hoffman, F.: Micronutrient Requirements of Cancer Patients. *Cancer 55*:295, 1985.

Jeevanandam, M., et al.: Cancer Cachexia and the Rate of Whole Body Lipolysis in Man. *Metabolism 35*:304, 1986.

Jepson, J., and Lampenfeld, M.: Nutrition in Patients Irradiated for Head and Neck Cancer. *NSS 5:*27, 1985.

Kern, K., and Norton, J.: Cancer Cachexia. *JPEN 12:*286,

Klatsky, A.L., et al.: The Relations of Alcoholic Beverage Use to Colon and Rectal Cancer. *Am J Epid 128:*1007, 1988.

Klimberg, V.S., et al.: Oral Glutamine Accelerates Healing of the Small Intestine and Improves Outcome after Whole Abdominal Radiation. *Arch Surg 125:*1040, 1990.

Kroes, R., et al.: Nutritional Factors in Lung, Colon and Prostate Carcinogenesis in Animal Models. *Fed Proc 45:*136, 1986.

Lane, H., and Carpenter, J.: Breast Cancer: Incidence, Nutritional Concerns and Treatment Approaches. *JADA 87:*765, 1987.

Loiudice, T., and Lang, J.: Treatment of Radiation Enteritis: A Comparison Study. *Am J Gastro 78:*481, 1983.

Lubin, F., et al.: Nutritional Factors Associated with Benign Breast Disease Etiology: A case-control Study. *AJCN 50:*551, 1989.

Lum, L., and Gallagher-Allred, C.: Nutrition and the Cancer Patient: A Cooperative Effort by Nursing and Dietetics to Overcome Problems. *Cancer Nursing* Dec., 1984, pp. 469–474.

Lundholm, K., and Drott, C.: Optimal Nutritional Indices in Cancer Patients. *JPEN 11*(5):135S, 1987.

Malayappa, J., et al.: Cancer Cachexia and Protein Metabolism. *Lancet 1;*1423, 1984.

Mansour, G., et al.: Guidelines for Nutritional Support of the Critically Ill Cancer Patient. *Cancer Bull 36:*152, 1984.

McArdle, A., et al.: Prophylaxis Against Radiation Therapy. *Arch Surg 121:*879, 1986.

Meguid, M., et al.: Letter to the Editor, Nutritional Support in Cancer. *Lancet 2:*230–231, July 23, 1983.

Meguid, M.: Nutrition and Cancer. *NSS 5:*8, 1985.

Menkes, M., et al.: Serum Beta-Carotene, Vitamins A and E, Selenium and the Risk of Lung Cancer. *NEJM 315:*1250, 1986.

Merrick, H., et al.: Energy Requirements for Cancer Patients and the Effect of Total Parenteral Nutrition. *JPEN 12:*8,

Miller, A., and Risch, H.: Diet and Lung Cancer. *Chest 96:*85, 1989.

National Dairy Council: Diet, Nutrition and Cancer. *Dairy Council Digest 54*(6), Nov.-Dec. 1983.

Newell, G.: Nutrition and Diet. *Cancer 51:*2420, 1983.

O'Connor, T., and Campbell, T.: The Influence of Nutrition on Carcinogenesis. *Nutrition 3:*155, 1987.

Ollenschlaeger, G., et al.: Nutrient Intake and Nitrigen Metabolism in Cancer Patients during Oncological Chemotherapy. *AJCN*

Ott, D.: Hospice Care: An Opportunity for Dietetic Services. *JADA 85:*223, 1985.

Patterson, B., and Block, G.: Food Choices and the Cancer Guidelines. *Am J Pub Health 78:*282, 1988.

Pezner, R., and Archambeau, J.: Critical Evaluation of the Role of Nutritional Support for Radiation Therapy Patients. *Cancer 55:*263, 1985.

Redd, W.: Control of Nausea and Vomiting in Chemotherapy Patients. *Postgrad Med 75:*105, 1984.

Ritenbaugh, C.: Carotenoids and Cancer. *Nutrition Today* Jan.-Feb. 1987, p. 14.

Rose, M.: Health Promotion and Risk Prevention Applications for Cancer Survivors. *Onc Nurs Forum 16:*335, 1989.

Russell, D., et al.: Effects of Total Parenteral Nutrition and Chemotherapy on the Metabolic Derangements in Small Cell Lung Cancer. *Cancer Research 44:*176, 1984.

Schottenfeld, D.: Epidemiology of Cancer of the Esophagus. *Sem Onc 11:*92, 1984.

Shamberger, R., et al.: A Prospective, Randomized Study of Adjuvant Parenteral Nutrition in the Treatment of Sarcomas: Results of Metabolic and Survival Studies. *Surgery 69*:1, 1984.

Shils, M.: Principles of Nutritional Therapy. *Cancer 43*:2093, 1979.

Shirley, R., and Minton, J.: Dietary Effects on Benign Breast Disease. *JAMA 255*:259, 1986.

Shizgal, H.: Body Composition of Patients with Malnutrition and Cancer. *Cancer 55*:250, 1985.

Shultz, T.D., and Rose, D.P.: Effect of High-fat Intake on Lactogenic Hormone Bioactivity in Premenopaual Women. *AJCN 48(Suppl.)*:791, 1988.

Silberman, H.: The Role of Preoperative Parenteral Nutrition in Cancer Patients. *Cancer 55*:254, 1985.

Singh, V., and Gaby, S.: Premalignant Lesions: Role of Antioxidant Vitamins and Beta-Carotene in Risk Reduction and Prevention of Malignant Transformation. *AJCN 53*:3865, 1991.

Snowden, P.: Diet and Ovarian Cancer. *JAMA 254*:356, 1985.

Sobala, G., et al.: Ascorbic Acid in the Human Stomach. *Gastro 97*:357, 1989.

Stevens, R., et al.: Body Iron Stores and the Risk of Cancer. *NEJM 319*:1047, 1988.

Symreng, T., et al.: Nutritional Assessment Reflects Muscle Energy Metabolism in Gastric Carcinoma. *Ann Surg 198*:146, 1983.

Szeluga, D.J.: Nutritional Support of Bone Marrow Transplant Recipients: A Prospective, Randomized Clinical Trial Comparing Total Parenteral Nutrition to an Enteral Feeding Program. *Cancer Res 47*:3309, 1987.

Van Eys, J.: Effect of Nutrition on Response to Therapy: *Cancer Research 42* (Suppl.):747s, 1982.

Vickers, Z., et al.: Food Preferences of Patients with Cancer. *JADA 79*:441, 1981.

Wade, E., and Sult, C.: TPN in the Cancer Patient. *NSS 3*:35, 1983.

Wall, D., and Gabriel, L.: Alterations of Taste in Children with Leukemia. *Cancer Nursing* Dec. 1983, pp. 447–452.

Watson, R.: Immunological Enhancement by Fat-Soluble Vitamins, Minerals and True Metals: A Factor in Cancer Prevention. *Cancer Detect Prev 9*:67, 1986.

Watson, R., and Leonard, T.: Selenium and Vitamins A, E, and C: Nutrition with Cancer Prevention Properties. *JADA 86*:505, 1986.

Welch, D.: Nutritional Consequences of Carcinogenesis and Radiation Therapy. *JADA 78*:467, 1981.

Wihawer, S., et al.: Declining Serum Cholesterol Levels Prior to Diagnosis of Conol Cancer. *JAMA 263*:2083,

Willett, W., et al.: Dietary Fat and the Risk of Breast Cancer. *NEJM 316*:22, 1987.

Willett, W., and MacFaden, B.: Diet and Cancer: An Overview. *NEJM 310*:633, 1984.

Willett, W., and MacFaden, B.: Diet and Cancer: An Overview, Part II. *NEJM 310*:697, 1984.

Williams, G.: Food and Cancer. *Nutrition International 1*:49, 1985.

Ziegler, M., et al.: Neuroblastoma and Nutritional Support: Influence on the Host-Tumor Relationship. *J Ped Surg 21*:236, 1986.

Ziegler, R.: A Review of Epidemiologic Evidence that Carotenoids Reduce the Risk of Cancer. *J Nutr 119*:116, 1989.

SURGICAL DISORDERS

Adler, W.: *Medical Evaluation of the Surgical Patient.* Philadelphia: W.B. Saunders Co., 1985.

Apelgren, K., et al.: Malnutrition in Veterans Administration Surgical Patients. *Arch Surg 116*:1059, 1981.

Bellantone, R., et al.: Preoperative Parenteral Nutrition in the High Risk Surgical Patient. *JPEN 12*:195, 1988.

Benabe, J., et al.: Disorders of Calcium Metabolism *In* Maxwell, M., et al.: *Clinical Disorders of Fluid and Electrolyte Metabolism*, 4th ed. New York: McGraw-Hill Book Co., 1987, pp. 759–788.

Bistrian, B., et al.: Cellular Immunity in Semistarved Status in Hospitalized Adults. *AJCN 28*:1148, 1975.

Bistrian, B., et al.: Protein Status of General Surgical Patients. *JAMA 230*:858, 1974.

Blackburn, G., et al.: Branched Chain Amino Acid Administration and Metabolism During Starvation, Injury and Infection. *Surgery 86*:1979.

Bristol, J., et al.: Nutrition, Operations and Intestinal Adaptation. *JPEN 12*:299, 1988.

Butterworth, C.: The Skeleton in the Hospital Closet. *Nutrition Today* March-April 1974, pp. 4–8.

Cerra, F., Upson, D., and Angelico, R.: Branched-Chain Support During Postoperative Protein Synthesis. *Surgery 92*:192, 1982.

Ching, N., et al.: The Outcome of Surgical Treatment as Related to the Response of the Serum Albumin Level to Nutritional Support. *Surg, Gyne and OB 151*:199, 1980.

Deitel, M., and Basi, S.: Indications for TPN in the Surgical Patient in the Community Hospital. *NSS 5*(8):25, August, 1985.

Duke, J., et al.: Contribution of Protein to Caloric Expenditure Following Injury. *Surgery 68*:168, 1970.

Elwyn, D.: Nutritional Requirements of Adult Surgical Patients. *Crit Care Med 8*:9, 1980.

Felson, D.T., et al.: Alcohol Consumption and Hip Fractures: The Framingham Study. *Am J Epid 128*:1102, 1988.

Fischer, J.: *Surgical Nutrition*. Boston: Little, Brown and Co., 1983.

Flink, E.: Magnesium Deficiency Causes and Effects. *Hosp Pract* February 15, 1987, p. 116A.

Freed, B., et al.: Initiation of an Admissions Nutritional Screening Program in a Community Hospital. *NSS 2*:19, 1982.

Gazzaniga, A., et al.: Endogenous Calorie Sources and Nitrogen Balance. *Arch Surg 111*:1357, 1976.

Greenhalgh, D., and Gamelli, R.: Is Impaired Wound Healing Caused by Infection or Nutritional Depletion? *Surgery 102*:306, 1987.

Grimes, C., et al.: The Effect of Preoperative Total Parenteral Nutrition on Surgery Outcomes. *JADA 87*:1202, 1987.

Hadley, S., and Fitzsimmons, L.: Nutrition and Wound Healing. *Top. Clin. Nutr. 5*:72, 1990.

Harken, D.: Malnutrition: A Poorly Understood Surgical Risk Factor in Aged Cardiac Patients. *Geriatrics 32*:83, 1977.

Hill, G.: Surgical Nutrition: Time for Some Clinical Common Sense. *Brit J Surg 75*:729, 1988.

Hill, G.: Surgically Created Nutritional Problems. *Surg Clin N Am 61*:731, 1981.

Hill, G., et al.: Malnutrition in Surgical Patients: An Unrecognized Problem. *Lancet 1*:689, 1977.

Holbrook, T.L., et al.: Dietary Calcium and Risk of Hip Fracture. *Lancet 2*;1046, 1988.

Jensen, J.: Nutrition and Orthopedia Surgery. *NSS 4*(2):27, Feb., 1984.

Law, D., et al.: The Effects of Protein calorie Malnutrition on Immune Competence of the Surgical Patient. *Surg, Gyne and OB 139*:257, 1974.

Levine, M., and Kueman, C.: Hypercalcemia: Pathophysiology and Treatment. *Hospital Practice* July 15, 1987, pp. 93–110.

McFadden, E., and Zaloga, A.: Calcium Regulation. *Crit Care Quarterly 6*:12, 1983.

McLaren, D.: Out of Sight, Out of Mind. *Nutrition Today* Jan.-Feb. 1985, pp. 4–9.

643

Mequid, M., et al.: Aggressive Perioperative Nutritional Support in the Major Surgical Patient (Symposium). *Contemp Surg* April, 1982.

Moss, G.: Postoperative Ileus is an Avoidable Complication. *Surg, Gyne and OB 148*:81, 1979.

Mullen, J., et al.: Implications of Malnutrition in the Surgical Patient. *Arch Surg 114;*121, 1979.

Mullen, J., et al.: Reduction of Operative Morbidity and Mortality by Combination Preoperative and Postoperative Nutritional Support. *Ann Surg 192*:604, 1980.

Mundy, G.: The Hypercalcemia of Malignancy. *Kidney Int 31*:142, 1987.

Neser, E., Fletcher, J., and Urban, E.: Short Bowel Syndrome. *Gastro 77*:572, 1979.

Randall, H.: Nutrition and Surgical Patients: Protein Metabolism and Requirements. *Contemp Surg 11*:17, Sept., 1977.

Randall, H.: Nutrition and Surgical Patients: The Need for Carbohydrates. *Contemp Surg 11*:17, Oct., 1977.

Randall, H.: Nutrition and Surgical Patients: The Value of Intravenous Fat. *Contemp Surg 11*:19, Nov. 1977.

Roubenoff, R., et al.: Malnutrition Among Hospitalized Patients. *Arch Int Med 147*:1462, 1987.

Ruberg, R.: Role of Nutrition in Wound Healing. *Surg Clin N Am 64*:705, 1984.

Schiller, W., et al.: Creatinine and Nitrogen Excretion in Seriously Ill and Injured Patients. *Surg, Gyne and OB 149*:561, Oct., 1979.

Schwartz, P.: Ascorbic Acid in Wound Healing—A Review. *JADA 56*:497, 1970.

Stevens, J.: Surgical Nutrition: The Fourth Coming. *JAMA 239*:192, 1978.

Studley, H.: Percentage of Weight Loss—A Basic Indicator of Surgical Risk in Patients with Chronic Peptic Ulcer. *JAMA 106*:458, 1936.

Thompson, J., et al.: Nutritional Screening in Surgical Patients. *JADA 84*:337, 1984.

Thompson, J., et al.: The Management of Perioperative Parenteral Nutrition. *NSS 6*(10):12, Oct., 1986.

Weaver, K.: Magnesium and Its Role in Vascular Reactivity and Coagulation. *Contemporary Nutrition 12*(3), Minneapolis: General Mills Nutrition Dept.

Welch, C., and Malt, R.: Surgery of the Stomach, Duodenum, Gallbladder and Bile Ducts. *NEJM 316*:999, 1987.

Wolfe, B., et al.: Experience with Home Parenteral Nutrition. *Am J Surg 146*:7, 1983.

Young, G., and Hill, G.: Assessment of Protein-Calorie Malnutrition in Surgical Patients from Plasma Proteins and Anthropometric Measurements. *AJCN 31*:429, 1978.

Young, G., et al.: Plasma Proteins in Patients Receiving Intravenous Amino Acids or Intravenous Hyperalimentation After Major Surgery. *AJCN 32*:1192, June 1979.

Young, M.: Malnutrition and Wound Healing. *Heart and Lung 17*:60, 1988.

Zaloga, G., and Chernow, B.: Magnesium Metabolism in Critical Illness. *Crit Care Quarterly 6*:22, 1983.

HYPERMETABOLIC, INFECTIOUS, TRAUMATIC AND FEBRILE CONDITIONS

Algert, S., Stubblefield, N., Grasse, B., et al.: Assessment of Dietary Intake of Lysine and Arginine in Patients with Herpes Simplex. *JADA 87*:1560, 1987.

Allgower, M., et al.: Infection and Trauma. *Surg Clin N Am 60*:133, 1980.

American Dietetic Association: Position of the A.D.A.: Nutrition Intervention in the Treatment of Human Immunodeficiency Virus Infection. *JADA 89*:839, 1989.

Barbul, A., et al.: Intravenous Hyperalimentation with High Arginine Levels Improves Wound Healing and Immune Fucntion. *J Surg Res 38*:328, 1985.

Barbul, A., Retturo, et al.: Arginine: A Thymotrophic and Wound-Healing Promoting Agent. *Surg Forum 28*:101, 1977.

Baue, A., and Chaudry, I.: Prevention of Multiple Systems Failure. *Surg Clin N Am* 60:1167, 1980.

Baue, A., Gunther, B., et al.: Altered Hormonal Activity in Severely Ill Patients After Injury or Sepsis. *Arch Surg 119*:1125, 1984.

Baxter, C.: Metabolism and Nutrition in Burned Patients. *Comp Ther 13*:36, 1987.

Beisel, W.: Magnitude of the Host Nutritional Response to Infection. *AJCN 30*:1236, 1977.

Beisel, W., Sawyer, W., et al.: Metabolic Effects of Intracellular Infections in Man. *Ann Intern Med 67*:744, 1967.

Beisel, W.: Role of Nutrition in Immune System Diseases. *Comp Ther 13*(1):13–19, 1987.

Bell, S., et al.: Adequacy of a Modular Tube Feeding Diet for Burned Patients. *JADA 86*:1386, 1986.

Bell, S., et al.: Prediction of Total Urinary Nitrogen for Burned Patients. *JADA 85*:1100, 1985.

Bell, S., and Wyatt, J.: Nutrition Guidelines for Burned Patients. *JADA 86*:648, 1986.

Bell, S., et al.: Weight Maintenance in Pediatric Burned Patients. *JADA 86*:207, 1986.

Bentler, M., and Stanish, M.: Nutrition Support of the Pediatric Patient with AIDS. *JADA 87*:488, 1987.

Bistrian, B.: Simple Technique to Estimate Severity of Stress. *Surg Gyne OB 148*:675, 1979.

Bistrian, B.: Interaction of Nutrition and Infection in the Hospital Setting. *AJCN 30*:1228, 1977.

Bistrian, B., Blackburn, G., et al.: Cellular Immunity in Semi-Starved States in Hospitalized Adults. *AJCN 28*:1148, 1975.

Blackburn, G., et al.: Branched-Chain Amino Acid Administration and Metabolism During Starvation, Injury and Infection. *Surg 86*:307, 1979.

Black, P., et al.: Mechanisms of Insulin Resistance Following Injury. *Ann Surg 196*:420, 1982.

Braude, A., et al.: *Infectious Diseases and Medical Microbiology*, 2nd ed. Philadelphia: W.B. Saunders Co., 1985.

Burdge, J., et al.: Nutritional and Metabolic Consequences of Thermal Injury. *Clin Plast Surg 13*:49, 1986.

Caldwell, F., et al.: The Effect of Occlusive Dressings on the Energy Metabolism of Severely Burned Children. *Ann Surg 193*:579, 1981.

Cerra, F., et al.: Septic Autocannibalism: A Failure of Exogenous Nutritional Support. *Ann Surg 192*:570, 1980.

Chandra, R.: Nutrition, Immunity and Infection: Present Knowledge and Future Directions. *Lancet 1*:688–691, March 26, 1983.

Chandra, R., and Scrimshaw, N.: Immunocompetence in Nutritional Assessment. *AJCN 33*:2694, 1980.

Chlebowski, R.: Significance of Altered Nutritional Status in AIDS. *Nutrition and Cancer 7*:85, 1985.

Del Salvio, N.: Nutritional Support for Thermally Injured Patients: The Role of the Dietitian. *NSS 4*:10, 1984.

Dempsey, D., et al.: Energy Expenditure in Acute Trauma to Head With and Without Barbiturate Therapy. *Surg Gyne OB 160*:128, 1985.

Dinarello, C., and Wolff, D.: Molecular Basis of Fever in Humans. *Am J Med 72*:799, 1982.

Frayno, K.: Hormonal Control of Metabolism in Trauma and Sepsis. *Clin Endo 24*:577, 1986.

Fry, D., et al.: Multiple System Organ Failure. *Arch Surg 115*:136, 1980.

Garre, M., et al.: Current Concepts in Immune Derangement Due to Undernutrition. *JPEN 11*:309, 1987.

645

Giovannini, I., et al.: Respiratory Quotient and Patterns of Substrate Utilization in Human Sepsis and Trauma. *JPEN 7*:226, 1983.

Gottschlich, M., et al.: Diarrhea in Tube-fed Burn Patients: Incidence, Etiology, Nutritional Impact and Prevention. *JPEN 12*:338, 1988.

Gottschlich, M.M.: Differential Effects of Three Enteral Dietary Regimens on Selected Outcome Variables in Burn Patients. *JPEN 14*:225, 1990.

Gump, F., and Kinney, J.: Calorie and Fluid Losses Through the Burn Wound. *Surg Clin N Am 50*:1235, 1970.

Harju, E., et al.: High Incidence of Low Serum Vitamin D Concentration in Patients with Hip Fracture. *Arch Orthop Tr Surg 103*:408, 1985.

Hegarty, M.T., Meara, P.A., and Burke, J.F.: Measured and Predicted Caloric Requirements of Adults during Recovery from Severe Burn Trauma. *AJCN 49*:404, 1989.

Holmes, et al.: A Cluster of Patients with EBV Syndrome. *JAMA 257*:229, 1987.

Ingram, W.: Role of Malnutrition in Multiple Organ-System Failure. *NSS 6*(5):12, 1986.

Ireton, C., et al.: Evaluation of Energy Expenditures in Burn Patients. *JADA 86*:334, 1986.

Kesler, S.: Nutrition Care of AIDS Patients. *JADA 88*:828, 1988.

King, N., and Goodwin, C.: Use of Vitamin Supplements for Burned Patients: A National Survey. *JADA 84*:923, 1984.

Kinney, J., et al.: Tissue Fuel and Weight Loss After Injury. *J Clin Path 4* (Suppl.):65, 1978.

Koop, E.: Surgeon General's Report on AIDS. *JAMA 256*:2784, 1986.

Kotler, D.P., et al.: Magnitude of Body-all-mass Depletion and the Timing of Death from Wasting in AIDS. *AJCN 50*:144, 1989.

Loggie, B., and Hinchey, E.: Effect of Iron Administration on the Outcome of Bacterial Peritonitis. *Surg Forum 35*:111, 1984.

Long, C.: Fuel Preferences in the Septic Patient—Glucose or Lipid? *JPEN 11*(4):333, 1987.

Meakins, J., et al.: Delayed Hypersensitivity: Indicator of Acquired Failure of Host Defenses in Sepsis and Trauma. *Ann Surg 186*:241, 1977.

Mechanic, H., and Dunn, L.: Nutritional Support for the Burn Patient. *Dimensions of Critical Care Nursing 5*:20, 1986.

Mochizuki, H., et al.: Optimal Lipid Content for Enteral Diets Following Thermal Injury. *IPEN 8*:638, 1984.

Moyer, E., et al.: Multiple Systems Organ Failure, VI. Death Predictors in the Trauma-Septic State. The Most Critical Determinants. *J. Trauma 21*:862, 1981.

Mullen, T., and Kirkpatrick, J.: The Effect of Nutrition support on Immune Competency in Patients Suffering from Trauma, Sepsis or Malignant Disease. *Surgery 90*:610, 1981.

Murray, M.J., et al.: Nutritional Assessment of Intensive-care Unit Patients. *Mayo Clin Proc 63*:1106, 1988.

Nanni, G., et al.: Increased Lipid Fuel Dependence in Critically Ill Septic Patients. *J Trauma 24*:14, 1984.

O'Sullivan, P., et al.: Evaluation of Body Weight and Nutritional Status Among AIDS Patients. *JADA 85*:1483, 1985.

Rabeneck, L., et al.: Acute HIV Infection Presenting with Painful Swallowing and Esophageal Ulcers. *JAMA 263*:2308, 1990.

Roger, J.: AIDS: An MD's Eye-View. *NSS 6*(4):24, 1986.

Saffle, J., et al.: Use of Indirect Calorimetry in the Nutritional Management of the Burned Patient. *J Trauma 25*:32, 1985.

Sherman, C.: Dealing with the Challenge of AIDS. *Top Clin. Nutr 4*:37, 1989.

Sherry, B.: The impact of *Haemophilus influenzae* type b meningitis on nutritional status.

Solomon, S.M., and Kirby, D.K.: The Refeeding Syndrome: A Review. *JPEN 14*:90, 1990.

Solomons, N.: Nutrition and Parasitic Disease. *Clinical Nutrition 2*(2):16, 1983.

Tramposch, T., and Hester, D.: Nutritional Management of the Elderly Burned Patient. *NSS 7*(9):26, Sept., 1987.

Wachtel, T.: Computer-Assisted Nutritional Management of Burned Patients. *NSS 3*(8):10, 1983.

Walsh, D., Griffith, R., and Behforoz, A.: Subjective Response to Lysine in the Therapy of Herpes Simplex. *J Antimicro Chemo 12*:489, 1983.

RENAL DISORDERS

Andress, D., et al.: Early Deposition of Aluminum in Bone in Diabetic Patients on Hemodialysis. *NEJM 316*:292, 1987.

Bannister, D., et al.: Nutritional Effects of Peritonitis in Continuous Ambulatory Peritoneal Dialysis (CAPD) Patients. *JADA 87*:53, 1987.

Bennett, N.: Urea Kinetics in the Nutritional Management of Patients with Renal Failure. *NSS 4*(3):21, March, 1984.

Borum, P., and Taggart, E.: Carnitine Nutriture of Dialysis Patients. *JADA 86*:644, 1986.

Brenner, B.: *The Kidney*. Philadelphia. W.B. Saunders Co., 1985.

Burton, B., and Hirschman, G.: Current Concepts of Nutritional Therapy in Chronic Renal Failure: An Update. *JADA 83*:359, 1983.

Consensus Conference: Prevention and Treatment of Kidney Stones. *JAMA 260*:977, 1988.

Cooper, K., and Bennett, W.: Nephrotoxicity of Common Drugs Used in Clinical Practice. *Arch Int Med 147*:1213, 1987.

Edwards, M., and Doster, S.: Renal Transplant Diet Recommendations: Results of a Survey of Renal Dietitians in the United States. *JADA 90*:843, 1990.

Eschbach, J., et al.: Correction of the Anemia of End-Stage Renal Disease with Recombinant Human Erythropoietin. *NEJM 316*:73, 1987.

Farrell, P., and Howe, P.: Dialysis-Induced Catabolism. *AJCN 33*:1417, 1980.

Feinstein, E., et al.: Clinical and Metabolic Responses to Parenteral Nutrition in Acute Renal Failure. *Medicine 6*:124, 1981.

Friedman, A., et al.: Animal Models of Chronic Renal Failure: Influence of Nutrition on Growth. *Am J Kid Dis 7*:335, 1986.

Fröling, P., et al.: Successful Pregnancy of a Woman with Advanced Renal Failure on Nutritional Treatment. *Nephron 44*:195, 1986.

Gillit, D., Stover, J., and Spinozzi, N.: *A Clinical Guide to Nutrition Care in End-Stage Renal Disease*. Chicago: The American Dietetic Association, 1987.

Giovannetti, S.: Answers to Ten Questions on the Dietary Treatment of Chronic Renal Failure. *Lancet* November 15, 1986.

Goldstein, D., and Frederico, C.: The Effect of Urea Kinetic Modeling on the Nutritional Management of hemodialysis Patients. *JADA 87*:474, 1987.

Hall, W.: Hypertension and Kidney Disease: Effects of Antihypertensive Therapy. *Pract Cardio 17*:45, 1991.

Hull, S.: Body Fluid and Electrolyte Balance. *Dietetic Currents*. Columbus: Ross Laboratories. *12*(1), 1985.

Klahr, S., et al.: The Progression of Renal Disease. *NEJM 318*:1657, 1988.

Krolewski, A., et al.: Predisposition to Hypertension and Suscept Ability to Renal Disease in IDDM. *NEJM 318*:140, 1988.

Losito, A.: Essential Hypertension and Renal Failure. *Comp Ther 17*:20, 1991.

Lucas, P., et al.: The Risks and Benefits of a Low-Protein-Essential Amino Keto-Acid Diet. *Kidney Int 29*:995, 1986.

Manske, C.: Lipid Abnormalities and Renal Disease. *Kidney 20:*25, 1988.

Miller, R., et al.: Indirect Calorimetry in Postoperative Patients with Acute Renal Failure. *Am Surg 43:*494, 1983.

Monteon, F., et al.: Energy Expenditure in Patients with Chronic Renal Failure. *Kidney Int 30:*741, 1986.

Moore, S., et al.: Protocol for Nutritional Intervention for the Adult-chronic Hemodialysis Patient. *Contemporary Dialysis Nephrology* May 1988.

Nahas, A.: Management of Progressive Renal Failure: The Role of Dietary Manipulations. *Postgraduate Medical Journal 63:*611, 1986.

Nahas, A., and Coles, G.: Dietary Treatment of Chronic Renal Failure: Ten Unanswered Questions. *Lancet* March 15, 1986, p. 597.

Piper, C.: Very-Low-Protein Diets in Chronic Renal Failure: Nutrient Content and Guidelines for Supplementation. *JADA 85:*1344, 1985.

Ramirez, G., et al.: The Plasma and Red Cell Vitamin B Levels of Chronic Hemodialysis Patients: A Longitudinal Study. *Nephron 42:*41, 1986.

Spreiter, S., et al.: Protein-Energy Requirements in Subjects With Acute Renal Failure Receiving Intermittent Hemodialysis. *AJCN 33:*1433, 1980.

Trang, J., et al.: Effect of Dietary Ascorbic Acid Restriction and Supplementation on Urine pH in Elderly Males. *JAMA 252:*2960, 1984.

Tsuru, N., and Chan, J.: Protein-Energy Metabolism in Children with Impaired Renal Function. *Nephron 43:*81, 1986.

Vahlquist, A., et al.: Vitamin A Losses During Continuous Ambulatory Peritoneal Dialysis. *Nephron 41:*179, 1985.

Van Duyn, M.: Acceptability of Selected Low-Protein Products for Use in a Potential Diet Therapy for Chronic Renal Failure. *JADA 87:*909, 1987.

Vitella, E., et al.: Abnormalities of Lipoprotein Metabolism in Patients with the Nephrotic Syndrome. *NEJM 323:*579, 1990.

Voigts, A., et al.: The Effects of Calciferol and Its Metabolites on Patients with Chronic Renal Failure. *Arch Int Med 143:*1205, 1983.

Williams, P., et al.: Amino Acid Absorption Following Intraperitoneal Administration in CAPD Patients. *Peritoneal Dialysis Bulletin 2:*124, 1982.

Wolk, R., and Swartz, R.: Nutritional Support of Patients with Acute Renal Failure. *NSS 6:*38, 1986.

ENTERAL AND PARENTERAL NUTRITION

Alverdy, J., Chi, H., and Sheldon, G.: The Effect of Parenteral Nutrition on Gastrointestinal Immunity: The Importance of Enteral Stimulation. *Ann Surg 202:*681, 1985.

American Dietetic Association: Position of the American Dietetic Association: Issues in Feeding the Terminally Ill. *JADA 87:*78, 1987.

American Medical Association Department of Foods and Nutrition: Multivitamin Preparations for Parenteral Use: A Statement by the Nutrition Advisory Group. *JPEN 3:*258, 1979.

American Medical Association Department of Foods and Nutrition: Guidelines for Essential Trace Element Preparations for Parenteral Use. *JAMA 241:*2051, 1979.

American Society for Parenteral and Enteral Nutrition: Guidelines for the Use of Enteral Nutrition in the Adult Patient. *JPEN 11*(5):435, 1987.

American Society for Parenteral and Enteral Nutrition: Guidelines for Use of Home Total Parenteral Nutrition. *JPEN 11*(4):342, 1987.

American Society for Parenteral and Enteral Nutrition: *Standards for Nutrition Support: Hospitalized Patients.* Bethesda, MD: ASPEN, 1984.

Anderton, A.: The Potentials of Escherichia Coli in Enteral Feeds to Cause Food Poisoning: A Study Under Simulated Ward Conditions. *J Hosp Infec 5:*155, 1984.

Askanazi, J., et al.: Respiratory Changes Induced by the Large Glucose Loads of Total Parenteral Nutrition. *JAMA 243*:1444, 1980.

Austin, C.: Water: Guidelines for Nutrition Support. *NSS 6*(9):27, 1986.

Bach, A., and Babayan, V.: Medium-Chain Triglycerides: An Update. *AJCN 36*:950, 1982.

Baker, S., Dwyer, E., and Queen, P.: Metabolic Derangements in Children Requiring Parenteral Nutrition. *JPEN 10*:279, 1986.

Bastow, D., Rawlings, J., and Allison, S.: Overnight Nasogastric Tube Feeding. *Clin Nutr 4*:7, 1985.

Bello, J., et al.: Oral Nutritional Supplementation: A Prospective Evaluation of Use, Compliance and Cost. *NSS 7*(8):16, August, 1987.

Berezin, S., et al.: Home Teaching of Nocturnal Nasogastric Feeding. *JPEN 12*:392, 1988.

Berner, Y.N., et al.: Low Plasma Carnitine in Patients on Prolonged Total Parenteral Nutrition: Association with Low Plasma Lysine. *JPEN 14*:255, 1990.

Bower, R., Kern, K., and Fisher, J.: Use of a Branched-Chain Amino Acid Enriched Solution to Patients Under Metabolic Stress. *Am J Surg 149*:266, 1985.

Bower, R., et al.: Postoperative Enteral Versus Parenteral Nutrition: A Randomized Controlled Trial. *Arch Surg 121*:1040, 1986.

Brody, H., and Noel, M.: Dietitians' Role in Decisions to Withhold Nutrition and Hydration. *JADA 91*:580, 1991.

Buzby, G., and Mullen, J.: Nutritional Assessment. *In* Rombeau, J., and Caldwell, M. (eds.): *Enteral and Tube Feeding*. Philadelphia: W.B. Saunders Co., 1984. pp. 127–147.

Campbell, S., et al.: Methods of Nutritional Support for Hospitalized Patients. *Am Fam Phys 29*:215, May, 1984.

Chen, M., et al.: A Decision Tree for Selecting an Appropriate Enteral Formula. *Nutrition 3*(4):257, Aug., 1987.

Delaney, R., et al.: Nutritional Support of the Acutely Ill Patient. *Heart and Lung 12*(5):477, 1983.

Dudrick, S., et al.: Long Term Total Parenteral Nutrition with Growth, Development and Positive Nitrogen Balance. *Surg 64*:134, 1968.

Evans, D., et al.: Comparison of Gastric and Jejunal Tube Feedings. *JPEN 4*:79, 1980.

Feitelson, M., et al.: Tube Feeding Utilization/A Quality of Care Review. *JADA 87*:73, 1987.

Frankenfield, D., and Beyer, P.: Dietary Fiber and Bowel Fucntion in Tube-fed Patients. *JADA 91*:590, 1991.

Hallberg, D., et al.: Parenteral Nutrition: Goals and Achievements, Part I. *NSS 7*(2):15, July, 1982.

Hardin, J., and Page, C.: Rapid Replacement and Maintenance of Serum Albumin in Patients Receiving Total Parenteral Nutrition (Abstract). *JPEN 8*:97, 1984.

Haynes-Johnson, V.: Tube Feeding Complications: Causes, Prevention and Therapy. *NSS 6*(3):17, March, 1986.

Heymsfield, S.: Enteral Nutrition Support: Metabolic, Cardiovascular and Pulmonary Interrelations. *Clin Chest Med 7*:41, March, 1986.

Hitz, M.: Medical Ethics and Nutritional Support: The Dichotomy of Decision. *NSS 6*(11):12, Nov., 1986.

Ho, C., et al.: Percutaneous Gastrostomy for Enteral Feeding. *Radiology 156*:349, 1985.

Houser, B.: Keeping Up With TPN. *NSS 3*(2):27, Feb., 1983.

Hutchins, E., et al.: Training for Dietitians Working in Critical Care. *Ross Roundtable on Medical Issues*, 6th Seminar. Columbus: Ross Laboratories, 1985.

Hyman, P., et al.: Effect of Enteral Feeding on the Maintenance of Gastric Acid Secretory Function. *Gastro 84*:341, 1983.

Imbrosciano, S., and Kovach, K.: Selecting the Optimal Enteral Feeding Pump. *NSS* 6:15, 1986.

Jhangiani, S., et al.: Clinical Zinc Deficiency During Long-Term Total Enteral Nutrition. *J Am Geriatric Soc* 24:285, 1986.

Jones, M., Bonner, J., and Stitt, K.: Nutrition Support Services: Role of the Clinical Dietitian. *JADA* 86:68, 1986.

Jones, T., and Moore, E.: Nursing Consultation for Needle Catheter Jejunostomy Feedings After Major Abdominal Trauma. *NSS* 6(10):16, Oct., 1986.

Josephson, R., Rupp, J., and Chanbers, J.: Needs Assessment of Enteral Nutrition Support Products. *JADA* 85:1485, 1985.

Just, B., et al.: Comparison of Substrate Utilization by Indirect Calorimetry during Cyclic and Continuous Total Parenteral Nutrition. *AJCN* 51:107, 1990.

Kalfarentzos, F., et al: Nasoduodenal Intubation with the Use of Metoclopramide. *NSS* 7(9):33, Sept., 1987.

Kaminski, M., and Freed, B.: Enteral Hyperalimentation: Prevention and Treatment of Complications. *NSS* 1:29, 1981.

Kaminski, M., et al.: *Intravenous Hyperalimentation in Modern Hospital Practice.* Tuckahoe, NY: USV Laboratories, 1977.

Katz, M., et al.: Comparison of Serum Prealbumin and Transferin for Nutritional Assessment of TPN Patients: A Preliminary Study. *NSS* 6(8):22, August, 1986.

Kelly, T., Patrick, M., and Hillman, K.: Study of Diarrhea in Critically Ill Patients. *Crit Care Med* 11:7, 1983.

Kresnowik, R., et al.: Does Nutritional Support Affect Survival in Critically Ill Patients? *Am Coll Surg* 32:108, 1984.

Lyman, B., Pendleton, S., and Pemberton, L.: The Role of the Nutritional Support Team in Preventing and Identifying Complications of Parenteral and Enteral Nutrition. *Quarterly Review Bulletin* July 1987, p. 232.

Mann, S., et al.: Measured and Predicted Caloric Expenditure in the Acutely Ill. *Crit Care Med* 13:173, 1985.

Marchand, S.P., et al.: Availability of Insulin from Total Parenteral Nutrition Solutions. *JPEN* 14:262, 1990.

Mauer, A.M., et al.: Special Nutritional Needs of Children with Malignancies: A Review. *JPEN* 14:315, 1990.

May W.: Economics and Ethics. *JADA* 86:1355, 1986.

McArdle, A., et al.: A Rationale for Enteral Feeding as the Preferable Route for Hyperalimentation. *Surg* 90:616, 1981.

McCauley, R., and Brennan, M.: Serum Albumin Levels in Cancer Patients Receiving Total Parental Nutrition. *Ann Surg* 197:305, 1983.

McCollough, M., and Hsa, N.: Metabolic Bone Disease in Home Total Parenteral Nutrition. *JADA* 87:915, 1987.

Mirtallo, J., and Fabri, P.: Assessment of Iron Requirements in Patients Receiving Parenteral Nutrition. *NSS* 5:45, 1985.

Mirtallo, J., Joch, L., and Fabri, P.: Caloric Requirements of Patients Receiving Total Parenteral Nutrition. *Hosp Form* 18:57, 1983.

Mirtallo, J.: Parenteral Therapy. *In* Lang, C. (ed.): *Nutritional Support in Critical Care.* Rockville, MD: Aspen Publishers, Inc., 1987, pp. 113–129.

Moss, G.: Malabsorption Associated with Extreme Malnutrition: Importance of Replacing Plasma Albumin. *J Am Coll Nut* 1:89, 1982.

Niemee, P., and Vanderveen, T.: Compatibility Considerations in Parenteral Nutrient Solutions. *Am J Hosp Pharm* 41:893, 1984.

Orr, G., Wade, J., et al.: Alternatives to Total Parenteral Nutrition in the Critically Ill Patient. *Crit Care Med* 8:29, 1980.

O'Sullivan-Maillet, J.: Calculating Parenteral Feedings: A Programmed Intruction. *JADA* 84:1312, 1984.

650

Paige, D., et al.: Enteral and Parenteral Nutrition. *In Manual of Clinical Nutrition.* Pleasantville, NJ: Nutrition Publications, Inc., 1983, Chapter 31.

Paige, D., et al.: TPN Issue. *Clinical Nutrition* 2(3):5. Pleasantville, NJ: Nutrition Publications, Inc. May-June 1983.

Pinchofsky-Devin, G., and Kaminski, M.: Visceral Protein Increase Associated with Interrupted Versus Continuous Enteral Hyperalimentation. *JPEN* 9:474, 1985.

Pinchofsky-Devin, G., et al.: Mortality Risk Index for Predicting Futility of Nutritional Support. *NSS* 6(3):14, March, 1986.

Rombeau, J., and Barot, L.: Enteral Nutritional Therapy. *Surg Clin N Am* 61:605, 1981.

Rombeau, J., and Caldwell, M.: *Enteral and Tube Feeding,* Vol. 1. Philadelphia: W.B. Saunders Co., 1984.

Sanders, S.: Nursing Home Problems In Tube Feeding the Geriatric Patient. *NSS* 7(7):21, July 1987.

Shatsky, F., and Kelts, D.: Blood Chemistry Considerations for Parenteral Nutrition, Part I. *NSS* 6(6):25, June, 1986.

Shils, M., et al.: Liquid Formulas for Oral and Tube Feeding. *Clinical Bulletin* 6(4):158, 1976. New York: Memorial Sloan-Kettering Cancer Center.

Silberman, H.: Total Parenteral Nutrition by Peripheral Vein: Current Status of Fat Emulsions. *Nutrition International* 3(2):145, May-June, 1986.

Sitzmann, J.V.: Nutritional Support of the Dysphagic Patient: Methods, Risks, and Complications of Therapy. *JPEN* 14: 1990.

Szwanek, M., et al.: Trace Elements and Parenteral Nutrition. *NSS* 7(8):8, August, 1987.

Tao, R., and Yoshimura, N.: Carnitine Metabolism and Its Application in Parenteral Nutrition. *JPEN* 4:469, 1980.

Wilson, J.: Gastrointestinal Dysfunction in the Critically Ill: Nutritional Implications. *Comp Ther* 11:45, 1985.

Worthley, L., Fishlock, R., and Snowswell, A.: Carnitine Deficiency with Hyperbilirubinemia in a Patient with Long-Term Parenteral Nutrition: Treatment with Intravenous L-Carnitine. *JPEN* 7:176, 1983.

Valentine, R., and Turner, W.: Pleural Complications of Nasogastric Feeding Tubes. *JPEN* 9:605, 1985.

Zurlo, F., et al.: Variability of Resting Energy Expenditure in Healthy Volunteers During Fasting and Continuous Enteral Feeding. *Crit Care Med* 14:535, 1986.